Saunders

Medical Office Management

Third Edition

Third Edition

Saunders Medical Office Management

Alice Anne Andress, CCS-P, CCP
Director of Physician Services
Parente Randolph, LLC
Harrisburg, PA

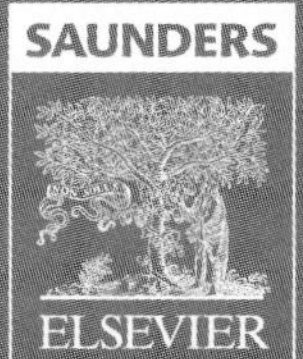

SAUNDERS
ELSEVIER

11830 Westline Industrial Drive
St. Louis, Missouri 63146

Saunders Medical Office Management, ed 3

ISBN-13: 978-1-4160-5668-3
ISBN-10: 1-4160-5668-8

Library of Congress Cataloging-in-Publication Data

Andress, Alice Anne.
Saunders medical office management / Alice Anne Andress. – 3rd ed.
p. ; cm.
Rev ed. of: Saunders textbook of medical office management / Alice Anne Andress. 2nd ed. c2003.
Includes bibliographical references and index.
ISBN-13: 978-1-4160-5668-3 (pbk. : alk. paper)
ISBN-10: 1-4160-5668-8 (pbk. : alk. paper) 1. Medical offices–Management. I. Andress, Alice Anne. Saunders textbook of medical office management. II. Title. III. Title: Medical office management.
[DNLM: 1. Practice Management, Medical–organization & administration. W 80 A561sa 2009]
R728.8.A56 2009
610.68–dc22 2008030864

ISBN-13: 978-1-4160-5668-3
ISBN-10: 1-4160-5668-8

Publisher: Michael Ledbetter
Developmental Editor: Jennifer Bertucci
Publishing Services Manager: Julie Eddy
Senior Project Manager: Celeste Clingan
Design Direction: Margaret Reid

Printed in Canada
Last digit is the print number: 9 8 7 6 5 4 3 2 1

I dedicate this book to Alex, my son, my reason for being.

REVIEWERS

Gerry A. Brasin, AS, CMA (AAMA), CPC
Education Coordinator
Premier Education Group
Springfield, Massachusetts

Jennifer Claire, CMA (AAMA), AA, BA, MSHS
Instructor, Course Lead
Schools of Health Sciences
Kaplan University
Fort Lauderdale, Florida

Mollie Banks, MPS, RHIT, CMS, CMRS
Billing and Coding Specialist, Lead Instructor
Draughons Junior College
Bowling Green, Kentucky

Judy Schlecht, BA, MAEd
Program Manager, Allied Health Courses
High Tech Institute
Phoenix, Arizona

PREFACE

Saunders Medical Office Management is a summary of 30 years of varied experience in health care. In the preparation of this text I have attempted to convey my commitment to the professionalism and overall high standards of health care. It is my firm belief that today, more than ever, medical office managers need to broaden their organizational, technical, personal, and leadership skills. Ongoing continuing education, both formal and informal, combined with innovative philosophies are critical for a successful office manager in today's environment. With this foundation, the committed office manager will be able to thrive and excel in his or her chosen managerial career.

Among the most important features throughout this text are the special insights contained in the *From the Expert's Notebook* boxes. These insights, obtained through years of practical experience, are intended to assist in daily decision-making. There are also other special sections throughout the text labeled *Manager's Alert!* These sections have been placed strategically throughout the book to caution the office manager about preventable difficulties.

This book was designed to provide a medical office manager with instant necessary information for immediate use or to educate students in the fine art of medical office management. I have presented this information in a logical format that can be incorporated into the daily activities of a medical office manager and can easily be understood by students at various levels of study. It is my belief that this book will assist the reader to obtain a greater understanding of the function of a medical office and the expertise necessary to be successful.

Alice Anne Andress, CCS-P, CCP

ACKNOWLEDGMENTS

A tender thanks is extended to my husband, Joe, who stood beside me, encouraged me, and shared my enthusiasm and commitment to this project; a tender thanks to my son, Alex, who continues to be an amazement to me. He is pure joy and makes my life whole; a special thanks must be extended to my many friends and family who are always there for me.

Alice Anne Andress, CCS-P, CCP

CONTENTS

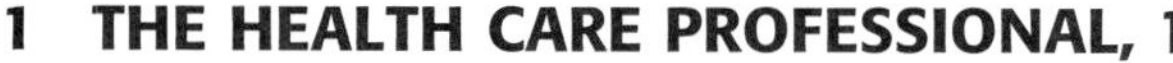

1

THE HEALTH CARE PROFESSIONAL

CHAPTER OUTLINE

CHAPTER OBJECTIVES

After completing this chapter, you will be able to do the following:

- Exhibit a professional appearance
- Comprehend the complexity of the health care system
- Explain the differences between primary and specialty care and recognize the various medical specialties
- Understand the life cycle of a medical practice
- Understand the interaction between health care professionals within a medical office
- Differentiate among the types of practice ownership

PROFESSION

If we look in the dictionary under the word *profession*, we find the following definitions:

> "an act of declaring a belief, faith, or opinion"
> "a calling requiring special knowledge and often long and intensive academic preparation"
> "a principal calling, vocation, or employment"

We then look up the word *professional* and find these definitions:

> "relating to or characteristic of a profession"
> "characterized by conforming to the technical or ethical standards of a profession"

If we check in our thesaurus under the word professional, we find such synonyms as *highly skilled, competent, knowledgeable, specialist, expert, experienced,* and *well-trained.*

These honorable words describe the health care profession and its members. Individuals are often encouraged to become more "professional" and to take a "professional" approach to their work. Professional standing cannot exist without training; practice administration; and recognition by qualified, state-approved agencies and governing bodies.

Professionalism can be thought of as a distinctive way of providing a service that has its own science of reasoning and practice. Many people confuse the term *occupation* with the term *profession,* but there *is* a difference. Professionals must have formal training, certification, or licensure and must demonstrate a high level of skill in the services that they offer, whereas individuals who are holding an occupation are simply providing either a product or a service in today's skill-driven market. Those involved in a profession are different from those committed to an occupation because of the use of judgment in their work and additional years of education and training.

Some experts believe that to be a professional, a person must possess the following traits:

- Commitment
- Education
- Service orientation
- Autonomy of judgment
- Honesty
- Integrity
- Dependability

The health care profession is committed to dealing with the problems of human functioning. Health care professionals deal with life-and-death matters and also aid individuals by helping them solve problems through counseling. They strive to maintain the dignity of all patients while advising them and their families in medical decision making. A bond forms between the health care professional and the patient. This bond is based on trust. Health care professionals have a duty to provide each and every patient with the information that is needed for decision making, and they must strive to protect the bond between themselves and their patients.

Anyone who takes a leap into the unknown for a career in health care may feel like Alice in Wonderland, falling headfirst into the profession and uncertain as to where the path is leading. Health care is different from other professions: while others may be making social plans, many health care professionals are arriving at a hospital or an office to perform clinical or administrative duties. In many cases, it is not a 9-to-5 job.

Most professions do not require the person to develop a given "set" of attitudes, but health care professionals must adopt behaviors, attitudes, and ethical guidelines to be able to do a good job. When individuals prepare for a profession rooted in health care, they should be prepared for a possible lifelong commitment that carries with it expectations, privileges, and responsibilities. There are three types of learning experience for health care professionals:

1. Basic concepts/theories
2. Skills
3. Attitudes

Each one of these will have its place in preparing a health care professional for interaction with patients.

Concepts

Individuals preparing for a life course in health care must possess knowledge in four basic areas:

1. Behavioral science: sociology, psychology, anthropology, and so on—to prepare one for an understanding of people's needs and behaviors and how they affect interaction
2. Mathematics: basic mathematics, statistics, computer, critical thinking, and so on—to provide a base in problem-solving techniques, critical thinking, and research
3. Liberal arts: philosophy, politics, religion, and so on—to have exposure to many ideas and to help formulate one's own ideas
4. Theoretic knowledge—to build on the techniques of the profession and to lay the foundation for applying specific professional skills

Skills

Health care professionals need the following skills:

1. Technical skills: the ability to use safe techniques to aid in diagnosing or conducting an evaluation of a patient
2. Teaching/administrative skills: the ability to instruct patients/family and other health care professionals; to organize and implement solutions; to communicate effectively

3. Research skills: the ability to collect and analyze data
4. Interpersonal relationship/communication skills: the ability to effectively interact with others, such as patients and families, other health care professionals, support personnel, business contacts, and so on.

Attitudes

The development of attitudes is highly important for health care professionals. Consider such areas as helping others, quality of life, and the role of your own convictions that help to form attitudes and effective ways to function. Do you like to help people? What feelings do you have regarding the physically handicapped patient? How do you feel about end-of-life decisions? All of these attitudes influence the professional's interactions with patients.

The term *medical care* encompasses the care an individual receives from physicians, technicians, dentists, nurses, medical office managers, and other health care professionals. People who lived many centuries ago were not blessed with having physicians and medicine; as a result, many died of diseases and conditions that are virtually nonexistent today. Progress and technology have no limits in the medical field as we know it now, and dramatic achievements are being made on an almost daily basis. Because of this, it is vitally important that medical office managers be well trained in running a medical practice. The physician, busy with "change," is free to concentrate on medicine while leaving the business side of medicine in the hands of a competent medical office manager.

HEALTH CARE CONTINUING EDUCATION

The health care profession requires continual learning. It is not a profession that is learned once; rather, it is a constant learning process. Changes in technical abilities and governmental regulations demand those in the industry to make a commitment to continual change. It is important to stay current, which will allow for both professional and personal success.

While preparing for a career in health care, it becomes evident that health care professionals have the potential for making a difference in people's lives. The realization of the value of a professional's future role becomes a great motivator for continued learning . . . continued learning with a zest!

THE HEALTH CARE SYSTEM

The United States has one of the most advanced health care systems in the world. The physicians in the United States, unlike those in some other countries, have the latest technology, medications, and training available to them. Technologic innovation causes the patient to expect better and more effective health care. However, this technology is expensive and results in pressures being placed on the physician that trickle down to the medical office manager. The pressures of cost containment, professional liability, continuing medical education, and federal intervention become the nightmare of not only the physician, but also the office manager. The office manager can monitor expenses, negotiate lower malpractice premiums, and ensure that the staff is attending continuing education courses to keep abreast of all changes. This process of continuous learning is a necessity not only for the physician, but also for the office staff. The office manager must realize that staff education is important to provide the physician with the support that is needed and to keep current with new technologic advances.

A type of "social contract" exists between the physician, the office staff, and the patient. This contract is a bond based on the patient's trust that the medical office will provide top-quality care in a compassionate manner. As the U.S. population continues to grow, more and more pressure is being placed on physicians for their services. We are seeing an aging population in the United States. It is estimated that by 2050, 30% of the population will be over age 65. As our population ages, our racial diversity increases. For example, the Hispanic population is expected to more than double between 1990 and 2010 and to be 11 times greater by 2050. The aging Hispanic population is growing faster than the aging African American population. The health care profession is constantly striving to provide better health care at an affordable price.

THE PATIENT AND THE HEALTH CARE PROFESSIONAL

The health care system must serve people. Nothing is more human and more personal than health. Many health care providers know a great deal about disease and illness but, if asked, cannot define the word *health*. The World Health Organization defines *health* as a state of complete physical, mental, and social well-being and not merely the absence of disease or infirmity. An individual is not only a statistic, but also a complex system of needs. It is important that the staff of a medical office realize this and approach the treatment of patients in a way that reflects this reality. A well-trained medical office staff, at the direction of the office manager, understands and meets the needs of each patient as an individual. This, in addition to the medical treatment provided by the physician, provides each patient with total quality care.

Although people are responsible for their own health, human nature is such that people are often in need of others to help them accomplish or maintain good health. The job of a medical professional is to deal with problems at the psychologic and biologic levels of individual functioning. The role of the health care professional is to assist individuals to make informed decisions regarding their health.

With all the knowledge and technology available in the medical field today, it is becoming more and more difficult for physicians to be experts in all areas of medicine. This has caused the need for the *specialist,* that is, a physician who is an expert in one particular field of medicine and confines her or his practice of medicine to the treatment and diagnosis of all disease falling under that specialty.

PATIENT PERCEPTIONS

Patients not only arrive with their illness or injury, they arrive with a perception of the situation. This perception is often very different from that of health care professionals. Patients are generally concerned with how their illness or injury affects their daily lives and activities. Does it keep them from going to play tennis? Does it keep them from playing with their grandchildren?

As professionals are trained to deal with the objective findings of the illness or injury, they must also be intuitive to understand the full effect of the condition as it relates to the patient. Patients' self-esteem plays a major role in how they feel.

THE PHYSICIAN

The word *physician* is a term used to describe a medical doctor. This is an individual who studies to be able to practice medicine by way of evaluation and treatment of patients. There are two types of physicians: the medical doctor (MD) and the doctor of osteopathy (DO). Both MDs and DOs are fully licensed to practice medicine in the United States, and both complete a 4-year undergraduate program before attending medical school. Their undergraduate program generally has more emphasis on science courses. They must then take and pass the Medical College Admissions Test (MCAT) and are generally subject to an extensive application process. Both then complete 4 years of medical education. Each doctor then chooses a specialty area (radiology, obstetrics, pediatrics, surgery, etc.) in which she or he would like to practice. Once they have completed their 4 years in medical school, they enroll in a residency program, which can last from 2 to 6 years depending on the specialty. MDs take the United States Medical Licensing Examination (USMLE), and DOs take the Comprehensive Osteopathic Medical Licensing Examination (COMLEX) and sometimes the USMLE examination also. Both are comparable. They must pass a state-licensing examination to be able to practice medicine. DOs receive extra training in the musculoskeletal system of the body. This provides them with a better understanding of how the nerves, muscles, and bones work together and how an injury or illness in one part of the body can affect another part. They perform a treatment called an osteopathic manipulative treatment (OMT) that improves circulation and blood supply to the injured or ill organs and promotes healing. Osteopathic medicine was developed in 1874 by Andrew Taylor Still. His philosophy focused on the fact that all body systems are interrelated and dependent upon one another for good health. He identified the musculoskeletal system as a key element of health and that by correcting its problems through manipulative treatment, the body's ability to function and to heal itself is greatly improved (American Osteopathic Association).

THE SUCCESSFUL PHYSICIAN

In his book *The Successful Physician* (W.B. Saunders, Philadelphia, 1923), Verlin C. Thomas, MD, passes on advice handed down from one generation of physicians to another during the previous century, including recommendations on how to instill confidence, faith, and gratitude in patients. The following is Dr. Thomas's advice on how to be a successful physician:

- Listen attentively and make written notes.
- Don't discuss finances with the patient until you have secured the patient's faith in you.
- Display friendliness and sympathy.
- Ask questions only about the case.
- Make verbal observations of patients' situations before they have a chance to tell you those things themselves.
- Explain what the diagnosis means.
- Show patients that similar cases have responded and that you assume their cases will respond as well.
- Live in a way that your life maintains your reputation for absolute integrity and honesty.
- Have exemplary personal habits and clean morals.
- Never let the fact that a patient was referred to you by another patient lead you to be careless or assume that you will keep the new patient.
- Cultivate the most desirable personal qualities: sincerity, tact, interest, enthusiasm, intelligence, and good judgment.

Dr. Thomas practiced at a time when the country doctor could move anywhere that a physician was needed (as most towns did), set up a small office, and expect that people would start walking down the road for care. The physician was a champion in those days, and patient gratitude was the supreme emotion that doctors craved. Dr. Thomas's book was written when medicine was still a cash business in which the physician and the patient negotiated fees at the time of the service. Many services would be paid for with chickens, apple pies, barn work, and so on. Besides the form of payment, has medicine really changed that much since Dr. Thomas practiced? Can we ignore Dr. Thomas's advice as old and outdated?

First impressions are as powerful today as they were 85 years ago. Essentially, the human nature of patients has not changed over the years.

THE PHYSICIAN-PATIENT RELATIONSHIP

Medical care is not an inalienable right that is guaranteed to every individual. The physician has control over the patients she or he chooses to treat. However, once the physician-patient relationship has begun, the patient has the right to expect it to continue unless the physician gives her or him suitable notice that it is going to end. Making an appointment does not constitute a physician-patient relationship, but once the patient arrives in the office, the relationship begins. Because there are no specific laws regarding the beginning of this relationship, most cases are decided by the state courts. For example, depending on the court, it is possible, though not probable, that the woman to whom the physician gave medical advice during open house at their children's school could view that encounter as a physician-physician relationship. It is important for the medical assistant to train the staff regarding giving advice to patients. When a staff member offers advice to a patient, the law views this as advice from the physician's agent, creating a duty on the physician's part to treat this patient.

There are a limited number of instances in which the physician can see the patient without being considered to have entered into a physician-patient relationship:

- Examining a patient for life insurance purposes
- Giving expert opinion in a workers' compensation or disability case
- Performing a preemployment physical
- Performing a court-ordered examination

Remember that any emergency treatment that a physician offers must be carried through by the physician. In other words, once a physician accepts an undertaking in an emergency situation, she or he is obligated to this patient. The physician may not neglect or withdraw her or his services unless there is another physician available to continue treatment of the patient.

Once a physician-patient relationship has been established, the patient becomes an established patient. If the patient is not seen by that physician or one of his or her associates of the same specialty within 3 years, the patient is then considered to be new for coding purposes. In this case, the new patient office visit codes 99201 to 99205 would be used instead of the established patient office visit codes 99211 to 99215.

PRIMARY CARE

Primary Care Physicians

Primary care physicians are general physicians such as family practitioners. Some also classify pediatricians and obstetricians/gynecologists in this category. For our purposes, we categorize pediatricians and obstetricians/gynecologists as specialists.

Family Practitioners

Family practice physicians are medical specialists who provide the comprehensive primary care of all members of the family, regardless of age or gender. A family practitioner can treat sunburn in one examination room and liver failure in another. The scope of their services is unlimited.

SPECIALISTS

Internal Medicine (Internists)

The *internist* is known as the "general specialist." Internists treat and diagnose internal diseases through nonsurgical methods. Often, patients are referred to a subspecialist for treatment of a particular illness. This frequently occurs after the internist has made the diagnosis of the disease. A *subspecialist* is an internist who confines his or her specialty to a particular organ or area of the human body.

Allergists

Allergists, for example, are internists whose subspecialty is the diagnosis and treatment of allergies. One of their major roles is to determine the cause of patients' allergic reactions to certain substances. These substances can be anything from medicine to foods, plants, pollens, animals, trees, and so on. People may be allergic to certain types of soap, clothing, or the stuffing in pillows and mattresses. People may also be allergic to certain inhalants, such as perfumes, hair sprays, and chemicals that are spread on lawns.

Cardiologists

Cardiology is another subspecialty of internal medicine. *Cardiologists* are experts in the diagnosis and treatment of the heart and the cardiovascular system. These specialists treat such conditions as heart attacks, irregularities of the heart muscle, defects in the vessels and valves of the heart, arrhythmias, and general cardiac dysfunctions. They order electrocardiograms (ECGs or EKGs), which are graphic tracings of electrical impulses given off by the heart. These tracings indicate what might have happened to the heart in the past and what is happening to the heart at the present time. With today's cardiac technologies, the replacement of clogged valves, heart transplants, and even the use of totally self-contained artificial hearts are becoming routine.

Dermatologists

Dermatologists are internists who specialize in diseases of the skin. Their medical education includes surgical training. Diagnosis and treatment are extended to a wide variety of conditions, ranging from a simple wart to skin cancer. There are treatments for wrinkles, face-lifts, and almost any type of cosmetic surgery a person may desire. They can make lips full and eyelids thin. Through the use of medications and surgery, they can slow down the effects of aging on a person's face. With the continual depletion of the ozone layer, there is a high risk of skin cancer, and dermatologists are continually explaining the hazards of the sun to their patients.

Gastroenterologists

Gastroenterologists are internists whose subspecialty is the diagnosis and treatment of any abnormal conditions of the gastrointestinal tract. This specialty covers a broad spectrum of the anatomy, including the esophagus, stomach, pancreas, gallbladder, liver, colon, and rectum. *Gastroenterologists* treat ulcers, excise polyps from the colon, remove food that is lodged in a person's esophagus, and diagnose and treat hepatitis.

Gerontologists

Because Americans on average are living longer, *gerontology* is an up and coming subspecialty of internal medicine. The *gerontologist* specializes in the treatment and diagnosis of diseases specific to the elderly. Alzheimer's disease, sleep pattern changes, decreasing physical capacity, and many other conditions are indicative of the aging process. In addition to understanding how the aging process affects the mind and body, the gerontologist must understand how aging affects both the patient and the caregiver.

Gynecologists

A *gynecologist* is an internist who attends to the particular concerns and illnesses of women. A gynecologist is also trained in surgery, even though she or he is considered a subspecialist in internal medicine. The treatment provided by a gynecologist can range from simple preventive medicine, such as Papanicolaou (Pap) smears and breast examinations, to major surgeries, such as hysterectomies and mastectomies. The gynecologist also helps keep women's complex hormonal systems in balance.

Neurologists

Neurologists specialize in the diagnosis and treatment of the nervous system. Their patients can have conditions such as strokes, multiple sclerosis, and dizziness. They also monitor the epileptic patient and treat diseases involving motor function.

Ophthalmologists

An *ophthalmologist* attends to the diagnosis and treatment of the eye and ocular system. This specialty is found in both internal (that is, nonsurgical) and surgical medicine. Patients may seek the services of an *ophthalmologist* for a simple eye examination, for cataract surgery, or for many other conditions related to the eye and ocular system. A patient with an abrasion of the eye as a result of a contact lens may seek out the expertise of this physician, as would a patient with glaucoma. This specialty has advanced to the replacement of the lens of the eye, so that after cataract surgery, the patient is able to regain vision in the affected eye.

Obstetricians

Obstetricians are physicians who attend to the needs of women during pregnancy and childbirth. Physicians generally specialize in both gynecology and obstetrics, so as to be able to handle all aspects of care related to a woman's reproductive system. Monitoring of the fetus and the mother during pregnancy is a very important function of this specialty. We are even able to obtain information on the unborn child through medical advancement in this field. We can know in advance whether the baby has a genetic abnormality and whether it is a boy or a girl. More and more women are starting their families late as a result of having careers. With the advancements in this field, older women are able to produce healthy babies with little risk to themselves or their child.

Orthopedists

Orthopedists are specialists who diagnose and treat conditions of the musculoskeletal system. They treat patients with ailments ranging from a sprained ankle to a herniated disk. These specialists treat athletic injuries of the muscle, bone, and tendon and perform joint replacement surgeries such as total knee and total hip replacements on patients.

Pediatricians

Pediatricians specialize in the diagnosis and treatment of children's diseases. Their practice generally spans birth to adolescence. They attend to the prevention of childhood diseases by vaccinating babies with vaccines for polio, measles, tetanus, mumps, and others. They diagnose and treat such common ailments as tonsillitis, earaches, measles, chickenpox, and mumps. They may even attend to children who have buried an eraser in their ear or pushed a raisin up their nose. They advise new mothers on how to care for their infants, when and what to feed them, how to deal with diaper rash, and many other childhood situations.

Physiatrists

A *physiatrist* specializes in the diagnosis of musculoskeletal conditions and their treatment by use of physical means. Treatments such as hydrotherapy, heat, massage, exercise, and electricity are commonly used in this specialty. This specialty is needed more and more as our aging population becomes plagued with the conditions associated with aging, such as gait dysfunction.

Psychiatrists

Psychiatrists are specialists who diagnose and treat patients suffering from emotional and mental disorders. Their patients range from the depressed patient to the patient with more severe diseases of mental and emotional climates. Counseling plays an important role in their work, and their ability to listen is one of their biggest assets.

Pulmonologists

A *pulmonologist* specializes in the diagnosis and treatment of the lungs. These physicians may care for patients with chronic obstructive lung disease, pneumonia, and emphysema, to mention only a few. They perform special diagnostic studies to aid in diagnosis and treatment of pulmonary conditions. These studies consist of oxygen saturation levels, pulmonary function tests, and more complex testing such as bronchoscopies.

Anesthesiologists

Anesthesiologists are physicians who administer all types of anesthesia necessary in the hospital setting. This can be as simple as a local anesthetic or as complex as general anesthesia. Some anesthesiologists also provide treatment in pain clinics for patients with moderate to severe pain.

Radiologists

Radiologists specialize in the diagnosis and therapeutic treatment of patients through the use of x-rays, magnetic resonance imaging (MRI), computed tomography (CT) scans, and radioactive materials. They monitor the activities of the technicians doing the tests and advise of any problems with patient positioning and film developing. They study the results of the tests performed and report to the referring physician both normal and abnormal findings. The referring physician then uses these findings to diagnose and treat the patient. Some patients require treatment with radioactive substances, which is also done by the radiologist.

Surgeons

Surgeons limit their practice to the diagnosis and treatment of diseases requiring surgery. They may confine their specialty to a certain area of the body, such as the chest, brain, or cardiovascular system. These surgical subspecialties are along the same lines as the subspecialties in internal medicine. Often, a surgeon's patients have already been diagnosed by another physician and are referred to the surgeon primarily for the surgery. A typical surgeon's day may include the following surgeries: removal of a gallbladder, removal of a benign or malignant growth, removal of a gangrenous limb, or repair required after a traumatic event.

Urologists

Urologists diagnose and treat diseases of the urinary system of the female and the genitourinary tract of the male. An examination of the bladder, called a *cystoscopy,* is done so that the physician can look directly into the bladder to check for abnormalities. Patients may consult a urologist for a urinary tract infection or for problems encompassing the testes or prostate.

SPECIALISTS BASED MAINLY IN HOSPITAL SETTINGS

Some specialties are practiced by physicians based at hospitals. These physicians work only in the hospital setting.

Emergency Physicians

Emergency department physicians have specialized training in emergency conditions of patients. Patients may arrive at an emergency department of a hospital with a severe earache, a kidney stone, a sprained ankle, a laceration of the face, and more critical situations such as heart attacks, strokes, and trauma.

Pathologists

Pathologists supervise the clinical laboratory located in the hospital. Their laboratory may include specialists in hematology, chemistry, bacteriology, serology, cytology, pathology, and urinalysis. It is the pathologist who examines *frozen sections* of tissue removed during certain surgical procedures to determine whether the tissues are malignant or benign. These physicians also perform autopsies on deceased patients to determine the cause of death. Pathologists may operate private laboratories outside the hospital.

Radiologists and anesthesiologists are mainly hospital-based, but some may have outpatient facilities.

OTHER SPECIALISTS

Chiropractor

Chiropractors are physicians that specialize in the diagnosis and treatment of diseases related to the functioning of the nervous system. Through manual manipulation of the spine, chiropractors restore and maintain overall health of patients by identification of condition, cause, and treatment by conservative noninvasive methods. A portion of their patient base is workers' compensation and motor vehicle accident patients.

Podiatrist

A *podiatrist* is a physician that specializes in the care of the foot. This includes diagnosis of disease and injury and the subsequent medical or surgical care. These physicians were once referred to as chiropodists. They provide foot care for diabetics, treat nail infections, and help patients to maintain good foot health.

Psychologists

Psychologists usually have their doctorate in clinical or counseling psychology. They specialize in diagnosis and treatment of psychologic disorders through interviews, psychologic testing, and psychotherapy. Although psychologists treat patients, they are not permitted to dispense prescriptions.

THE LIFE CYCLE OF A MEDICAL PRACTICE

Because of the economic restraints put on health care today, it has become increasingly important for the medical office manager and the physician to seek out and use any management tools they believe will increase their practice's effectiveness. In 1960, Kotler and Levitt devised a method to forecast a product's life cycle. It has since been taught in all management and marketing courses as the most crucial way to monitor the growth of a product. The method identifies the various stages in the life cycle of a product in the market:

Stage 1: Introduction
Stage 2: Growth
Stage 3: Maturity
Stage 4: Decline
Stage 5: Revitalization

Introduction

The office is newly established, waiting for patients to call for appointments. Physicians are attending community functions in an effort to become known.

Growth

Word is out. Patient volumes are building. The practice is hiring more employees and perhaps even more physicians.

Maturity

The practice is well established. Physicians and patients are "settled in." Physicians believe that it is not necessary to market practice. They are very busy.

Decline

There has been no marketing for several years. New physician offices of the same specialty have opened in town. Patient volumes are starting to decline. Many established patients have passed away. Some physicians are retiring.

Revitalization

New physicians are hired, and employees have either been remotivated or replaced. The practice finally realizes that marketing can never stop. New, fresh ideas for marketing are evolving. Perhaps new procedures are being offered to patients. The practice is reborn!

Dale and Gombeski, from the Cleveland Clinic Foundation, showed that this product life cycle could be applied to physician services (Figure 1-1). Physicians have since used this method to find out how their specialization has been affected by their competitor's practices. They can also

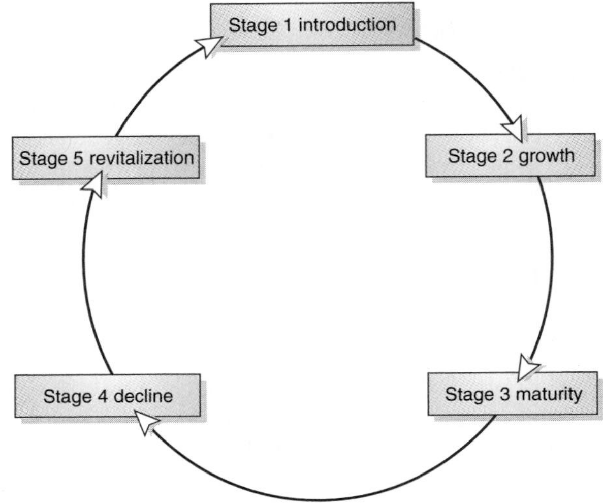

FIGURE 1-1. Life cycle of a medical practice.

determine what they can realistically expect in terms of volume of patients and total revenues. This method also allows a medical office to plot the time period before a new associate must be added and identify what ancillary personnel are needed. It can aid in practice decisions. Medical office managers can also use the product life cycle concept. Once the demographics regarding the practice have been collected and the philosophy of the established physician(s) is known, this cycle has allowed medical office managers to better understand the needs of the practice at which they work.

TYPES OF MEDICAL BUSINESS ORGANIZATIONS

There are three types of medical practices: sole proprietorship (solo), partnership, and corporation (Figure 1-2). A solo practice is a medical practice consisting of one physician only. A partnership practice consists of three or more physicians practicing as a group. A corporation can be one physician or two or more physicians practicing as a group. Each form of medical business ownership has advantages and disadvantages. In a study released by the Center for Studying Health System Change (HSC), there has been a shift away from small practices. In 1997, the percentage of physicians in solo and two-physician practices was 41%. This figure had decreased by 2005 to 33%. In 2005, the percentage of solo/2-physician practices was 33%; the percentage of practices with 3 to 5 physicians was 10%; the percentage of practices with 6 to 50 physicians was 18%; the percentage of practices with more than 50 physicians was 4%; the percentage of medical school physician practices was 9%; the percentage of health maintenance organization (HMO) physician practices was 5%; the percentage of hospitalist physician practices was 12%; and the percentage of all others was 9%. More and more physicians are practicing in mid-sized, single-specialty groups of 6 to 50 physicians. Changes in physician organizations have important implications for the practice of medicine and the care that patients receive. Current trends in the U.S. health care system are rapidly changing the career opportunities of patient care physicians and, hence, physicians' choice of practice arrangement.

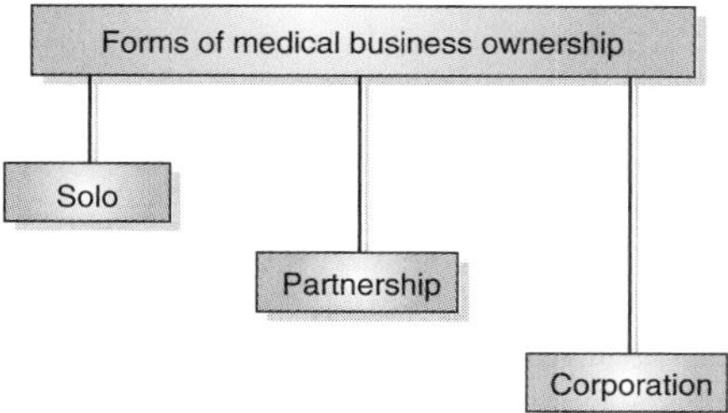

FIGURE 1-2. Three types of medical business organizations.

Sole Proprietorship

In a sole proprietorship (Figure 1-3), the physician owner employs needed personnel, collects all revenues, and assumes responsibilities of all financial obligations of the practice. There is no formal formation as with the formation of a corporation, but the physician owner must register the name of the practice. All revenues are reported as personal income of the physician owner. *No* legal documents are necessary for this type of ownership.

The advantages of a sole proprietorship are as follows:

- It is easy to form as a legal entity.
- The physician has a certain amount of independence.
- There is flexibility in the organization and management of the practice.
- There is a certain amount of privacy in a solo practice.
- There are tax advantages: the physician pays taxes only on personal income from the practice.

The disadvantages of a sole proprietorship are as follows:

- There is limited potential for profit.
- There can be management problems.
- There can be financial problems.
- There exists *unlimited liability,* which means that any damages or debt incurred by the business can also be

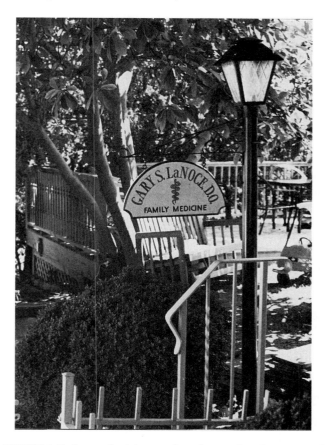

FIGURE 1-3. Some physicians prefer solo practice. (Courtesy of Gary LaNoce, DO.)

attached to the owner of the practice. The life of the practice is limited; when the physician dies, the practice ends or can be bought by another physician.

Partnership

A partnership consists of two or more physician owners, who, regulated by certain laws, can vary in size from two physicians to an unlimited number. Physician co-owners usually share equally in all revenues, and each co-owner assumes joint responsibility for all obligations of the medical practice. Under the Uniform Partnership Act (UPA), partners have an equal right to manage the practice. Most issues are resolved by majority vote. The legal documents necessary for a partnership are a partnership agreement, a buy-sell agreement, and employment agreements.

The advantages of a partnership are as follows:

- There is the potential to create more profit than can be obtained from a solo practice.
- There are incentives for motivated employees.
- There are legal and financial advantages.

The disadvantages of a partnership are as follows:

- There can be interpersonal problems between partners in the practice.
- There can be management problems.
- The life of the practice can be limited; when the last partner dies, so does the practice.
- There is unlimited liability for the partnership's debt, obligations, and acts of fellow partners in the partnership.

A *limited partnership* is the same as a general partnership except that each partner is confined to that partner's capital contributions as long there is no participation in daily operations. There must be one general partner, and there can be an unlimited number of limited partners. Income is considered to be stable to the individual partners. A *limited liability partnership* can be formed in 19 states in the United States. The difference in this partnership is that debt and obligations can be modified so that there is not individual liability. Partners, however, are individually liable for their own malpractice. A *limited liability company* (LLC) has owners, which are called "members," and the liability is limited to each one's investment in the practice. Although all states recognize this type of ownership, not all states recognize single-member LLCs. Taxation laws are different depending on the state in which the partnership exists. The legal documents necessary for an LLC are articles of incorporation, an operating agreement, and an employment agreement.

Corporation

A corporation is a simulated person or entity that is separate from the owners. It has a life of its own. The legal documents necessary for a corporation are articles of incorporation, bylaws, employment agreements, and stock purchase and redemption agreements.

The advantages of a corporation are as follows:

- There is *limited liability;* damages/debt can be applied only to the practice, not to the physician.
- The practice can readily raise cash by issuing stock.
- The life span of the practice is unlimited.

The disadvantages of a corporation are as follows:

- The practice must publicly disclose its finances and operations.
- It is expensive to incorporate.
- High taxes are associated with corporations.

Although there are several types of corporations, generally only a few are found in the medical field. An *open corporation* is a corporation that makes a profit for the owners and has shareholders. It is a public corporation. A *closed corporation* is also a profit-making business but has only a few owners and does not have an open market for shares of stock. *Nonprofit corporations* are service institutions that are incorporated mainly for the advantage of limited liability. A *single-person corporation* is an individual who incorporates to avoid paying high personal income taxes.

TYPES OF MEDICAL PRACTICE

There are two types of medical practice: solo and group. Group practices are further broken down into single-specialty and multispecialty groups and small and large groups.

A *solo practice* is a physician who practices alone or with others, but does not pool income or expenses. A *group practice* consists of three or more physicians in practice together. Over the past 25 years, there has been an increase in group practices, largely due to the evolution of managed care. A *physician network* differs from the traditional solo practice and group practice. A physician network can be any of the following:

- An integrated provider network
- A management services organization
- A physician-hospital organization

Integrated provider networks can be a great "marriage" between hospitals and physicians. This type of physician practice is sometimes called a "clinic without walls." It allows physicians to become part of a single practice organization while maintaining their individual practices. *Management services organizations* provide management and administrative support services to physicians and hospitals. These organizations provide a high degree of independence. *Physician-hospital organizations* are a conglomeration of physicians and hospitals that maintain a separate identity. These organizations can be beneficial in negotiating managed care contracts.

A *single-specialty* medical office is a group practice that is limited to one specialty (for example, surgery or internal medicine). A *multispecialty* medical office contains physicians with different specialties practicing together; an example is an office with a cardiologist, a hematologist, and a gastroenterologist.

The advantages of a small group practice are as follows:

- Physician coverage of the practice is sometimes available.
- Other physicians are available for consultation and assistance if needed.
- Revenues may be enhanced.
- It is easier to take vacations and sick days.

The disadvantages of the small group practice are as follows:

- The physician cannot always take off when desired; there are others to consider.
- Large amounts of capital are sometimes necessary for investment, and then cannot easily be retrieved (not liquid).

The advantages of a large group practice are as follows:

- It offers more free time for the physicians.
- Consultations with colleagues are readily available.
- Some physicians may not want to be in charge of daily operations, in charge of investments, in charge of marketing and practice growth, and so on; other physicians can take over these tasks.

The disadvantages of the large group practice are as follows:

- The physicians must conform to the rules of the practice and lose some of their independence.
- It can take time to become a full partner in a partnership or corporation.

According to the American Medical Association (AMA) definition, group practice is a group of three or more physicians who are formally organized as a legal entity in which business and clinical facilities, records, and personnel are shared (Figure 1-4). Income from the group medical services is divided according to a prearranged plan. In single-specialty groups, more than one third are made up of the following specialties: obstetrics/gynecology (OB/GYN), anesthesiology, radiology, pediatrics, and orthopedics. Most single-specialty physician practices that are solo physicians can be found in dermatology, endocrinology, rheumatology, and allergy. In multispecialty groups, the most common specialties are internal medicine and family practice.

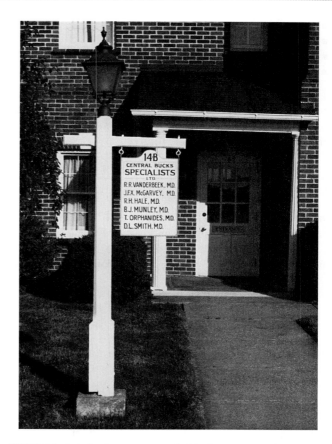

FIGURE 1-4. It is often more profitable for a group of specialists to form a partnership than for a specialist to go into practice alone. (Courtesy of Central Bucks Specialists.)

RETAIL CLINICS

Some medical groups are entering into the world of retail by opening clinics in pharmacies, department store chains, and supermarkets. These minimalistic clinics enhance primary care and are the answer for patients who do not have a family doctor or for patients whose family doctor offices are closed. Some clinics limit their patients to those who are over 2 years of age, have a temperature of over 103 degrees, have a trauma from an accident, have an injury that may require an x-ray, or take more than seven medications.

All patients are sent back to their primary care physicians if they have one, and if not, are given a listing of several primary care offices within the area who are accepting new patients. Many of these retail clinics employ midlevel providers who attend to rashes, earaches, coughs, and so on but have physician oversight. Most of the physicians involved in these clinics come from an urgent care or emergency department background and are accustomed to "24/7 medicine." These clinics began in 2006, with 62 operating around the country. By the end of February 2007, the number had grown to 150 and in early 2008, there are over 900 clinics in this country (*Managed Care Magazine*, March 2008). The costs associated with these clinics are as follows:

- Leased space from the retailer (approximately 225 to 250 square feet)
- Construction costs

- Equipment (minimal)
- One midlevel provider or physician
- Marketing
- Supervising and managing

Physicians who are considering stepping into the retail marketplace should be prepared for a sizable outlay of cash to carry the operations for approximately 2 to 3 years. Is this the medical office of the future?

TYPES OF HEALTH CARE PROFESSIONALS

Many new health care professions, such as nurse practitioners, physician assistants, and certified nurse specialists, to name a few, have been developed to meet health care needs (Figure 1-5). By using these providers, physician practices can shift some patient care and provide it at a lesser cost. There is also a shift of health care services from the inpatient setting to the outpatient setting. This shift allows for less expensive health care as more and more procedures are performed on an outpatient basis.

Various physician specialties were described earlier in this chapter. The following is a partial list of some of the other health care professionals with whom the medical office manager will come in contact:

Cardiovascular technician: performs physician-ordered electrocardiograms on patients for interpretation by the physician.

Clinical social worker: provides services to patients with psychologic disorders through interviews and counseling.

Coders: provide coding expertise to physician practices by having a thorough understanding of coding with

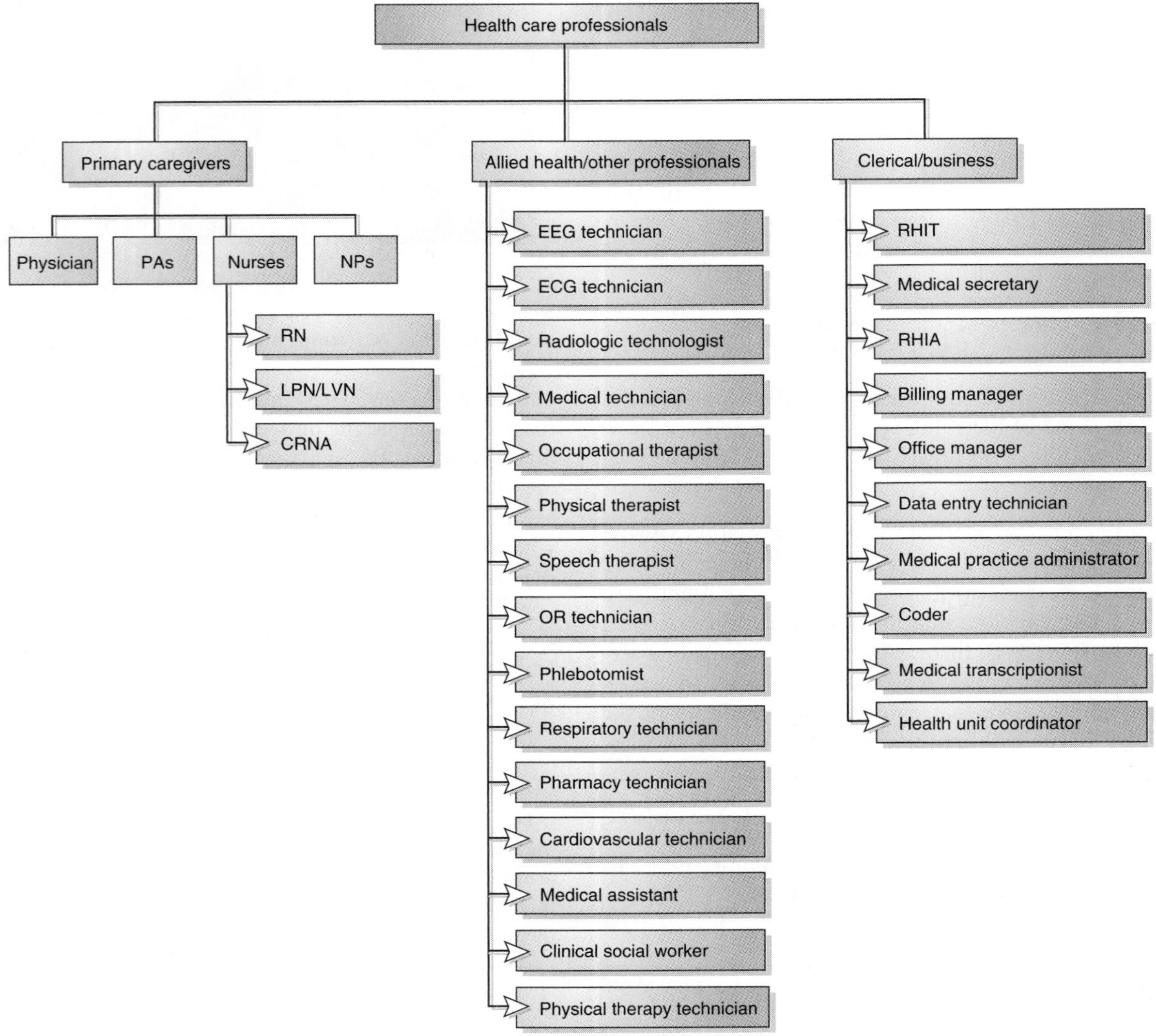

FIGURE 1-5. Health care professionals.

CPT, HCPCS, and ICD-9-CM codes. Some coders have taken an examination to further define themselves as Certified Procedural Coders. These individuals are greatly sought after in the job market.

Electroencephalogram (EEG) technician: performs EEGs on patients for interpretation by a physician.

Health unit coordinators: perform administrative duties for nurses, physicians, and patients.

Licensed practical nurse/licensed vocational nurse (LPN/LVN): a nurse with a vocational degree who aids physicians in the treatment of patients in the office or hospital setting (or both).

Medical assistant (MA): medical professional graduated from a certificate program who is trained to aid physicians in patient care by performing clinical and clerical duties.

Medical laboratory technician (MLT): performs venipuncture laboratory tests on patients.

Medical secretary: trained in medical terminology to handle telephones and correspondence for physicians. May act as a liaison between physician and patient.

Medical technologist (MT): performs the same function as the medical laboratory technician but has a bachelor's degree.

Medical transcriptionist: transcribes all types of dictation, including reports, letters, progress notes, and so on.

Nurse anesthetist (certified registered nurse anesthetist [CRNA]): performs anesthesia services under the direction of the anesthesiologist.

Nurse practitioner (NP): a highly trained nurse who has a master's level of education and board certification. Nurse practitioners provide both nursing and medical services to patients in all settings. They provide diagnosis and treatment of illnesses through ordering and interpreting tests, counseling, and appropriate prescription therapies.

Occupational therapist: assists patients when needed in relearning such daily activities as tying shoes, brushing teeth, buttoning clothing, and so on.

Operating room technician: assists the surgeon during operations, both major and minor.

Phlebotomist: draws blood from patients when laboratory tests have been ordered.

Physical therapist (PT): provides care to patients with disabilities or changes in their physical function that affect their ability to engage in normal activities of daily living.

Physical therapy technician (PTT): provides care to patients requiring therapy for physical function. This care is provided under the direction of the physical therapist.

Physician's assistant (PA): provides health care to patients under a physician's supervision and diagnoses and treats the same types of conditions as physicians. About 50% of all physician assistants can be found in primary care settings.

Radiologic technologist (RT): performs physician-ordered radiology examinations on patients for interpretation by a radiologist. These examinations include diagnostic studies, CT scans, MRIs, ultrasounds, nuclear medicine, mammography, interventional therapies, and so on.

Registered health information administrator (RHIA): administers regulations and supervises the medical records department.

Registered health information technician (RHIT): maintains, audits, codes, and transcribes patients' medical records.

Registered nurse (RN): a college-educated and board-certified individual who, by license, is able to perform higher levels of nursing care under the direction of the physician.

Respiratory technician: performs pulmonary function studies and treatments on patients.

Speech therapist: helps patients regain speech patterns after they have suffered a stroke or other event that has affected speech.

Most of these professions have a direct line of communication with the physician's office. Everyone who is employed in a medical office is part of the "big picture" and recognizes the vital importance of teamwork. Many of these professionals can be found on a daily basis working hand-in-hand with physicians to provide the best medical care possible.

THE FUTURE OF HEALTH CARE

Health care is changing rapidly in all areas involving health care systems, insurance carriers, government, physicians, and health care professionals. The three most important factors in health care are

1. Costs
2. Quality
3. Access

There has been a constant movement to improve access to health care for the entire population, with special emphasis on low-income individuals and the elderly. Managed care was to be the answer; however, with managed care, there are constant concerns of quality and access to care. There is growing discontent with our health care system because it does not deliver health care to all individuals. The major challenges of health care are stated by S. M. Shortall and U. E. Reinhardt in *Creating and Executing Health Policy in the 1990s, Improving Health Policy and Management: Nine Critical Research Issues:*

1. Growing number of uninsured
   a. Creation of basic benefit packages
   b. State-level experimentation
   c. What can the country afford?

2. Demand for greater accountability
   a. Search for value (greater quality for less cost)
   b. Focus on patient safety
3. Technologic growth and innovation
   a. New diagnostic and treatment modalities
   b. Growth of outpatient care population
   c. Stem cell research
   d. Demand for faster service
4. Changing population: increase in elderly and ethnically heterogeneous populations
   a. Changes in demand for care
   b. Increased number of ethical issues
   c. Increased social morbidity
5. Changing professional labor supply
   a. Shortages of key professionals
   b. Redefinition of professional roles
   c. Productivity and quality issues
6. Globalization of the economy
   a. Increased focus on costs
7. Changing delivery systems: consolidations, mergers
   a. Increased potential for providing care to defined populations
   b. Increased potential for managing a continuum of care
   c. Increased practice area by providing services at a distance, for example, telemedicine
8. Information management
   a. Facilities accountability
   b. Tools for increased productivity
   c. Direct clinical applications
   d. Opportunity to actively manage clinical care
   e. Management of medical informatics
   f. Electronic medical record implementation

According to *Futurescan 2000, A Millenium Forecast of Healthcare Trends 2000-2004,* there were five major forces that would affect health care. The report was based on a study of 400 health care leaders. The top two trends for each category were as follows:

- *Society*
  - Aging baby boomers: baby boomers become America's most powerful consumer of health services.
  - Internet-informed consumers: consumers are flooding cyberspace, creating an industry to serve them.

The forecast for this major force, society, came true. As of 2006, baby boomers were still using the majority of health care resources. These Internet trends have continued and have become an even greater force.

- *Science and technology*
  - Biomedical devices: new biomedical devices such as body-drug dispensing devices.
  - Electronic medical records: use of electronic medical records will increase.

The forecast for science and technology certainly came true. Electronic medical records have been implemented, and the number of practices adopting this paperless initiative is steadily growing.

- *Economics and finance*
  - Bankruptcies: because of decreasing revenues, more hospitals and health systems will be forced to close their doors.

This forecast for economics and finance was certainly accurate. Hospitals are closing, or merging in an attempt to remain solvent. The number of Medicare and Medicaid patients is increasing.

- *Health policy*
  - Medicare/Medicaid HMOs: because of decreasing government payments, growth of Medicare HMOs and managed care Medicaid will grow at a slower rate.
  - Medicare pharmacy benefit: Medicare reform will add a pharmaceutical benefit.

This health policy forecast has been right on target, with decreasing reimbursements and Medicare Part D.

- *Health care organizations*
  - Staffing shortages: nursing shortages will increase despite higher wages.
  - Complementary medicine: alternative medical services and products will increase as a result of patient interest.

Health care organizations continue to experience nursing shortages. Alternative medicine and homeopathic medicine are slowly growing.

No one knows if the future will bring shortages or overabundances of health care professionals, but the impact of all of these changes will be considerable. Flexibility and transition will be key.

THE FUTURE OF THE PHYSICIAN

During this age of health care reform, there has been a major reduction in power, control, prestige, and independence of physicians. The demand for primary care physicians continues to grow, with more and more patients enrolled in managed care. There continues to be a growing need for physicians to practice in inner cities and rural areas. Pressure is being placed on medical schools to limit the number of physicians they graduate. By 2010, the estimated number of physicians will rise from 450,000 to 600,000. The oversupply of physicians in 2010 is estimated to be mainly specialists, but by 2030, it is estimated that the specialists will again be needed.

THE FUTURE OF THE HEALTH CARE PROFESSIONAL

Many hospitals are merging or even closing their doors. Many physician practices are merging in an effort to increase their "bottom line," negotiating power, and purchasing power. This force is creating constant disruptions in health care employment. The key here is flexibility. We have seen an increase in flexibility in work schedules and the birth of job sharing. Forecasters expect that there will be even more experimentation and variation in staffing patterns, both in the hospital and in the physician practice as there is an attempt to "tighten the belt" to increase profitability. Technology can be either friend or foe. On one hand, technologic advances can be substituted for human labor. For example, white cell counts that had to be performed manually are now completed in seconds by machine. On the other hand, technologic advances create needs for new types of personnel. For example, the development of new cardiac imaging technologies has created the need for specially trained technologists to perform the procedures.

No one knows if the future will bring shortages or overabundances of health care professionals, but the impact of all these changes will be considerable. Flexibility during this transition will be key.

EXERCISES

MULTIPLE CHOICE

Choose the best *answer for each of the following questions.*

1. If a patient is having stomach problems, he or she would seek care from which of the following specialty physicians?
   a. Gerontologist
   b. Gastroenterologist
   c. Gynecologist
   d. Dermatologist
2. Which of the following is not considered by Dr. Thomas to be a trait of a successful physician?
   a. One who listens attentively
   b. One who asks questions about the case
   c. One who orders several studies
   d. One who explains the diagnosis
3. This type of physician practice is called a "clinic without walls":
   a. Solo practice
   b. Open corporation
   c. Integrated provider network
   d. Management service organization
4. A neurologist treats which of the following?
   a. Pancreatic conditions
   b. Cerebrovascular accident
   c. Chronic obstructive lung disease
   d. Nail avulsion
5. Which does *not* describe a profession?
   a. A principal calling
   b. A group membership requiring expertise
   c. Act of declaring belief
   d. A calling requiring special knowledge
6. Which is *not* a type of corporation?
   a. Single-person
   b. Group
   c. Open
   d. Nonprofit
7. When a patient is referred to a pain clinic, what type of physician specialty would the patient expect to see?
   a. Pulmonologist
   b. Psychiatrist
   c. Physiatrist
   d. Podiatrist
8. What is a type of learning experience for a health care professional?
   a. Skills
   b. Attitudes
   c. Basic concepts
   d. All of the above
9. The AMA definition of a group practice is
   a. Two physicians
   b. Three or more physicians
   c. One physician
   d. All of the above
10. Which individual would *not* be found assisting a physician in the operating room?
    a. Coder
    b. CRNA
    c. RN
    d. Operating room technician

MATCHING

Match the specialty with the description provided.

1. _____	Neurologist	A. Psychologic disorder therapy
2. _____	Pulmonologist	B. Pregnancy and childbirth
3. _____	Pathologist	C. Laboratory medicine
4. _____	Surgeon	D. Emotional/mental disorders
5. _____	Podiatrist	E. Primary care
6. _____	Family practitioner	F. Treatment of allergies
7. _____	Chiropractor	G. Illnesses/conditions of women
8. _____	Allergist	H. Treatment of the nervous system
9. _____	Gynecologist	I. Musculoskeletal conditions
10. _____	Psychiatrist	J. Treatment of lungs
11. _____	Gerontologist	K. Diseases requiring surgery
12. _____	Psychologist	L. Care of the foot
13. _____	Physiatrist	M. Diseases of the elderly
14. _____	Obstetrician	N. Functioning of the nervous system

Match the profession with the description provided.

1. _____	Assists in the operating room	A. Radiologic technician
2. _____	Assists with anesthesia	B. Occupational therapist
3. _____	Performs electroencephalograms	C. Operating room technician
4. _____	Teaches patients daily activities	D. Nurse anesthetist
5. _____	Performs x-ray examinations	E. EKG technician
		F. EEG technician

TRUE OR FALSE

1. ______ A closed corporation sells shares of stock.
2. ______ A corporation is inexpensive to establish.
3. ______ A group practice consists of two or more physicians.
4. ______ In a group practice, the physician can take time off whenever she or he wants.
5. ______ A registered nurse has a higher level of education than a nurse practitioner.
6. ______ Many allergy practices are solo physicians.
7. ______ Dermatology is the treatment of foot problems.
8. ______ A large group practice offers physicians more free time.
9. ______ Unlimited liability can affect the owner of the practice.
10. ______ Some physician specialties are hospital based.
11. ______ A gastroenterologist treats patients with bladder problems.
12. ______ A cardiologist would order an EEG to check on a patient's cardiac condition.
13. ______ To be a professional, it is important to have autonomy of judgment.
14. ______ Most professionals have a certification or license.
15. ______ Emergency physicians have practices that are office based.

THINKERS

1. List five stages of a medical practice life cycle.
2. List the disadvantages of a partnership.
3. What terms best describe the word *professional*?
4. Provide an example of how technology has created a need for a type of health care professional.
5. Provide an example of how technology can be substituted for human labor.

REFERENCES

Clarkson, K., Miller, R., Jentz, G., & Cross, F. *West's Business Law.* New York: West Publishing Company, 2006.

Dale, W., & Gombeski, W. "Better Marketing through a Principles-based Model." *Marketing Health Services.* Chicago: American Marketing Association, 1998.

Day, J. C. *U.S. Bureau of the Census, Population Projections of the United States by Age, Sex, Race and Hispanic Origin: 1993 to 2050, Current Population Reports.* Washington, DC: Government Printing Office, 2005.

Futurescan 2000. *A Millennium Forecast of Healthcare Trends 2000-2004.* San Francisco: American Hospital Association Health Forum, 2000.

Kotler, P., & Levitt, T. "A Critical Assessment of Marketing Theory and Practice." *Diffuse Marketing Ideas.* Champaign, IL: The University of Illinois Press, 1978.

Proportion of Physicians in Solo/Two Physician Practices Drops, Center for Studying Health System Change. News release, August 16, 2007. Retrieved from www.hschange.com/CONTENT/942/

Shortall, S. M., & Reinhardt, U. E. "Creating and Executing Health Policy in the 1990s." *Improving Health Policy and Management: Nine Critical Research Issues for the 1990s.* Ann Arbor, MI: Health Administration Press, 1992.

Sultz, H., & Young, K. *Health Care USA: Understanding Its Organization and Delivery.* Gaithersburg, MD: Aspen Publishing, 2001.

2

PERSONNEL MANAGEMENT

CHAPTER OUTLINE

CHAPTER OBJECTIVES

After completing this chapter, you will be able to do the following:

- Define and differentiate among the various employee benefits
- Define *cafeteria plan*
- Recognize the differences between full-time and part-time employees
- Identify the most common fringe benefits offered in medical practices

HUMAN RESOURCES

Human resources are a combination of administrative personnel functions, employee relations, and management of employee performance. Most large companies, firms, and hospitals have human resource departments that handle the key functions of hiring, employee compensation, management of performance, promotions, and employee relations. In most physician practices, however, the human resource function is performed by the office manager. The three major areas that an office manager must address are

- Demographics
- Diversity
- Qualifications and skills

Demographics are the characteristics of the workforce, such as gender, age, marital status, and so forth. Demographics have a direct correlation to employee benefits, such as health insurance, disability insurance, time off, and so on.

Diversity is the variation that is found within the workforce. Recent changes in the workforce show an increase in the number of female employees and an increase in the number of employees from different cultures.

Qualifications and skills are necessary for employment and advancement in today's workplace. When more than one individual is being considered for a position, history shows that the individual with the highest skill set will be the one chosen for the position. All three areas are of major importance to the office manager when performing the duties of human resource director.

UNDERSTANDING EMPLOYEES' PERSONALITIES

Because we are all human, we share certain characteristics. Yet each of us has a distinct personality and unique life experiences. There are several types of employee operating types, each with its own assets and liabilities. Having a thorough understanding of these personality types will aid the office manager to be more effective and efficient. The following are some personality types the office manager will encounter:

- Rational
- Intuitive
- Feeler
- Doer
- Pragmatist
- Conservator
- Controller

Rational employees think logically, live their lives in an orderly fashion, and expect right-or-wrong, yes-or-no answers. Rational people tend to be skeptical and are often perfectionists. They are not interested in experimentation; they prefer to have a good plan, which they will follow through to the end. Delegating responsibility makes them uncomfortable. Thus they often end up with an excessive amount of work, which leads to stress and burnout.

Intuitive employees rely on their instincts and are somewhat introverted. Although they may appear to be lazy and ineffective, they are not; this is simply their work style. An office manager should not measure intuitive workers by partial accomplishments, only by final results. Their partial work may appear fragmented, but the final result is usually thorough and complete. They are process oriented, enjoying each procedural step without particular concern for the final goal, and are likely to question each step along the way. Intuitives must be treated with care, because they tend to try to read between the lines and may misconstrue what you are telling them. Their demeanor is sometimes misunderstood by other employees as rebellious or arrogant. They do their best work when given specific assignments. They are not practical and do not like to deal with the bottom line.

Feelers are people who are adept at nonverbal communication. They listen intently and empathize with others. Because of their extroverted nature, they prefer personal involvement and like to be helpful. Feelers tend to focus on other people's strengths, rather than on their faults, thus lowering workplace anxiety. They are tolerant of mistakes and are not critical. One disadvantage of the feelers' work style is impulsiveness, and frequently their first idea becomes their final one. Feelers are very effective in solving personal problems and often impress others with their warmth and understanding.

Doers are action oriented and refuse to be confined or obligated. They are impulsive and do what they want to do when they want to do it. Doers live for the here and now and have been known to cause crises just to liven things up. Doers have an "easy come, easy go" attitude and wander off when bored. They generally do not develop solid, in-depth friendships and feel that values are not important. During a crisis, they can be of real help because the situation allows them to direct their energies and really get into the thick of things. These individuals have the energy to get things done; however, they need the constant attention of the office manager for guidance.

Pragmatists are task-oriented individuals who direct their action to an immediate goal. They are known for their belief in the trial-and-error method and take calculated risks when necessary. Pragmatists often act on principle and are excellent negotiators. They have a real need for achievement and are assertive and controlling. Their coworkers often perceive them as manipulative and exploitive. Pragmatists usually do not work well with others and may have difficulty with interpersonal relationships.

Conservators are traditionalists. Generally, they follow a set of rules and regulations to the letter and are stable, reliable, and organized. They look for respect and recognition and value status and position. Conservators can be preoccupied with a personal problem (for example, a sick child or financial problems), but they can still maintain excellent quality control in the workplace and look to the past for direction.

Controllers want power and control. They crave responsibility and structure and are strong willed, decisive, and always interested in the bottom line. As goal-driven people, they are seen by other workers as tough skinned and will make decisions on an impersonal basis. Controllers pride themselves on being objective and look for well-ordered, scheduled plans. Controllers are apt to seek power over other workers as a way of controlling their working environment. Often, they will make rigid plans that do not fit into the scheme of things.

Once the office manager realizes the differences among work styles, she or he can integrate employees into an effective, innovative office staff.

"SIZING UP" THE MEDICAL OFFICE STAFF

"Hiring and training are costly, but it is definitely more costly to have a marginal employee."

—GORDON WHEELING, BECKMAN & WHITLEY

Having the proper personnel is the greatest asset of an office manager. Therefore the responsibility of the office manager is to evaluate the staff on a regular basis and identify the employees who will help the practice achieve the physician's goals. The office manager must understand how each employee functions in her or his job and must then identify the strengths and weaknesses of each employee. Evaluating the employees can be done by talking to them, meeting with them on a regular basis, helping them set combined goals, observing them on a daily basis, and conducting regularly scheduled performance reviews to assess their efficiency and workload. Most employees will be on their best behavior if they think they are being observed for evaluation.

Judgment regarding an employee's suitability for the office should be withheld until a specified time has been established. This is a process that should not be rushed. As already stated, recognizing the different personality types enables the office manager to see beyond first impressions and understand how each employee operates. Every staff has employees who fail to meet the standards of the office and thus no longer contribute. It is sometimes possible to motivate an employee of this type; however, if a stated time has gone by and the employee is still not performing adequately, the manager may have to consider terminating this employee. One of the keys to motivating employees is to allow them to participate in decision making. This is discussed further later in the chapter in the section titled "How to Remotivate the Staff."

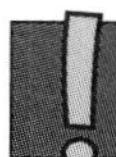

MANAGER'S ALERT

Keep in mind that it is in the best interest of the practice to retain employees, because hiring and training are costly. It is in everyone's best interests to remotivate and communicate openly with existing employees rather than to hire new ones.

Rebel

The office manager knows that the rebel employee can be both devious and manipulative. She or he may even be described as a good worker with special talents. This may be why this employee has been able to get away with rebellious behaviors such as constantly coming to work late, inappropriate dress, and sometimes bucking authority. This individual does not usually benefit by being given more flexibility in scheduling, because her or his reasons for being late are not always related to the hours the office maintains. The office manager does not want to create negative employer/employee relationships, but knows that all employees must abide by office standards. The best way to deal with a rebel employee is to be open and direct. In being direct, the manager tells the employee how much her or his work is valued but also explains the problems and their impact on others. Because the notice is preceded by positive feedback, the response is accepted more easily and the rebel employee generally is found to comply. Rebel employees also tend to sway others to follow suit, therefore creating more office havoc.

Houdini

One concern of the office manager is the employee who is the "disappearing act." When employees leave their work area without mentioning to anyone where they are going, problems can occur. It should be a common practice in the office that employees inform each other, or the office manager, when they are leaving, where they are going, and when they expect to return. All employees should be held responsible for this, even if they are leaving their area for only a minute. "A minute" sometimes stretches to 15 minutes, and office flow should not be interrupted while someone frantically searches for the missing employee.

It is a good idea for the office manager to adopt this practice also. The employees should always be able to locate the manager in case of a problem. If the manager is not going to be readily available, she or he should specify to the employees certain times when she or he will call to check on the office and review messages. By adopting this call-in plan, the office manager will keep up to date on the pertinent events of the day and earn the respect of the employees.

Jekyll and Hyde

Employees will almost always be polite and well mannered in front of the boss. They will treat the office manager just as Emily Post would, with the most impeccable manners. Now, imagine that this employee, who treats the office manager and physician with respect, treats co-workers and patients with disrespect. This type of employee might see herself or himself as more of an equal with the office manager than with the rest of the staff and convey an air of superiority to other employees.

The manager should watch and listen to identify signs of rudeness or other inappropriate behavior by the staff. Do patients avoid dealing with a particular employee? Are the employees planning an outing and leaving someone out? Maybe the position that was filled five times in the past 2 years is not a problem with that particular position, but a problem with the personality of a specific employee. Here are four common ways to discourage rudeness and negative behavior in employees:

- Stress courtesy.
- Set the right example.
- Act immediately to compliment courteous behavior.
- Recognize and correct the problem immediately.

COURTESY IN THE MEDICAL OFFICE

The importance of being courteous to all patients and co-workers should be stressed to each employee at the time of hire. A new employee should be instructed that courtesy is a major part of her or his position and that the lack of it will not be tolerated. Long-time personnel may also need to be reminded with gentle pep talks on an occasional basis. They should be reminded that without satisfied patients, there would not be work. Patients today are consumers. They will choose their physician on the basis of the service provided by both the physician and the staff. Patients will always return to a medical office that has a friendly, polite, and caring staff.

Compliment Courteous Behavior

Performance reviews should include evaluation of employees' courtesy. Employees who go out of their way to be courteous to patients, physicians, and co-workers should be commended, both verbally and in writing. Compliment them on their grace under pressure. Positive reinforcement strengthens employees' recognition of the importance of good manners. It boosts office morale and productivity.

There is no excuse for rudeness or bad manners. Physicians, patients, and co-workers will respond in a positive manner if they are complimented for their handling of a situation.

SETTING THE RIGHT EXAMPLE

Many office managers do not realize how important their function as a role model is on an everyday basis. Everyone has a bad day now and again; however, the office manager should put on her or his best face for patients, the physicians, and the employees. Inconsistent behavior by the office manager is not advised.

Temper tantrums should be kept out of the office. This type of behavior should not be permitted in an office setting and should be discouraged immediately. If an employee does have a temper tantrum, remove her or him from the office and settle the matter away from other employees. Only "out-of-control" children throw tantrums.

TEAMWORK

There is no "i" in teamwork! —ANONYMOUS

A team is a set of interpersonal relationships serving to achieve established goals. They function as individual members that interact together as a team. The essential elements of effective teams are

- Positive interdependence
- Individual accountability
- Face-to-face interaction
- Collaborative skills
- Group processing/brainstorming

Positive interdependence is when team members are linked together in such a way that each member cannot succeed unless the others do, and vice versa. One person's work benefits the others', and the others' work benefits that person. It is the belief that everyone sinks or swims together.

Individual accountability is present when the performance of each team member is assessed to inform the group and increase the others' perceptions.

Face-to-face interaction is the perception that a team member's efforts and participation are needed, and this perception increases as the size of the team decreases.

Collaborative skills must be taught just as technical skills must be taught. Team members must be taught the precise social skills for high-quality collaboration and must be motivated to use them.

Group processing is the group's ability to make decisions and describe what member actions were helpful.

Six Processes Necessary for Teamwork

There are six processes that must take place for teamwork to be effective:

1. The team is given the opportunity to create and identify issues that are important. It must have the collective knowledge to envision the office's needs.
2. The team members gather information regarding these issues.
3. The team analyzes the information and prioritizes it.
4. The team plans a course of action.
5. The team leader implements the plan.
6. The process is evaluated to ensure that the goals have been met.

Teamwork ensures the delivery of quality service, efficiency of operations, decreased stress, and confidence. Don't forget to include the physician in the practice team. She or he is the team's owner, and you are the coach. It is important to stress to the employees that all members of the team must work together, from clinical personnel to billing personnel to front-desk personnel. They must form a cohesive bond whereby everyone strives to work together as efficiently as possible.

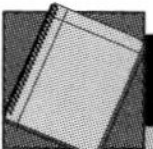

FROM THE EXPERT'S NOTEBOOK

When an office lacks teamwork–the result is CHAOS! An office manager should work to foster teamwork among the employees.

Benefits of Teamwork

Teamwork yields high gains in both productivity and social areas. It is one of the most important factors in creating a friendly office. It has been proven that patients are happier in an office where all staff members work together toward a common goal. Employees working together accomplish so much more than employees working independently of one another. When two employees join together, they can create an effect greater than what is predicted by working separately. This is known as *synergy*, where the whole is greater than the sum of the parts. The benefits of teamwork are listed in Box 2-1.

BOX 2-1 Benefits of Teamwork

Increased office morale
Easier cross-training
Increased revenues
Positive working environment
Decreased staff turnover
Increased productivity
Increased quality of work
Open communication
Happier physicians
Better organization and scheduling
Satisfied patients

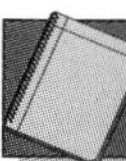

FROM THE EXPERT'S NOTEBOOK

"Snowflakes are one of nature's most fragile things, but just look at what they can do when they stick together!"

—Anonymous

Dealing with the Employee Who Is Not a Team Player

If you find that an employee refuses to be a team player, give serious consideration to replacing that employee with one who will be a team player. The last thing an office needs is a negative attitude among employees . . . replace that person quickly! There is something about negativism; it seems to spread quickly throughout an office, turning a hard-working, happy office into a waking nightmare.

Rallying and Rewarding Team Members

Make your employees feel needed and reward them for a job well done. Everyone—the patients, the physicians, and the employees—likes to feel important. If the employees and physician feel important, it will trickle down to the patients, providing them with satisfaction. Show the employees that you care about them. Recognize their individual accomplishments and their contributions to the team. Listen to them, support their ideas, and value what they contribute to the general working of the office. Don't make them feel that they are working in a threatened environment. Don't use threats to get jobs done . . . you won't like the results! Remember, it's nice to be nice. A good office manager manages without resorting to threats. She or he rallies employees to work together; motivates them; encourages them; and, most of all, believes in them. A good manager stresses the common thread among them: the desire to achieve. The last thing a manager should hear is "That's not my job" or "Well, we've always done it this way." These are the phrases that send office managers through the roof. Help employees build confidence in themselves and each other. Show them that a little effort to adapt to change will lead to big rewards. Give them clear expectations, guidance, and the resources to be able to effect change. Be a cheerleader, cheering your team on to success!

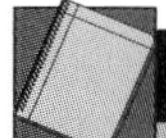

FROM THE EXPERT'S NOTEBOOK

As a manager, you must be a cheerleader, leading not dragging them on to success.

Foundation for Teamwork

The foundation for teamwork comes from the employees having a clear understanding of what is expected of them. From this, solid working relationships are built. The staff and office manager are able to work together to reach common goals. In clarifying what she or he expects from employees, the office manager may find that the subject of lunch hours is a good place to start. In every practice, large or small, the telephone must be monitored at all times, a factor that influences whether and when employees can take lunch breaks. The office manager must make sure that all staff members understand the office's policy regarding lunch hours.

The office manager who is managing a large staff may find it necessary to initiate set lunch periods, whereby each employee is assigned a regular lunchtime in which to eat lunch, run errands, do banking, and so on. To ensure that the phones are managed at all times, the manager of a small office has two options. Lunch breaks can be staggered, which allows for telephone coverage at all times. If the flexibility is not there to allow each employee to have a set lunch period, the best solution is to stagger the lunch periods so that the employees get a break and the telephones are still answered. It is important that the office manager decide how flexible she or he is going to be about the length and time of lunch breaks. Employees should be made aware of the office policy regarding lunch hour at the time of hire, and this should also be addressed in the office policy and procedure manual.

The second option would be to close the office for an hour to ensure that the employees and physician are able to eat without interruption. It must be emphasized that each employee is part of a greater whole. Something as trivial as being late getting back from lunch can affect others and alter the day's workflow.

Cliques

It is almost inevitable that some employees will group together to make a clique. A clique is a narrow, exclusive social grouping of people with the same interests, objectives, or goals. Cliques can be based on tenure, profession, social or economic class, ethnicity, gender, or any factor that differentiates one person from another. The exclusionary nature of a clique hampers effective teamwork in the office. However, human nature being what it is, cliques do exist and can be powerful and difficult to deal with. A skilled office manager will recognize a clique and will take the necessary steps to defuse the power it has. Cliques are a "high school" leftover and do not belong in the workplace! The following warning signs indicate that a harmful clique exists:

- Critical decisions may be taking place without appropriate input.
- Employees of the clique get a different ratio of promotions, incentives, bonuses, and other perks in the office.
- Employees of the clique get a different ratio of disciplinary action or warning.

Professional cliques are common. In health care, there are physicians versus the nursing staff. This results from individuals with a different knowledge base and skill set, and people who perceive themselves as having invested more in their careers than others. Once you have determined that a clique exists, it needs to be dissolved. Individuals will act defensively when they feel threatened. Groups that are facing uncertainty are especially prone to cliques. For example, if there are tenured employees forming a clique, it may be necessary to ask their opinion of ongoing events within the practice and make them feel included and valuable. It is important to recognize the value of each employee and the importance of her or his role within the practice.

PERSONAL TELEPHONE CALL PLAGUE

"Alexander Graham Bell did not invent the telephone, he invented a source of entertainment!" —ANONYMOUS

Office policy regarding personal telephone calls should also be discussed at the time of hire. Giving employees a lot of leeway regarding personal phone calls will result in problems for any office. However, the occasional personal telephone call is certainly permissible, and always in the case of an emergency. It is good to have a certain amount of flexibility in each office, because it builds a productive office environment. However, care must be taken to make sure the privilege is not abused. This personal telephone call problem is even more exaggerated now that most employees have cell phones. It is important to have a cell phone policy in the office policy and procedure manual. Cell phones are discussed in detail in Chapter 3.

PERSONAL PROBLEMS AND THE EMPLOYEE

Although we are at the threshold of humanizing the workplace by meeting employees' needs for day care, counseling, fitness, and so on, personal problems most be left at home. Nasty divorces, disobedient children, family drug abuse, car problems, and other personal issues do not belong in the workplace. One of the most important reasons for requesting that employees keep their personal problems out of the workplace is that employees who reveal personal issues in the office may find that they come back to haunt them at a later date. The story of a personal crisis will linger in an individual's mind. It has been found that long after the crisis is over, the employee is still perceived as preoccupied or impaired.

When one employee confides in another, she or he is placing a burden on the other not to mention the situation to the rest of the staff. However, co-workers have been found to use this information against each other for personal gain. This can easily happen in a competitive environment, be it a small, single-physician practice, or a large, multi-specialty practice.

There may come a time when an employee finds it necessary to mention a personal problem to the office manager. This may be affecting the employee's productivity, or the employee might be receiving an excessive number of personal phone calls. Even in this case, the less said the better. The office manager should ask for the minimal amount of information, and that only of a factual nature. The manager should maintain a distance and give no opinion one way or another. The only crisis that warrants more detail is a true personal tragedy, such as a death in the family or a family member with a severe illness, such as cancer. In this instance, sympathy tends to outweigh stigma. If the personal problem becomes substantially intrusive, the manager might suggest a leave of absence to the employee in order to get matters resolved.

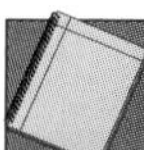

FROM THE EXPERT'S NOTEBOOK

Talking about personal problems over and over again can get "old" fast. Fellow employees will initially show empathy, but after a while, will "scatter" as you begin to repeat your "monologue of woe." Leave it at home!

RECOGNIZING THE POWER OF THE GRAPEVINE

The effective medical office manager never underestimates the power of the grapevine. Gossip networks exist at every level of every office and company. Yes, even physicians are sometimes guilty of gossiping. Attempts to quell the flow of information through the grapevine are usually a waste of time; however, the effective office manager tries to ensure that at least some of the information being passed around is on the positive aspects of the practice. There are five ways the office manager can influence the nature of the grapevine:

1. Informed communication
2. Give-and-take policies
3. Performance reviews
4. Trusted employees
5. Formal responses

Informed Communication

Informed communication starts with better-informed employees. Employees who are kept well informed are less likely to turn to the grapevine for information. Whenever possible, the office manager should discuss issues with the employees so that they will not have the need to gossip. If there are no office secrets, there are generally no office problems. Informed employees also make better employees. Regularly sharing information and distributing memos will create less need for an office grapevine and will positively convey the office's position.

Give-and-Take Policies

Give-and-take policies are much more effective than policies set in stone. It is good practice to be known as an office manager who is fair and flexible and open to negotiations. The office manager is often the person to whom the employees turn for confirmation or denial of information traveling through the grapevine. It is good to establish an open and truthful relationship with the employees. Employers with open door policies can provide positive feedback for employee problems.

Performance Reviews

Performance reviews are done on a quarterly, a semiannual, or an annual basis and are good opportunities to exchange information with employees. When an employee hears through the grapevine that she or he may be in hot water, the office manager should be truthful with the employee during the performance review. Sensitive issues should be confronted "head on" with a positive attitude and not be avoided. The manager should state the information available to her or him and suggest that any further information will be passed on to the employee as it becomes available. If the office manager does not know the information or is not aware of the problem, she or he should tell the employee that the appropriate source will be checked and feedback will follow in a timely manner.

Trusted Employees

It is helpful for the office manager to have a trusted employee to whom she or he can turn when in need of an intermediary. This employee can act as the eyes and ears of the office manager and should be someone in the practice who is highly regarded and can be trusted. A written formal response should be considered only as a last resort, but may sometimes be necessary to quiet some of the more egregious rumors. A written response does give a degree of credence to the rumors; however, it also allows for a resolution of the matter.

Formal Responses

The grapevine can be addressed by issuing a formal response to the rumor. For example, if the rumor is that the practice is going to be hiring a new physician, it is sometimes best to send a memo, which either confirms or denies this rumor. It is always best to keep the employees "in the loop" with open communication. The walls have ears, and even the lowest whispers can be heard by some. A memo issued to address the rumor can work well.

STAFF SUPERVISION

"Leadership is the ability to get men to do what they don't want to do and like it!" —DWIGHT D. EISENHOWER

Some office managers have a difficult time understanding the difference between being a manager and being a policeman. Good office managers realize that the people in their office come first. This means they know that employees do their best work when they are not afraid to make decisions and feel free to express their opinions. It is not necessary to become an ogre to supervise staff. Office managers should not act as spies or dictators. More can be accomplished by creating an environment of enthusiasm, commitment, respect, and trust. The slightest lean toward spying and bullying will sabotage this environment every time.

Down-to-earth leadership will show that well-managed employees are more productive and responsible than scared employees. A well-trained office staff will be more productive when provided with structure and clear expectations of the task. Good training is designed to build confidence in employees, confidence that is reflected in the way they do their jobs and treat patients. Training is not about standing near employees and pointing out what they are doing wrong. It is about motivating them to do it right; you not only give them an example, you give them reason. As mentioned previously, teamwork is the answer to a well-run office. Studies have shown that medical offices that use teamwork approaches to their tasks are more organized, efficient, and flexible than are offices ruled by the heavy-handed practices of the past.

How to Remotivate the Staff

Motivation is a constant concern of the good office manager. Dealing with sick patients, demanding doctors, and cranky co-workers can quickly wear down even the best employees. When this happens, it is time to reenergize the staff. Offering good salaries is an important factor in obtaining and keeping good employees, but that alone will not necessarily be the only way to motivate them. It is important for employees to feel in control of and secure in their jobs, respected by their co-workers and superiors, and hopeful about their professional futures. Building trust and morale in a medical office is an art and can be accomplished by encouragement, enthusiasm, and loyalty. There are several tried and true ways of motivating the staff:

- Don't issue commands.
- Delegate, don't dump.
- Set goals with staff.
- Listen, really listen!
- Let staff share in decisions.
- Offer constructive criticism.
- Provide continuity and consistency.
- Avoid hasty judgments.
- Provide rewards and incentives.
- Lend a friendly ear.
- Follow through with promises.
- Monitor without smothering.

Instead of issuing commands, effective office managers sell a course of action to their employees. They know that persuading and rewarding will get them further than shouting orders like an army sergeant. Many managers feel that it is necessary to be in control and to be firm, but when they give quick, harsh orders, they can easily start to lose the support of their employees. A manager can be firm without being harsh or demeaning.

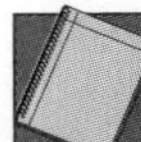

FROM THE EXPERT'S NOTEBOOK

Be careful not to micromanage your personnel. Treat them like the professionals that they are. Give them a task, and monitor from afar. Most employees will appreciate the opportunity to work on a project and will rise to the occasion.

Delegating is essential to successful medical office management, yet many office managers do not understand what it means or how it works. By delegating certain tasks, the office manager is free to do other tasks. The office manager who delegates only unpleasant tasks is "dumping," and employees view it as an abuse. Delegating gives an employee the responsibility and authority to complete a task, which will enlarge her or his area of expertise. *Hint:* Make sure the employee is capable of performing that task before you delegate it!

Setting goals with the staff improves motivation more than any other technique mentioned here. By sitting down with employees and defining their work in terms of goals and objectives, the manager shows employees that she or he has confidence in them and is counting on them.

In times of low morale, listening to what the employees are saying is a valuable tool. If necessary, the manager should schedule a one-to-one talk with each employee. The manager should listen to what the employees have to say and let them know it is important. Although the manager does not have to agree with everything employees say or suggest, it shows that she or he respects their opinions.

Allowing the staff to make some of their own decisions gives the staff a sense of authority over their own jobs.

It is better if they are allowed to make some decisions on their own than if they have to ask the office manager about every single decision. This creates a feeling of ownership and responsibility. Allowing employees to participate in decision making that relates to their jobs allows them to develop their decision-making ability. As Woodrow Wilson said, "I use not only all the brains I have, but all I can borrow."

Private, constructive criticism is much better than public ridicule. The office manager should *never* criticize any employee in front of others. Neither should the manager get into the habit of telling employees to come into her or his office only when the intent is to criticize them. It is necessary to be fair to everyone, even those in trouble. Yelling, public criticism, gossip, and personal feuds are self-indulgent. Set clear rules and stick to them.

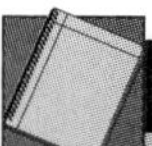

FROM THE EXPERT'S NOTEBOOK

Always try to couple a criticism with a compliment on a job well done. It takes away the bitter taste of the criticism.

Employees need continuity in all aspects of their position. They expect the office manager to remember what they told her or him yesterday and the day before. They expect consistency in what they are told, and they expect that if a change in policy occurs, they will be notified as soon as possible. The manager tries to insulate the employees from inconsistencies in the physician's actions and policies. If the manager passes them on, the staff feels as though nobody is in control. The manager must weed out any inconsistent information from the physician before passing it on to the staff. Change can be difficult. It is very important to notify each employee of all changes. This will make the change more positive.

Avoid hasty judgments about employees' work styles. The office manager who expects employees to work exactly as she or he does is many times disappointed. It is crucial that the manager recognize that employees have different ways of handling different tasks and that the manager's way is not always the *only* way. The office manager's disapproval of any decisions that are not identical to her or his own could erode any free flow of ideas that could be coming from the employee. In a productive medical office, the manager is flexible, recognizes different work styles, and avoids hasty judgments.

Rewards and incentives should be provided. The office manager's praise for a job well done immediately after an employee did something well is just as important as a paycheck the following week. People respond to praise; when it is used as often as possible, it will provide the office manager with positive results. The ratio of praise to punishment should be four to one. Some offices choose to issue bonuses to employees who have performed beyond what is expected of them.

The manager should be sociable and encourage office camaraderie. Employees who are allowed to socialize at work generally stay on their jobs because they like the people they work with. Teamwork is easier among co-workers who have developed friendships. If employees are allowed to be sociable, they become more energized and creative. This positive atmosphere will be felt by the patients and create a pleasant office environment.

Promises of action must be kept. Employees need to know that matters are being responded to. When the office manager tells employees that she or he will check on something for them, it is imperative that the office manager follow through. The manager's credibility will be lost each time employees' expectations are not met. If a decision from the physician is being awaited, the manager should let the employees know that she or he is still working on the problem and hasn't forgotten it.

Monitoring the staff on a daily basis without smothering them is a good way for the office manager to keep problems from becoming major. The manager should talk with each employee regularly and ask for a summary of her or his projects and what her or his work entails. The office manager should create a list of employee projects and provide the physician with updates of this list on a regular basis (Figure 2-1). If the office manager has a regular monitoring system in place, employees will expect the manager to check on them and will not see this as being an intrusion. The manager should make sure that all employees are monitored on a regular basis so that no one feels singled out or persecuted.

The Art of Instruction

As mentioned earlier, the delegation of responsibility is essential to effective medical management. However, delegated projects can come back to the office manager below the standard that the office manager was expecting. Many office managers

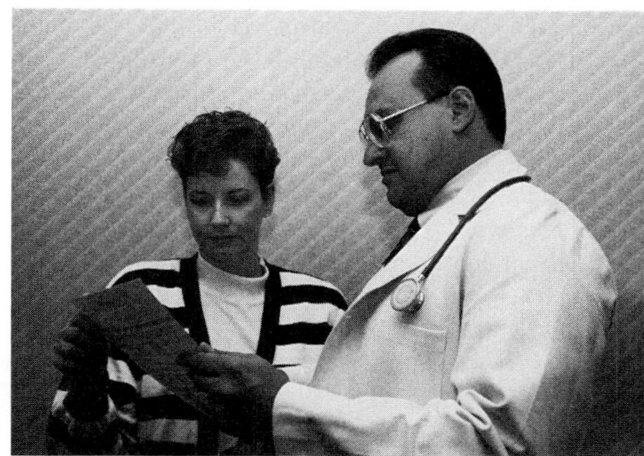

FIGURE 2-1. The physician and the office manager discuss a new policy.

find themselves saying, "I should have done it myself." In a frustrated state, they point the finger at an employee, saying that she or he is incompetent. However, the problem may very well lie in the instructions that were given by the office manager, not the inadequacies of the employee. Clear and thorough instructions must be given for each delegated responsibility. When delegating work, the office manager needs to do the following:

- Be specific and clear
- Avoid jargon
- Explain to the employee why she or he is being asked to handle this task
- Ask for feedback
- Understand when to give instructions and when to give directives

The manager needs to be specific, explain exactly what is to be done, and specify when it is to be completed. If the employee is given the latitude to make some decisions, the manager needs to specify which areas of the project should not be changed. The instructions should be presented in easy-to-understand steps. Everyone has a different learning style. Some people like to read directions, whereas others like to be shown. It is a good idea to assess the learning style of the new employee, so that the training period is easier on both parties. Regardless of whether they give instructions in writing or verbally, office managers must never assume that employees will know what they mean. Therefore it is important not to leave out any steps in the directions. Office managers should check their directive skills by writing down the steps of a certain task from start to finish and then asking someone to perform the task by following only the written directions. This is a proven way of determining whether the manager's directions are clear or vague.

One key to giving clear directions is avoiding jargon. Employees may not understand some terminology and may be afraid to ask for explanations. Ask employees to repeat instructions to eliminate confusion.

When employees are asked to handle a specific project, they need to be told why they must complete it in a certain manner, so that they understand and comply with the directions. Certain projects require specific details and procedures. For example, if the employee is asked to copy and mail patient records, it is important to follow the office protocol for this activity. Is there a patient-signed records release form? Have all procedures for this type of release been followed? This is not the place to be an independent thinker . . . just follow instructions.

FROM THE EXPERT'S NOTEBOOK

Avoid NIH syndrome—"Not invented here." If it is not the manager's idea, it is not a good idea.

Feedback is important to employees. They need to know when the office manager is pleased with their work. If an employee did not follow the instructions given, the manager should find out why. Communication problems should be identified so that the employee will be able to correct the problem in the future. The office manager needs to know when to give verbal instructions and when to give written directives. The manager may want to use a written directive for a task when an employee has successfully handled similar projects in the past or when the office manager is confident that the employee understands her or his expectations. As already mentioned, some people perform better with written instructions than with verbal instructions.

PERSONNEL CREDIBILITY

Individuals with good reputations are sought out and respected. The medical office staff should be concerned about how people, particularly patients and their families, perceive them and the role they play in the health care setting. If patients were asked to describe their physician's office personnel, would they describe them as problem solvers, advice givers, counselors, bookkeepers, physician helpers, teachers, form filers, or obstacles in getting to the doctor? The image of the medical office staff is critical to the patient-physician relationship. If the patient has doubts about the professionalism of the office staff, these concerns are generally transferred to the physician.

The image that medical office personnel present should be professional and compatible with a medical office environment. A good reputation must be earned, and the need to maintain this good reputation must be continuously reinforced by the medical office manager. Each interaction between the staff and patients and their families should be looked on as an opportunity to enhance the positive professional image of the office.

People are generally influenced more by negative experiences than by positive ones. It has been found that 11 positive experiences are required to neutralize 1 negative experience. One mistake, one incident of inaccurate information, or one instance of rude treatment may negate all of the positive experiences that a patient has had with the physician's office. The patient could start looking for a new physician. Many patients in a physician's office are friends, relatives, or co-workers of other patients, which can cause a mass exodus from the medical practice. A bad reputation can be difficult to overcome, and thus mistakes that may give rise to one are to be avoided at all costs. The physician's staff can be a detriment if they are not expressing a solid professional image of the physician and her or his practice.

THE VALUABLE EMPLOYEE

"Loyalty is like love. You have to give some in order to get some."

—ANONYMOUS

Most physicians don't understand the value of a good employee until that employee has left. A good office manager should recognize the value of each employee and do everything possible to make the employee feel appreciated and valued. The departure of an employee immediately throws the office into a state of confusion, which usually results in less productivity from everyone. Studies have shown that during a transition period, a medical office can lose $5,000 or more. This figure includes the hidden costs involved from a typical "downtime" period, such as the cost of temporary employees; the cost of work delays, which, depending on the position vacated, can be high; the cost of obtaining a new employee (the cost of a classified ad or a fee to an employment agency); and the loss of the office manager's time during the interview process. To prevent the loss of a good employee, the office manager should address the concerns of all employees. These concerns may be conflicts between co-workers, conflicts between the manager and an employee, unclear understandings of job descriptions, and personal crises. It should be the number one objective of each office manager to attempt to know each employee, to interact with her or him, and to communicate with the employee on a daily basis. This will minimize future problems. The number one reason for employee turnover is that the correct person was not hired in the first place. Careful selection of all employees can help the practice to retain experienced employees.

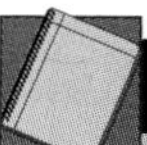

FROM THE EXPERT'S NOTEBOOK

Cross-training employees in positions other than their own helps alleviate some of the stress created by the loss of an employee.

CROSS-TRAINING

An employee absence can cripple a medical practice. If the practice has its employees cross-trained, it becomes less of a problem to "plug" those holes created by an employee absence. Whether or not it is planned, it is still problematic for the practice. To be able to cross-train effectively, it is important to hire the right personnel who are able to multitask and learn new things quickly. Some of the benefits of cross-training are as follows:

- There is consistency in the operation of the office.
- It provides the office manager with options that would otherwise not be available.
- It identifies hidden talents among employees.
- It is a morale booster.
- Patients may have fewer problems with insurances and appointment scheduling, and will be reassured when there is a familiar face or voice.
- It promotes fresh thinking and ideas about the position.
- It increases empathy and promotes teamwork.

THE EMPLOYEE LIFE CYCLE

The *first stage* of the employee life cycle is the search for candidates for a position. The *second stage* is selection of the best-qualified employee after interviews with several people. The *third stage* is the training stage. If employees are not properly trained, their productivity will be low. The office manager will ultimately be blamed for this, so it is imperative that the manager take the time to train an employee well or appoint an appropriate person to oversee the training.

The *fourth stage* is the directional stage. At this point, the employee is given direction as to her or his performance and the expectations of the medical practice. Proper direction opens many doors into a solid employee/employer relationship. A person cannot be expected to start a position without being informed of the goals of the practice. Orienting a new employee through philosophies of the medical practice by way of a mission statement is just as important as informing her or him of the technical aspects of the job. The mission statement is printed in the office policy and procedure manual, but it also needs to be discussed with the new employee. How well this mission statement is explained to the employee affects the overall character and assertiveness with which the employee will approach the position. Simply handing a new employee an office policy and procedure manual with no explanation is like giving someone a car full of gas and telling the person to drive, without ever telling her or him the destination. The priorities of the office, the benefits of productivity, and the reason for the practice of medicine in that particular area must be explained. This stage can prevent the loss of good employees and should never be overlooked.

The *fifth* and final stage of the employee life cycle is termination. By properly using the first four stages, most office managers can prevent this unpleasant stage. The employee life cycle is illustrated in Figure 2-2.

THE THREE BASICS OF A SUCCESSFUL "BOSS"

All managers want to be a successful "boss" and have the support of quality staff. There are three basic rules to remember

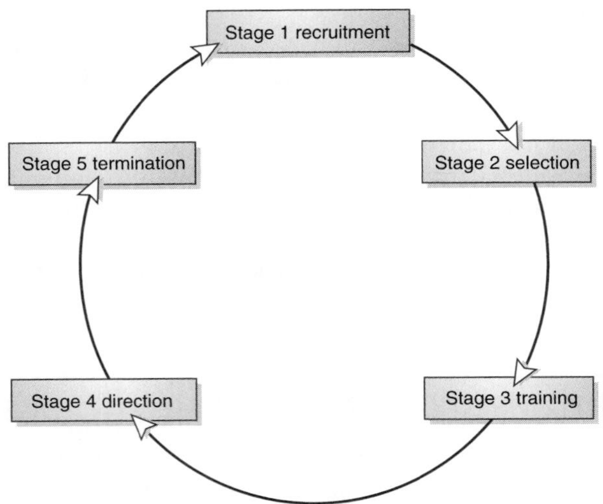

FIGURE 2-2. The employee life cycle.

to become successful. Follow these rules, and success will follow:

1. Hire the best qualified for the job . . . check references very carefully.
2. Pay the person what she or he is worth—have a salary range table.
3. Explain the expectations of the position . . . no surprises. If the office manager is expected to work late one night a week to meet with the physician, this should be discussed during the interview process.

THERE'S ONLY ONE BOSS . . . THE PATIENT!

Sam Walton of Wal-Mart Stores once said, "There's only one boss—the customer." In health care, there is only one boss, the patient. Employees need help to understand that they are key in making the practice successful. They need to take ownership in the practice and treat it as if it were their own. Make the connection for each employee that their personal performance is directly tied to the success of the physician's practice. Office managers should act like model employees showing them that you are not above stopping in the hallway to pick up a piece of paper that fell on the floor. At Disneyworld in Florida, they provide management training. During that training, they tell participants that it is part of the job description of a manager at Disneyworld to stop and pick up trash if they see it. At Google, employees can use 20% of their workday developing ideas outside of their actual job descriptions. These are just a few examples of empowering employees to think outside the box, to learn by mistakes, to have pride in the medical office and their specific jobs, and to take ownership of the practice.

An office manager can help employees invest in the practice and show that management maintains a sense of ownership. To this end, the office manager will create a positive, productive, patient-oriented employee. **An empowered employee = a successful medical practice = a happy patient!**

JOB DESCRIPTIONS

Job descriptions provide an effective guide for selection and employee placement. The American Disabilities Act addresses the lack of job descriptions in small offices and states that even small medical practices should have formal job descriptions.

It is essential to keep a list of up-to-date job descriptions in a file that is easily accessible. A job description is nothing more than a list of the duties and expectations of each position in the medical office. A job description should contain the following elements:

- Title of the position
- Responsibilities of the position
- Specific duties of the position
- Educational requirements
- Amount of supervision needed
- Experience needed
- Skills needed
- Accountability statement

The list of duties should be prioritized so that new employees are not found tidying up the lunchroom when they should be confirming patients for the next day. Most employees will welcome the direction that a job description gives them because it clarifies their roles and provides specific guidelines.

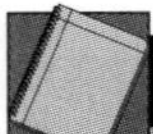

FROM THE EXPERT'S NOTEBOOK

It is always a good idea to ask an employee to provide a list of his or her functions. This will give the manager an overview of how the job is actually being done.

Job descriptions can be used when hiring a new employee, when interviewing and selecting a new employee, for training purposes, for employee evaluations, for salary evaluations, and for termination. Box 2-2 shows a sample job description that can be used as a model.

HIRING THAT "RIGHT" EMPLOYEE

It is important to hire an employee with the exact mix of characteristics that a position requires. In the medical office, employees' performance in their job is directly related to patient satisfaction. The right person for the job is the one

BOX 2-2 Job Description Sheet

Job Title: Transcriptionist
Supervisor: Lauren Casey
Date of Original Description: May 31, 2007
Date of Updated Description: June 2, 2008
Skill Requirements: Use of Word, Excel, Power Point; knowledge of medical terminology
Educational Requirements: High school diploma, advanced degree a plus
Experience Requirements: At least 3 years of experience in medical transcription
Duties:

- Transcribes from physician dictation to patient's chart by using typewriter or computer.
- Maintains a correspondence file of all letters dictated.
- Maintains a list of temporary employment agencies in event of absence of any member of the secretarial pool.
- Sorts and opens mail and distributes it to the appropriate persons.
- Answers the telephone when others are busy.
- Posts checks from mail in absence of secretary, who usually does this job.
- Prepares all physicians' copies of dictation and manuscripts.
- Performs special duties when asked.
- Is in charge of lunchroom cleanup schedule.

who smiles; is polite to co-workers, patients, and supervisors; and is responsive to the needs of the office.

When looking to fill a position in a medical office, the office manager should be aware that a person who is effective in a certain environment might become unglued in a hectic medical office environment. Picture the telephones ringing off the hook, a patient waiting to make an appointment, and a patient contesting her or his bill and Medicare coverage; this scenario can turn a calm, cool, and collected person into a frazzled, quick-tempered individual. Most patients are not happy to be at the physician's office to begin with and therefore are not in a good mood. They feel anxiety, pain, apprehension, and all varieties of other emotions. These are the people who need empathy from the medical staff. When patients walk into the office, they should always encounter a friendly and caring receptionist who is eager to greet them and welcome them to the office. After all, the receptionist is the window to the medical practice. The clinical staff of the office should also consist of warm, empathetic, and concerned individuals who give the patient a sense of security. Knowing that the individuals in the office *care* means a lot to a patient. Caring is not a taught behavior; caring is a deeply personal individual trait, and it is a truly valuable commodity in a health care employee.

When faced with the dilemma of searching for a new employee, the office manager may want to consider the following methods to find applicants:

- Contacting an agency
- Placing an ad in the newspaper or on the Internet
- Contacting a technical school or college for intern programs
- Using a headhunter
- Word of mouth or e-mail
- Posting notices on bulletin boards in a hospital

EMPLOYEE HANDBOOK

Each medical office should have an employee handbook. At the time of hire, each employee should receive her or his own copy of the employee handbook, which outlines the do's and don'ts of the employees of the practice. Have all employees sign a form within 2 weeks of the first day of their employment that acknowledges they have read and understand the handbook. This handbook should be written in clear, concise language that sets the ground rules for employment with the practice. Once the handbook is prepared, it should be given to the practice attorney to review for any issues with employment law. Each employee handbook should cover the following topics:

- A short welcome message from the physician and the office manager
- The office hours of the practice, discussion of breaks and lunch periods, flexible schedules
- Tardiness and absences (bereavement, jury duty, family and medical leave, sick time)
- Compensation, discussion of confidentiality of salaries, overtime pay, salary increase structure, employee evaluations, bonuses (if applicable)
- Vacation time (calculation of vacation time, structure)
- Benefits, including holidays, health insurance, disability insurance, life insurance, retirement plans
- Licensing and certification requirements
- Continuing education credits
- Personal use of cell phones, pagers, personal phone calls, the Internet, e-mail, fax machines, copiers
- Patient confidentiality, Health Insurance Portability and Accountability Act (HIPAA) privacy regulations
- Discrimination
- Personal conduct, courtesy, respect for co-workers and patients, disruptive behavior, substance abuse, offensive language, sexual harassment
- Termination; at-will employment; causes for termination include, but are not limited to, the following: . . .

Employment Agencies

Many medical office managers have hectic schedules and do not always have the proper amount of time to allot to the interviewing process. They should not be swayed by fancy clothes or pretty faces. They are trained to dig deep into the employment history of the individual and extract the qualities of that individual.

When they do not have the time to do this, the employment section of the telephone book provides them with a list of employment agencies. These agencies hire trained employment counselors who know just the right questions to ask of the individual seeking employment. They are experienced in what to look for and are familiar with certain behaviors that will trigger "red flags." Some agencies specialize in finding temporary personnel, whereas others specialize in finding permanent staff.

Such agencies greatly benefit a medical practice. A prospective employee can be hired as a temp for a set amount of time and then be brought on board as a permanent employee. If the temp is not exactly what the office is looking for, she or he can be exchanged for a different one. There is a great deal of flexibility in this type of system; however, this type of system can also be costly. When hiring an employee through an agency, the medical office is then responsible for a fee, which is commonly called a "buyout" figure. The longer the temporary employee works for the office, the more costly the buyout figure is. For many agencies, the buyout figure for a temporary employee is less at 3 weeks of employment than it is at 3 months of employment.

There is a fee for this service that may be paid by the person seeking employment. It can be a good show of faith if paid by the employer. This shows the employer's commitment to an employee. An employee whose fee has been paid by the employer tends to start the job with a reservoir of good will toward the new job. Many times, a medical office will reimburse a new employee two thirds of the fee after a reasonable probationary period has been met and satisfactory work has been completed. If the physician is willing to allow the office manager to use an employment agency, it can be a definite plus to the office manager!

The Employment Application

"The closest to perfection a person ever comes is when he fills out an employment application!" —STANLEY RANDALL

Several different formats can be used for an employment application. A preprinted employment application form may be used, but some offices prefer to design their own form, integrating important subjects that uniquely apply to their office. Once the office manager has designed an employment application that suits the particular needs of the practice, it can be either typeset and printed at a local print shop or formatted on the practice's computer and copied onto a better grade of paper. Formatting the form on the office computer and printing it out and making photocopies is much less expensive than having it typeset and printed by the local printer and is done by many offices today in an effort to contain costs. The following important issues should be addressed in the employment application:

- Education history
- Employment history
- Salary from last employment
- Special qualifications
- Reason for leaving previous position
- Current salary requested
- Long-range professional goals
- Flexibility of applicant
- Date of availability

A sample employment application is shown in Figure 2-3. If an interviewee arrives with a resume, she or he should be instructed to fill out the application in full even though there are areas of redundancy.

The Art of the Interview

There is a certain art involved in the interview process. As Figure 2-4 shows, the two main areas to assess during the interview are technical skills and people skills. Managers should listen to their gut feelings; only they know their needs. However, coupled with this gut feeling should be a systematic approach to the decision to hire.

The first thing the office manager should do before beginning an interview is to have a tablet in which to jot down notes during the interview. Some office managers use a form that has been designed to be completed during an interview. Later, these notes will be invaluable to the process of remembering and rating the applicants.

The manager should remember to let the prospective employee talk and should listen intently to everything that is said. Some applicants will offer much more information than is asked for and should be listened to, because this information can be very helpful later. Answers to the questions will help to determine the best applicant. Their overall demeanor and body language can also be helpful.

First impressions are not always the right ones. *Never, ever* hire an applicant on the first interview. Many times, the second interview provides a completely different picture of the applicant than the first. During the first interview, all aspects of the job should be covered, along with the nuts and bolts of office policy, such as vacation time, benefits, salary, and so on. The applicant should always be allowed time to ask questions.

Second interviews should be scheduled for applicants who possess the qualities that are necessary for the position. In the second interview, the manager talks with the applicants about a trial period of employment and why the applicant wants this particular position.

It is then time to check the references on the final applicants. More information will be obtained by calling the person given as a reference than by sending her or him a letter. Always have the applicant sign granting permission

Name: ______________________________
Address: ______________________________
Phone: ____________________ E-mail: ____________________
SSN: ______________________________

Education: (List most current first)
1.
2.
3.

Experience: Name, address, telephone number, supervisor (list most current first)
1. ______________________________
____
Hourly rate: ____________________ Reason for leaving: ____________________
Position Held: ______________________________
May we contact your supervisor? ______ Y ______ N
Supervisor's name: ____________________ Phone number: ____________________

Experience: Name, address, telephone number, supervisor
2. ______________________________
____
Hourly rate: ____________________ Reason for leaving: ____________________
Position Held: ______________________________
May we contact your supervisor? ______ Y ______ N
Supervisor's name: ____________________ Phone number: ____________________

Experience: Name, address, telephone number, supervisor
3. ______________________________
____
Hourly rate: ____________________ Reason for leaving: ____________________
Position Held: ______________________________
May we contact your supervisor? ______ Y ______ N
Supervisor's name: ____________________ Phone number: ____________________

Are there any physical problems that could keep you from performing the duties of this position? ____Y ____N
If yes, what are they? ______________________________
Have you ever been convicted of a crime? ______ Y ______ N
If yes, explain: ______________________________
____

Are you willing to be bonded? ______ Y ______ N
As in most physician offices, there may be days where employees are asked to work later than usual. Is this a problem? ______ Y ______ N
What qualities do you possess that might make you more qualified than others?
____
What computer skills do you possess? ____ Word ____ WordPerfect ____ Excel ____ Lotus ____ Access
____ PowerPoint ____ Quicken ____ Quick Books ____ Microsoft Money ____ Peachtree Accounting
____ Other (List): ____________________

FIGURE 2-3. Employment application form.

(Continued)

Do you have an understanding of medical terminology? ______ Y ______ N

List any commitments you have that might interfere with your work:

____

What are your long-range career plans? ____

____

List three **professional** references: Name, address, telephone number

1.

2.

3.

What salary/hourly rate are you seeking for this position? $______________

Date of availability: ______________ Date of interview: ______________

FIGURE 2-3. (CONTINUED) Employment application form.

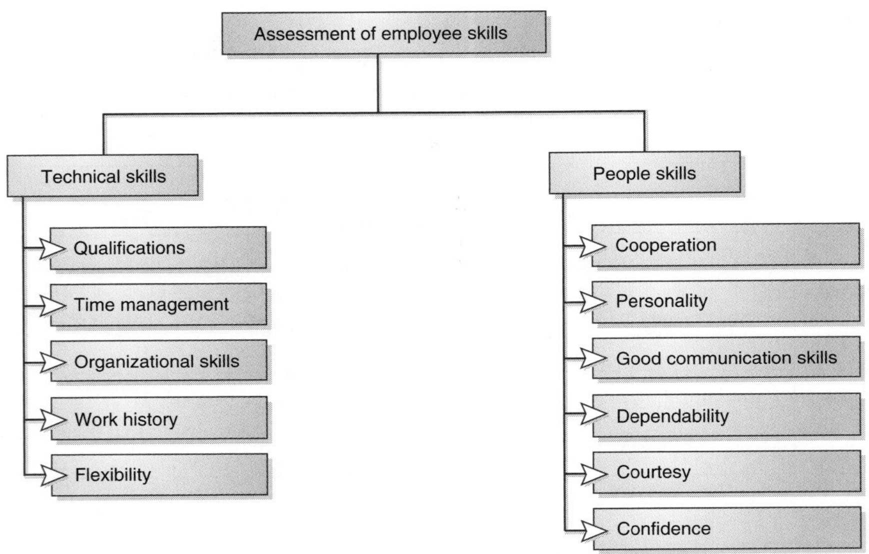

FIGURE 2-4. Assessment of employee skills.

to call the references that were provided. When speaking with an applicant's past employers or professional references, the manager should always ask the million-dollar question: "Would you hire this person again?" In addition, information should be obtained on the applicant's health history, dependability, general personality traits, and compatibility. It is a good idea to give applicants only salary ranges until an applicant has been chosen. At that point, a starting salary may be offered. All details of office policy should be explained to the individual at that time, such as the lunch policy, whether there is a lunch room (microwave, refrigerator, etc.), when the applicant should start, and who will be training the applicant.

The office manager should be well versed in the job requirements of the position available. The manager should thoroughly evaluate the demands of the position before beginning to conduct interviews for the position. At this time, the office manager might want to make some long overdue changes in the job description. The position should be carefully analyzed as to the specific personality traits it demands, the physical capabilities it requires, and the mental and emotional demands associated with it. Be sure to not only discuss the positive aspects of the job, but also include any negative aspects that may arise.

Most physicians do not want to be involved in the interviewing process and give their office manager a "green light" in the hiring department. Some physicians want the office manager to do all the preliminary interviewing and choose the best applicants to interview with the doctor. In a group practice, one physician may handle personnel matters, and it may not be necessary for all of the physicians to interview the applicants.

Issues to Consider during the Interview

The medical office manager needs to consider the following issues when interviewing an applicant:

- Where does the applicant live in relation to the location of the office? This is an important concern. In conjunction with this, it needs to be determined whether the applicant has her or his own transportation or will be using public transportation.
- Does the applicant's job history indicate job stability?
- In what type of practices has the applicant worked? Are they close to the type of practice that contains the available position?
- What is the applicant's educational background? Does the applicant have a teaching degree along with any other medical office certification? Experience has shown that this type of applicant will generally not stay, and is probably just using this position as a "stepping stone." However, to deny someone a position for this reason might be considered discriminatory, so care must be taken when interviewing this type of individual.

Fair and Sensitive Questioning of Applicants

Beware of questions that could promote a lawsuit down the road. Federal and state laws protect individuals from job discrimination, and what an office manager might think is an innocent question can result in a discrimination suit! Hiring employees used to be an easy task; find the person you like and hire her or him. Not any more! There are many laws in place to protect individuals against discriminatory questioning. The manager must be careful not to ask any questions that might relate to the applicant's credit history. Care must be taken to avoid any questions that might constitute an invasion of privacy or discrimination. The following are some questions to avoid. These questions may seem harmless enough, but they are not. A medical office may be slapped with a lawsuit before it knows what happened.

Instead of "Will you have any difficulty obtaining child care?"
Ask "If you have to work late some days, will that be a problem?"
Instead of "Will you be using public transportation, or do you have a car?"
Ask "Will you have any difficulty in getting to work?"
Instead of "Do you have any plans for a family in the next few years?"
Ask "Where do you see yourself in the next five years?"
Instead of "Are you a U.S. citizen?"
Ask "Are you legally permitted to work in the U.S.?"

Before asking a question, office managers should always ask themselves, "How does this relate to the job?" They must stick to asking questions regarding the job; after all, that is what the applicant is there for. Education, work history, and technical skills should be important areas of discussion. They should not try to slip any trick question to the applicant in an effort to obtain information. They should always check with the state laws, because each state has different guidelines to be followed.

Even after a person has been hired, care must be used. For example, an office manager should never say, "Keep up the good work, you have a future here!" This simple phrase can come back to haunt you. If down the road it becomes necessary to fire that employee, those simple words spoken a year ago can make it difficult for the manager to prove that she or he has a legitimate reason for letting that individual go. Words can be a dangerous thing and can create situations that may not have been intended.

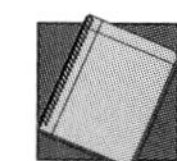

FROM THE EXPERT'S NOTEBOOK

Always use open-ended questions during an interview.

EMPLOYEE BENEFITS

BENEFITS AS A FORM OF EMPLOYEE COMPENSATION

An *employee benefit* is any benefit or service (other than wages for time worked) provided to an employee in whole or in part by his or her employer (Figure 2-5). Employee benefits became an important issue during World War II and the Korean War when wage freezes were in effect. Today, many offices offer a variety of employee benefits in lieu of higher salaries, and benefits for employees can usually be secured at a lower cost through group arrangements than on an individual basis. The employer reaps tax benefits for offering certain types of employee benefits. Employee benefits are often used to improve employee performance, increase job satisfaction, and reduce employee turnover. If the benefits offered are not competitive with other positions in the area, employees may seek employment with another practice. Employee benefits are an expensive component of the total compensation package.

Most office managers know that employees believe their benefits package is just as important as their salary. In our fast-paced, competitive society, we are always looking for more benefits. We need plans that reimburse child-care expenses and provide tuition assistance. We need flexible schedules to balance our family lives with our professional lives. Although it is not easy, medical offices should recognize the needs of their staff and meet those needs when possible. This recognition makes for happy employees, which makes for a happy office.

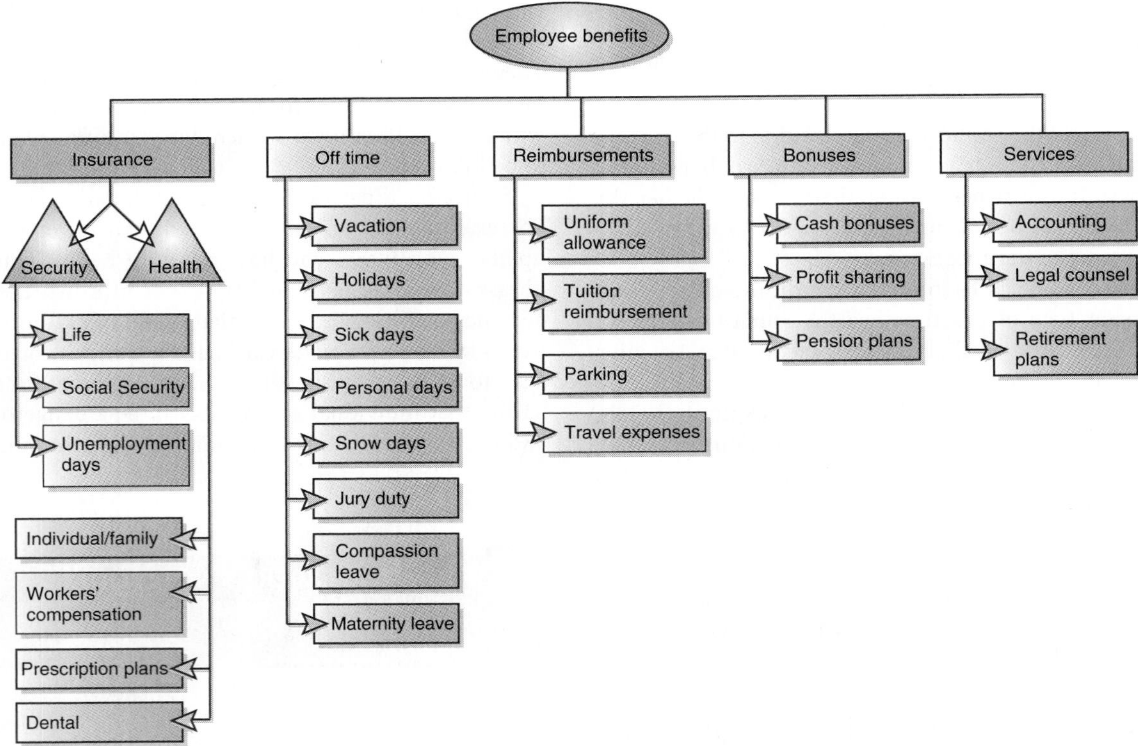

FIGURE 2-5. Types of employee benefits.

The major employee benefits offered are medical and retirement plans. The costs of medical and retirement benefits have risen consistently by about 2% per year. The cost of health care benefits for an employee in a medical office ranges from $2,000 to $9,000 per year, depending on the size and type of the medical practice. Because of the steady increase in costs, more and more employers are raising the deductibles of their medical plans. A government survey showed that there is a definite trend toward flexible benefits plans, or *cafeteria plan benefits*. Cafeteria plan benefits allow the employee to choose from a variety of benefit options to meet his or her specific needs.

CATEGORIES OF BENEFITS

Employers may offer five categories of employee benefits:

1. Private insurance plans
2. Bonus cash payments
3. Social insurance plans
4. Services
5. Payments for time off

Private insurance plans include life insurance, disability insurance, health insurance, and retirement plans.

Bonus cash payments consist of payments made in addition to salary or wages, such as tuition reimbursement, holiday bonuses, profit-sharing plans, and savings plans.

Social insurance plans include Social Security, workers' compensation coverage, and unemployment insurance.

Services include van pools, free parking, day care, clothing or uniform allowances, and wellness/fitness programs.

Payments for time off include sick time, compassion leave, maternity leave, vacation time, holidays, and jury duty.

Private Insurance Plans

LIFE INSURANCE

The oldest and most common life insurance plan is term insurance. This type of life insurance provides death benefits only and does not build up any cash value. Most group life insurance plans are designed to provide coverage during an employee's tenure at work and are usually canceled on termination of employment. Section 162 of the Internal Revenue Code allows employers to deduct payments made to group term insurance companies. This is considered an ordinary business expense for the employer, and therefore it is rewarded with favorable tax treatment. The employee cannot deduct any contribution he or she makes as an individual. Any payroll deductions for group term insurance are included in the employee's taxable income.

DISABILITY INSURANCE

Group disability insurance supplies employees with partial or total replacement of income while they are out of work as a result of a qualified disability. In a medical office, disability insurance is the most common omission from the benefits package, yet it is probably one of the most important benefits to the employee. During a recent survey, it was found that three quarters of American businesses offer short-term disability benefits and approximately two thirds of them offer long-term disability benefits.

HEALTH INSURANCE

Health insurance is the most significant type of group insurance in terms of the number of employees it covers and the dollar amount it takes to cover them. With the exception of very small medical practices (generally solo practices), most physician offices offer some type of medical insurance coverage to their employees. At one time, group medical insurance was provided at no cost to the employee. However, with the skyrocketing cost of health care today, most offices now require employee contributions. Today's employers are providing more extensive health insurance coverage to employees than in the past. The three basic benefits provided are as follows:

1. Hospital expense benefits
2. Surgical expense benefits
3. Physician expense benefits

Other benefits that are often included are as follows:

- Long-term care
- Home health care
- Ambulatory care
- Extended care
- Hospice care
- Birthing center care
- Vision care
- Prescription drug benefits
- Preventive care
- Dental care

RETIREMENT PLANS

Retirement plans are another commonly offered employee benefit, accounting for the largest portion of expenditures for each employee. Retirement income can come from employment earnings after retirement, individual savings accounts, Social Security, or employer-sponsored retirement plans. The federal government offers incentives in the way of tax benefits to physicians who sponsor retirement plans for their employees.

PROFESSIONAL LIABILITY INSURANCE

Some more innovative offices are offering to reimburse employees for the cost of professional liability insurance. Personnel such as nurse practitioners, physician assistants, registered nurses, and medical technicians are now maintaining this insurance. It is generally obtained by the employee and reimbursed through the office.

Bonus Cash Payments

Some compensation plans include cash bonuses to be paid to employees immediately after achieving a goal, at an employee's date-of-hire anniversary or birthday, or after they have worked a certain amount of time. Many of these bonus payment plans are based on merit or practice growth. For instance, a billing manager who has achieved the objective of decreasing aged patient account balances of over 90 days by $20,000 might be rewarded with a $500 bonus. Bonuses have been found to increase revenue, productivity, and morale.

Social Insurance Plans

A large portion of money employers spend on employee benefits is used to make legally required payments to social insurance programs. For medical offices with small benefits programs, this contribution may account for the majority of each employee's total benefit package. The term *Social Security* refers not only to payments people receive when they retire, but also to survivors' benefits, disability benefits, unemployment benefits, Medicare hospitalization benefits, and supplementary medical insurance benefits provided by federal government insurance programs.

WORKERS' COMPENSATION

Workers' compensation laws were enacted to require employers to provide employee benefits for losses resulting from work-related injury or illness. These laws are based on liability without fault, and benefits are subject to statutory maximums. Workers' compensation benefits include medical care, disability income, death benefits, and rehabilitative services. Because workers' compensation plans are state run and regulated, they vary from state to state. Office managers should be aware of state regulations regarding work-related employee injury or illness. Employers must purchase coverage through an insurance company that handles workers' compensation insurance. In most states, employers must pay the full cost of this insurance for their employees.

UNEMPLOYMENT

Before the Social Security Act of 1935, few people had any protection for lost wages during a period of unemployment. The Social Security Act provided for a payroll tax to be paid into a government fund to cover citizens during such a time. This act has two objectives: to provide individuals with income during unemployment and to help them search for new employment. To be eligible for unemployment benefits, individuals must meet the following requirements:

- They must have a previous working record within a certain base period. In most states, this period is either 52 weeks or four quarters before the time of employment.
- They must be physically and mentally able to work and must be available for work.
- They must be actively seeking work. Most states require that an individual make an honest effort to obtain a job.
- They must comply with a 1-week waiting period before benefits start.
- They must be free of any disqualifications that would result in cancellation, postponement, or reduction of benefits. These disqualifications include the following:
  - Voluntarily leaving a position
  - Being discharged for misconduct
  - Refusing to accept a suitable job
  - Being involved in a labor dispute

Employment regulation books from each state outline state rules and regulations on employment. This information is also available online. The books contain more information than is actually needed, but they are an invaluable resource for every office manager.

Services

An optional benefit that can be offered to employees is medical care. W-2 employees (paid employees who are not independent contractors) can be provided with free medical care for themselves and their families. This courtesy cannot be offered to employees who are not W-2 employees because of anti-kickback regulations. More about these regulations can be found in Chapter 8.

Payments for Time Off

Being paid for days not worked is a welcome benefit for any employee. Paid days off may include holidays, sick days, personal days, and inclement weather days. Some physician offices give the Friday after Thanksgiving as a paid holiday. Others pay for time off for immediate family medical emergencies. This practice establishes instant goodwill between employees and employers.

CAFETERIA PLANS AND FLEXIBLE BENEFITS PLANS

Although the terms *cafeteria plan* and *flexible benefits plan* are sometimes used interchangeably, for present purposes the following distinction will be made: Flexible benefits plans allow employees to choose which employer-funded benefits are most important to them. Benefits offered under these plans can be wide ranging and can include anything to which employees attach value. Cafeteria benefits plans are operated under the rules of Section 125 of the IRS code, and provide employees and employers with certain tax benefits. The choices available to employees under these plans are limited to those defined under Section 125.

How Cafeteria/Flexible Benefits Plans Work

The flexibility of cafeteria/flexible benefits plans allows employees to choose benefits based on their needs at different times of life. For example, young employees may benefit from a tuition reimbursement program, parents may choose reimbursement for child-care expenses, and employees who take care of their parents may prefer adult daycare benefits. An expansion of these plans can also include benefits that are provided to same-sex domestic partners. (Same-sex partners have not become an issue in most practices, but may be found in the hospital setting.) An increasing number of physician's offices are adopting the cafeteria/flexible benefits plans for their employee benefits program. Each employee is presented with a list of available benefits from which to choose and a specific dollar amount to spend on benefits. With a cafeteria plan, the employer defines a specific dollar amount for employer-funded benefits, and employees decide how much pretax income they want to divert into the plan to supplement the employer's contribution. The financial advantage of this plan is that the benefits employees choose are deducted from their salary (thus reducing the employees' taxable income) and are not an added expense for the business. If the plan operates under Section 125 (a cafeteria plan), there is an additional benefit to the employer; deductions for a Section 125 plan reduce employee's taxable income on which FICA taxes are computed, so employers' FICA contributions are also reduced. In a typical cafeteria/flexible benefits plan, one person may choose a disability plan as part of his or her benefits package, whereas another staff member may choose child-care benefits. Depending on how much they were willing to spend, staff members could actually choose both. Employees are also given the option of additional salary equal to the cost of the benefits package. If they take this option, employees are responsible for paying taxes on these dollars. The office manager must understand that certain employee benefits, such as workers' compensation, are the financial responsibility of the employer and are not to be included in a cafeteria/flexible benefits package.

Some people criticize cafeteria/flexible benefits plans because they fear that employees may choose their benefits unwisely, and there is concern about employers' moral and legal obligation to prevent financial injury to their employees. This concern has been incorporated into the design of the plan, which specifies that certain basic benefits must be offered, providing a certain degree of security for each employee. A selection of optional benefits is then presented, from which employees can add to their plan.

The basic benefits provided in a cafeteria/flexible benefits plan are generally as follows:

- Medical insurance
- Disability income insurance
- Term life insurance
- Travel accident insurance (when an employee is on a business trip)
- Pension and profit-sharing plans

Optional benefits are generally equal to 3% to 6% of the employee's salary. They can include the following (entries followed by an asterisk are not available under the Section 125 regulations):

- Additional life insurance
- Accidental death insurance (when basic travel insurance does not apply)
- Term life insurance on dependents
- Dental insurance
- Annual physical examinations for the employee
- Tuition reimbursement
- Wellness and fitness programs
- Child-care program
- Adult daycare program
- Vacation time*
- Cash (bonuses)*
- Personal days*
- Free parking*
- Transportation*
- Moving expense reimbursement*
- Paid jury days*
- Financial planning*
- Legal services*
- Accounting services*

If an employee does not have enough credits to purchase optional benefits, the costs of the desired benefits can be paid via payroll deductions.

Part-Time Employees

Part-time employees are not eligible for the same range of benefits received by full-time employees. Each office must establish a policy for part-time employees that complies with state employment laws. Some practices have developed a tier system based on the number of hours an employee works. This system is written in the policy manual and does not change or allow for exceptions. For example, employees working 80 hours in a 2-week pay period may be classified as Status 1, employees working 60 to 79 hours as Status 2, employees working 40 to 59 hours as Status 3, and employees working less than 40 hours as Status 4. The office manager must meet with the physician to determine what benefits will be provided to the various levels within the tier system.

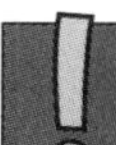

MANAGER'S ALERT

When establishing a cafeteria plan, the office must do it on a strictly nondiscriminatory basis. All full-time employees must be included!

RATIONALE FOR A CAFETERIA PLAN

Many employers believe that employees are unaware of the cost of benefits they receive and that a cafeteria plan makes employees more aware of these costs. Once employees are educated to the costs of benefits, they are often more appreciative of the benefits being offered to them.

The inflexibility of conventional benefits plans usually causes them to fall short of meeting the needs of some employees. For example, an employee with no children cannot get excited about a benefit for child care. Employee dissatisfaction over benefits contributes to employee turnover. Cafeteria plans improve employee satisfaction, which results in better employee retention and an increased ability to attract qualified employees. There is a great deal to be said for promoting goodwill between the employer and employee. Everyone wins in this situation.

Many employers use cafeteria plans as a way to contain escalating costs of benefits programs. Between federal and state regulations and the inflation rate, employee benefits can become quite costly. Because a cafeteria plan is a "defined contribution" plan rather than a "defined benefit" plan, it helps control costs.

Drawbacks of the Cafeteria Plan

The office manager should realize that if a cafeteria plan is adopted, it will be a complex and time-consuming project to put it in place. The costs of designing and adopting such a plan are slightly higher than for a conventional plan, primarily because of expenses associated with plan development and administration. Continuing costs of the plan depend on such factors as what benefits are involved, the number of options presented, the frequency with which employees are allowed to change benefits, and the number of employees covered by the plan.

FRINGE BENEFITS

Following are the 10 employee fringe benefits most commonly offered by medical practices today:

1. Paid vacations
2. Paid holidays
3. Paid sick days
4. Medical insurance
5. Prescription plans

6. Dental insurance
7. Personal days
8. Inclement weather days
9. Pension plans
10. Profit-sharing plans

Paid Vacations

Vacations can be granted in a variety of ways. Vacation options should be described completely in the office's procedure and policy manual. The following are models that the office might use to grant vacations.

MODEL 1

First year: No vacation
Second year: 1 week of vacation
Third year: 2 weeks of vacation
Fourth year: 3 weeks of vacation
Fifth year and beyond: 4 weeks of vacation

MODEL 2

First year: No vacation
Second to fourth years: 2 weeks of vacation
Fifth to ninth years: 3 weeks of vacation
Tenth year and beyond: 4 weeks of vacation

MODEL 3

After 6 months: 3 days of vacation
After 12 months: 1 week of vacation
After 3 years: 2 weeks of vacation
After 5 years: 3 weeks of vacation
Vacation caps at 3 weeks

MODEL 4

One vacation day for every 60 days worked
Vacation caps at 18 days

These models are for full-time employees only. Part-time employees typically follow a rated schedule commensurate with the number of days they work per week. For instance, in an office that follows Model 1 for its full-time employees, a part-time employee working only 2 days a week will receive no vacation pay the first year, 2 days in the second year, 4 days in the third year, 6 days in the fourth year, and 8 days in the fifth year.

Paid Holidays

The six paid holidays most commonly observed in the medical office are New Year's Day, Memorial Day, July Fourth, Labor Day, Thanksgiving Day, and Christmas Day. Other holidays that may be given to employees include Martin Luther King Jr. Day, Presidents' Day, Columbus Day, Good Friday, Easter Monday, the day after Thanksgiving, Christmas Eve, and New Year's Eve. Some offices may also elect to give employees their birthday off as a paid holiday. Offices with employees of Jewish, Muslim, and other religious persuasions will wish to observe their religious holidays in addition to the six most common holidays.

Paid Sick Days

The office manager and physician must determine how many paid sick days will be allotted to full-time employees. Medical offices generally provide from 5 to 12 paid sick days. Some offices grant a minimum number of sick days, but also give personal days. Many offices today allow employees to "bank" sick time in case of catastrophic illness. In other words, an employee may be allowed to carry over 40 hours of unused sick time per year with a cap of 30 days. This time can be used should an employee have an accident, undergo major surgery, or contract a debilitating illness such as pneumonia. Some offices also allow for paid sick days if an employee needs time off to tend to a sick parent, spouse, or child.

Medical Insurance

Medical insurance is the most important fringe benefit that a medical office can offer. This insurance can be a Blue Cross/Blue Shield plan, a managed care plan, or a commercial insurance plan. There are also some fee-for-service carriers out there, but they are few and far between because of cost. When thinking about employee medical insurance, the office manager should investigate many different plans to compare their benefits and costs. Some offices offer employer-paid coverage for family members as well.

Prescription Plans

Prescription plans are becoming more popular as a medical office benefit. Many managed care plans provide a reasonable rate for prescription plans. With prescription prices continuing to soar, employees are most appreciative of this benefit.

Dental Insurance

Although dental insurance is not provided as often as medical insurance is, it is still among the top 10 benefits. Dental insurance can become quite costly, and most employers attempt to keep costs down. As with medical insurance companies, the office manager should investigate various companies that provide dental insurance and compare the benefits of the plan and the costs. An office might provide employees a managed care plan for their medical insurance and a different plan for their dental insurance. Shop around to get the most for the office's money!

Personal Days

The number of personal days given as a benefit in medical offices ranges widely—from none to 10 or more. Some offices do not provide personal days to their employees; however, these offices are the exception, not the rule. Most offices recognize employees' need for personal days to tend to matters such as medical or dental appointments, family illness (if paid sick days are not allowed for this purpose), car repair, and financial business. Personal days are a much needed and much appreciated benefit. Many office employees work full time, which does not leave time for much else. By providing these days as a benefit, the physician and office manager will promote goodwill.

Inclement Weather Days

Weather can sometimes prevent employees from getting to the office. In such cases, it is best to have an inclement weather policy in place. Some offices grant a set number of days per year for which they will pay employee wages when weather keeps them home. Other offices never close in bad weather and feel that their employees should be able to get to work no matter what. They deduct any days lost from employee pay. Other practices pay employees if the office is closed because of snow, ice, extreme storms, and the like, but not if the office is open and the employee cannot make it to work. In this case, the office must have a policy as to whether the employee will be docked for this time, or whether he or she will be allowed to make the time up at a later date. In any case, it is best to have an inclement weather policy in place before you need it. It should be included in the office's procedure and policy manual so that employees are aware of it ahead of time. An example of an inclement weather policy is shown in Box 2-3.

Pension Plans

To recognize the hard work and good effort of employees, an employer may wish to establish a money purchase pension plan for the exclusive benefit of all eligible employees and their beneficiaries. In this plan, the employer makes a contribution to the employee's pension every year. This retirement benefit is provided totally at the employer's expense and does not consist of any contributions from the employee. When the employee retires or leaves the practice, he or she receives the value of this account. These plans are developed to the specifications of the Employee Retirement Income Security Act of 1974. A sample plan is shown in Appendix A.

BOX 2-3 Sample Inclement Weather Policy

If the office is officially closed because of inclement weather, employees who are scheduled to work will be paid. If the office is open on a day of inclement weather and the employee either cannot make it to work or chooses not to come to work, the employee will be paid but will be expected to make up this time at a later date.

Profit-Sharing Plans

A profit-sharing plan is designed to allow a relatively short-term deferral of income; it is a somewhat more tentative benefit because the employer's contribution is based on profits. This plan differs from the pension plan, which is designed to provide income at retirement. A profit-sharing plan can provide for a totally discretionary employer contribution. This means that even if the office makes a profit in a certain year, the employer does not necessarily have to make a contribution to the plan that year. There is no minimum-funding rule; however, there must be a substantial and recurring contribution, or the plan will be considered terminated. A profit-sharing plan is viewed more as an incentive than a predictable source of income. Employees may be permitted to withdraw from the plan before retirement; however, early withdrawals may be subject to a substantial penalty. A sample employee benefits booklet for a small practice can be found in Appendix F.

Additional Benefits That Some Offices Offer Their Employees

LIFE INSURANCE

An employee benefit that is not commonly offered is life insurance. Some medical insurance plans come with a piggyback life insurance policy. This is generally a small life insurance policy that is provided to all employees subscribing to medical insurance.

TUITION REIMBURSEMENT

Most offices encourage continuing education for their employees, and many pay for educational expenses. Employees can deduct from their taxes un-reimbursed educational expenses if the education maintains or improves a skill related to their position or is directly related to maintaining their position. If the office reimburses employees for this education, the payment can be claimed as a tax-free form of compensation.

UNIFORM ALLOWANCE

Occasionally, one will find a small medical office that offers its employees uniform allowances. This is generally not found in larger practices, where it becomes too costly. Employees can deduct the cost of uniforms required for their position from their taxable income. Some offices require a specific uniform and provide an allowance toward its purchase. For instance, a physician might want her or his office staff to dress in blue scrubs with white jackets. Employees generally prefer wearing colors, as opposed to traditional whites.

"AT-WILL EMPLOYMENT"

The employment-at-will doctrine states that any employee can be terminated by the employer at any time and for any reason. The only time this does not apply is if there is a contract that exists between the two parties, which would prohibit such an action.

In more recent years, however, individuals and the court systems have become more sophisticated, and employers must be very careful of what they do and how they do it. Congress has expanded employees' rights and, with that, taken away employers' rights. In today's litigious society, employers must follow the guidelines of each state and make sure that everything is in order.

During performance reviews, employees should always be asked if there is a comment they want to make regarding their performance, or whatever it is that is negative. Sometimes, an office manager will find extenuating circumstances that may warrant another look at the situation. When considering termination, the manager must make sure that there are documented memos to track an employee who has been given warnings about the problem. Documentation is the key. The termination should not come as a surprise. Experience shows that one of the easiest ways to avoid a discrimination suit may be to keep employees informed about their performance. If termination follows, a severance package may be offered depending on the circumstances. More information on this doctrine can be found in Chapter 8.

GIVING EMPLOYEE REFERENCES

The threat of a lawsuit also makes it tricky to give a reference for a former employee with a negative work history. The medical office manager must know the state laws regarding conditional privilege (that is, some degree of protection against a claim of defamation of character) in giving employment references. Each state handles this differently. If an office manager gives an employee whom she or he fired a very good reference, that employee may decide to file a wrongful-discharge suit against the office, and the employer does not have a leg to stand on, since the office manager gave such a glowing reference. If the office manager gives a detailed, derogatory reference about an employee who was fired, the office could be sued for slander (i.e., defamation of character).

If the office manager discloses little to no information about a former employee, the office could be sued for defamation under the self-publication act. For example, if a receptionist was fired for stealing from the daily receipts and the office manager does not tell a prospective employer calling for a reference the reason for dismissal, the prospective employer could sue the office if she or he hired the individual and the individual did not disclose this to the new employer. It is best to consult the office attorney when dealing with a reference on a former employee with an unfavorable work history. Many medical offices and hospitals have adopted the policy of providing only the dates of the individual's employment and verification of the position held. The state labor board could be contacted if the office manager is unsure in this area. This protects the office and the office manager from any problems down the road.

THE FRAZZLED EMPLOYEE

No matter how much a patient complains to a health care giver, the patient must be treated with respect and understanding at all times. Various levels of employee stress are found in medical offices, and the office manager must be able to identify and deal with them. An employee who argues with a demanding patient not only upsets the patient more, but also becomes just as tense and out of control. An employee must be able to adapt to various situations that might arise in a medical office. The employee must show this adaptability when relating to patients, physicians, co-workers, and any ancillary services that they might be using.

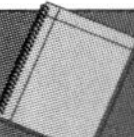

FROM THE EXPERT'S NOTEBOOK

When choosing between an individual with excellent technical abilities and an individual with a genuine caring ability, consider choosing the individual with the genuine concern for others. Most skills can be taught, but caring and concern can't!

THE ENTHUSIASTIC EMPLOYEE

One very important lesson for the office manager to learn is the power of positive reinforcement. There is an old saying that goes, "You can catch more flies with honey than you can with vinegar!" Your employee turnover will decrease, productivity will increase, negativism will decrease, and even illnesses seem to abate. It has been proven that employees will go the extra mile for the office manager if they are receiving some positive reinforcement. For example, by simply stopping by an employee's workstation and thanking her or him for doing such a good job on a report, the office manager increases the confidence of that employee. Confidence, coupled with genuine appreciation, gives a benefit to the employee, which in turn means more productivity for the office. Everyone benefits from a compliment from time to time, and medical office personnel are no exception. They possess a certain amount of pride in their work, and for many a word of appreciation is just as important as a weekly paycheck. Give your employees enough latitude to be creative with their ambition. Bad attitudes are contagious, but enthusiasm can be just as contagious or even more so!

EMPLOYEE PERFORMANCE EVALUATION

The size of a medical office does not dictate whether there should be a performance review system in place—*every* medical office needs a review system. It is of vital importance to evaluate staff performance on a scheduled basis (Figure 2-6). If there is not some type of systematic review in place, unproductive employees may "coast" for years, and "prized" and productive employees will look for new positions where they will be recognized and appreciated. There are three basic steps to employee evaluation:

1. For each employee, maintain a file that contains the employee's performance evaluations; an employee data sheet (Figure 2-7); a copy of the employee's resume; and records of vacation days, sick days, raises, and promotions.
2. On a quarterly basis, review and assess the information that has been inserted into the file.
3. Meet with the employee at an appointed time to discuss her or his performance (a note with details of this meeting should be inserted into the file). Both the manager and the employee should sign the employee evaluation form at the end of the review. Recognize that taking care of the employee is just as important as taking care of the patients!

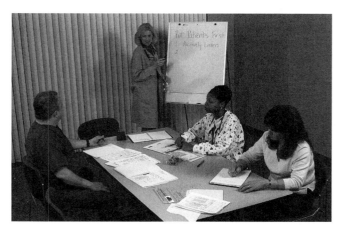

FIGURE 2-6. The physician, office manager, and supervisory staff discuss employee evaluations.

Some physicians do not want to be involved in employee performance reviews and leave their office managers in charge of this task. If there is an impending problem with an employee, the office manager may want to ask the physician to sit in on the review session. Some offices use an evaluation sheet to evaluate each employee. Only the office manager may complete this sheet, or it may be a collective effort between the office manager and the physician or physicians in the group. Irrespective of who completes the evaluation sheet, it is important that it be completed as objectively and affirmatively as possible. New hires should receive a review at 1 month and then again at 90 days; thereafter, reviews should be conducted on a yearly basis. Yearly reviews should be scheduled by seniority so that no one will think there is a specific pattern in the way in which the reviews are scheduled. The most logical time to schedule a review is on the anniversary date of the employee. Offices that do not raise salaries on anniversary dates may conduct reviews at the time of year at which the salaries are raised. It is generally best to start off the evaluation with any problems that may have arisen and need to be addressed. The end of the interview should address the strong points of the employee and should end with a statement of whether the employee will receive a raise and how much. When reviews are conducted in this way, employees leave the evaluation session feeling confident and good about themselves.

When there is a problem that needs to be addressed with an employee, the office manager will explain the problem and set a certain time period in which the matter must be corrected. The time period granted must be fair—30 to 60 days is more than fair for an employee to correct the situation. If it is not resolved by the end of 60 days, this can be used as a step toward the employee's dismissal. The manager must be sure to document the conversation held at the end of 60 days and insert the documentation into the employee's file, especially if she or he gave the employee a warning that if the situation is not rectified, termination will occur. The manager always allows the employee to participate in the evaluation and to express any concerns or ideas on how to improve a specific situation or task. The office manager listens intently and remains objective. In fact, the office manager might learn something about the managerial aspects of the office that might not be apparent but may need reworking. Medical offices that use the performance evaluation system find that it improves productivity and morale. Employees feel that someone cares about their work and recognizes their accomplishments. A sample evaluation sheet is shown in Figure 2-8.

Name: ______________________

Address: ______________________

____

____

Phone: ______________________

E-mail Address: ______________________

Social Security number: ______________________

Number of exemptions: ______________________

(Please attach copy of W-2)

Spouse/life partner name: ______________________

Spouse/life partner work phone number: ______________________

Person to notify in case of emergency: ______________________

Relation to employee: ______________________

Daytime phone number: ______________________

FIGURE 2-7. Employee data sheet.

The "SIPS" Way to Avoid Errors in Employee Evaluation

Many office managers make mistakes during an employee evaluation that can be costly to both them and the practices for which they work. The *SIPS* method helps the office manager identify and avoid these common errors and prevents turmoil in the office. SIPS identifies these common errors (Box 2-4):

Softness
Influence
Particularity
Strictness

Softness refers to an office manager's tendency to overrate every aspect of the employee. Such a manager wants to be nice and therefore gives all employees higher ratings than perhaps they deserve. This might win them a popularity contest, but it often hinders the practice. Employees do not get an accurate accounting of their work and therefore do not know how to correct certain aspects of their performance.

Influence refers to an office manager's becoming friends with one or more of the employees. When this situation arises, the office manager cannot help but show favoritism toward these employees. All office managers have favorites among their employees; however, this favoritism should never be shown.

Particularity is probably the most common error in employee evaluation. The office manager tends to focus on one particular task that was done well and rate the employee's entire performance according to that single task. The manager can avoid this by, first, being aware of the potential problem and, second, carefully evaluating each area on the employee evaluation slowly and accurately.

Strictness refers to using the position of office manager to exhibit power. Strict managers are managers who boast that no employee deserves the highest rating on the evaluation.

The Employee Self-Evaluation Form

"Only the mediocre are always at their best." —ANONYMOUS

The office manager might want to use employee self-evaluation as a tool for reviewing employees' productivity and work habits. One way to obtain employee self-evaluations is to provide employees with the Employee Task Sheet (Figure 2-9) 2 weeks before their scheduled evaluation. They should be instructed to take their time and fill out the form carefully. It must be returned to the office manager 1 week before the evaluation appointment. It is often interesting to find out how employees view their jobs.

A tool that can be used in conjunction with the Employee Task Sheet is the Employee Self-Evaluation Form (Figure 2-10). Again, employees should take the time to judge themselves carefully. Many managers will find that the employees are harder on themselves than they are.

Employee name: ____________________

Position: ____________________

Date of review: ____________________

Date of last review: ____________________

Reviewer: ____________________

CONFIDENTIAL

[1] Excellent [2] Good [3] Adequate

[4] Needs work [5] Poor

(Enter the evaluation figure that best suits the area being rated)

________ Attendance

________ Cooperation

________ Dedication

________ Dependability

________ Disposition

________ Flexibility

________ Initiative

________ Job perception

________ Quality of work

________ Quantity of work

________ Versatility

Total ____________________

Total from last review ______________

Raise _____ Y _____ N Percent ______________

Comments:

FIGURE 2-8. Employee evaluation sheet.

BOX 2-4 Common Errors in Employee Evaluation: SIPS

Softness
Influence
Particularity
Strictness

The Employee Task Sheet and Employee Self-Evaluation Form can be altered to suit a particular office's needs, or they can be copied and used as is straight from this book. All office managers will find these tools to be invaluable in evaluating the employees. The Employee Task Sheet can be given to each employee midyear so that the office manager can gain an understanding of the tasks the individual performs and her or his goals. This has been found to be a valuable tool in increasing productivity and job satisfaction.

RAISES

Medical offices handle raises in many different ways. The three most common ways of handling pay increases are merit, fixed, and variable raises. One thing is certain: If good employees are to be kept, they must be paid a median

Name:

Date:

The tasks that I perform now are:

1.
2.
3.
4.
5.
6.
7.
8.
9.
10.

Other tasks that I feel I could do are:

1.
2.
3.
4.
5.
6.
7.
8.
9.
10.

FIGURE 2-9. Employee task sheet.

Name:

Date:

I feel my weaknesses are

I feel my strengths are

Individual Rating Factors: (5 = Superior, 4 = Good, 3 = Adequate, 2 = Needs work, 1 = Poor)

________ Quantity of work done

________ Quality of work done

________ Understanding of job

________ Cooperation

________ Dependability

________ Productivity

________ Neatness

________ Organizational skills

Areas in which I feel I need improvement:

1.
2.
3.
4.

FIGURE 2-10. Employee self-evaluation form.

salary or better. If they do not get the salary they deserve, they will begin to look elsewhere for employment. Economic conditions such as flat inflation and virtually full employment across the nation can combine to create a very tight job market for physician practices. The ongoing trend is that there is a very high turnover in lower-paying positions. Employees will leave one position for another for a raise of just 50 cents per hour. Should that employee leave, the costs of recruitment and downtime are much greater. Some employers give 5% to 7% increases to keep good employees.

Merit Raises

Merit raises are usually a direct result of employee evaluations. Merit raises, generally awarded in addition to cost-of-living raises, can be an invaluable tool in boosting morale and increasing performance. When the merit raise approach is used, the employee who performs beyond the call of duty is rewarded. It also provides incentives for others to increase work performance so that they might increase their salaries as well. For example, if Jill is doing commendable work and is staying late on occasion to finish projects, the office manager might want to increase her pay, say, an additional 4% on top of her cost-of-living raise. At the same time, if Julie has slacked off on collecting overdue accounts and the accounts receivable figures are beginning to soar, she might receive only the cost-of-living increase. Ned, who is performing at an adequate work level and doing only the amount of work that is expected, might receive a 2% merit raise in an effort to boost his work performance by renewing his morale.

Fixed Pay Raises

Fixed pay raises are generally given in smaller offices. These raises are generally a cost-of-living increase or the cost-of-living increase plus a small percentage. The difference between the fixed pay raise and the merit pay raise is that in the fixed pay raise, everyone in the office receives the same percentage of increase. For example, the cost-of-living increase may be 3% for the year, and because the physician feels that all the employees are doing a good job, he adds an additional 2% to that figure to give everyone a 5% raise for the year. Because one percentage is the same for everyone, employees who draw a larger salary, of course, will receive more of an increase. For instance, Mary makes $8.00 per hour and Ann makes $12.00 per hour. With the 5% raise, Mary's new hourly rate would be $8.40 per hour, whereas Ann's new rate would be $12.60 per hour.

Flexible Pay Raises

Flexible pay raises are generally not a good idea in any office. This type of raise has been used in small, one-physician offices, but it is not without its problems. If a physician has two employees, a medical assistant and a receptionist, she or he might choose to increase their salaries by different amounts. For example, the medical assistant's salary might be increased 7%, whereas the receptionist's salary might be increased only 4%. A word to the wise: people talk! They always want to talk about their salaries, and in a close-knit office such as this the medical assistant and receptionist probably know what one another had for breakfast that morning! The issue of favorites comes into play in a situation like this, and enough problems can occur in a medical office without creating new ones. To save a lot of headaches and gnashing of teeth, the office manager should advise the physician to avoid a flexible pay raise system in favor of a fixed pay raise system.

DISCIPLINE

The wise office manager makes all employees aware of the various infractions that can result in disciplinary actions. When a list of disciplinary actions is made available to each and every employee, it may be presumed that all employees understand the seriousness of certain types of behavior (Box 2-5). During the hiring of an individual, the disciplinary action form should be reviewed and signed by the employee to acknowledge her or his understanding of the policy. It is far better to have typed a "Levels of Disciplinary Actions" list than to discipline an employee and hear "I didn't know that!" In addition to making all employees aware of behaviors that

BOX 2-5 Levels of Disciplinary Actions

Secondary Offenses That Require Disciplinary Action
Excessive tardiness
Inappropriate dress
Conducting personal business during work hours
Smoking
Minor damage to office property
Uncontrolled emotional outburst

Primary Offenses That Require Disciplinary Action
Excessive absenteeism
Conduct unbecoming a professional
Obscene language or behavior
Insubordination

Severe Offenses That Require Disciplinary Action
Use of obscene/abusive language to patients or co-workers
Lying or stealing
Loss of temper with patients or co-workers
Fighting with patients or co-workers
Drug or alcohol use
Falsifying records
Violation of confidentiality
Any other behavior deemed inappropriate by the office manager
Employee Reviewed:__________________
Date:__________________

may result in disciplinary action, the list provides the office manager with a paper trail that can be referred to should termination be necessary. Some offices include this list in every employee's personnel manual. Other offices post it in a common area, such as a lunchroom or lounge.

Wherever this sheet is placed, it will be most helpful during employee warning sessions, where it can be referred to for a policy backup. The list shown in Box 2-5 can be customized to suit a particular office, but it should include every type of scenario that might arise in a medical office.

MANAGER'S ALERT

Use care when citing the "any other behavior deemed objectionable by the office manager" item on the Levels of Disciplinary Actions list. Many loopholes can be associated with this item. If it becomes necessary to cite this item, be sure to document and verify all information. Offenses described by this item must be highly objectionable in nature.

Managers who use this technique for discipline must realize that it is most important that a follow-through occurs. An office manager who merely threatens and does not follow up is not an effective manager. She or he will not be respected by any of the employees, making future managing very difficult. The purpose of the employee warning notice is to create a paper trail, in other words, a record of infractions by the employee that were severe enough to warrant written confirmation. The office manager should use common sense when choosing between verbally reprimanding and completing an employee warning notice that would become part of the employee's permanent record. When the office manager chooses to use an employee warning notice, she or he has made the decision that the problem was highly serious. A sample warning notice is shown in Figure 2-11. It may be altered to suit a particular practice's needs.

As a general rule, the first warning becomes a "W," or warning. The second becomes a "P," or probation, and the third becomes a "T," for termination. This form is for use only with employees who appear to need discipline on a regular basis or

Employee name: ____________________

Type of incident: ____________________

_______ Attendance

_______ Tardiness

_______ Rudeness

_______ Unsatisfactory work

_______ Disregard of policies and/or procedures

_______ Insubordination

_______ Working on personal matters

_______ Other ____________________

_______ Other ____________________

1st Occurrence: ____________ Date ____________ Letter Code

2nd Occurrence: ____________ Date ____________ Letter Code

3rd Occurrence: ____________ Date ____________ Letter Code

W = Warning P = Probation T = Termination O = Other

Employer statement:

Signature of office manager ____________________

Signature of employee ____________________

FIGURE 2-11. Employee warning notice.

when the office manager feels that an employee has the potential to become a problem employee. It is not intended for use as a daily tool, for every reprimand or incident. This form should be placed in the employee's file and kept confidential in a locked drawer in the office manager's office.

TERMINATION

Poor job performance, violation of an office policy, or illegal activities may make it necessary to terminate an employee. It is important for the office manager to document all conversations and dealings with the employee. She or he should keep in mind that this documentation might end up in a court of law. Therefore all notations must be clear, concise, objective, and properly dated. The number of times the employee's work habits were discussed must be documented.

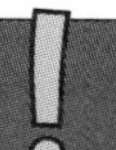

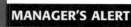

MANAGER'S ALERT

The manager must keep all information strictly confidential! It is not appropriate to share with others.

In confronting the employee, the manager reviews the job description and compares the employee's strengths and weaknesses to this description. It is important that strengths not be forgotten. During the conversation with the employee, the manager points out dates and times of incidents and information that was reviewed for improvement or change. This type of interaction is known as an "exit interview" and is very important to the practice. Many times the feedback received by the exiting employee is valuable to the office manager and may result in future changes to be made within the practice. Exit interviews can also be helpful in compliance issues, which are discussed in Chapter 7. At the end of the conversation, the office manager may suggest ways in which the employee could improve in her or his next position. Ideally, the employee will be able to learn from this experience. It is usually best to have this conversation at the end of a workday, preferably on the last day of a workweek. The manager must make sure that the employee understands that the termination is a fact and must explain clearly, with no emotional involvement, the basis for this decision. All keys, pass cards, and ID cards are returned on the last day of employment. If the office computer is password protected, ask the employee to provide his or her password before leaving. In fact, it is a good idea for the office manager to maintain a listing of all passwords of the employees.

As mentioned, the use of employee warning notices is a good way for the office manager to create a paper trail for a termination. The employee warning notice is signed by the employee; therefore there can be no accusations of miscommunication about the problems.

EXIT INTERVIEWS

One of the most important reasons for exit interviews is to establish an opportunity for employees to vent their feelings or thoughts regarding their employment at the practice. It will identify the "real" reason the employee is leaving. If the employee is resigning against the wishes of the practice, it can be a final attempt to keep her or him. The office manager can obtain information that may identify problem areas within the practice, including duties of the position, co-worker issues, supervisors, and so on. During this interview, the proper documents, if any, are signed and the parting employee is advised of any severance or vacation pay that is due him or her. Pension and profit sharing can also be discussed. Remember that the main reason for this interview is to maintain a good parting relationship. It may prevent a whistleblower suit in the future!

ORIENTING THE NEW EMPLOYEE

Introductions

New employees have a certain level of skill; however, they need to be taught the system of the new office and to be oriented in a manner that makes the transition from the old employer to the new employer as smooth as possible. Well-oriented employees are more likely to stay; since there is a certain amount of cost associated with rapid turnover of employees, it is advisable to orient all new employees as effectively as possible.

The best approach to orienting a new employee is the team approach. The transition period is faster and smoother when everyone on the staff helps in the training process. Just as important as training the employee in the aspects of the new job is explaining the rules and regulations of the practice. Explaining the mission statement of the practice, and its goals and philosophies, is essential in establishing a solid relationship with the new employee. The bonding that must take place between the existing staff and the new staff member is an important part of the orienting process. Co-workers should be introduced to the new staff member and should make a special effort to ensure that she or he feels comfortable. One way to do this is to have each member of the staff spend a few minutes chatting with the new employee.

The office manager should give the new hire some information about her or his manager's role in the medical office and how the new hire will interact with her or him. Volunteering a little personal information may help ease the situation and will help the new employee to better understand the office manager. Training should also include explanation of how the new employee's position interacts with all others on staff.

The office manager should also introduce the new employee to the building security guards, maintenance workers, parking lot attendants, and housekeepers. This will be valuable if the new employee needs any of their services. If the bookkeeping is not done by the office manager, the new employee should be introduced to the bookkeeper and accountant when they come to the office. Depending on the new employee's job responsibilities, the office manager might want to take her or him to the bank or hospital to introduce her or him to staff there.

Showing the New Employee the Ropes

The new employee needs to be given a thorough tour of the office so that she or he doesn't have to waste time looking for certain areas. It is helpful to show the new employee where coats are hung and where personal belongings can be kept during working hours. Because of security problems, some offices have a designated area for such items.

Explaining lunch procedures and breaks is also very helpful. Many offices have lunchrooms equipped with refrigerators, microwaves, and coffee pots. Some offices send out for lunch, and some take a lunch hour in which they can leave the office to get lunch or do errands.

All of these regulations must be explained to a new employee either at the time of hire or on the first day of work. The office policy and procedure manual will help to explain these procedures and should be given to the new employee on the day of hire. Although their contents vary from office to office, procedure manuals can be helpful in explaining telephone and scheduling techniques, billing procedures, physicians' schedules, and so on.

Both clinical and logistical procedures vary from office to office, so it is imperative that the new employee be oriented properly to how the office works: the closest person to the phone when it rings answers it, only the receptionist can call the answering service at the beginning and end of each day, only the data entry employee is allowed to turn on the computer in the morning, and so on.

It will take time for the new employee to feel at home in this new environment, and anything that the office manager or staff can do to help is always appreciated. The manager should remind all employees and physicians to be patient with the new employee during this transition period and that a kind word or gentle suggestion is better than impatience and snarling.

If the new employee is new to the area, the office manager should have the local Chamber of Commerce send materials on churches, community services, and other activities to the office for her or him. Many of the other employees may want to suggest entertainment possibilities, reputable car repair shops, good bakeries, dry cleaners, and so on. This will help to make the new employee feel at ease in unfamiliar territory. If parking at the office is not possible, the office manager should acquaint the new employee with the closest, cheapest, and safest off-site parking lot available. If there is a parking garage, the new employee should receive a parking card on her or his first day at work and be reimbursed for any parking expense she or he had for that day.

A final word about orienting the new employee: Care should be taken not to overload her or him with too much information about all the quirks of the practice or the employees.

Job Awareness and Feedback

The office manager should encourage the new employee to express any ideas she or he might have for improving current procedures. Many times, employees will bring ideas with them from other practices that can be useful to the new practice. Feedback from the new employee after the first week on the job is very important. It is important to learn of any concerns the new employee might have; however, she or he may feel reluctant to speak out. The manager can make the new hire feel invited to express her or his concerns by asking some very nonthreatening questions, such as "Is there anything you need help with?" The manager may want to ease into the conversation by saying, "The first month in a large practice like this can be very hectic and stressful. It took me a few months to . . ." This becomes a sharing situation between the office manager and the new employee, the basis for a bond. Remember, the office is looking for loyal and dependable individuals, and a little bit of kindness and caring will go a long way toward this end.

THE APPEARANCE OF THE MEDICAL PROFESSIONAL

The best steam to have is self-esteem. —ANONYMOUS

The image that an employee presents to patients and their families is another important factor that will influence others. Appearance, posture, vocabulary, tone of voice, and manners are all part of the medical office employee's image and have been found to influence patients and their families. Some physicians require office staff to wear crisp, white uniforms that will inspire trust and suggest credibility. Others prefer a low-key, relaxed atmosphere and allow colored scrubs and uniforms in the office. The common theme in both of these offices is professionalism. More and more offices today allow the staff individuality in their attire as long as it is *appropriate.* Depending on the type of medical office, some office managers allow clinical personnel to wear street clothes under white laboratory coats to show an air of warmth and confidence. Dressing for a professional role in a medical office has become increasingly important and must always be neat and clean. Each individual physician's office will establish a dress code, which should be part of its office policy and procedure manual. Jewelry should be kept at a minimum and should be in good taste. Body piercing such as pierced tongues, eyebrows, noses, and so on should not be allowed! This is a major distraction to patients and may make many patients uncomfortable, not to mention co-workers! Tattoos should not be above the shoulders or on forearms. In other words, unsightly tattoos should not be in an area where they can be seen by patients. Small ankle tattoos should be allowed. Hairstyles should not border on the extreme, and makeup should be on the light side. It is a good idea to refrain from wearing perfumes, colognes, or aftershaves, because some patients have allergies and other respiratory infections that could be aggravated by the smell. Employees with facial hair such as mustaches and beards should keep them neatly trimmed and clean. A patient does not want to see remnants of today's lunch in someone's mustache!

Shoes and sneakers should be in good condition and should be cleaned or polished on a regular basis. Sandals and open-toed shoes should not be worn in a medical office. T-shirts, shorts, jeans, hats, clothing with advertising logos (e.g., sports teams, beers, or a favorite race car driver), sweatsuits, short skirts (shorter than 2 inches above the knee), low-cut tops, and any clothing that is acid-washed, faded, stained, ragged, dirty, or wrinkled do not belong in a medical practice. If you want respect, you have to look the part.

An office manager should always convey a sense of authority in her or his attire, whether it is a uniform or street clothes. With image playing such a big role in the medical office, the staff should be guided by the patients', the patients' families', sales representatives', and physicians' reactions to their appearance. First impressions of a medical office are important and are generally long lasting. As in other professions, such as the military and law enforcement, appearance that commands respect and authority has a very positive effect on individuals.

Name Badges

By adding name badges to the attire of the office personnel, you add professionalism and efficiency. It becomes easier for patients to relate to office personnel when they can address them by name. These badges should be supplied by the office and should be a mandatory part of the uniform.

EMPLOYEE-TO-PHYSICIAN RATIO

Four factors affect the number of employees a medical office has on staff (Figure 2-12):

1. The type of medical practice
2. The type of physician practice
3. The location of the practice
4. The style of the practice

The most widely used method of determining the number of staff that a medical office needs is allowing three employees per physician. As the number of physicians increases, so should the ancillary staff. For instance, because of the variety of treatments involved in family practice, a family practitioner may require slightly more staff than a general surgeon. A recent study by National Association for Home Care/Practice Management Group showed that, on average, the staff to physician ratios for the following specialties:

Specialty	*Staff-to-Physician Ratio (Full-Time Employees [FTEs])*
Cardiology	3.74
Dermatology	4.30
Family practice	4.06
Gastroenterology	3.75
Hematology/ oncology	4.19
Internal medicine	3.51
Neurology	2.78
Obstetrics/ gynecology	4.35
Ophthalmology (dispensing)	5.80
Ophthalmology (nondispensing)	5.19

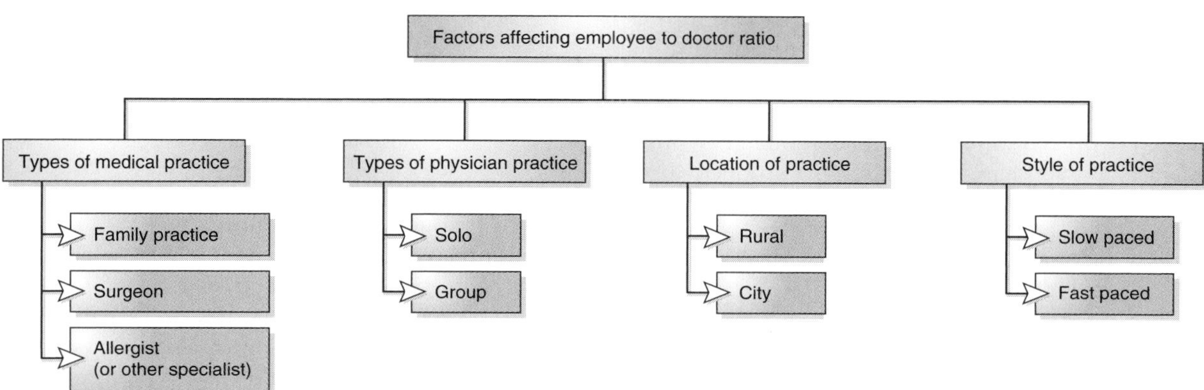

FIGURE 2-12. Factors that affect the employee-to-doctor ratio.

Otolaryngology	4.22
Pediatrics	3.79
Pulmonary	2.86
Surgery (general)	2.50
Surgery (orthopedic)	4.12
Urology	3.29
Overall average	**3.73**

Many physicians make the mistake of thinking that if profits are down, they must decrease their expenses, with payroll being the most likely place to start. This could be a big error in judgment on the physician's part. It has been proven that medical offices that employ three people see 50% more patients in a typical week than the medical office that employs only one person. The problem is getting the physician to believe in this statistic! If hiring another employee allows the physician to see just two more patients a day, the system is working. This figure will grow, constantly increasing the patient volume and subsequent income of the office.

Some physicians become overzealous and add too many employees as the practice grows. A surplus of employees can also result when two medical practices merge, because neither physician wants to let her or his employees go. What should be done if the office finds itself overstaffed? The solution to this problem is easy. The situation should be viewed as an opportunity to get rid of "deadwood" and trim the staff down to the employees who are necessary for the office to run efficiently. Those employees who have just been along for the ride for the past year will be let go and, in the case of a merger of two practices, replaced with employees from the other practice who are doing top-notch work. This might sound harsh, but many consultants asked to evaluate the size of a practice's staff will take this approach and decisively make changes in personnel as they see fit, without consideration of the employees. This is a business decision and is not based on the employees personally, but duties and responsibilities.

An effective way for the office manager to establish whether the office is overstaffed is to have each employee list, in order of importance, the 10 most important tasks she or he does. The manager then collects all the lists and compares them to see if any of the tasks are repeated on any lists. If a task appears on two or more lists, the office manager might want to take this time to revise the job description and responsibilities of each employee. The addition of new office equipment might also have an effect on the productivity of the office. Reorganization can be very helpful in making the staff more efficient and in determining the amount of staff necessary for a particular medical office.

OFFICE ROMANCES

Romances between physician-bosses and employees or between office managers and employees can turn into living nightmares for everyone involved. In the first place, the people involved may think that no one knows what's going on when, in fact, everyone knows and the couple has become the topic of conversation in the lunchroom. Romances can also lead to embezzlement in the blink of an eye. For example, an office nurse was having an affair with a physician-boss and, during this fling, decided to help herself to monies from bank deposits every day. Because the physician had become partial to the nurse, he gave her more responsibility, which included making all the bank deposits from the office. Because the nurse was always working late, she was the last employee to leave the office, and it became increasingly easy for her to change bank deposit slips. This office did not have an acting office manager, and when the receptionist spoke with the doctor about the suspected problem, the receptionist was immediately labeled a troublemaker and asked to leave. The doctor finally saw the error of his ways, $35,000 later, when the nurse moved out of state unexpectedly.

An office manager should always be aware of personal relationships that might be brewing and attempt to put a stop to them. Of course, if one of the players is the physician, the office manager might have a difficult time. There is no way an office romance can go on without its hurting the practice. It is not uncommon to hear from job applicants that their reason for leaving their last position was that "the doctor was having an affair with the receptionist and I just didn't want to deal with it any more!" Office romances give rise to irreversible morale problems and complaints about favoritism. Office romances have been the start of divorces, dissolutions of partnerships, and embezzlement proceedings.

SEXUAL HARASSMENT

Sexual harassment can be as open as a physician's or supervisor's offering an increase in salary in return for sexual favors or as elusive as making a comment about an employee's dress. Every office should have a policy in place regarding sexual harassment issues. The Equal Employment Opportunity Commission (EEOC) defines sexual harassment in a very loose manner that can, however, be translated into *trouble* for the medical office. Some feel that sexual harassment is merely an issue between the two people that it involves. This is incorrect! The office manager should recognize that sexual harassment not only affects those involved, but also creates tension, low morale, and reduced productivity in the office.

Fewer than 10% of harassed individuals file formal complaints. Those in the medical profession tend to feel that we are immune to such nasty issues as sexual harassment, when, in fact, sadly, there is much of it going on. A survey conducted by *Nation's Business* magazine showed that 9 out of 10 medical professionals had either witnessed or been involved in sexual harassment on the job.

The Equal Employment Opportunity Commission's Definition of Sexual Harassment

Since 1963, Congress has passed a series of laws protecting the rights of each individual with respect to employment. These laws place responsibilities on employers by specifying certain job requirements. For example, when an employer or a manager is interviewing an applicant for a job or considering whether to continue to employ a particular person, she or he can consider only job-related criteria. For instance, an employer or manager cannot ask questions during an interview that are not job related. A person's sex and race are not job related. Whether the person is married or has children is not job related. Whether a person is gay or straight is not job related. A person's qualifications and experience . . . *are job related!* These are the issues that should be discussed.

The EEOC defines *sexual harassment* as follows: unwelcome sexual advances, request for sexual favors, and other verbal or physical conduct of a sexual nature. These constitute sexual harassment when the following exist:

- An individual surrenders to a conduct that was made either explicitly or implicitly a term or condition of the individual's employment.
- An individual surrenders to or rejects a conduct that is used as a basis of employment decisions affecting the individual's employment.
- Such conduct has the purpose or effect of unreasonably interfering with an individual's work performance or creating an intimidating, hostile, or offensive working environment.

To understand how sexual harassment cases are defined, it is necessary to understand that the standard used to determine the validity of sexual harassment acts is that of a "reasonable person." The law views the case from the victim's perspective. There is a lot of latitude in the interpretation of what constitutes sexual harassment. This means that everyone must be very careful of how they act in their place of employment.

Types of Sexual Harassment

The three types of sexual harassment as shown in Figure 2-13 are physical, verbal, and nonverbal. *Physical sexual harassment* is just as stated: being touched, rubbed against, pinched, or assaulted or receiving *any* unwanted physical contact. *Verbal sexual harassment* consists of innuendos, sexual jokes, foul and unacceptable language, sexual comments, and threats. *Nonverbal sexual harassment* consists of obscene gestures, leering, whistling, and suggestive objects or pictures. The legal system recognizes sexual harassment by "quid pro quo" (demanding sexual favors for economic compensation, such as a promotion or money) and "hostile work environment." Each medical office should compose a policy statement regarding sexual harassment. A sample statement provided by the Medical Group Management Association is shown in Box 2-6.

The Sexual Harassment Complaint

The costs of a sexual harassment suit can be substantial, whether the medical office wins or loses. Sexual harassment suits increase absenteeism, tardiness, and employee turnover; result in low productivity; and ruin the image of the office in general. If the suit is lost, the physician could be responsible for paying back wages, punitive damages, and reimbursement for pain and suffering of the victim.

Every complaint should be handled with dignity and proper documentation, whether it is a small incident or a serious one. Any other employee who might have witnessed the act should be interviewed. The person committing the act should also be interviewed and advised of the allegations against him or her. Disciplinary actions can be oral; however, it has been found that written disciplinary actions are much more effective. A copy of this action should be made a part of the employee's personnel file. It is important to obtain correct and accurate information before taking any action against the employee. Failure to do so can result in a wrongful-termination suit against the office. A sexual harassment

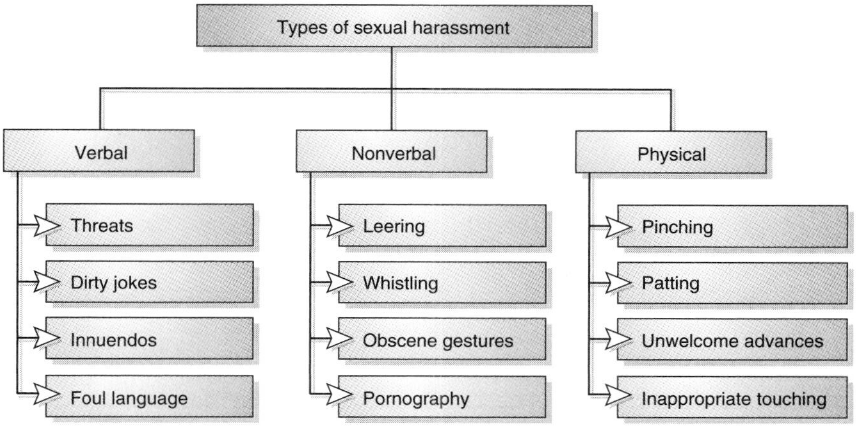

FIGURE 2-13. Types of sexual harassment.

BOX 2-6 Sexual Harassment Policy Statement

Community Medical Clinic is committed to providing a working environment in which its employees are treated with courtesy, respect, and dignity. Community Medical Clinic will not tolerate or condone any actions by any persons that constitute sexual harassment of any employee.

Sexual harassment is defined as unwelcome sexual advances; requests for sexual favors; and other verbal, written, or physical conduct of a sexual nature by employees or supervisors where such conduct is either made an explicit or implicit term or condition of employment, is used as the basis for employment decisions affecting employees, or has the purpose or effect of unreasonably interfering with an employee's work by creating an intimidating, hostile, or offensive working environment.

Deliberate and repeated comments with sexual overtones, sexual jokes or ridicule, physical gestures or actions of a sexual nature, and solicitations for sexual favors are examples of violations of this policy and will subject the offender to discipline, including discharge. A sexual harassment complaint should be directed to the medical office manager or practice administrator, who will promptly and fully investigate. Confidentiality will be maintained to the maximum extent possible, consistent with the need to investigate the complaint fairly and thoroughly.

form can be implemented to resolve sexual harassment complaints; the one shown in Figure 2-14 can be revised to fit the personal needs of each office.

LIABILITY AND THE MEDICAL OFFICE

The physician is responsible for any acts of her or his managers or administrators. If a co-worker is responsible for the act of sexual harassment, the employer can still be held liable, especially if the employer knew about the act and did nothing to prevent it. Physicians can also be held responsible for the actions of individuals not in their employ, for instance, pharmaceutical representatives, patients, and delivery people. The best way to avoid problems is to create an atmosphere of loyalty and positive employee relations.

EMPLOYEE COUNSELING

Office managers may occasionally find themselves in the position of confidant or counselor. Employees may look to them for advice on various matters from personal to

Alleged victim's name and position: ______________________

Date and time of alleged incident: ______________________

Location of alleged incident: ______________________

Date and time reported: ______________________

Individual reported to: ______________________

Allegation:

Action requested:

Alleged harasser's name and position: ______________________

Alleged harasser's statement:

Action taken:

Witnesses:

	Name	Position
1)	______________	______________
2)	______________	______________
3)	______________	______________

Date: ______________

FIGURE 2-14. Sexual harassment complaint form.

Date: ______________________________

Employee name: ______________________________

Problem:

Employee response:

Corrective steps taken:

Signature of office manager: ______________________________

Signature of employee: ______________________________

FIGURE 2-15. Employee counseling report.

professional. A good office manager always has time for the staff and has excellent listening skills. If the employee is experiencing a problem involving the office, the personnel, or the employee's role in the practice, it is important to use an employee counseling report (Figure 2-15). This should be filled out and placed in the employee's permanent file.

VIOLENCE IN THE WORKPLACE

In today's society, we listen to the news to hear that an individual has fallen victim to violence in the workplace. This can be caused by a spouse, an ex-spouse, a lover, an ex-lover, a family member, or a co-worker, or one could simply become a victim of others' problems. When the violence is attributed to an external factor, unfortunately, there is not much that can be done to prevent it. When the violence is the result of a disturbed co-worker, it is the responsibility of the office manager to recognize the signs that may point to a potential problem. Certain warnings can identify potential problems:

- Excessive tardiness or absences
- Increased need for supervision
- Reduction in productivity
- Inconsistent or unusual behavior
- Inability to concentrate
- Changes in health or hygiene
- Substance abuse
- Fascination with weapons or violence
- Stress or depression
- Excuse their actions by blaming others for their problems

Identification of any of these signs in an employee should be taken seriously and dealt with accordingly. Observe and be aware!

EXERCISES

MULTIPLE CHOICE

Choose the best *answer for each of the following questions.*

1. Which of the following is considered a form of sexual harassment?
   a. Pinching
   b. Dirty jokes
   c. Innuendos
   d. All of the above
2. Which of the following is a warning sign of potential violent behavior?
   a. Tardiness
   b. Depression
   c. Change in health or hygiene
   d. All of the above
3. Violence can be caused by
   a. A spouse
   b. A family member
   c. An ex-boyfriend or an ex-girlfriend
   d. All of the above
4. Which of the following specialties usually requires the largest number of employees in the office?
   a. Anesthesiology
   b. Pathology
   c. Family practice
   d. Surgery
5. Which question should *not* be asked during an interview?
   a. "Where do you see yourself in the next five years?"
   b. "Will you have any difficulty working late occasionally?"
   c. "We love children in this office; do you have any?"
   d. "Are you legally permitted to work in the United States?"
6. Which is *not* an element of an effective team?
   a. Positive interdependence
   b. Collaborative skills
   c. Brainstorming
   d. Marchand thinking

7. Which of the following is *not* a way to remotivate the staff?
   a. Set goals
   b. Share in decisions
   c. Provide continuity
   d. Issue formal responses
8. Which of the following is the best way to delegate?
   a. Use slang
   b. Use a formal request
   c. Relay the message through others
   d. None of the above
9. The directional stage of the employee life cycle is stage
   a. One
   b. Four
   c. Three
   d. Five
10. Which of the following should *not* be found on an employment application?
    a. What is your national origin?
    b. Educational history
    c. Employment history
    d. Reason for leaving last position
11. Which of the following is *not* a major area of human resources?
    a. Demographics
    b. Efficiency
    c. Experience
    d. Skills
12. Which of the following is a task-oriented personality type?
    a. Conservator
    b. Doer
    c. Rebel
    d. Pragmatist
13. Which of the following personality types is adept at nonverbal communication?
    a. Feeler
    b. Houdini
    c. Controller
    d. None of the above
14. Which of the following is *not* a benefit of teamwork?
    a. Easier cross-training
    b. Decreased revenues
    c. Satisfied patients
    d. Increased office morale
15. Which of the following is a way to motivate the staff?
    a. Listen
    b. Gym membership
    c. Unilateral decisions by management
    d. Make hasty judgments
16. What is the number one reason for employee turnover?
    a. Personal problems of employee
    b. Not enough paid vacation time
    c. Incorrect person hired
    d. Lack of communication
17. Which of the following should *not* be included in a job description?
    a. Title of position
    b. Skills needed
    c. Specific duties of position
    d. Salary
18. Which of the following is *not* an issue to consider when hiring a new employee?
    a. Where the applicant lives
    b. Where the spouse works
    c. If history illustrates employment stability
    d. The educational background of the applicant
19. When an office manager focuses on one thing an employee did well during the employee's evaluation, it is called
    a. Peculiarity
    b. Projection
    c. Praise
    d. Particularity
20. Which of the following is the best approach to orienting a new employee?
    a. Team approach
    b. Managerial approach
    c. Solo approach
    d. None of the above

MATCHING

Match the offense with the category provided.

1. _____ Smoking
2. _____ Stealing
3. _____ Falsifying records
4. _____ Emotional outburst
5. _____ Inappropriate dress
6. _____ Obscene language in general
7. _____ Obscene language to patients
8. _____ Obscene language to co-workers
9. _____ Tardiness
10. _____ Violation of confidentiality
11. _____ Drug/alcohol use
12. _____ Excessive absenteeism
13. _____ Fighting with co-workers
14. _____ Insubordination

A. Secondary
B. Primary
C. Severe

TRUE OR FALSE

1. _____ New employees should not be asked for input into their positions.
2. _____ Flexible pay raises are the most commonly found type in a medical practice.
3. _____ New hires should be evaluated 6 months after their start date.
4. _____ Use jargon when giving explanations to office personnel; they understand it.
5. _____ Cliques do not belong in the workplace.
6. _____ During an employment interview, ask the applicant how many children she or he has.
7. _____ One should avoid office romances.
8. _____ Delegating is bad. An office manager should never delegate.
9. _____ A controller is generally considered a traditionalist.
10. _____ It is cheaper to replace employees rather than to correct situations and retain them.

11. _____ Employees should be allowed as many personal calls as necessary.
12. _____ Informed communication is key in "defusing" the office grapevine.
13. _____ Everyone has the same learning style.
14. _____ Sexual jokes are classified under nonverbal sexual harassment.
15. _____ The fourth stage of the employee life cycle is training.
16. _____ A good office manager should not talk with employees regularly. Let them do their work.
17. _____ A small office does not need employee job descriptions.
18. _____ In solo practice, it is not necessary to check applicants' references during the interviewing process.
19. _____ Exit interviews are important for all medical practices.
20. _____ A mission statement should provide information about office hours.
21. _____ Workers' compensation laws are the same in every state.
22. _____ Dental insurance is an inexpensive benefit to provide employees.
23. _____ An employee who has injured herself horseback riding with her family on Sunday can file for workers' compensation benefits.
24. _____ Most employers provide employees' families with health insurance coverage.
25. _____ Child daycare is commonly provided to employees through health coverage benefits.
26. _____ Cash payments are sometimes awarded to employees for a "job well done!"
27. _____ Most offices offer at least six paid holidays per year.
28. _____ It is common practice for offices to provide a uniform allowance to employees.
29. _____ Employees are always compensated for days they cannot get to work because of inclement weather.
30. _____ Cafeteria plans are time consuming to implement.

THINKERS

1. Describe "pragmatists" and how they work with other personality types.
2. List three elements of an employment application and the reason for their importance.
3. Describe "Houdini."
4. List four articles of clothing that would not be acceptable in a medical office.

REFERENCES

Caplan, C. "A Guide to Hiring and Keeping Good People." *Physician's Management*, March 1993, pp. 122-138.

Coleman, D. "What You Must Know Before You Hire or Fire an Employee." *Physician's Management*, May 1992, pp. 60-70.

Curry, G. "Temporary Help Market Continues to Grow." *The Office*, July 1993, pp. 8-10.

Davis, M. "Hiring the Overqualified." *Management Review*, August 1993, pp. 35-38.

Employee Benefit Research Institute. *Current Populations Surveys.* Washington, DC: Employee Benefit Research Institute, May 2001.

Farber, L. *Encyclopedia of Practice and Financial Management.* Oradell, NJ: Medical Economics Company, 1988.

Gray, R. "How to Deal with Sexual Harassment." *Nation's Business*, December 1991, pp. 28-32.

Hirsh, R. "Office Romance: A Sure Way to Shatter a Practice." *Medical Economics*, February 1991, pp. 118-120.

Holley, W.H., Jennings, K.M., & Wolters, R. *The Labor Relations Process*, 7th edition. Hinsdale, IL: South-Western, 2001.

Martocchio, J.J. *Employee Benefits: A Primer for Human Resource Professionals.* New York: McGraw-Hill, 2002.

Price, C. *Group Practice Personnel Policies Manuals.* Englewood, CO: Medical Group Management Association, 2001.

Prince, T., & Mayberry, E. *Physician Office Policies and Procedures.* Reston, VA: St. Anthony's Publishing, 1995.

Regel, R., & Hollmann, R. "Gauging Performance Objectively." *Personnel Administrator*, June 1987, pp. 74-78.

Schneier, C., Beatty, R., & Baird, L. "Creating a Performance Management System." *Training and Development Journal*, May 1986, pp. 74-80.

Sevel, F. "The Most Effective Ways to Train a New Employee." *Physician's Management*, November 1992, pp. 97-115.

3

THE FRONT OFFICE

CHAPTER OUTLINE

CHAPTER OBJECTIVES

After completing this chapter, you will be able to do the following:

- Choose a proper phone system for a medical practice (equipment and available features)
- Understand the importance of proper telephone techniques, triage, and message taking
- Identify the various types of appointment scheduling
- Handle emergency appointments and keep the physician on time
- Configure a warm and friendly reception area
- Differentiate among the types of mail and handle various types of correspondence
- Recognize and avoid roadblocks to patient flow

WHY BAD THINGS HAPPEN TO GOOD OFFICES

The patient who walks into a medical office today is quite different from the patient of the past. In today's hectic society, many physicians find themselves so busy that they do not have the luxury of developing a rapport with the patient, as physicians in the past did. Decades ago, physicians knew all the family members by name and often had delivered them. In our busy urgent care facilities today, the physician generally deals with demanding, hectic schedules that preclude the opportunity for closeness.

When patients walk into a medical office today, they walk in as consumers, knowing what they need, looking for the right price, and knowing how they plan on getting it. There are some potential danger zones into which a medical office can fall. The following is a list of potential problems that the medical office manager should be aware of and try to correct before they occur:

1. Patients rarely understand that some problems do not have easy answers.
2. Patients seldom understand that delays in scheduling occur despite the best efforts of the office staff.
3. Some patients are "doctor hoppers" and arrive at your office with a history of conflicts with other physicians. They're in your office simply to put you to the test.
4. Patients never fully understand their insurance coverage and usually think they have much more coverage than they do.
5. Patients are consumers. They believe they know what they need and are there to get it.
6. Newspapers and television programs may sometimes pass along incorrect information to patients and may be biased about how the physician *really* feels about the patients. Patients are exposed to book titles such as *Drugs That Don't Work,* magazine articles such as "How to Demand the Most from Your Doctor," and local news broadcasts such as "Mammograms: Are They Helpful?"
7. Patients may believe that they require intensive treatment when, in fact, they do not.

Some patients are more interested in whether they are entitled to a particular service under their insurance plan than in whether they really need that service. One important factor to remember is that if the office excuses itself to patients who are angry, this may be seen as a weakness. Patients have a right to sound off about their grievances; however, if the medical office overreacts, it only makes the situation worse. Many patients feel better if they make an issue out of a delay, a bill, or whatever might be bothering them on that particular day. The office staff should be trained to remain unruffled and to allow these difficult patients to vent, but let them know that the office staff will do what they can to correct it.

INTERPERSONAL SKILLS FOR PATIENT INTERACTION

Interpersonal skills are the way we interact with one another. Being a "people person" involves listening to and caring about what others are saying. The following is a list of communication skills that can help the health care professional during interactions with patients.

- Acknowledge others communicating with you. When someone is speaking to you while you are reading a chart, acknowledge that the person was heard and ask him or her to please wait just a minute.
- Rephrase what is being said so that you are sure you understand what the person is saying.
- Give an example to further explain information you are relaying to the patient.
- Use good diction. Speaking clearly and distinctly (especially with the elderly) is extremely important.
- Make sure the patient sees your face and lips.
- Maintain a positive attitude when communicating with patients. Most patients are not feeling well, and your positive attitude may "catch on."
- "Read between the lines" of what is being said. Many patients will not be straightforward about their symptoms.
- Build trust with each patient. There will be a more free exchange of ideas if there is a bond between you and the patient.
- Try to find some common ground or a common interest to open the way to good conversation.

Angry Patients

Now that medical professionals must view patients as consumers, the old adage, "the customer is always right," applies in the medical office just as it does in any other place of business. Even the rude and angry patient should be handled with a certain degree of respect and friendliness. Office personnel can accomplish more at a faster rate by disarming the angry patient than by feeding the patient's anger with their own. Patients should be allowed to vent their problems, and staff should refrain from interrupting them.

Some patients need to talk out their problems and feelings. Letting patients verbalize their problems gives staff time to assess the situation and come to the appropriate perception of exactly what the problem is and what the patient wants the office to do about it. Allowing the patient to witness your notation of his or her complaint can also be helpful. Empathy works very well in situations like this;

an example of an empathic response is, "I'm sorry that this happened to you, Mr. Brown." Agreeing with the patient can also be helpful. For example, a good response to a patient who is angry about a delay in getting x-ray results is, "I would be upset too if I had to wait a week for the result of my x-ray." The staff member then asks the patient where the test was done, what was done, and when. She or he then calls the appropriate hospital or laboratory to obtain these results. The office procedure and policy manual should be referred to for guidelines for looking for test results. Generally, the physician reviews these results, and then the staff is directed as to how to handle each specific case. Patients requiring prescription renewals should also be handled according to the guidelines in the manual. Staff must *never* renew a prescription without first checking with the physician, no matter how much they know about the patient.

Patients become angry when they are made to wait for what they perceive to be long periods of time. This occurs in traffic (road rage), in airport terminals (flyer rage), and in medical office and emergency department reception areas (patient rage). Adrenaline rises, and patients (in our case) become angry—sometimes very angry. It is better to allow patients to remain in the reception area where they can talk with others, read a magazine, and perhaps watch videos or television, as opposed to placing patients in examination rooms by themselves with the door shut. The "old-school" method of letting patients think that they are "getting somewhere" by removing them from the reception area to an area within the inner office is not really the best solution to this problem. Patient rage can result in a loss of that patient, plus the possible loss of other patients, due to word of mouth.

At times, patients will give nonverbal cues that illustrate that they are not happy. The majority of all communication is through nonverbal cues. When dealing with an angry patient, the use of open palms with hands turned upward creates a gesture of openness. The voice of an angry or excited individual is loud and continues to increase in volume as the conversation progresses. The response to that volume should be a gentle, calm, and soothing tone. This will show the individual that you are not in competition with her or him. If you talk in a low voice, you force the other individual to become a better listener. Head tilting is another way to show that you are not threatening. Just as animals instinctively minimize exposure to their neck, because it is a vital area, humans can show, by tilting their head and exposing their neck, that they are not going to be combative or argumentative.

Noncompliant Patients

The office staff can be invaluable in interactions with the physician's noncompliant patients. They can coax them into compliance when the physician has exhausted all efforts. Patients who will not cooperate with the physician may cooperate with office staff. One of the most common reasons for compliance with the staff is very simple. The office nurse or health care professional might favor the patient's grandchild, whom the patient loves dearly. When an office assistant shows caring, the patient feels secure and trusts that person. Don't forget: staff builds relationships with patients just as much as or more than the physician does. The office manager should recognize this and attempt to use it in a positive fashion. Much can be accomplished!

COMMUNICATION DURING REGISTRATION

The staff at the front desk become key personnel in building the patient-physician relationship. Once the telephone appointment has been made, they are the next in line to show off their excellent communication skills. Once the patient arrives at the office, she or he should be greeted within 20 seconds. If the receptionist at the front desk is busy on the phone, the practice should reevaluate its staffing to allow opportunity for staff to be free to handle patients who are checking in.

It is at this step that the practice begins to build on this relationship. The receptionist should always provide his or her name when greeting the patient. Using the patient's name during the greeting also makes the patient feel special and promotes a positive experience. An example of this greeting would be, "Hello, Mrs. Wilson? Welcome to our practice. My name is Barbara. Did you have any trouble finding our office today?"

The patient is then handed any forms that are necessary for completion. Simple, clear instructions should be provided. New patients may be nervous and may confuse easily. Help them through the process and advise them to return the forms to you once they are completed. If they require help, personally assist them in completing these forms. Continue to use the patient's name frequently. Explain the Health Insurance Portability and Accountability Act (HIPAA) policy to them, and ask them to sign to acknowledge that they were informed of this policy. Provide reassurance if the patient seems anxious. Remember, all interactions with the patient should be positive! Explain to the patient that she or he should take a seat and someone will call for the patient soon. If the patient seems to be in distress, it may be necessary to notify the clinical personnel so that they can assess the patient and perhaps place her or him in an examination room.

Gentle Nudge

Not all patients are willing to adjust to policies regarding office scheduling. Most of them do not care about the events of the day—they just want to see the doctor! Once a medical office establishes an appointment scheduling policy, it is important to make every attempt to stick to it. Patients must be dealt with in a firm yet tactful manner. If they are late for an appointment, they can be told politely when they check in that they have arrived late, but they will be seen as soon as possible. Positive reinforcement is just as important. Patients who arrive on time should always be told how much their promptness is appreciated. Gentle nudges such as these can do a world of good in getting the office policy on promptness across without offending patients.

Some patients want appointments on certain days and at certain times. They must be told of the office hours and that the physician has the following openings available. This should be done in a pleasant yet firm manner. Offices should try their best to accommodate both the patient and the physician.

Every receptionist's motto should be "Firm and controlled, yet tactful." These situations can be very difficult when dealing directly with a referring physician.

Patience, Patience, Please!

One key characteristic of a health care professional is patience. Patience is the number one characteristic that should be found in all health care professionals. Patients are generally not feeling well when they are in a physician practice and therefore may be a little "out of sorts." They don't want to be sick, they don't want to wait, and they don't want to have to do paperwork so the physician gets paid; they just want to get better! Let's face it . . . everyone has bad days, but when dealing with patients, the health care professional must always be in control. Understanding how to deal with impatient patients will help. Examples of this type of impatient behavior found in health care personnel include the following:

- Eating lunch too fast
- Interrupting people when they are speaking
- Finishing others' sentences
- Answering questions quickly and abruptly
- Trying to do two things at once

Receptionist

The position of receptionist is the key position in the practice. This position affects the physician-patient relationship and the billing. The receptionist is the first person to come in contact with patients as they walk into the reception area. The receptionist is often the first person to speak to the patient via the telephone. The receptionist's information gathering should be complete and accurate because it is absolutely key to getting the patient's bill paid. Many insurance company claim denials are due to incomplete demographics, incorrect insurance company information, incorrect date of birth or health insurance number, and so on. Each patient should be greeted immediately on her or his arrival at the office. The receptionist should not have so many other responsibilities that he or she cannot immediately greet and check in the patients.

Lifeline of a New Patient

A new patient is one who has not been seen in the office or hospital by the physician, or one of her or his colleagues of the same specialty, within the last 3 years. This distinction is not based on the diagnosis or the reason for the visit.

1. The patient arrives at the office.
2. The patient is not asked to sign in. Many offices have discontinued the use of a sign-in sheet because of patient confidentiality and HIPAA issues.
3. The patient is handed the medical office HIPAA policy and the new patient paperwork. The patient is asked to read the HIPAA policy.
4. The patient is asked to complete the new patient paperwork, which consists of a patient information form, a past history form, and the insurance and billing form.
5. The patient is asked to sign the consent-to-treat form, the authorization of medical benefits form (which allows the practice to release information necessary for payment of the claim and to request that payment be made directly to the practice), and the HIPAA acknowledgment form.
6. If the form is returned and it is not completed in its entirety, one of the health care professionals should help the patient to complete the forms.
7. The patient is asked to present her or his insurance cards. The cards are copied, both front and back, and then returned to the patient. The copies are used to enter the insurance information into the computer and they are then placed in the patient's chart.
8. Depending on the insurance, verification of coverage may be necessary. This may or may not be performed by the receptionist.
9. If the practice is a specialty practice and the patient has managed care insurance, it will be necessary to obtain a referral for evaluation and treatment.
10. If the patient has a managed care plan, he or she is responsible for payment of a co-pay. This co-payment may be anywhere from $2.00 to $20.00. The co-payment can be collected when the patient checks in, or it can be collected at discharge.
11. Other insurance plans, such as Medicaid, also require a co-payment. It is important to read the back of the patient's card to identify if any co-payment is required.
12. If the patient is a child, the health care professional must be aware of the *birthday rule.* If both parents

carry insurance, the child will be covered under the parent whose birthday is first in the calendar year. For example, if the mother's birthday is in March and the father's birthday is in June, the mother's insurance would be primary for the child.

13. A medical chart is created with inclusion of the completed forms. All forms should contain patient identification.
14. Other forms used by the practice should also be added to the medical chart at this time. Such forms might include medication logs, progress note forms, office visit templates, history forms, problem lists, and so on.
15. Appropriate labels should be affixed to the outside of the patient's chart. These labels would include the following: allergies, type of insurance, year of the visit, and alphabetic labels indicating the patient name (assists in filing).
16. A patient account is created in the computer with the information obtained at check-in. This may or may not be performed by the receptionist.
17. A patient encounter form is generated and placed on the front of the patient's chart.
18. The patient is now ready to see the clinical staff of the practice.

Lifeline of an Established Patient

An established patient is one who has been seen by the physician within the last 3 years. This distinction is not based on the diagnosis or the reason for the visit.

1. The patient either returns for a previously scheduled appointment or has called for an appointment to be seen.
2. The patient is not asked to sign in. Many offices have discontinued the use of a sign-in sheet because of patient confidentiality and HIPAA issues.
3. All patient information is verified for accuracy. If the patient has not been seen in the past year, he or she is asked to complete an updated patient information form.
4. Insurance cards are collected, copied, and placed in the patient's chart.
5. Depending on the insurance, verification of coverage may be necessary. This may or may not be performed by the receptionist.
6. If the practice is a specialty practice and the patient has managed care insurance, it will be necessary to obtain a referral for evaluation and treatment.
7. If the patient has a managed care plan, he or she is responsible for payment of a co-pay. This co-payment may be anywhere from $2.00 to $20.00. The co-payment can be collected when the patient checks in, or it can be collected at discharge.
8. Other insurance plans, such as Medicaid, also require a co-payment. It is important to read the back of the patient's card to identify if any co-payment is required.
9. The chart is checked to see if there is room to document the office visit on the progress note form. If not, a new form is added to the chart.
10. A patient encounter form is generated and placed on the front of the patient's chart.
11. The patient is now ready to see the clinical staff of the practice.

Patient Registration Form

The patient registration form is one of the most important documents in a medical practice. It contains all of the necessary information required for billing for services and procedures. It also contains patient demographic information.

COMPONENTS OF THE PATIENT REGISTRATION FORM

- Date
- Patient's name
- Patient's age
- Patient's date of birth
- Patient's Social Security number
- Guarantor's name, address, and phone number
- Employer's name, address, and phone number
- Spouse's name
- Spouse's employer name, address, and phone number
- Insurance company name, address, and phone number
- Insurance identification and group numbers
- Emergency contact
- Referred by
- Patient signature

Some forms also contain the following information:

- List of current medications
- Past illnesses/surgeries
- Allergies

This form should be reviewed by the health care professional for completeness, because it is critical to the billing process. Any information that is missing should be obtained from the patient.

This form should be updated on a yearly basis or more frequently if the patient's information changes. Each time the patient visits the office, the patient should be asked if any of her or his information has changed. Questions such as the following can be asked:

- "Are you still at 1 Versailles Circle?"
- "Is your phone number still 111-123-4567?"
- "Is your employer still Miller and Associates?"

- "Is your wife still working at Hanes Department Store?"
- "Do you have a cell phone number?"
- "Do you have a cell phone number for your wife?"
- "Do you still want your emergency contact to be Mrs. Peters?"
- "Is her number still 111-432-9876?"
- "Is your insurance still Blue Shield?"
- "Can you verify the numbers for me?"
- "May I please see your insurance card so that I can make a copy?"

Patient Encounter Form

The patient encounter form is an integral part of the billing process. It is imperative that it be comprehensive and accurate, because much of the billing information is keyed from this document. Once the information on the patient registration form is complete, it is entered into the computer and a patient account is created. From this patient account a patient encounter form will be generated. This form will follow the patient throughout the office and will contain the following information:

- Date
- Patient's name
- Patient's address
- Patient's age
- Patient's phone number
- Patient's date of birth
- Gender of patient
- Patient's Social Security number
- Guarantor's name
- Insurance company name, address, and phone number
- Insurance identification and group numbers
- Provider's name
- Listing of CPT codes
- Listing of ICD-9-CM preprinted codes
- Area for written diagnosis codes if not preprinted
- Return visit area
- Space for special instructions

Some forms may contain the following information:

- List of current medications
- Past illnesses/surgeries
- Allergies

PHARMACEUTICAL REPRESENTATIVES

Some offices see pharmaceutical representatives ("reps") by appointment only. Allowing pharmaceutical reps to walk in at any time and be seen can be problematic for the practice. Such a policy will ruin even the best of schedules. The pharmaceutical reps will take as much time with the physician that you, as the office manager, will permit. This is where a firm, but tactful, receptionist or office manager will come in handy. She or he must be instructed to adhere to the policy that the office has set up.

Most pharmaceutical reps understand the hectic schedule of the physician and will abide by the office policy. Occasionally, if the pharmaceutical rep has seen the physician recently, but the office called for more samples, the pharmaceutical rep will simply leave the samples and ask for a physician signature in return (Figure 3-1). Some offices schedule pharmaceutical reps on certain days and at certain times, which helps in planning not only the physician office schedule, but also the schedule of the pharmaceutical rep.

Some pharmaceutical reps provide lunch for the office and, while everyone is eating, attempt to corral a physician or two to talk with them about their drugs. Some practices enjoy taking the time to lunch and speak with the reps about their drugs, while others simply do not have the time.

Speaking with pharmaceutical reps today becomes both an ethical and a time management issue. The pharmaceutical industry estimates that it spends $5.7 billion a year on marketing to physicians, which means about $6,000 to $7,000 per physician. The pharmaceutical rep was not only known for free lunches, but for note pads, pens, clocks, gadgets, and toys. In the past, physicians were even treated to lush weekend getaways and tickets for concerts and sporting events. Now, we are questioning the ethics of accepting these "freebies" because they can be seen as a violation of anti-kickback statutes. A few years ago, the state of Vermont enacted a groundbreaking law that required pharmaceutical companies to publicly report all freebies. The University of Pennsylvania, Yale Medical Group, and Stanford University have developed a policy prohibiting physicians from accepting industry gifts of any size. These policies also prohibit the dispensing of drug samples. Each practice should decide how to handle this issue and should develop and implement a policy.

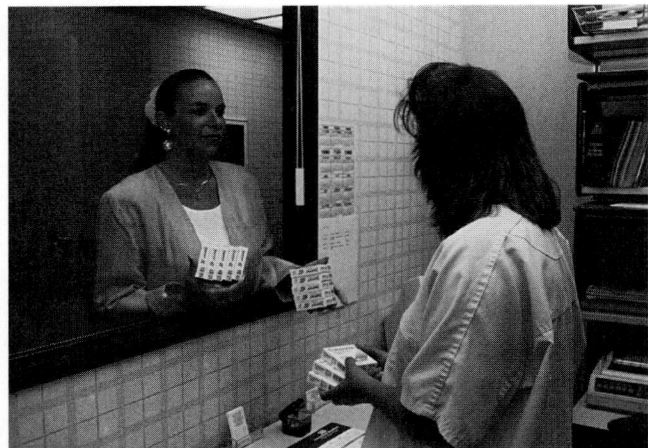

FIGURE 3-1. A pharmaceutical representative brings samples to the office.

In terms of time management, are the pharmaceutical reps' visits worth the loss of patient time? One physician decided not to take appointments with pharmaceutical reps any more and was able to see a few more patients each week, which translated into approximately $6,500 more per year in income. When questioned, physicians fell on two sides of the fence when it came to pharmaceutical rep visits. Some physicians feel that they are a strain on the practice and that they attempt to persuade physicians to "lock in" their patients to new drugs that may or may not be better than the ones they are currently taking. Other physicians feel that the samples are helpful for their patients and welcome them to leave samples and, sometimes, lunch! It is estimated that there are approximately 100,000 pharmaceutical reps on the streets calling on 10 physician offices per day. Some physicians report that they may see an average of 29 pharmaceutical reps in a week, whereas others report 2 visits per week. It was reported that in 2005, 85% of pharmaceutical rep visits were "drop-ins," 5% were appointments, and 10% were lunch dates. The office manager should discuss this topic with the physician(s) to establish a policy of rep or no rep!

RECEPTION AREA . . . THE HEART OF THE PRACTICE

Reception rooms should be warm, friendly places (Figure 3-2). It is up to health care professionals to maintain a calm and tranquil setting for the patients while performing the many other projects for which they are responsible. Many patients in the reception area are ill or upset, and need a quiet, calm environment in which to wait. Noisy children playing should be asked to play quietly, loud patients should be asked to talk quietly, and patients should be reminded that there is no smoking, eating, or drinking in the office.

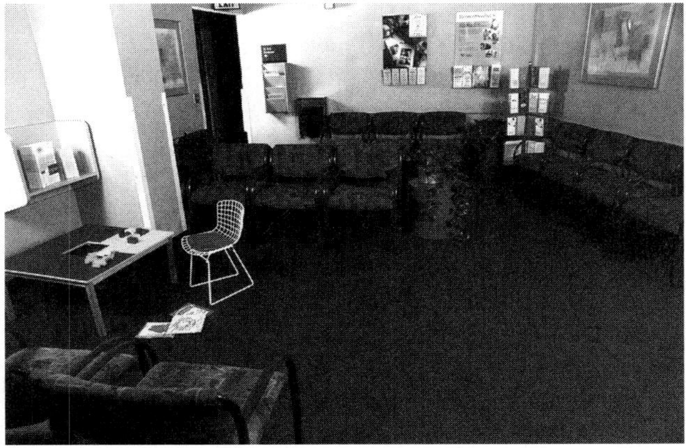

FIGURE 3-2. The waiting room should be bright, clean, and cheerful.

A Happy Reception Room

This area should be a reflection on the practice and should not be cluttered or dirty. Although there are no tried and true cures for the reception room "blues," there are some things you can do to reduce anxiety as patients wait for their name to be called.

Many offices have installed a television, and some even show movies throughout the day. Even though the physician is late in seeing the patient, the patient becomes engrossed in a television program or movie and does not realize the time. Other practices, such as some ophthalmology practices, use low lights and soft music. Whatever the preference of the physician, it should be a pleasant area.

For patients who like to become better acquainted with their illnesses, or even read about what their friends have, it is a good idea to keep various educational brochures available in the reception room. For instance, a pamphlet on toilet training is of interest to new mothers and might be found in a family practice, an obstetrics/gynecology office, or a pediatric reception room. A family practice or an internal medicine office might display brochures on hypertension, diabetes, arthritis, or high cholesterol. These brochures are sometimes provided by pharmaceutical companies, or they can be purchased at a nominal price per copy. Some physicians like to personalize them by writing up their own pamphlets. Other practices develop information sheets on various types of illnesses or injuries. They then print across the top, "RECEPTION ROOM COPY. DO NOT REMOVE." They print them on brightly colored paper and have them laminated. Patients can pick them up and read them while they wait. By having them laminated, it provides a more durable sheet. Keep in mind that some of these information sheets may "grow legs and walk away." It is a good idea to make a few sets of them.

Pamphlets are also available from various organizations explaining what they are all about and the people to contact should patients wish to become active in them. Examples of these organizations are the American Liver Foundation, the American Diabetes Association, the Alzheimer's Association, and other organizations, such as daycare centers, transportation services, and senior centers.

All magazines should be arranged neatly and should be easily accessible to all patients. It may require the health care professional to make several trips to the reception area throughout the day to straighten them up. The amount of light in a reception area is important. The room needs to have adequate lighting so that patients can read without straining their eyes. Some ophthalmology offices have low lighting because of the nature of the specialty. Many patients in the reception area have received eye drops that dilate their eyes, and bright lights can be uncomfortable. In these reception areas, there are generally televisions that play movies continually, because patients with dilating drops have a difficult time reading. Some community pharmacies sponsor magazines for a physician's waiting room if the physician is willing to put them in plastic covers advertising the pharmacy. This saves the office that added expense.

If the reception room has plants, they should be watered regularly. Choose plants that will thrive in the environment that you have, such as low lighting, direct lighting, indirect lighting, full sun, and so on, and that are not poisonous or toxic to humans. Be sure to "groom" your plants weekly, discarding any dead leaves or stems.

It has been found that individual chairs are better in a reception area than benches, loveseats, or rows of attached chairs. Generally, patients do not want to sit directly next to another person. Chairs should be comfortable (not metal or wooden), yet firm enough so that elderly patients can get up out of them. It is helpful if the chair has arms so that patients who have difficulties in getting up can use the arms for support. Some practices prefer leather or a less expensive leather substitute, so that the chairs can be cleaned easily. Wiping off leather or leather substitute is easier than cleaning fabric seats.

Place boxes of tissues on the tables in the reception area, especially during cold and flu season. Don't forget to also place waste cans there, otherwise dirty tissues may be left on the tables. All ophthalmology offices should have tissues because of the eye drops that they use with patients.

If the practice has hard floor surfaces (tile or hard wood), it is not a good idea to place throw rugs on the floor. Elderly patients who tend to shuffle as they walk will trip over loose carpets and fall. Some offices have a coffee machine on a counter and provide powdered cream and sugar packets. This can be messy, and the staff may end up cleaning up messes and shampooing carpets on a regular basis.

Allergy problems are on the rise. Keeping the reception area clean and dust free will be appreciated by the patients. The reception area should be dusted daily to ensure that there is as little dust as possible. Some offices place air purifiers in the reception area to help ward off dust particles and unclean air. Do not place air fresheners in the reception area because the perfumes in the fresheners can contribute to allergy problems as well.

Having an aquarium installed in the reception room has a calming effect on patients. Patients will sit and watch the brightly colored fish without consideration of the time that has passed. If you do not have the time to keep the tank clean, either hire someone to provide aquarium maintenance, or don't have a fish tank!

Arrange the seating so that patients will chat with each other. Place good reading lights next to some chairs for those who wish to sit and read.

Patients love to read about health problems, whether their own or their Aunt Myrtle's. Having educational materials available in the waiting room has been found to be helpful and also keeps the patients busy while waiting. Installing a bookcase and filling it with hardbound books and pamphlets is a great way to start. By stocking books (acquired through discount bookstores or from pharmaceutical reps), the office introduces patients to a variety of issues that they might find they are interested in learning about further. Topics can range from Alzheimer's disease, to parenting tricks, to how to deal with rheumatoid arthritis. All books should be stamped with the office's name and address and should be allowed to be taken home by patients. Index cards can be used to track the location of borrowed books. The office can set a deadline as to when they want the books returned. A library generally allows 2 weeks for lending of books, but the office staff can set up any deadline they think is appropriate. The office can also accept books donated by area businesses and individuals. This idea can also be expanded to educational videos. For instance, patients with Crohn's disease might appreciate a video on how they can adapt their lifestyle to their disease. The lending library is a great public relations tool!

Young Visitors

For practices with children or young parents, it is a good idea to have some children's books and toys that are easily accessible in the reception area. Children need to be occupied; whether they are the patient or with an ailing adult, they get bored quickly. Many pediatric offices have little tables and chairs, blackboards, and whiteboards for children to use. Offices that have "little visitors" should have quiet toys, puzzles, and books to keep everyone entertained. Offices should consult the working mothers employed by the practice, because they are generally experts on what is considered a dangerous toy. Don't buy coloring books and crayons unless you want colored walls and ground crayons in the carpet! There have been instances of an office manager buying what was thought to be innocent toys for the waiting room and later finding that Mr. Potato Head had many small pieces that children could easily swallow, put in their ear, or push up their nose. Health care professionals who do not have experience with children's toys should consult the mothers they have working for them; they will be experts on dangerous toys.

Most pediatric offices split the reception area into SICK and WELL sides (Figure 3-3). Parents find this split reception area appealing. If their child is scheduled for a "well visit," that is, for a routine checkup and immunization, the child is not exposed to ill children. Puzzles, books, and quiet toys are a good choice and will be appreciate by the parents, other patients, and office staff. Toys should be picked up several times a day in an effort to keep the reception room neat.

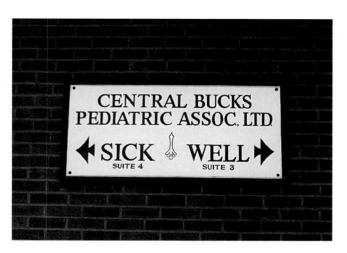

FIGURE 3-3. One pediatrician divides his waiting room into sick children and well children areas.

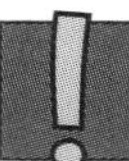

MANAGER'S ALERT

Never have toys smaller than the tube of a toilet paper roll because they are choking hazards. If the toy fits inside a toilet paper tube, it does *not* belong in the office.

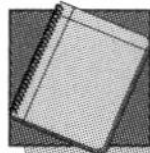

FROM THE EXPERT'S NOTEBOOK

Don't let the doctor tell you that she or he has a lot of magazines at home and will bring them in to the office for the waiting room. This is fine as an addition to the subscriptions, but the office managers with happy waiting rooms are those with current office magazine subscriptions available. Remove the "blow-in" cards from the magazines before placing them in the reception area, or they may scatter all over the floor, tables, and chairs.

The office manager should take the time to address the magazine issue with sincerity. It is an old joke that if you're looking for an older issue of a particular magazine, go to a doctor's office—that's all they have. Because patients can spend some serious time in a waiting room, it is a good idea to keep current with various magazines to accommodate various tastes. Along with general magazines such as *Time, Newsweek, People, Family Circle,* and *Sports Illustrated,* more specialized magazines that parallel the specialty of the office might be provided. *Arthritis Today* and *Parents' Magazine* are good examples of specialty magazines that might be found in a medical office. Magazines older than 2 months should be discarded. They should be arranged in a neat, orderly fashion that is easy for all patients to access. The goal is to try to keep the patients happy. This makes everyone's day a little easier.

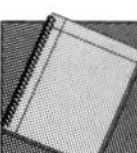

FROM THE EXPERT'S NOTEBOOK

Some community pharmacies will sponsor magazines for a physician's waiting room if the physician is willing to put them in plastic covers advertising the pharmacy. This saves the office that added expense.

It may be necessary for the office staff to continually visit the reception room to "tidy up." Straighten the magazines, straighten the lamp shades, and straighten the toys!

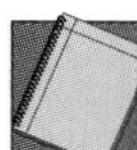

FROM THE EXPERT'S NOTEBOOK

As a courtesy to the patients, place a box of tissues in the reception area. Don't forget the waste can!

PATIENT FLOW

In a group practice, it is sometimes difficult to find a system to direct each doctor to her or his next patient. When there is more than one physician in an office at a time, "traffic jams" are common. One way in which to handle this problem is to use a color-coded flag system. In this system, a set of different-colored flags is mounted on the wall outside the examination room. Each doctor is assigned a different flag. When a patient is taken to an examination room, the appropriate flag is manually raised to indicate which physician has a patient in that room. These flags can be purchased from any office supply store.

A simple method is to position the chart in such a manner that it becomes a code for the physician. This type of system works well only for a small group office, but it does the job effectively and inexpensively.

A more sophisticated system from a company such as Veratronics can also be used. Veratronics designed a system of lights that enables the physician to ascertain which room her or his patient is in. The system is programmed to represent each physician as a different color. When a staff member takes a patient into the examination room, she or he pushes the color button representing the physician whose patient is in the room. Outside the room, that physician's light will flash, showing which patient is ready for the physician. (A light that is not blinking indicates that there is a patient in the room but the patient is not ready for the physician at this time.) When the physician finishes with the patient, she or he turns off the light. This is also helpful in aiding the staff when they are looking for a physician and might not be sure which room she or he is in.

Many physicians get behind in their daily schedule of patients and by the end of the day, the delay may be an hour or more depending on the physician and the specialty. Some physicians just don't realize that they are running behind. To avoid having patients "stack up" in the waiting room, use the signal on the telephone and buzz once each time a patient is ready and waiting. Three buzzes over a period of 5 to 10 minutes notifies the physician to pick up speed. If there are no buzzes, the physician knows she or he can chat with the patient and will not get behind.

COMMUNICATION

Communication That Reflects Patient Awareness

It is important for the office manager and other staff members to develop strong communication skills. Patients are concerned with the following areas when coming to the medical office: what is wrong with them, will they be all right, and did they cause this problem to occur? Because of this, it is important to remember that patients are generally upset when they are at the physician's office, which causes confusion and lack of understanding.

The office manager and other members of the staff must be carefully trained in patient awareness and patient instruction so that they can provide clear and concise explanations (Figure 3-4).

The outcome of a patient's medical treatment depends on effective communication. Effective communication takes place best when the office staff "connects" with the patient, that is, enables the patient to understand something by speaking to the patient on a level that he or she can understand. Office managers and other staff members must conduct themselves with an air of self-confidence. It is important to look the part and to be confident in your interactions with patients. They will respond better to an office manager and other staff members who have high self-esteem, and handle themselves in a professional manner, than to those who act unsure of themselves. To be effective, communication must acknowledge the cultural and religious beliefs that patients bring with them to the office. For example, Jehovah's Witnesses cannot receive blood or blood products from another person. Many Jehovah's Witnesses believe that it is a sin to accept a blood transfusion, because the Bible states that they must abstain from blood. The Christian Scientists are another religious group who do not believe in preventive vaccines for measles, mumps, tetanus, and so on and therefore refuse to be immunized.

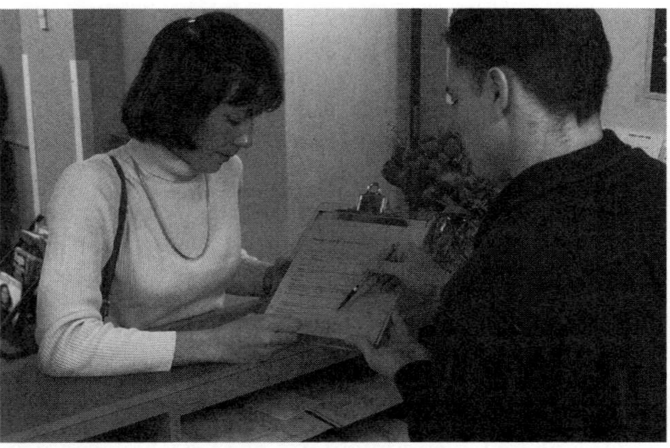

FIGURE 3-4. The receptionist helps a patient with a form.

Levels of Communication

There are two types of communication: distance and closeness. In most interactions distance and closeness are subjective, meaning that at one end of the spectrum you will find a total lack of interaction (distance) and at the other extreme complete intimacy (closeness). At any point within this spectrum, there are certain combinations of professional and personal characteristics that will be put into play. The interaction of the health care professional and the patient will thus vary accordingly.

There are four levels of communication in which health care professionals can engage:

1. *Superficial involvement:* This is a superficial level. "How are you?" "Have a good day." "It's good to see you again." There is no genuine personal sharing. This level protects people from each other and decreases the likelihood of any further personal involvement.
2. *Facts:* Almost nothing personal is discussed at this level. An example is when the patient arrives at the office and relays the name to the administrative medical assistant and provides her insurance card to the health care professional. Some sharing may take place, but on a very limited level, such as sports, good books, local news, and so on.
3. *Personal ideas and opinions:* At this level an individual provides some limited personal information. This may be an expression of an idea or a judgment, which is usually determined by the other's response. If the listener looks bored or disinterested, the person will cease conversation. An example of this is when the patient comments on the interesting fish tank in the waiting room.
4. *Emotions:* This is the last and most intimate level of communication. Simply put, it is known as gut-level communication. Individuals who share a deep trust will communicate at this level. In the medical office this communication often occurs with long-time patients of the office.

These communication styles describe various levels of involvement. There are times, however, when situations arise in which interpersonal distance should be created.

In situations where this occurs, the office staff is creating distance to help the patient. Patients may have problems that cannot be solved by the office staff and therefore it is best to keep a bit of distance. There are three main circumstances in which interpersonal distance should be created:

1. *Loneliness:* Often the office manager, in a desire to help the patient overcome loneliness, will end up in a companionship role and begin to interact with the patient outside the office environment, for example, shopping or dinner together after hours.
2. *Pity:* In an attempt to respond well to a patient, the office manager gets so entangled in the futility of the patient's plight that it is impossible to act rationally toward the patient. It is important to maintain a professional distance from the patient so that there is a clear understanding of the patient's plight without getting too involved. Too much involvement may cloud the issue at hand.
3. *Projection:* The patient is seen as someone else and therefore is unable to see the patient for who he is. Perhaps the office manager's beloved grandfather has a similar condition as the patient. This projection regarding the condition of the grandfather causes the focus on the patient to be lost.

Communication plays an important role in malpractice issues. Creating good relationships with patients decreases the possibility of being involved in malpractice litigation. Typically, patients who are happy with their care, and like and respect their physicians, will not institute a suit against them. In circumstances where the outcome of the treatment may not have been what was expected, having a good relationship between the patient and the physician is key. Feedback, both good and bad, coupled with effective communication helps to make a solid physician-patient relationship.

Communication Tips

Certain behaviors are exhibited during communication. The following are some common behaviors that are necessary for open communication:

- Let patients speak. If you are speaking more than 40% of the time, you are talking far too much.
- Give the patient your full attention. Don't look out the window or become preoccupied by something in the hallway.
- Don't rush patients. Give them the time necessary to explain their thoughts and concerns. Don't act like you need to be somewhere else.
- Explain everything. Use easy-to-understand words and phrases.
- Be aware of your nonverbal language, such as shrugging or avoidance of eye contact. Body language often speaks louder than words. Never point or shake your finger at a patient or co-worker. This message will cause communications to break down.
- Seek patient understanding. Ask if the patient understands and if he or she has any questions.
- Ask questions. If you are not sure you understand what the patient said, ask for clarification.
- Let the patient finish talking before you begin to talk. Interruptions can be perceived as not listening. Interruptions can also cause patients to forget to tell you an important fact.
- Ask the patient how he or she prefers to be addressed. For example, the patient may prefer to be addressed by her last name rather than her first name. Use of the patient's first name may be considered inappropriate or insulting by some patients.
- Incorporate a warm smile when communicating with patients, which relays care and concern.
- Be professional, yet competent.
- Keep a balance between professional services and personal attention.
- Give respect to the patient.
- Realize that listening consists of these components: hearing, understanding, and judging. When listening, one must not only be involved in the physical act of hearing, but must also comprehend what is being said, and be knowledgeable enough to judge accordingly.

The Bad and the Good: Communication Guidelines

Only 25% of listeners grasp what the patient is really saying. In the following exercise, we consider changing from a "bad" listener to a "good" one:

The Bad Doesn't look at the patient, shows no interest, tunes out the patient.

The Good Maintains eye contact, nods, and helps the patient with her or his explanation.

The Bad Listens for facts.

The Good Listens for central ideas.

The Bad Gets "caught up" on phrasing and focuses more on the words used than on the meaning behind them.

The Good Understands phrasing and doesn't get hung up on it. Listens, and interprets the meaning and content well.

The Bad Takes tedious and exhaustive notes, tries to capture every word.

The Good Jots down only short phrases and key words in order not to miss anything.

Communication Barricade

"I like to listen, I have learned a great deal from listening carefully. Most people never listen." —ERNEST HEMINGWAY

Nothing is simple . . . not even communication. There are many barricades that prevent effective communication. Simple things such as noise, for example, impede good communication. Machinery noise can prevent both parties from hearing each other and therefore miscommunication can arise. When we tend to focus on ourselves, "What have you done for me lately . . ." becomes a barricade to good communication. Stimuli may provide a distraction; therefore our communication is less than best. Stress plays an important factor in how people give and receive information. Our frame of mind is key to effective communication. How we perceive others will influence what we hear and say. If the individual is perceived as important, the message is perceived as important—whether it is or it isn't. The opposite holds true: if the individual is thought of as being unimportant, the message is also deemed unimportant and therefore some may not listen. Incorrect use of words, grammar, and perhaps accent may distract from the message. Dismiss these factors and concentrate on the message being conveyed.

Inevitably, people struggle with effective communication. In health care, as in other professions and businesses, there is sometimes a failure in communication. For example, one barrier to effective communication is the use of slang or "professional language" (jargon), which can result in a breakdown in communication. The speaker must think of the audience to whom he or she is speaking. Using specific and technical terminology that a patient may not understand becomes problematic and can even result in a malpractice suit. Another barrier to communication is the timing of the message. If the message is received at a time when the receiver is preoccupied, the information being sent may not be processed correctly. If the speaker and the receiver are involved in a conflict at the time the message is being given, the information may not be received as it should. The following list illustrates communication barriers that health care professionals must be familiar with:

- A patient with a hearing, speech, or vision problem
- A discussion that takes place in an area that is noisy
- A patient who is known to have comprehension difficulties
- A patient who is fearful, aggressive, or prejudiced, or who feels threatened
- A patient who does not speak English

Good communication skills are imperative in health care. They are especially critical when advising patients, discussing their medications, discussing their condition and prognosis, and discussing preventive medicine issues. Good communication becomes important between health care professionals when they are discussing patients and their care. It is also important when speaking with insurance companies to discuss the reason for a referral or for a specific treatment plan.

Tact

Tact is the ability to speak and to act skillfully and considerately in difficult situations or with difficult people. It is sometimes necessary to be diplomatic and use good judgment when working with patients. With tact, it is not what you say, but how you say it. As an example, perhaps there is a mother and her 8-year-old son in the waiting room. The child, Tommy, is jumping around screaming loudly when he is speaking to his mother. You look around the waiting room and see patients shaking their heads and sighing. You need to be nice to Tommy's mother, but you have other patients to consider. You tactfully and quietly ask Tommy if he could please speak quietly so that he does not disturb the other patients.

Another situation requiring tact is patients who complain about their insurance company and the amount of payment the insurance company has made or not made on their bill. It is important to recognize that insurance companies are sometimes difficult to deal with and do make mistakes. Offer to take a look at what the insurance company has paid to see if you can explain it to the patient. Do not lose your temper with patients. Instead, kill them with kindness!

The Voice

When patients hear the health care professional's voice on the telephone, they imagine what that person looks like. When the health care professional is speaking with someone face-to-face, the person immediately attaches that face to the sound of that voice. Everyone is born with a voice that is personal. If patients like the sound of that voice, they will perceive that person as a knowledgeable and confident person. If they can't seem to "connect" with the voice, they will immediately be "turned off." It is not what health care professionals say, but how they say it. The way we use our tone of voice influences how we will be perceived by patients.

The office manager should instruct the staff to have a caring, clear (not mumbling), friendly, and in-control voice. A voice sells patients and colleagues on the knowledge level and professionalism of the individual who is speaking. It is possible to improve the sound of a voice by using a few tried and true techniques:

- Be sure to add pauses and breathing; this improve the voice.
- Keep good posture; sit up straight.
- Keep properly hydrated; it keeps the vocal cords lubricated.
- Avoid caffeinated products, because they are a diuretic and can affect your voice.
- Use gestures to emphasize energy.
- Smile; it goes great with a nice, confident voice.
- If your voice is high, it can be lowered by practicing (lower voices have more credibility).

Pitch also affects the voice. Pitch is an average mix of the many frequencies of the voice. A higher pitch in the voice may make you sound like a cartoon character, and a lower pitch in the voice makes you sound like a radio announcer. Find a midrange that is good and practice it. The human voice is a wonderful instrument and can carry meaning not only through words, but through its volume, rhythm, and pitch. When someone is angry or scared, the pitch of the voice automatically rises, just as the heart beats faster.

Timbre is the distinctive property of a complex sound (a voice or noise or musical sound). It is known as the sound "color," the characteristic quality of sound. Emphasis is another factor relating to voice. Placing emphasis and inflection on different words within a sentence can vary the meaning of what the person is saying. It is important to be aware of one's voice and to make any changes in pitch, tone, timbre, or inflection that may be necessary to portray a competent, caring health care professional.

Empathy

Empathy is the understanding of someone's feelings and being able to respond in a sensitive manner. Empathy is not only important for the patient, but also for the patient's family members, who are worried and concerned for their loved one. Empathy and sympathy are often confused. *Empathy* is the recognition of someone's feelings, whereas *sympathy* is the recognition of someone's grief or loss. You would provide empathy to someone who was experiencing a lot of pain. You would provide sympathy to someone who lost a spouse.

The office manager should be aware of the importance of empathy and should instruct the staff in its recognition and understanding. *Empathy* is defined as "the quality or process of entering fully, through imagination, into another's feelings or motives." Empathy is putting yourself in another person's shoes and understanding her or his concerns, fears, and pain. The opposite of empathy is invalidation. In *invalidation,* someone presents an idea or a feeling and it is rejected or contradicted. Invalidation fosters feelings of anxiety and fear in the patient.

Maintaining Emotional Distance

Health care professionals can express genuine care for patients by maintaining distance, as well as becoming close. When a close relationship has developed with a patient, it becomes necessary to avoid further development of that relationship. This can be handled by limiting conversation with the patient to small talk and to matters involving the patient's health care. Maintaining distance does not mean that one should become cold and impersonal with the patient. This may only increase the patient's loneliness or self-pity. If the relationship prevents the office manager from seeing the patient objectively, another professional should provide some insight into the situation. A careful structured and fostered relationship maintains the dignity of both the staff and the patient.

Listening

Hearing is the act of perceiving sound. It is physiologic in nature, meaning that it is arises from a physical body part. Listening involves that physiology plus the interpreting of that sound into meaning. There are two types of listening:

- Active
- Passive

Passive listening is a step above hearing and occurs when there is very little context to the message. The second type of listening is *active listening.* This involves listening with a purpose. The listener may need to obtain directions, solve a problem, get or give advice, show support, and so on. Active listeners spend more time listening than talking. They do not finish the sentences of others and do not answer questions. People speak 100 to 175 words per minute, which is why dictation in a medical practice is invaluable! It has been noted that providers who dictate their medical records provide more information regarding the patient visit than those who handwrite their notes. Also, people can listen to 600 to 800 words per minute and still be able to understand what is being said. The health care professional who may be transcribing those dictations can perform this task very efficiently. As you can see, communication is a wonderful tool!

BECOME A BETTER LISTENER

Speak comfortable words! —William Shakespeare

Most people think that listening is the same as hearing. It is not. Listening, or lack thereof, has been the cause of many family feuds, disgruntled employees, and probably even some higher diplomatic conflicts. Most people can hear, or get help by use of a hearing aid to hear. But most people do not listen, and do not know how to get help for that.

Becoming a good listener takes skill; it is not something you are born with, as hearing is for most. Being a good listener takes practice, lots of practice. The health care professional should learn to listen and to develop this skill. When speaking to patients, the health care professional should be friendly, and should use verbal cues to show that he or she is listening to and interested in everything the patient is saying. It is important to make the patient feel comfortable.

Don't let your mind wander when listening to a patient. While the patient is tediously explaining an ailment, are you thinking about what you are having for dinner? If your spouse will remember to pick up your son from soccer? If that special guy or girl will call tonight? Instead, listen to the patient and listen hard. The patient needs to have your full attention, because this is a very important subject to her or him. The comments made to the patient when she or he is done speaking should reiterate some of what the patient said, if for no other reason than to be sure that you understood the patient correctly. Give the patient your undivided attention! Even on a phone call, if your mind is wandering, when the patient stops talking there is dead silence as you realize the patient is no longer speaking and you are trying to find something to say. The patient thinks that you have been disconnected. You may have been disconnected mentally, but not by the phone line!

Taking notes can be helpful. You don't have to write word for word, just jot down some notes as the patient is speaking. Be sure to maintain eye contact as much as possible. If you are too busy writing, you may not be listening and may miss an important fact that the patient is relaying. Be sure not to bring your "baggage" into the conversation; stay open-minded, which is what the patient needs. Always review your notes with the patient to ensure that you have not improperly written a note or misunderstood what the patient said. Be sharp, be there, be listening.

TALKING VS. LISTENING: KNOWING THE DIFFERENCE

Listening to others helps others to listen. —AUTHOR UNKNOWN

When the health care professional is doing the talking...

- Think about what you are going to say before you say it.
- Think about the needs of the person who is listening.
- Use empathy at all times.
- Ask for feedback.
- Speak at a level that the patient can understand.

When the health care professional is doing the listening...

- Give the patient undivided attention.
- Listen to what is said.
- While listening, think of the person who is speaking.
- Be patient when necessary.
- Repeat what has been said to be sure that you understand.

ROADBLOCKS TO LISTENING

Certain behaviors constitute ineffective listening. Beware of falling into these traps!

- **Roadblock #1:** Your attention is on preparing your next comment. You look interested with an occasional nod, but your mind is actually thinking about what you are going to say next.
- **Roadblock #2:** You have labeled this patient as uninformed and therefore you are not paying much attention to what the patient is saying.
- **Roadblock #3:** Something a patient says reminds you of an incident that you personally experienced. Before the patient can continue, you interrupt, and begin your story.
- **Roadblock #4:** You suddenly change the subject because you were bored listening to the patient go on and on.
- **Roadblock #5:** You feel like such an informed individual that you really don't need to hear any more about what the patient is saying. You know what to do next without hearing the patient's entire conversation.
- **Roadblock #6:** You want to be nice and supportive to patients. You want them to like you, so you agree with everything. You placate them with phrases such as, "Oh, I know . . . ," "Absolutely . . . ," "Of course you are . . . ," and so on.

To learn to be an effective listener, it is important to understand some of the roadblocks that may be present. Identifying and correcting these listening roadblocks will allow for better communication.

Nonverbal Cues

Body language and nonverbal cues are a key component of effective communication. To be a good listener, you must act like one. Although many people have "information overload," it is necessary to recognize when we must listen. Our faces do a lot of listening, not only our ears, through hearing, but our face tilts and our eyes make contact. The health care professional must be an active participant in the communication for it to be successful. One of the first key indicators of nonverbal communication is posture. How you carry and present yourself tells a story. Stand up straight with stomach in, chest out, shoulders back and head up. . . . sound like your mother? Slouching, shoulders drooping, head forward, and stomach out tells people that you are not sure of yourself. Command the respect that you deserve by planting your feet about 8 inches apart with one slightly in front of the other. You will feel "grounded and secure" in this posture. One rule of thumb: do not turn your upper body away from the patient. . . it looks like you are disinterested and unfriendly.

THE FACE

Nonverbal cues are also fraught with meaning. Let's take continually touching oneself, for example. We unconsciously touch our face to release stress that we may be feeling. Rubbing your hand, arm, or wrist may be a sign of deception or uncertainty.

The face is an ever-changing canvas of nonverbal expressions. Our facial expressions reveal our true emotions and are the window into who we are, our attitudes and our moods. Remember the old phrase, "You could never be a poker player?" Some individuals wear their emotions on their face, whereas others do not.

The following facial characteristics identify the emotion of an individual:

- Smile: happiness, contentment
- Grimace: fear
- Lip knitting: frustration, thinking, anger
- Pout: sad, uncertainty
- Raised brow: intensity, interest
- Brow frown: anger, sad, thinking
- Wide eyes: anger, surprise

Eye contact is a powerful aid to nonverbal communication. Eye contact is important because it cuts the physical distance between you and others and creates a personal connection. Eye contact can be intimidating, so do not stare! Eye contact should be broken into segments consisting of approximately 5 seconds per segment.

It has been stated by Professor Albert Mehrabian, Ph.D., University of California, Los Angeles (UCLA), that 55% of the meaning of communication is body language, 38% is the tone of your voice, and 7% is the content of what you are saying. To be perceived in a positive, light manner by patients, you should smile, nod occasionally, lean slightly forward, and tilt your head to the side as you are listening. Since we react to what we think the other person said, it is good to think about whether your body language matches the words you are saying.

TRUTH

Sometimes people will stretch the truth a bit for various reasons. To be able to recognize untruths, there are signs that may provide insight.

When individuals stall for more time, it generally means that they need to formulate a response. If they answer quickly without much thought, they are probably telling the truth. Someone who is caught off guard will need time to compose an answer and therefore will use such phrases as, "Can you repeat the question?" "What do you think?" "Could you be more specific?" Questions such as these provide enough of a delay to buy some time to formulate the answer.

Look for words that are absolutes. Absolutes are words such as "always," "never," "every time," and so on. Absolutes are used when individuals are trying to persuade the person to do something or when the individual is defensive about something. Since we all end up using absolutes at one time or another, we must try to avoid using these words. Absolutes are always associated with deception because they are untrue to begin with.

Beware of using the expression "Just kidding!" Almost all of us have used this phrase in conversation; however, the phrase is considered a "minimizer" phrase and has the ability to smooth things over. It is used to downplay what came before it. Generally, when someone uses this phrase, she or he believes in what was said before the "minimizer."

OTHER NONVERBAL CUES

A shoulder shrug may be construed as a sign of uncertainty or submissiveness. When eyes move sideward after a question is posed, this nonverbal action is significant for reflection of thought and information processing.

Believe it or not, even hairstyles speak volumes about a person. A Procter & Gamble study was performed at Yale University in 2000 by Marianne LaFrance. She found that a person's hairstyle plays a major role in how people view him or her. For women, a short, tousled hairstyle speaks of confidence and a person who is extroverted. A medium-length hairstyle speaks of intelligence and a person with a good nature. A long, straight hairstyle speaks of affluence and sexuality. For men, a short, flip front hairstyle speaks of confidence and a sort of self-centeredness. Medium-length hairstyles that are parted on the side speak of intelligence, affluence, and narrow-mindedness. Long hair speaks of carelessness and a good nature. This information may be useful in not only your personal hairstyle, but in reading other people with these hairstyles.

Throat clearing can also be a nonverbal cue, because there are no actual words being spoken. Throat clearing by a speaker can mean uncertainty, whereas throat clearing by the listener may mean disagreement or anxiety.

Verbal Communication

Just as important as listening is being able to ask the right questions. Having a grasp of this skill will enable the staff to gain more information and insight into what the patient is trying to say. Avoid asking the patient questions that can be answered with a "yes" or a "no" because it leaves the staff in a passive state and limits conversation with the patient. Use open-ended questions whenever possible to create communication between two parties. An open-ended question is one that cannot be answered with a yes-or-no answer. For example, instead of asking, "Does your knee hurt?" you would ask, "Where does your knee hurt?" For staff at the front desk, instead of asking, "Do you still live at 1 Versailles Circle?" you would ask, "What is your current address?" Create motion by asking the patient, "How can we . . . ?" or "How can you . . . ?" Create options by saying, "Where would you . . . ?" or "Why haven't you . . . ?" Delve deeper by asking, "What needs to be changed? What do you think this means?" Put the patient in the driver's seat by asking, "What would you like to do about this? What would you like us to do about this?" Sitting quietly and listening to the patient will prompt additional conversation from the patient. If there is a lull in communication, one of the parties involved will begin to speak. If the office professional sits quietly, it will give the patient more time to discuss his or her needs and wants.

The Handshake

Another component of interpersonal communication is the handshake. Understanding handshakes can help understand the other person. Handshakes can tell a story; there are power shakes, sandwiches, dead fish handshakes, and wilted lettuce handshakes.

A power shake is when a person extends his hand to you and then maneuvers it on top to show that he is in control.

The sandwich is only used between two people who know each other very well. For this handshake, your hands envelope the other person's hand, which is a personal stance expressing tenderness and should not be used in a business environment.

The dead fish handshake comes from someone who is either nervous or has been holding a cold beverage just before the handshake. This handshake is wet!

The wilted lettuce handshake comes from someone who gives a light and tentative handshake, usually by extending only the fingers, not the whole hand. To correct this type of handshake, one should extend the hand fully (not cupped) and hold the other person's hand firmly. The elements of a good handshake are as follows:

- Hold the person's hand firmly and fully.
- Shake, whole hand, three times maximum.
- Maintain eye contact.
- Show a positive posture.

Personal Space

A misconception regarding medical professionals is that being "professional" also means being aloof and coldly competent. Professional abilities and personal traits can and should be integrated into one set of complementary qualities in order to achieve professional success. Those who are successful in establishing social relationships and adapting to changes in their everyday lives are also more effective in their therapeutic relationships. Each individual must define what personal space means to her or him.

Proxemics is the study of personal space and territory. What we refer to as our *comfort zone* varies heavily depending on whom we are speaking to and where we are. Proxemics provides us with another form of nonverbal communication and allows us to better understand the individual with whom we are interacting.

In 1959, anthropologist Edward Hall discovered that humans are very aware of their personal space. He conducted numerous experiments and concluded that Americans have four comfort distances: 0 to 18 inches, 18 inches to 5 feet, 4 to 12 feet, and 12 feet to line of sight:

0 to 18 inches	Intimate distance	Reserved for personal relationships
18 inches to 4 feet	Personal distance	Reserved for personal conversation
4 to 12 feet	Social distance	Reserved for business meetings or interviews
12 feet to line of sight	Public distance	Reserved for public speaking

When communicating with patients, the most appropriate personal space should be 18 inches to 4 feet. The goal for successful communication is to attain the closest distance without making the other person feel uncomfortable.

Body Language in Other Cultures

Body language (nonverbal cues) can mean very different things depending on what country and culture you are from. Our military personnel receive training in reading body language before they are deployed overseas. Politicians take courses in it, and now, since the terrorist attacks of September 11, 2001, airport and transit police are trained in how to "read" people. More than 500,000 forms of body language are used in communication around the world.

The most perceptive culture to body language is the Asian people. They come to rely more heavily on body language than they do the spoken word. The people of Asia are taught to practice self-control and therefore appear to exhibit a lack of emotion. Smiling in Asia does not mean happy, it means "yes." Eye contact is a sign of disrespect and challenge. These individuals believe that their head is where their spirit resides and therefore they never touch one another on the head. Although a handshake is accepted in Asia, the Southern and Southeastern Asian countries still prefer a bow with their hands together as if in prayer. Asians and Middle Easterners prefer a handshake. Be careful with handshakes, however, because a strong handshake is a sign of aggression. Sitting with your legs crossed in Asia is a sign of disrespect, and resting your ankle over the other knees risks pointing the sole of your shoe at another person. This is considered to be an extremely rude gesture.

In Greece, Yugoslavia, Bulgaria, and Turkey, a nodding head means "no." Eye contact in Africa, as in Asia, is considered to be a sign of disrespect. In Europe, people tap their nose, which in England means "confidential," but in Italy it means "watch out!" Italians like to wave their arms freely when they speak, but the Japanese are very reserved and it is considered impolite to use arm movements when speaking. A goodbye wave in North America can mean "no" in Latin America and Europe. The Italian wave for goodbye can be interpreted by North Americans as the gesture of "come here." The North American gesture for "come here" is an insult in Asia, where they would use the gesture to call an animal. The "okay sign" in North America means "fine" in some cultures, but it means "zero" or "worthless" in France and many European countries and is an insult in Greece, Brazil, Turkey, Russia, Italy, Australia, New Zealand, and most African countries.

It is good to be aware of the meaning of body language in other countries because it helps with more effective communication. Health professionals are able to understand what patients are saying without the utterance of words.

Communication with Special Groups

COMMUNICATING WITH THE MULTICULTURAL COMMUNITY

The United States is becoming increasingly multicultural, and health care has to adjust to patients who do not speak English, or at the very minimum, do not speak it well. In New York City, 1.7 million people (one in four) are not proficient in English. The inability to speak the English language can cause problems with obtaining a consent form, advising patients of their condition, discussing medications, and so on. Because of this influx of non–English-speaking patients, federal and state laws have been adopted to protect patients and provide access to health care for them. Many patients bring family members with them who can speak English. Sometimes, however, these family members are children or others who themselves do not speak English well. There was case where a misinterpretation of a single word led to delayed care for the patient with a result of quadriplegia. This, of course, became a malpractice suit with a $71 million settlement tied to it. The English language that we speak in the United States is very difficult to understand. We use many slang words and jargon that make comprehension impossible. Many hospitals are now printing their signs in two languages, English and a second language that is spoken in the neighborhood in which the hospital is located. Physician practices are faced with communication challenges as they deal with language barriers in their practice. They also use a language assistance telephone line, but most often all interpretations are performed by the patient's family or friends. Hospitals now have standards that they must follow for the use of interpreters, foreign-speaking volunteers, and language assistance telephone lines where qualified individuals can be reached via telephone when necessary. These individuals generally are required by law to be available within a certain amount of time, generally 20 minutes for an inpatient and 10 minutes for an outpatient. Many employment applications now contain a section for any additional languages that prospective employees may speak.

COMMUNICATING WITH THE ELDERLY

When communicating with an elderly patient, several things must be kept in mind:

1. Most elderly patients are poor historians of their problems and may omit important facts. They may not think it important to tell you about their fall yesterday, or their dizzy spell last week.
2. The greatest fear of most elderly patients is the fear of loss of independence. They need to feel in control and that they can take care of themselves.
3. The differences in sensory or motor acuity (this may affect a response). It is important to keep in mind that many elderly patients require the assistance of glasses, hearing aids, dentures, and so on. This may affect the way the patient interacts with the health care professional.

The most important factor to remember when working with an elderly patient is to not stereotype him or her. Intellectual changes and patient needs vary widely from one elderly patient to the next. In addition, each elderly patient comes to the office with a different set of problems and must be dealt with in an appropriate manner.

COMMUNICATING WITH CHILDREN

Showing interest in what children are saying is key to open communication. At times, the best communication is when parents are not around. When speaking with children, it is important not to tower over them. The health care professional should get down to their level! It is also important to listen carefully to what they are saying and don't interrupt them while they are speaking. This may cause them to lose their thought process, and valuable information may be lost.

Nonverbal communication can be helpful in putting children at ease. A simple smile or nod will show them how you feel and that you are open. At the end of the visit, ask the child for his or her input into the suggested diagnosis and treatment plan. Be certain to ask children, in age-appropriate language, if they have any questions or if they understand what was discussed.

EFFECTIVE COMMUNICATION WITH COLLEAGUES

Medical practices are goal oriented. All members of the staff want the same end . . . quality patient care. It is not only important that communications between the patients and the staff and physician are good, but also communication among the office personnel is key to mobilizing effective communication and quality care. There are seven ways in which one can avoid communication errors with colleagues:

1. *Keep it simple*—Keep sentences and phrases simple. Unfocused, run-on sentences are confusing. Avoid the use of slang and unnecessary words.
2. *Use metaphors*—Metaphors (his mother said he is a couch potato) and analogies (coronary artery disease is like a clogged pipe) can be helpful when communicating complex ideas. Use of colorful words (I can give Dr. Smith a glowing recommendation) can often help to portray ideas more effectively.
3. *Use different forums*—There are many ways to get the message across. For example, an idea may be shared at a staff meeting of the entire staff, or maybe just at the departmental level. Perhaps it is best shared with only the supervisor on a one-to-one basis. Bringing up an idea in various different ways and different places will ensure that it is heard.
4. *Repeat important messages*—Phrases such as *quality service* and *quality care* should be part of everyday language in the office and become the essence of what the office staff should be focusing on.
5. *Address concerns about change*—Any changes within the practice should be addressed, and all employees should understand the reason for those changes.
6. *Listen and be listened to*—Communication is a two-way street. Explain and then ask for feedback. This is key for good communication not only among colleagues, but with everyone throughout the practice.
7. *Be a team player*—There is no "i" in the word "team." Staff members working together as a team will accomplish more than each member of the staff working individually. One snowflake will do nothing, but put a lot together and see what happens. If everyone cooperates with one another, the office will run more efficiently. If the health care professionals working in the clinical area of the hospital or office have completed their work for the day, but the front office health care professionals are still working on end-of-day procedures, the clinical staff should volunteer to help in the completion of those procedures. Everyone will then be finished and will be able to leave the office at the same time. The physician will be happy, the patients will be happy, and the staff will be happy.

FOUR GENERATIONS

There are four groups that span the generations: Traditionalists, Baby Boomers, Gen-Xers, and Millennials. The first generation is the *Traditionalists* (or *Veterans*), who were born between 1922 and 1945. These individuals are now retired or getting ready to retire. Traditionalists as patients are often found to be stubborn, yet their respect for health care professionals is refreshing. They come from the "old school" where the physician was like a "god." They are very compliant, except when they forget things. They want to take their medications, but sometimes they forget.

The *Baby Boomers* come next. They were born between 1946 and 1964. They are the largest group. Many of these "boomers" can be found in management positions. Communicating with the Baby Boomers is a pleasant experience. Overall, Baby Boomers are caring and personable and are often "people" people. They are good at forming relationships and try to avoid conflicts. Generally their technology skills are self-taught. Baby Boomers are concerned about their personal growth within the workplace and exist well in a democratic one. They work well with recognition, and their favorite reward is money. Baby Boomers as patients are a delight! They are compliant with their patient instructions and medications and are easy to interact with when dealing with such issues as appointments and waiting times.

The next group of people are the *Gen-Xers*, who were born between 1965 and 1980. This is a smaller group and can be found just moving into management positions. Gen-Xers don't like to be micromanaged and to be "bossed" around. They want to do everything their own way and in their own time. Gen-Xers are movers and shakers and work well in a well-balanced workplace. They are concerned with quality of life and therefore want balance between job and family. They want flexibility and freedom. Gen-Xers as patients can be a bit difficult, because they are the ultimate consumers, expecting quality and efficiency at every turn. They do not like to wait and think that their time is just as important as the providers'. They try to bend the rules in the office and hospital setting and often want the freedom to do it their way.

The *Millennials* are the last group. These people were born between 1981 and 2000. This is a large group. All groups bring varied experience to the workplace. The Millennials are positive and engaging people. They are great workers because they are ambitious and loyal. However, they are impatient and want everything now, like the Gen-Xers, and need to learn patience. This can be a communication challenge.

Millennials as patients are stressed with everyday issues of jobs, children, and caring for their elderly parents. They are loyal, but expect a lot in return. They are more impatient than the Gen-Xers and often need to be intimately involved in their parents' medical care. They feel that they don't have time for their own care, let alone taking time off from work to take a loved one to the physician.

Since the Gen-Xers and Millennials are more interested in getting the job done rather than following the rules, communication must be clear and precise when communicating with these two groups. They must be reminded to slow down and take their time. Quality of work should be stressed. Millennials are brainstormers. They love to collaborate and work well in a creative and positive workplace with supervision and structure.

It is important to understand the nuances of each group so that you are able to effectively communicate with them.

Involving the Family

"I think one lesson I have learned is that there is no substitute for paying attention." —DIANE SAWYER

When considering whether to involve family members in the care of the patient, staff must assess the wishes of the patient. This can be done by observing the patient's age, sex, and culture. The patient's family plays a major role in her or his welfare. Some patients do not want their family members involved in their care or, for that matter, in any of their business! One must be careful of patient confidentiality in certain cases, and the health care worker should be careful to "read" the patient in order to determine whether to involve the family (see Chapter 7). Some patients are hesitant to inform the staff that they want patient confidentiality. The physician can be most helpful in many of these cases, and the health care workers can take their cues from her or him.

Some patients want and need the support of their family. The office staff must be cognizant of this process of involving the family in their care. In this case, it is sometimes necessary to invite family members to the examination room during the patient visit. Diagnoses, medications, and treatment plans can be discussed with them at this time.

TELEPHONE SYSTEM

There are many manufacturers of telephone systems today. After reviewing the information obtained on the top five companies, the health care professional should invite four or five of the top companies to come in and present their products and service. Once it has been narrowed down to two companies, the health care professional should ask if there are local practices that are currently using the product so that he or she can observe the system in use. The telephone company should also provide the health care professional with a list of references that he or she may contact before making a decision. Before contacting these companies, the office manager should try to determine how many phone lines and phone sets are going to be needed.

It is important to keep in mind the anticipated growth of the practice in the next 5 years. Expansion capabilities are an important part of this purchase. It is not easy to predict the growth of a practice, but a basic rule in purchasing a telephone system should be that the system purchased today should be large enough to allow for double the amount of lines and units over the next 5 years. Many systems have growth modules that can be purchased to expand the system as the time draws near.

The office manager can determine how many telephone lines the office needs by asking the telephone company to conduct a traffic study, or what they call a "busy study" on the lines. This study shows how many times a patient got a busy signal instead of the office staff. If the last line regularly rings busy, the general rule is to add two additional lines. The sales representative will need the following information from the office:

- About how many calls the office receives
- About how many local calls the office makes
- About how many long-distance calls the office makes
- Whether the office wants customized calling, whereby certain lines are designated to certain individuals (for instance, the office manager might want a certain number to ring directly at the billing department or at the appointment secretary's desk)
- Whether there is a need for any special features

Special Features

A variety of special features offered by telephone companies may be useful to the medical office. The office manager needs to think about the needs of the office ahead of time so that they can be discussed with the sales representative. An office's needs may require certain telephone equipment or may require certain services that the company provides. The following are some of the special features available:

Caller ID: A screen message that identifies the caller, either by name, number, or both, before you answer the phone. When the message reads the state you are in along with a number, it signifies that the call is coming from a cell phone. Most medical offices use this service.

Caller ID with name: Lets you see the telephone number and main listed name of the person who is calling before you answer the phone.

Call trace *57: In an emergency, the phone company can trace the number of the last call received. This function could be used to locate the origin of life-threatening or harassing calls.

Call direct: Provides an automatic transfer without announcement of the new referral number. This is an excellent service for physicians who might be using a back line or private number to call patients. It works well for physicians to use on their home phone also.

Call direct plus: Provides an announcement with the number's status and the referral number, then offers to transfer and connect the call.

Call waiting: Lets you know when someone is trying to reach you while you are on the phone. A tone will notify you that someone is trying to call. This can be helpful to the practice if it uses a private line that the physicians use to call the office. Call waiting for the public lines in the practice does not work well.

Call blocking: You can block your name and phone number from the person you are calling if the person has the caller ID function. This service is good for physicians using a private, back line at the office to call patients and can be very helpful on their home phones also.

Call gate: Allows the practice to monitor calls by allowing or not allowing outgoing calls from a specific line. This can be helpful with personal phone call problems.

Conference calling: Three-way phone calls can take place. This can be a big help if the physician wants to speak with a patient and the patient's family member who resides out of town. All three parties can be placed on the call. This will save the physician time and provide continuity in what has been said. This prevents any miscommunication that may occur as a result of separate phone calls between the patient and the patient's family.

Distinctive ring: This service provides a distinctive ring to certain lines so that when they ring, you know that it is a particular line that is ringing. This service can be used on the line the physician calls in on.

Toll restrictions: Any attempts to call toll numbers are rejected.

Direct inward station dialing: Direct access to a particular extension is provided.

Call cost display: A running total of the cost of a call is displayed as the call goes on.

Privacy buttons: With the press of a button, the physician can ensure that the conversation she or he is having on one of the phones on a line cannot be overheard by someone picking up the receiver of another phone on that line.

Intercom: One employee can summon another through a buzzer; they can then talk on the intercom.

Display messaging: Some phones have a screen on which a message can be left, for example, "I'm at lunch until 2:00 PM."

Secure off-hook voice announcement: Co-workers can interrupt phone conversations with important messages and without the other party hearing the conversation.

Battery backup: This ensures the availability of telephones that are plugged into outlets.

Repeat call: The last number dialed is redialed for up to 30 minutes.

Busy redial: Redials the last number you dialed; if the number is busy, it will continue to dial for 30 minutes and will ring back with a special ring if the call becomes available.

Return call: The person who called can be called back, regardless of whether the phone was answered or not.

Speed dialing: Regularly used numbers can be preprogrammed for faster dialing.

Call trace: This mechanism traces the number of the last call and sends it to the telephone company's annoyance department.

Select forward: Up to six calls can be transferred to another location.

The office manager must be careful not to buy features that the office doesn't need. An array of features and fluff should not sell the product. The knowledgeable office manager buys the system that allows for growth, provides the necessary features, is easy to use, and demonstrates the most service for the money.

Why Not Used Equipment?

With technology changing as rapidly as it does, there is a great deal of used equipment available for purchase. This equipment can be purchased at anywhere from 30% to 70% of the original price. There are several things to keep in mind about buying used equipment. First, the company selling the used equipment must be a reputable one. It's a good idea to ask for a list of references and call them. Second, what is the warranty on the used equipment, and who will provide repairs if needed? Remember, you get what you pay for!

TELEPHONE SAVVY

Importance of the Telephone

The government's creation of diagnosis-related groups in the 1980s has resulted in competition among physicians and decreased the censuses of many hospitals. This increased competition has required that both hospitals and physicians market their services more effectively. The medical field has been able to step back and view patients as consumers. This new breed of patients will shop around for their physician, just as they would shop around for a new car.

The upshot of this is that patients today expect to be treated in a courteous, friendly, and professional manner by both their physician and their physician's staff, and if they are not treated in this way, they'll go elsewhere. Often, it is the staff member on the phone who gives the patient her or his first impression of a physician's office. When a business depends on the person answering the phone, it is important to have employees who are trained in the courteous and productive use of the phone. No one gets a second chance to make a good first impression.

The professional treatment should not stop when a patient is no longer new to the practice. The physician works hard to establish a relationship of mutual trust and confidence, and this must not be destroyed by staff blunders or unprofessional treatment of patients. The overall tone of the office is set by the office staff, and the personal interactions patients have with the staff will color their view of the physician.

Telephone Impressions

Telephone personality is an important asset of a health care professional because it reflects the personality of the medical practice. It is important to recognize the importance of having a good telephone personality. When using the phone, slow down and enunciate. Do not speak fast, especially to the elderly. Telephone conversations must stand on verbal etiquette, since the all important nonverbal cues are nonexistent on the phone. This makes it imperative to employ the LISTEN tips to achieve telephone effectiveness:

Let others speak
Intend to hear what they are saying
Speak when the caller has finished
Talk *with* them, not *at* them
Empathetically respond to patients with a problem
Never speak when the other person is talking

A bad experience with someone on the phone may cause the patient to find another physician. The telephone is the lifeline from the patient to the physician; therefore it is necessary to understand the seven basic principles of proper telephone technique:

1. *Attitude*—Be friendly, yet empathetic. Portray a happy office that is interested in helping the patient. Put a smile in your voice.
2. *Response*—Provide answers to the patient's questions. When you don't have the answers, advise the patient that you will find out and get back to him or her. Give the patient a reasonable time period in which he or she can expect your call. Don't get angry, even if the patient is! Let the patient vent, and then take a deep breath and show the patient that you care. Don't add to the patient's aggravation; just be a good listener.
3. *Projection*—Project a positive attitude and use good manners when speaking with the patient. Maintain a low pitch to your voice because a voice in a high register can sometimes be disturbing to patients. Don't project emotional overtones, don't sound impatient, and don't sound like you are being interrupted by the call. Don't sound like an announcer on TV or radio; use less exaggerated tones.
4. *Follow-throughs*—If you tell a patient you or someone else in the practice will call the patient back, someone needs to call the patient back! Some practices follow up on earlier calls to be sure that the patient has been taken care of appropriately.
5. *Transfers*—Keep transfers to a minimum. If it is necessary to transfer the call to another extension, for example, the scheduling desk or the nurse, transfer only once. Make sure the person you are transferring to is available; don't place the caller on hold, transfer, then hold again, transfer, and so on.
6. *Hold*—Control that HOLD button! If you are going to place someone on hold, let the person know how long she or he may have to wait (that is, once you have determined that this is not an emergency). If it looks like the caller will be on hold a long time, ask the person if you can call them right back. A minute on hold is like a lifetime!
7. *Jargon*—Avoid use of jargon. Talk at the patient's level. The patient is probably upset about not feeling well, and you need to keep things simple and understandable.

A Major Source of Discontentment

The telephone has the potential to be a major source of discontentment for patients. The telephone is an important part of the medical office, and skilled personnel should be answering it. Receptionists and secretaries spend more than 50% of their day dealing with patients on the telephone. They are the key individuals in creating the initial bond between the prospective patient and the physician's office. Once the patient is in the office, the receptionist or secretary can communicate the office's environment by nonverbal means, such as projecting a welcoming personality and a friendly, caring, professional appearance. Over the phone, however, the responsibility lies in the way the office staff talks to the patient. The telephone should always be answered after no more than three rings. The office that is too busy to be able to adhere to this rule on a regular basis might have a need for additional personnel. If a delay occurs, it is appropriate to answer the telephone and say, "Hello, Dr. Miller's office, Jan speaking. Sorry for the delay. May I help you?" If a delay of 2 minutes or less is anticipated, it's okay to ask the caller for permission to put her or him on hold. The conversation should always resume with a "thank you" to the caller for waiting. "Thank you" should also end every conversation, regardless of the nature of or reason for the call.

The Secretary Has a Secretary . . . Automated Phone Systems

Most offices today use technology to help with their busy telephone. The patient calls the office and receives a greeting followed by a menu of options that the caller may choose from. A sample answer is as follows:

Hello, you have reached the office of Dr. Babinetz. The office is closed and will reopen tomorrow at 9:00 AM. *If this is an emergency, please go to the nearest emergency room. If this is not an emergency, but you need to speak to the doctor before tomorrow, please call our answering service at 111–222–3333. If this call is routine, please call back during normal business hours of 9:00* AM *to 5:00* PM.

Or you may call during office hours and hear this type of recording:

Hello, you have reached the office of Dr. Babinetz.

- *If this is an emergency, press 1 now.*
- *If you know the extension of the person you are calling, please dial it now.*
- *If you are calling for an appointment, please press 2 now.*
- *If you are calling for a prescription renewal, please press 3 now.*
- *If you are calling to schedule your surgery or have a question about a surgery, please press 4 now.*
- *If you are calling for test results or to speak with a nurse, please press 5 now.*
- *If you are calling with any other question or would like to speak with the receptionist, please press 6 now.*
- *If you are calling with a billing question, please press 7 now.*
- *If you are calling from a rotary phone, please stay on the line and a receptionist will be with you as soon as possible.*

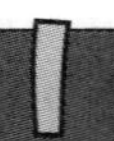

MANAGER'S ALERT

When using an automated answering system, be sure to make the first option an emergency option.

The emergency line may dial directly to an answering service, a beeper, or an individual in the office. Some physicians do not like automation, stating that it is too impersonal. One problem with automated systems is that if the patient population of the office is elderly, the patients may have a difficult time using this type of system and often will simply press the last number that they heard in the menu. Each practice needs to evaluate what system works best for it.

Staff should be instructed to follow the **PHEE** principle:

Positive
Helpful
Empathetic
Efficient

If patients complain that they can never get through to the office because of busy signals, it is time to call the local telephone company and have it do a study to evaluate what the practice needs. This study generally takes 2 weeks. Anxious patients only become more anxious as the telephone rings repeatedly. Even if the patient simply wants to set up an appointment, the constant ringing of the telephone can convey an impression of a disorganized, chaotic practice. This could cause the patient to hang up and call another physician. Prompt answering of the telephone builds a reputation of efficiency.

Many telephone companies hold "Improving Telephone Skills" workshops. They usually offer group discounts and on-site training for larger office staffs, and often there is no cost for these workshops. The education services department of your local phone company will provide information regarding these workshops. It will also send newsletters on a regular basis, which helps the office manager keep abreast of new services and seminars and offers helpful hints.

What one patient feels is an emergency may not be an emergency to another patient. However, no matter what the problem is, if the patient feels it's an emergency, it is the office staff's responsibility to take the time to listen and advise the patient according to the guidelines established by the office manager or the physician. The patient on the other end of the telephone neither knows nor cares that you had an emergency patient walk into the office first thing this morning; that the physician was an hour late for office hours; that the first five patients of the day were staring holes through you from the waiting room; and that it looks like you will not get any lunch today! All the patient cares about is her or his problem and when the physician's office will solve it.

The Voice of a Friendly, Competent Medical Office

Tone of voice is the key factor in handling the patient on the telephone. The staff should practice the technique of smiling with their voices. If they are thinking with a friendly smile on their face, they will present a caring, pleasant image. Niceness is almost always contagious. Killing with kindness works in many cases and diffuses the most difficult of situations. When attempting to solve a patient's problem, be it medical or clerical, office staff will find that their chances greatly increase if the patient perceives them as competent and caring (Figure 3-5). It is important to portray an impression of interest in the patient's problem and efficiency in attempting to solve it. Staff must guard against representing themselves through their voices as having had a busy day and being tired. Since moods are contagious, an employee's negative tone of voice can easily be adopted by the patient, resulting in the patient's becoming unpleasant and uncooperative. Situations like this have no happy ending.

The voices of the office staff reflect their thinking. Canned enthusiasm doesn't fool anyone. Staff's voices should be natural and well modulated and should contain the appropriate inflections. One way to answer the telephone that is a very effective icebreaker is to say, "Hello, Dr. Smith's office, Ann speaking. How may I help you?" Having personnel automatically give their name projects a familiarity that allows the patient to become better acquainted with her or his physician's office. It forms a bond between the patient and the staff and adds a personal

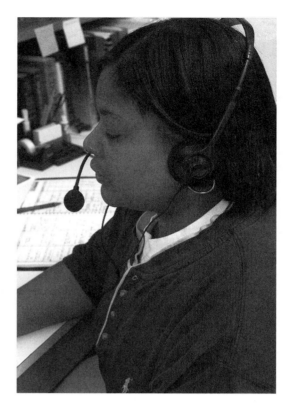

FIGURE 3-5. The medical office receptionist should be a friendly voice on the phone.

flavor to the staff's professionalism. Saying the patient's name several times during the conversation implies that the office recognizes the patient and is familiar with her or his problems. This personal touch puts the patient at ease and sends the message that she or he is special. Each patient wants to be thought of as the only patient the office has, and saying the patient's name is an effective and simple way of conveying this.

Staff should *never* be allowed to answer the telephone and, before asking who is calling, say, "Can you hold please?" This technique is guaranteed to provoke a negative response from the caller when the employee returns to the line—either angry words or, worse yet, a dial tone. Many patients feel that they have an emergency, or are at the very least the most important case of the day, no matter what their ailment. The liability involved with putting a caller on hold before asking her or his name is great. Suppose the patient *does* have an emergency! In a busy office setting, it is possible to have more than one telephone line ringing at the same time. Staff should be instructed that in this situation, they should answer the telephone by saying, "Hello, Dr. Smith's office, Rob speaking. May I ask who is calling? Mrs. Johnson, I'm on a call on the other line. May I ask you to hold the line for a minute?" This courtesy allows the patient to understand the situation and to voice any emergency that might be taking place. This ensures cooperation from the patient and is another way of saying that the office cares about the patient.

Office managers need to decide whether they will take all calls that come in for them or would like to have their calls screened. It is up to the office manager to instruct the receptionist or secretary of her or his preference.

Telephone Etiquette

Follow these simple rules:

1. Don't put the patient on hold until you know why the patient is calling.
2. Assess the patient's need (e.g., to talk to the physician or make an appointment).
3. Avoid "why" questions if possible; ask open-ended questions.
4. Do not express your opinion.
5. Clearly understand the patient's use of words and phrases.
6. Always express concern and empathy for the patient—be reassuring.
7. If instructions are given, have the patient repeat them to you to ensure clarity.
8. Document the call in the patient's medical record, the message book, or the triage form.
9. When answering the telephone, say, "Cardiovascular Center, Melinda speaking."
10. Identify who is calling. Is it a patient? Another physician? The hospital?
11. Don't put the patient on hold until you know why he or she is calling; then, if it is not an emergency, ask the patient if you can place him or her on hold.

The Chosen Few

Constant interruptions to take phone calls can disrupt the work of any physician or staff member and should be kept to a minimum; however, there are exceptions. Every office has some patients who have special privileges and require special treatment. The office manager needs to give the receptionist or secretary the names of the people who fall into this category so that the receptionist knows how to handle the call. Possible options include the following:

- Whether to interrupt the office manager or physician.
- What questions to ask the patient.
- Where to route the call in the event the party with whom the patient wishes to speak is absent.

Employees should not be expected to know which patients get special privileges. The manager should provide them with a list of such patients and should update the list periodically.

Correct Handling of Telephone Messages and Responses

If a telephone call requires an answer from the physician, it can be handled in two ways. If it is not an emergency situation, it is best for staff to advise the patient that they will check with the physician and get back to her or him. This way, staff does not hinder the patient care that is currently being handled in the office. The physician can be asked the question at a more convenient time, and then the return call to the patient can be placed by the staff.

Staff should be instructed that if the patient feels that it is necessary to talk directly with the physician, they should say, "May I take the message and have the doctor return your call later today?" They should always ask the patient how long she or he will be at that particular number, and that information should be noted with the message. It is always a good idea to assign a staff member to be responsible for checking the physician's messages intermittently, so that if there is a message that needs urgent attention, the staff member can direct it to the physician sooner. The telephone triage form can be used for patient messages if the patient is not requesting an appointment. It will provide the physician with specific information to be able to better assist the patient.

According to a study released by the Medical Group Management Association (2001), physicians may spend more time on the phone than is realized:

Number of minutes physicians spend on the telephone	*Percentage of physicians*
0–30 minutes	34%
30–60 minutes	31%
60–90 minutes	15%
90+ minutes	20%

Message Book

Messages taken for the physician should be kept in a telephone logbook. This is a must for every office because it maintains a record of each call. This is helpful for many reasons—for example, when the physician wants to talk to a family member from out of town who called last week and when a medical-legal issue arises—as well as preventing the loss of scraps of paper with messages written on them. All messages for the physician should contain the following information:

- The patient's name
- The date and time of call
- The caller's name and relationship to the patient, if the caller was not the patient
- The patient's/caller's phone number and how long she or he will be at that number
- The reason for the call
- The result of a laboratory test, if the patient is looking for a result (if the result has not yet come in, call for it)
- The pharmacy's phone number, if the call is for prescription renewal
- Signature of the person taking the message

Telephone message books can also be used by the office staff as a reference. These books allow the staff member taking the call to fill in the blanks of the message form, pull off the physician's copy, and leave a hard copy in the book for reference at a later date. Many physicians prefer this system and like the messages put on a spindle on their desk for them. The patient's chart should be pulled and handed to the physician along with the patient's phone message. In some offices clinical personnel (nurse, physician's assistant, nurse practitioner, etc.) will handle a call back to the patient. The patient, as a consumer, is important to the business. Patients who are happy with their physician's practice are an excellent source of referrals for new patients.

To make sure that telephone messages are complete, make a list of questions that should be asked when each patient calls. This list will provide the information needed to determine the urgency of the call and is helpful to all staff members, clinical and nonclinical. (Note the information regarding specific telephone area codes in Box 3-1.)

Triage

All patient telephone calls should be triaged in order of importance. The health care professional should be trained in how to triage patient problems in order to properly address them. A policy on how to triage patients in the practice should be part of the policy and procedure manual for the practice. In 1987 the American Medical Association classified medical problems into three categories (Mancini & Gale, 1987):

- Emergent
- Urgent
- Nonurgent

An *emergent problem* is defined as one that requires immediate attention. This problem is of an acute nature and may be life threatening. An *urgent problem* is defined as one that requires medical attention in the near future. This problem is also acute in nature, but is not as severe as an emergent one. A *nonurgent problem* is defined as a problem that is not an emergency and does not require immediate care. This problem is not acute and usually is minor in nature.

When patients call the office to request an appointment, the staff can better assist the physician by asking the patient the right questions. The patient should first be asked, "Have you seen Dr. Babinetz before, either in the hospital or in one of our offices?" This is asked first so that as the

Telephone Triage Form

Patient Name:______________________________

Date:________________Time called:____________________

Number at which patient can be reached:____________________

Physician: ______________________________

Symptom	Patient Questions	Patient Answers
Location	Where is it? Can you put your finger on it? Does it go anywhere?	
Quality	What does it feel like? Is it sharp? Dull? Crushing? Achy?	
Severity	On a scale of 1 to 10, how bad is it? How much does it immobilize you? Can you sleep?	
Timing	When did you first notice it? Is it constant? How long does it last?	
Modifying factors	What were you doing when it occurred?	
Context	Does anything make it better or worse? What seems to cause it?	
Aggravating conditions	What makes it worse?	
Alleviating conditions	What makes it better?	
Associated signs and symptoms	Have you noticed any other changes?	

FIGURE 3-6. Telephone triage form. (From Matherly, S., & Hodges, S. *Telephone Nursing: The Process.* Englewood, CO, The Medical Group Management Association, 1992.)

BOX 3-1 Area Codes

All calls made that are out of your local calling area must contain an area code. This number must be dialed in front of the seven-digit number that you are dialing. Certain cities in the United States that have more than one area code for that region require that the area code be dialed even for local calls. The listing below provides area codes for regions across the country.

Alabama
- Birmingham 205
- Huntsville 256
- Mobile 251
- Montgomery 334

Alaska
- 907

Arizona
- Flagstaff 928
- Phoenix 602
- Sun City 623
- Tempe 480
- Tucson 520

Arkansas
- Fort Smith 479
- Little Rock 501
- Pine Bluff 870

California
- Anaheim 714
- Bakersfield 661
- Beverly Hills 310/424
- Big Bear Lake 909
- Burbank 818
- Chico 530
- Concord 925
- Florence 323
- Fresno 559
- Irvine 949
- Long Beach 562
- Los Angeles 213
- Modesto 209
- Monterey 831
- Norwalk 562
- Oakland 510
- Palm Springs 760
- Palo Alto 650
- Pasadena 626
- Redding 530
- Sacramento 916
- San Diego 619
- San Francisco 415
- San Jose 408
- Santa Ana 714
- Santa Barbara 805
- Santa Rosa 707
- Temecula 951

Colorado
- Aspen 970
- Colorado Springs 719
- Denver 303/720

Connecticut
- Bridgeport 203
- Hartford 860

Delaware
- 302

Florida
- Bradenton 941
- Daytona Beach 386
- Ft. Lauderdale 954/754
- Ft. Myers 239
- Gainesville 352
- Jacksonville 904
- Key West 305
- Lakeland 863
- Miami 305/786
- Orlando 407/321
- St. Petersburg 727
- Tallahassee 850
- Tampa 813
- Vero Beach 772
- West Palm Beach 561

Georgia
- Albany 229
- Atlanta 404/770/678
- Columbus 706
- Macon 478
- Savannah 912

Hawaii
- 808

Idaho
- 208

Illinois
- Aurora 630
- Chicago 312/773
- East St. Louis 618
- Elgin 847/224
- Joliet 815/779
- Lansing 708
- Peoria 309
- St. Charles 630
- Springfield 217
- Waukegan 847/224

Indiana
- Evansville 812
- Fort Wayne 260
- Gary 219
- Indianapolis 317
- Kokomo 765
- South Bend 574

Iowa
- Cedar Rapids 319
- Des Moines 515
- Dubuque 563
- Mason City 641
- Sioux City 712

Kansas
- Dodge City 620
- Kansas City 913
- Topeka 785
- Wichita 316

Kentucky
- Ashland 606
- Bowling Green 270
- Frankfort 502
- Lexington 859

Louisiana
- Baton Rouge 225
- Houma 985
- Lake Charles 337
- New Orleans 504
- Shreveport 318

Maine
- 207

Maryland
- Annapolis 410/443
- Baltimore 410/443
- Rockville 301/240

Massachusetts
- Boston 617/857
- Brockton 508/774
- Salem 978/351
- Springfield 413
- Waltham 781/339

Michigan
- Ann Arbor 734
- Battle Creek 269
- Detroit 313
- Escanaba 906
- Flint 810
- Grand Rapids 616
- Jackson 517
- Kalamazoo 269
- Lansing 517
- Muskegon 231
- Pontiac 248/947
- Saginaw 989
- Sault Ste. Marie 906
- Warren 586

BOX 3-1 Continued

Minnesota
- Bloomington 952
- Duluth 218
- Maple Grove 763
- Minneapolis 612
- Rochester 507
- St. Cloud 320
- St. Paul 651

Mississippi
- Biloxi 228
- Greenville 662
- Jackson 601/769

Missouri
- Jefferson City 573
- Kansas City 816
- Marshall 660
- St. Charles 636
- St. Louis 314
- Springfield 417

Montana
- 406

Nebraska
- Lincoln 402
- North Platte 308

Nevada
- Carson City 775
- Las Vegas 702

New Hampshire
- 603

New Jersey
- Elizabeth 908
- Hackensack 201/551
- New Brunswick 732/848
- Newark 973/862
- Trenton 609
- Vineland 856

New Mexico
- 505

New York
- Albany 518
- Binghamton 607
- Buffalo 716
- Hempstead 516
- Huntington Station 631
- New York City
- Bronx 718/917/347
- Brooklyn 718/917/347
- Manhattan 212/917/646
- Queens 718/917/347
- Staten Island 718/917/347
- Niagara Falls 716
- Poughkeepsie 845
- Rochester 585
- Syracuse 315
- White Plains 914

North Carolina
- Asheville 828
- Charlotte 704/980
- Fayetteville 910
- Raleigh 919
- Rocky Mount 252
- Winston-Salem 336

North Dakota
- 701

Ohio
- Akron 330/234
- Ashtabula 440
- Cincinnati 513
- Cleveland 216
- Columbus 614
- Dayton 937
- Portsmouth 740
- Toledo 419/567

Oklahoma
- Lawton 580
- Oklahoma City 405
- Tulsa 918

Oregon
- Astoria 503
- Medford 541
- Salem 503/971

Pennsylvania
- Allentown 610/484
- Erie 814
- Harrisburg 717
- New Castle 724/878
- Philadelphia 215/267
- Pittsburgh 412/878
- Scranton 570

Rhode Island
- 401

South Carolina
- Columbia 803
- Charleston 843
- Greenville 864

South Dakota
- 605

Tennessee
- Chattanooga 423
- Columbia 931
- Jackson 731
- Knoxville 865
- Memphis 901
- Nashville 615

Texas
- Amarillo 806
- Austin 512
- Brownsville 956
- Bryan 979
- Corpus Christi 361
- Dallas 214/972/469
- Del Rio 830
- El Paso 915
- Forth Worth 817/682
- Galveston 409
- Houston 281/713/832
- Huntsville 936
- Midland 432
- San Angelo 325
- San Antonio 210
- Tyler 903/430
- Waco 254
- Wichita Falls 940

Utah
- Cedar City 435
- Salt Lake City 801

Vermont
- 802

Virginia
- Abingdon 276
- Arlington 703/571
- Harrisonburg 540
- Lynchburg 434
- Richmond 804
- Virginia Beach 757

Washington
- Everett 425
- Olympia 360
- Seattle 206
- Spokane 509
- Tacoma 253

Washington, DC
- 202

West Virginia
- 304

Wisconsin
- Eau Claire 715
- Green Bay 920
- Madison 608
- Milwaukee 414
- Racine 262

Wyoming
- 307

patient is talking, her or his medical record can be looked up on the computer. If staff does not ask about the hospital, they could spend hours looking for an office chart that doesn't exist. This also helps in determining how much time to allot for this patient's appointment. A list of questions that should be asked of each patient who calls the office with a problem should be kept by the telephone. Better yet, design a telephone triage form to be filled out for each caller with a problem. A sample triage form is shown in Figure 3-6.

It is also important to check the type of insurance patients have to be sure that their coverage will allow for treatment by your practice. Some carriers require the use of certain physicians within a network for the care of their patients. Ask them to bring their cards with them if they are told to come to the office to be seen. If their insurance requires a referral from a primary doctor, make sure they have a referral with them. The office will not be able to treat the patient without a referral.

Voice Mail

Along with all this new technology, came voice mail. Many businesses have used voice mail systems for years, but it took some time for it to find its way into a medical office. Voice mail is another time saver and will allow the office to become more efficient. Callers who know the extension of the person they wish to speak to can dial directly, or, after speaking with the secretary or receptionist, they can be transferred to that person's voice mail box. Why is this a good thing? It saves time and lost messages, that's why!

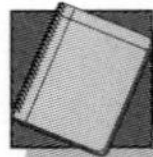

FROM THE EXPERT'S NOTEBOOK

Some medical offices put together a "New Patient Packet" and send it to all new patients who schedule an appointment on the telephone. This packet specifies the routine laboratory tests that the physician orders on all new patients and asks the patients to have them done before the initial visit. At the time of the visit, the physician already has the laboratory results in the new patient's chart. It saves a lot of time, and the patients and physicians are grateful!

Cell Phones

Cell phones are the new pagers. Although pagers are still used, most people have switched to cell phone use. These mobile phones were introduced in the 1980s and were so large that it was like holding a brick to your head. Martin Cooper is credited with the invention of the cell phone in 1973, while he was a manager in Motorola's communications division. Cell phones are like sophisticated radios, only better. Before the popularity of cell phones, radio phones were installed in cars, but were very limited because they required a powerful transmitter to transmit 40 to 50 miles. The cell phones that we use today use "cells" in which to operate. Each area of the country is divided into cells, which provides an incredible range for each cell phone.

Many people have a cell phone; even 50% of the children in the United States own a cell phone. In fact, it has been estimated that in 2005 there were 2.14 billion subscribers of mobile phones, and 80% of the world's population had mobile phone coverage in 2006. By 2020, this figure is expected to rise to 90%. That is why it is important for the practice to include a policy on cell phones in their policy and procedure manual. This policy should be reviewed with each new hire and may need to be reviewed with established employees as well. Most offices will not permit the use of personal cell phones within the practice. It becomes difficult to control and is disruptive to the practice and its patients.

Cell phones can provide a great deal of flexibility, as the following list of functions indicates:

- Storage of important names (other physicians' numbers, patients, hospitals, etc.) and phone numbers
- To-do lists that can remind physicians of tasks that need to be completed (e.g., stop by the nursing home on the way from the hospital)
- Appointment tracking (can be set to remind physicians of such things as personal dentist appointments, staff meetings, etc.)
- Calculator to calculate dosages of medications (or the tip at lunch)
- E-mailing can be performed on some cell phones, providing greater flexibility for physicians and staff
- Internet access to obtain stock quotes, news, and so on

Cell phones for physicians are a different story. They are very helpful when trying to contact the physician. Some hospitals do not allow the use of cell phones anywhere inside the building, whereas some allow them everywhere but the intensive care and cardiac care departments. Even with limited usage within some hospitals, it is easier to use cell phones than pagers. The office manager should inquire as to how each physician would like her or his cell phones used and place this information in a policy for all employees. It is important not to overuse them just because it is convenient. Some people experience problems with unwanted calls coming through their cell phones. Using the physician's cell phone, the office manager can call the National Do Not Call List to register that physician's cell number with this agency. This will prevent some unwanted calls, especially from telemarketers. The phone number for this service is 1-888-382-1222, or this can be done online at https://www.donotcall.gov/.

Individuals using cell phones should maintain a degree of "cell phone etiquette." This means turn off cell phones at concerts, lectures, plays, weddings, funerals, doctor's offices, hospitals, churches, libraries, movies, restaurants, schools, and any other place where people talking on a cell phone may disturb others nearby. When it comes to cell phones, be considerate.

Pagers have been replaced by cell phones in many instances. Some physicians still use pagers because of hospital regulations. Certain hospitals and certain areas within hospitals do not allow the use of cell phones because of interference with medical equipment. To be able to get in touch with physicians while they are in the hospital setting, pagers become necessary.

Slamming and Cramming

Slamming occurs when your long distance or local telephone service provider is changed without your knowledge and approval. It is a federal and state crime for a company to "slam." If the practice is a victim of slamming, call the company associated with the charge. You are entitled to be switched back to the company of your choice. You cannot be billed for this service, so be sure to check the bill when it comes in. If the company refuses to switch you back, write a letter to the Federal Communications Commission (FCC) for assistance in resolving the issue. Their address is

Federal Communications Commission
Common Carrier Bureau Consumer Complaints
445 12th Street, SW
Washington, DC 20554

Send a copy of your bill and a record of all communications you have had with the rogue company.

Cramming is when an unexpected and unauthorized charge suddenly appears on your phone bill. These charges may include such items as pagers, calling cards, voice mail, and so on. Most state laws prohibit the cramming of services onto your phone bill. If you believe you're a victim of cramming, call your carrier to report the erroneous charge.

Always review the phone bill carefully to be sure that all charges are correct and have been incurred by the practice or an authorized person in the practice. Keep a file in the office of all phone services that have been ordered. Don't accept collect calls in the office from people that you do not know, and don't return a call to an unfamiliar area code unless you are told it is a family member of a patient or the patient himself or herself who may be away. To prevent future slamming, ask your carrier to put a "freeze" on your phone line so that slamming cannot occur without your acknowledgment.

INCOMING CALLS

There are various types of incoming calls. Health care professionals who are assigned to answering the telephones in a medical office should be trained in how to answer these calls. Other calls, such as patients looking for test results, patients requiring a prescription renewal, patients needing their records forwarded, and patients with billing and payment questions, require individual attention.

Depending on the policy of the office, a patient calling for a test result can be handled in several ways. Some offices instruct their patients that if the office does not call them within 5 days, the results were normal or satisfactory. Some offices have a call-in service where a patient enters her or his pass code and is able to get her or his detailed results. Some offices take messages and have the clinical staff address the call. Patients with normal studies are called by the health care professional, and patients with abnormal studies are called by the physician at the end of office hours. Calls from the hospital or another physician wishing to speak with the physician are immediately transferred to the physician. A call from the hospital with a routine result is handled by the staff. Most hospital results are now obtained via computer, because most offices have software that enables them to dial into the hospital system to obtain laboratory results, x-rays, and other information.

Patients calling with requests for referrals should be transferred to the person in the practice that handles this task. Some primary care practices have a large volume of patients requesting referrals. In these practices, patients are transferred to a message line where they leave pertinent information such as name, date of birth (used for further identification of the patient), and the type of referral that they are requesting. Most practices have a policy that referral requests require a 48-hour turnaround time. A request for medical records can be handled in the same way and by the same person or by someone working in medical records.

It is common for medical practices to have a prescription renewals extension. If the practice has an extension that handles prescription renewals, all calls for renewals should be transferred to that extension. If not, the call should be transferred to whomever within the practice handles that type of call. Sometimes this task is rotated through the office along with other similar tasks. When a patient calls for a prescription renewal, use the following procedure:

1. Advise the patient that renewals are handled throughout the day. Generally it is the policy of the office to place a 24-hour waiting time on all renewals.
2. Ask the patient if he or she wants to pick up the prescription or have it called in.

3. Pull the patient's chart.
4. Verify the pharmacy number that is listed in the patient chart, if there is one. If not, ask the patient for his or her pharmacy number.
5. Ask if the patient has prescription insurance. If so, there may be limitations as to how many pills can be called in at one time.
6. Write the request on paper and attach it to the patient's chart.
7. Give the request to the physician for approval.
8. If the prescription is to be written, the physician will write the prescription and give it to the health care professional to either place in the pickup bin or to mail to the patient.
9. If the prescription is to be called to the pharmacy, the physician will either call it in or instruct the health care professional to do so. The health care professional will write out the prescription in the patient's chart exactly as it is to be called in. *For example:*
   4/10/08 4:15 PM
   XYZ drug 10 mgs.
   # 30
   Take one tablet daily.
   Renewals x3.
   LAJ, M.A.

Once the physician reviews the written request, the health care professional will then call it in to the patient's pharmacy. It is important to include the date and time the prescription was called in.

How to Handle Callers

As discussed earlier under "The Chosen Few," the physician should set up guidelines on how to handle certain callers. Callers who do not identify themselves or refuse to provide their name and reason for calling should be told that their call cannot be handled properly without that information. Angry patients should be spoken to in a quiet, calm manner. The health care professional should speak slowly and ask what the problem is. Depending on the problem, the call will be "routed" to the appropriate person. For example, a patient who calls about a bill should first speak to a person in the office billing department or the office manager. If it appears that the physician may have to get involved, the health care professional should write a brief summary of the reason for the call and give it to the physician at the end of office hours. Family members and personal friends fall into the category discussed under "The Chosen Few." Some physicians leave instructions that if their children call, to put them through. Others leave instructions that they will not speak to family and friends unless it is an emergency. The physician instructs the health care professional to tell the caller that the physician will return the call as soon as he or she gets a break and to take the telephone number of where the caller can be reached.

Physicians who call should be immediately transferred to the physician. It is considered a professional courtesy to not make them wait. Ask them if they are calling about a specific patient so that you can pull the chart and hand it to the physician before she or he picks up the telephone. If a patient calls with a medical problem, the problem should be triaged immediately (see the triage section of this chapter). All other problems should be transferred to the office manager. Pharmaceutical representatives and salespersons call the office all day. It is best to have someone in the office be the designated person to handle such calls. If the office requires that pharmaceutical representatives make appointments, perhaps those calls can be answered by the health care professional who is in charge of appointment scheduling for the day. It is a good idea to write down these callers and how to handle them in the policy and procedure manual. Employees can then access the policy any time they may have questions.

Transferring the Call

After it has been determined that the call needs to be transferred, be sure to transfer it to the correct extension. Patients become disgruntled when they have to call back because they were placed into the wrong person's mailbox. Always announce the caller and the reason for the call when transferring so that the person receiving the call is aware of who is calling. This can be accomplished by saying, "Maryann, when I hang up, you will have Mrs. Saunders on the line," or, "Maryann, Mrs. Saunders is on the phone for you; can you speak with her now, or would you rather call her back?" When you place the patient on hold before the transfer, tell the patient you are placing him or her on hold. For example, "Mrs. Saunders, I am placing you on hold to see if Maryann is available. Can you hold?"

Answering Machines and Services

Some answering machines have been replaced by voice mail available as a service through the telephone company. Answering machines contain a prerecorded message from someone in the office. For example,

Hello, you have reached the office of Dr. Babinetz. Our office is now closed. Our office hours are Monday through Friday, 9:00 AM to 5:00 PM, and Saturdays from 8:00 AM to 12 noon. If you have an emergency, please call our emergency number at 111-222-3333. If you wish to leave a message for the office, please leave your message at the sound of the beep. Thank you.

This same type of message could also be placed on a voice mail system. The messages left on the answering machine are retrieved and handled appropriately when the office opens.

Answering services are companies that are paid a monthly fee to answer the telephone when the office is not open. When hiring an answering service, instruct the supervisor on how the phone should be answered and what parameters should be used for taking a message. Some physicians ask that the answering service hold all calls and only call once per hour, unless it is an emergency. Give the answering service instructions on how to handle emergencies. It is a good idea to have a spouse or other family member call occasionally so that the answering service can be checked against the instructions that it has been given.

TELEPHONE APPOINTMENTS

"There cannot be a crisis next, my schedule is already full!!"
—HENRY KISSINGER

When patients call for an appointment, it is often their first impression of that practice. It is an excellent opportunity to provide each patient with a snapshot of the staff and their interactions with the patients. The following list provides guidance for the front office staff to provide quality communication:

- Answer the call by the second ring. A ring is actually just a matter of seconds, but to a patient, it seems like an eternity.
- Always be courteous. Patients are generally not feeling well and need an empathetic person to answer the phone and address their needs.
- Be sure to obtain all necessary information to provide the patient with the correct amount of time for his or her appointment.
- All questions that cannot be answered by the receptionist should be addressed to the appropriate person and answered in a timely fashion.
- Be sure to transfer all calls to the correct extensions.
- Be positive in all responses to the patient.
- Give patients clear instructions as to what they should bring with them for their office visit (e.g., a listing of medications, insurance cards, any medical records from other physicians).
- Obtain demographic information to begin creating a patient account. Ask the patient for his or her name (spell it for the patient to be sure that you have spelled it correctly), address, phone number, type of insurance, and so on.
- If the patient has managed care insurance, discuss the practice's access policy for services and procedures under the patient's insurance. Discuss the policy for obtaining referrals and your policy on co-pays.
- Provide the address of the office and offer directions if needed. Explain any special directions that the patients would need, such as where to park. Is the building easily recognizable? Is the front door easy to find?
- Discuss the cancellation policy with the patient. If the practice has a cancellation policy that includes a charge, be sure to explain this policy to the patient.
- Be sure to keep all communications with the patient positive.

This first encounter with the patient provides the office staff the opportunity to provide caring yet efficient service.

TAMING THE APPOINTMENT BOOK

The medical office appointment schedule is the lifeblood of the office. The duties of all members of the staff revolve around it. Physicians find themselves slaves to it. It commands the respect of everyone and is the most difficult part of the practice. It changes like the weather and therefore forces change around it. It is a powerful tool and should not be taken lightly. Making patients wait for their appointments is bad for any practice. Patients will become agitated if making an appointment with the physician turns into a small project. They will easily become dissatisfied and turn to another physician for care. Surveys on patient satisfaction have shown that the main complaint is excessive waiting. The appointment schedule that handles all situations has not been designed yet. A seasoned medical office manager knows that the number of patients scheduled for a particular day is not necessarily the number of patients seen on that day. It is important to remember that the appointment book is the key factor in the office manager's day. It should be used as efficiently as possible to maximize the physician's time.

It is important to set up the appointment schedule based on the needs of the practice (i.e., patient volumes, physician availability, number of new patients, etc.). It is also important to take into consideration seasonal variation. Fall and winter bring flu season. Spring and fall bring allergies. Summer brings injuries due to increased activity—lawn and garden work, sports, swimming, home improvements, and just plain having fun! August is the time for school and college physicals, and children away at college may need appointments during their school breaks in the spring or at holidays. Scheduling routine physicals for patients during these times is not a wise use of appointment scheduling.

General Scheduling Rules

1. Don't expect a flawless system.
2. Staff and physicians should be present to begin office hours on time.
3. Schedule the first patient about 15 minutes before the office opens.
4. Prepare a schedule that is individualized to each physician's or physician extender's (nurse practitioner,

physician assistant, clinical nurse specialist, etc.) style of practice.

5. Don't prepare a schedule that cannot be kept; keep it as stress free as possible.
6. If volumes increase, revisit your scheduling approach and make any modifications that are necessary.
7. Calculate the patients per hour before beginning your new scheduling system.
8. Recalculate about 6 months into the new scheduling system.
9. Compare the patient per hour rate and make any changes necessary.
10. Have new patients arrive at the office 15 minutes before their appointment to complete any paperwork that is necessary.

New Patients

When a new patient calls for an appointment, several important pieces of information should be obtained:

- The reason for the visit
- The name of the person or physician who referred the patient to the practice
- The patient's name, address, and home phone number
- The patient's work and cell phone number
- The patient's e-mail address, if applicable
- The patient's date of birth
- The patient's insurance company with identification numbers
- A referral if necessitated by the insurance company

Established Patients

When established patients call for an appointment, it is good to check the demographic information in addition to the reason for the visit. The patient may have moved, changed jobs, or changed insurance companies since her or his last visit to your office. Always remember to remind the patient of needed referrals when the patient's insurance dictates.

Appointment Scheduling Types (Figure 3-7)

1. Standard (stream approach)
2. Wave
3. Modified wave
4. Open access

The standard appointment schedule consists of nonflexible appointment times issued in equal intervals every 10 to 15 minutes based on the flow of the practice and physician needs. Some longer appointment slots are "earmarked" for new patients. These slots may be anywhere from 30 to 60 minutes long, depending on the physician, the specialty, and the patient problem. The drawback to this type of appointment scheduling is that it soon becomes easy for the physician to fall behind. Patients call with emergencies, patients do not keep their appointments, and scheduled patients may take more time than what was allotted. In an attempt to lessen the appointment delays, add a nonpatient into the schedule in the morning and afternoon sessions. This patient can be called Patient X.

The wave appointment scheduling approach is characterized by the scheduling of multiple patients in each hour. All patients are assigned at the top of the hour, that is, 10:00 AM, 11:00 AM, and so on. There may be four patients scheduled for 10:00 AM, another four patients may be scheduled with an appointment time of 11:00 AM, and so on. This type of scheduling creates a more even flow for the physician and staff. This scheduling approach is not as affected by no-shows as the standard or stream approach. If three of the four patients scheduled at 10:00 AM arrive at the same time, there are always patients to be prepped and seen. The fact that the fourth patient did not show for an appointment does not affect the staff or the physician. This approach is not always the best for the patient, however, because many patients have to wait longer for their appointment since it is on a first come, first serve basis. The fourth patient to arrive for a 10:00 AM appointment will have to wait a significant period of time before he or she is seen. By loading all the patients at the front end of the hour, the office schedule runs very efficiently.

The modified wave scheduling approach takes the wave scheduling and makes it better. It not only works well for the office, but is also more patient friendly. In a modified wave schedule, two patients are scheduled at the top of the hour, two at the quarter hour, and one at the half hour—for example, two patients at 10:00 AM, two patients at 10:15 AM, one patient at 10:30 AM, and none at 10:45 AM (this is used as a catch-up slot). With this type of schedule, the physician can see more patients with only a small wait.

Each office should identify the correct modified wave schedule for its practice. Because wave scheduling is so flexible, it can be used for portions of the day, hours in the day, or for all day every day. To determine the right scheduling for your practice, discuss the schedule with the physician to identify how it will be set up. First, decide how many patient can be seen per hour. Begin by scheduling half of the patients at the beginning of the hour and then the remaining patients through the second half of the hour.

Open access scheduling is characterized by leaving a certain amount of slots open for patients who need to be seen urgently. This type of scheduling helps the practice to balance the needs of the patient and the demands on the physician. In this approach, patients with emergencies can be seen without a major disruption to the days events. Practices with specialties whose patients require intense workups and practices that perform procedures should not use this approach.

SAMPLE STANDARD OFFICE SCHEDULE

Dr. Quinn **July 11, 2008**

9:00	Alexander James	12:00-1:00	>>>>*LUNCH*<<<<
9:15	Fran Szabo	1:00	Dana Gleason
9:30	Charlene Cyr	1:15	Sarah Salvateri
	Ref: Dr. Babinetz	1:30	Marci Toms
	NP (MC & BS)	1:45	**PATIENT X**
10:00	Justin Kilganon	2:00	Jean Safin
10:15	Carole Saunders	2:15	Albert Roye
10:30	**PATIENT X**	2:30	Elmer Segear **NP**
10:45	Deb Hinton		Consult-Ref. by Dr. Hale
11:15	George Casey	3:00	Arthur Roberts
	Police PE	4:00	***Staff Meeting at***
11:45	Gilly Conklin		***hospital***

SAMPLE WAVE OFFICE SCHEDULE

Dr. Quinn **March 24, 2008**

9:00	Andrew Quince	12:00-1:00	>>>>*LUNCH*<<<<
	Marilyn Miller	1:00	William Miller
	Natalie German		Thomas Kent
	Michael Dean		Maria Lucas
	NP (MC & BS)		Larry Conklin
10:00	Patrick McCreedy	2:00	Jean Helens
	Alexis Manahan		Sherrie Shalob
	Tony Bullis		Kate Winters
	Nancy Battle		Carrie Williams
11:00	Karen Wolcott	3:00	Rob Zelinger
	Janet Rumsey		Josh Bok
	John Jacobs		Marnie Chilner
	William Stevens		Lee Elery

FIGURE 3-7. Sample scheduling types.

SAMPLE MODIFIED WAVE OFFICE SCHEDULE

Dr. Quinn **July 21, 2008**

9:00	Alice Guinther	12:00-1:00	>>>>***LUNCH***<<<<
9:00	Jasmine Harvey	1:00	Michael Murphy
9:15	Harry Stauffer	1:00	Ruby Carson
9:15	Rachel Ragar	1:15	Hilary James
9:30	Amanda Ragar	1:15	Frank Mesteros
9:45	***Catch up***	1:30	Kelly Sharpe
10:00	Hazel Hershey	1:45	***Catch up***
10:00	Marc Monaghan	2:00	Gabriella Garrison
10:15	Dora Kolbe	2:00	Joan Reynolds
10:15	Russel Whittaker	2:15	Josh Camburn
10:30	Cary Hamil	2:15	Brendan Bowers
10:45	***Catch up***	2:30	Brenda Lingle
11:00	John Fraley	2:45	***Catch up***
11:00	Rebecca Snyder	3:00	Adrian Darnell
11:15	Ronald Snyder	3:00	Oliver Skidmore
11:30	Lynn Rohrer	3:15	Jake Stallworth
11:45	***Catch up***	3:15	Collette Kasper
		3:30	Kathleen McWilliams

SAMPLE OPEN ACCESS OFFICE SCHEDULE

Dr. Quinn **October 16, 2008**

9:00	Helen Brown	12:00-1:00	>>>>***LUNCH***<<<<
9:15	Frank Burns	1:00	***Emergency***
9:30	James Weiss	1:15	Julian Brostoni
9:45	***Emergency***	1:30	Lee Pugh
10:00	Brenda Ace	1:45	***Emergency***
10:15	Richard Scott	2:00	Katie Goldberg
10:30	Brie Nesbitt	2:15	Janice Jacobs
10:45	***Emergency***	2:30	Drake Besse
11:00	Maria Marchese	2:45	***Emergency***
11:15	Brittany Doyle	3:00	Sharon Fielding
11:30	Danny Packard	3:15	Jim O'Brien
11:45	***Emergency***	3:30	Hunter Zartman
		3:45	***Emergency***

FIGURE 3-7. (CONTINUED)

Computerized Appointment Scheduling

Computerized appointment scheduling can provide speed, flexibility, and staff efficiency. It is easy and fast to make and change appointments, add notes, and track examination room schedules. It is easy to find appointments for patients who have lost their appointment cards, by simply searching the appointment database. Finding a lost appointment in an appointment book can take time that office staff may not have. The computerized appointment templates can be set up to accommodate a scheduling approach, and most allow for each provider in the practice to have her or his own customized schedule. Appointments can be viewed by day, week, or month. An appointment can be searched by using either the patient name, date of birth, social security number, or phone number. Parameters can be entered to look for the next available time slot. For example, the staff can search for any Monday morning with Dr. Babinetz.

The computer can generate a list of the appointments for each day (Figure 3-8). This list can be used to call the patients with reminders. It can also be used by the physician so that she or he can review the list of patients for the day. The clinical staff can also maintain a copy of the list in their area so that they can monitor the day's activities. The appointment software is also used to generate the patient encounter forms for each day. Areas within the software template can be color coded to delineate spaces for new patients, consultations, emergency patients, procedures, and so on. The practice may also want to develop an appointment "shorthand" to note and identify the type of appointment; for example, NP for new patient, C for consultation, MC for Medicare, HMO for patients with managed care (who might be in need of a referral), MA for Medical Assistance, BS for Blue Shield, and so on (Table 3-1).

Patients per Hour

One way to take the pulse of the practice is to measure the number of patients per hour by each provider. This calculation can be used for physicians and physician extenders.

TABLE 3-1 Appointment Scheduling Shorthand

ABBREVIATION	DESCRIPTION
NP	New patient
EP	Established patient
OV	Office visit
C	Consultation
PE	Physical
LAB	Lab work
X	X-ray
MTG	Meeting
MC	Medicare
MA	Medicaid
HMO	Managed Care
COMM	Commercial
BS	Blue Shield
TRI	Tricare

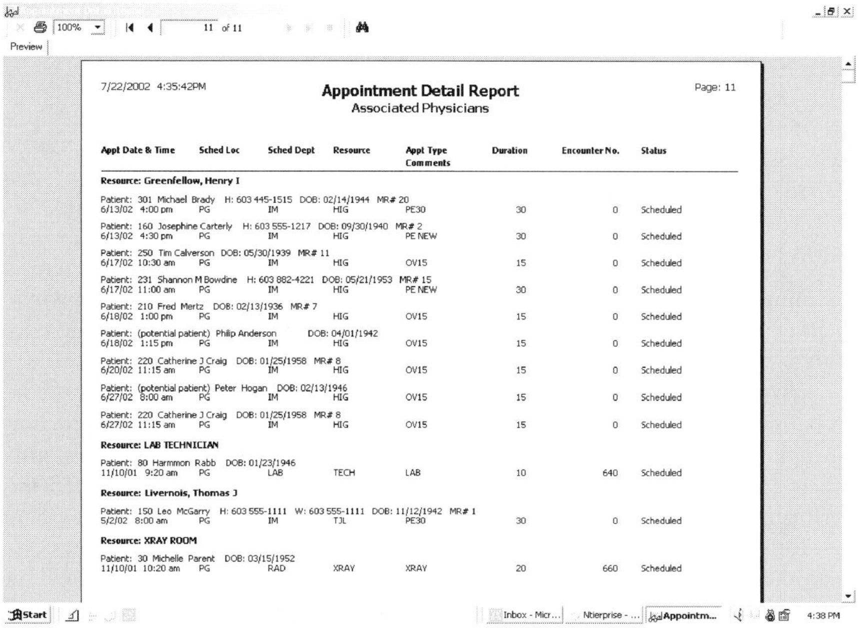

100% 11 of 11

Preview

7/22/2002 4:35:42PM

Appointment Detail Report
Associated Physicians

Page: 11

Appt Date & Time	Sched Loc	Sched Dept	Resource	Appt Type Comments	Duration	Encounter No.	Status
Resource: Greenfellow, Henry I							
Patient: 301 Michael Brady H: 603 445-1515 DOB: 02/14/1944 MR# 20							
6/13/02 4:00 pm	PG	IM	HIG	PE30	30	0	Scheduled
Patient: 160 Josephine Carterly H: 603 555-1217 DOB: 09/30/1940 MR# 2							
6/13/02 4:30 pm	PG	IM	HIG	PE NEW	30	0	Scheduled
Patient: 250 Tim Calverson DOB: 05/30/1939 MR# 11							
6/17/02 10:30 am	PG	IM	HIG	OV15	15	0	Scheduled
Patient: 231 Shannon M Bowdine H: 603 882-4221 DOB: 05/21/1953 MR# 15							
6/17/02 11:00 am	PG	IM	HIG	PE NEW	30	0	Scheduled
Patient: 210 Fred Mertz DOB: 02/13/1936 MR# 7							
6/18/02 1:00 pm	PG	IM	HIG	OV15	15	0	Scheduled
Patient: (potential patient) Philip Anderson DOB: 04/01/1942							
6/18/02 1:15 pm	PG	IM	HIG	OV15	15	0	Scheduled
Patient: 220 Catherine J Craig DOB: 01/25/1958 MR# 8							
6/20/02 11:15 am	PG	IM	HIG	OV15	15	0	Scheduled
Patient: (potential patient) Peter Hogan DOB: 02/13/1946							
6/27/02 8:00 am	PG	IM	HIG	OV15	15	0	Scheduled
Patient: 220 Catherine J Craig DOB: 01/25/1958 MR# 8							
6/27/02 11:15 am	PG	IM	HIG	OV15	15	0	Scheduled
Resource: LAB TECHNICIAN							
Patient: 80 Harmmon Rabb DOB: 01/23/1946							
11/10/01 9:20 am	PG	LAB	TECH	LAB	10	640	Scheduled
Resource: Livernois, Thomas J							
Patient: 150 Leo McGarry H: 603 555-1111 W: 603 555-1111 DOB: 11/12/1942 MR# 1							
5/2/02 8:00 am	PG	IM	TJL	PE30	30	0	Scheduled
Resource: XRAY ROOM							
Patient: 30 Michelle Parent DOB: 03/15/1952							
11/10/01 10:20 am	PG	RAD	XRAY	XRAY	20	660	Scheduled

Start Inbox - Micr... Ntierprise - ... Appointm... 4:38 PM

FIGURE 3-8. An example of a physician appointment schedule. (Courtesy of Allscripts, Practice Management Software, Chicago, 2008.)

To perform this calculation, choose 10 half-day sessions at random. Choose from various times of year to capture busier times in the office. Total the number of patients seen during those sessions and divide by the number of hours elapsed. The number of elapsed hours consists of the number of hours in the sessions adjusted for late arrivals. This will give you the number of patients per hour per provider. For example:

Dr. Smith saw a total of 140 patients in the 10 sessions that were chosen. He spent 40 hours in those 10 sessions.The number of patients seen per hour is 3.5.

This calculation can be helpful when negotiating contracts with physicians because it is a good measurement of physician productivity.

Appointment Reminders

Appointment cards should be used to provide patients with a reminder as to when they are to return to see the physician. They may say that they will remember, but it is always good for them to have a written reminder that they can take home and tape to the refrigerator or transfer the appointment data to their own personal calendar. Some practices print the next appointment on the bottom of the patient encounter form receipt that is handed to the patient at their departure. Whatever the method, an appointment reminder should be given to each patient.

Appointment "No-shows"

The average number of no-shows per practice is about 5%. There are many different excuses, such as the following:

- "I had a family emergency."
- "I had a work emergency."
- "I forgot."
- "My family doctor would not give me a referral."
- "I had car trouble."
- "Traffic was so bad that I totally missed the appointment."
- "The weather was too bad."

No-shows cause scheduling dilemmas because they may leave gaps in the schedule where the physician has no patients. These patients then need to be rescheduled, which can be problematic for a busy physician practice. Many no-show appointments can be prevented by sending reminder letters, sending e-mails, or having the staff call to remind patients 2 days before their appointment (Box 3-2). There are also services that perform this task.

Patients should be informed that they may incur a charge if they do not keep their appointment without canceling it. Most practices require 24-hour notice for cancellation of all appointments. This will allow space in the schedule for patients who need to be seen that day. If the practice develops a patient brochure, this policy should be clearly stated in the brochure. Some practices charge a $25 fee for missed appointments; however, many do not charge, because they believe that this will annoy their patients.

BOX 3-2 Appointment Reminder Codes

N/A—no answer
L/M—left message with person
L/MM—left message on machine
Checkmark—a confirmed appointment
RS—rescheduled

Cancellations

When cancellations occur, refer to a cancellation list to schedule patients into those available appointment slots. A cancellation list is prepared when there are no immediate appointments available for routine visits. Patients are placed on the cancellation list and provided with appointments as their name rises to the top of the list. This list can be kept on the computer or in a notebook. All employees who work at the front desk or in scheduling should be aware of the list. It is important to understand that long lists translate to missed appointments, lost income, and lost opportunity to care for the patients of the practice. This can be both inefficient and frustrating for the physician and his or her staff. One thing to remember is to do today's work today. If you put it off, the list will continue to grow and patients will become unhappy.

Charges for Missed Appointments

In June 2007, the Centers for Medicare and Medicaid Services (CMS) issued Article 5613, which addressed missed appointments. According to CMS, as of October 1, 2007, physicians, providers, and suppliers can charge Medicare beneficiaries and non-Medicare beneficiaries for missed appointments. To be able to do this, the missed appointment policy must apply equally across all patients and all patients much be charged the same.

This charge represents a missed business opportunity, not a charge for a service rendered.

All physician practices should develop a policy for missed appointments and maintain it with all other policies and procedures for the practice. The important thing to remember is that this policy must apply to all patients and all patients must be charged the same amount.

Medicare does not make payments for missed appointment charges to patients by physicians, and any claims sent to Medicare for these charges will be denied. Hospital outpatient departments may charge a beneficiary for a missed appointment, but cannot charge the beneficiary if he or she is also a hospital inpatient.

EXERCISES

MULTIPLE CHOICE

Choose the* best *answer for each of the following questions.

1. Which of the following is *not* a type of appointment scheduling?
   a. Watch
   b. Wave
   c. Modified wave
   d. Standard
2. Which of the following is *not* a general scheduling rule?
   a. Prepare schedules that cannot be kept
   b. Begin hours on time
   c. Schedule the first patient 15 minutes before the first appointment
   d. Calculate the patients per hour
3. When four patients are scheduled at 10:00 AM and then four at 11:00 AM, what type of scheduling is this?
   a. Watch
   b. Wave
   c. Modified wave
   d. Open
4. What type of appointment scheduling finds the physician falling behind rather easily?
   a. Open
   b. Wave
   c. Standard
   d. Modified wave
5. What type of appointment scheduling leaves 45 minutes after the hour (9:45 AM, 10:45 AM, 11:45 AM, etc.) as a catch-up spot?
   a. Standard
   b. Wave
   c. Modified wave
   d. Watch
6. What piece of information would *not* be obtained when making a telephone appointment?
   a. Patient cell phone number
   b. Person to call in case of an emergency
   c. Insurance information
   d. Patient's home phone number
7. Which of the following is *not* a level of communication?
   a. Personal ideas
   b. Emotions
   c. Skills
   d. Facts
8. Which is *not* an important factor to remember when dealing with the elderly?
   a. They may have difficulty hearing.
   b. They are terrible historians.
   c. They are afraid of losing independence.
   d. They go to the senior citizens' center.
9. Which of the following is *not* a tip for good communication?
   a. Tell patients to ask their children to explain their medicines to them.
   b. Let the patient finish before you begin to talk.
   c. Give the patient your full attention.
   d. Try to limit interruptions.
10. Which of the following is *not* an interpersonal skill that promotes good patient interaction?
   a. Build trust with each patient
   b. Use good diction
   c. Use slang
   d. Give examples
11. Which of the following refers to social distance?
   a. 12 feet to line of site
   b. 4 feet to 10 feet
   c. 2 feet to 4 feet
   d. 4 feet to 12 feet
12. Which is *not* an example of an absolute?
   a. Never
   b. Always
   c. Everybody
   d. Some
13. Which of the following is *not* an important thing to keep in mind when purchasing a phone system?
   a. Price
   b. Growth rate
   c. Color
   d. Available features
14. What does call blocking do?
   a. Shows the telephone number of who is calling
   b. Provides an announcement with the number's status
   c. Prevents name and phone number from appearing
   d. None of the above
15. What is *not* an acceptable amount of time to wait before greeting a patient?
   a. 20 seconds
   b. 10 minutes
   c. 10 seconds
   d. 20 minutes
16. If the patient remains agitated and the doctor is still behind schedule, what should the receptionist do?
   a. Kick the patient out of the office.
   b. Tell the patient that she or he would have to wait this long in any other office.
   c. Tell the patient nicely that she or he will have to leave.
   d. Check with clinical personnel to see if the patient can be moved back to an examination room.
17. Which of the following is *not* a form that a patient is asked to sign?
   a. HIPAA acknowledgement form
   b. Consent-to-treat form
   c. Authorization for medical benefits form
   d. Prescription blank
18. Which of the following is *not* a form that the patient is asked to complete?
   a. Patient registration form
   b. Patient encounter form
   c. Patient history form
   d. Flow sheet
19. The birthday rule applies to health insurance coverage for
   a. Children

b. Husband
c. Wife
d. None of the above

TRUE OR FALSE

1. _____ Referring physicians are important to most medical practices.
2. _____ Conference calling involves two-way calling.
3. _____ The telephone company offers a service that will track the last number that is called in.
4. _____ A key indicator of nonverbal communication is posture.
5. _____ One should not take notes when listening to the patient; it is distracting.
6. _____ Patients should be double-booked whenever possible to maintain the flow.
7. _____ A new phone system should allow for double the amount of lines in 6 years.
8. _____ Tact is the ability to speak and act skillfully and considerately.
9. _____ In a busy office, answer the phone and immediately ask the caller to hold.
10. _____ It is good to take the name of the caller (if not the patient) when taking a message.
11. _____ The most common time frame for patient scheduling is every half hour.
12. _____ It is not necessary to call no-shows.
13. _____ New patient "blocks" are important for good flow within the office.
14. _____ With an automated phone system, the first option presented to the caller should be, "If this is a physician, press 1 now."
15. _____ It is good to save money by bringing old magazines into the reception area.
16. _____ Crayons are a great toy for the reception area.
17. _____ Patients find reception area fish tanks agitating.
18. _____ Pitch affects voice.
19. _____ Don't tower over children when speaking with them.
20. _____ Most elderly patients are fearful of a loss of their independence.

MATCHING

Match the nonverbal message with the movement.

	Movement		Message
1. _____	Rubbing your hand, arm, or wrist	A.	Uncertainty
2. _____	Slouching, head forward, stomach out	B.	Disagreement
3. _____	Turning upper body away from patient	C.	Fear
4. _____	Raised eyebrow	D.	Frustration
5. _____	Pouting	E.	Happiness
6. _____	Grimace	F.	Sadness, uncertainty
7. _____	Smile	G.	Unsure of yourself
8. _____	Lip knitting	H.	Disinterested and unfriendly
9. _____	Throat clearing by the listener	I.	Deception or uncertainty
10. _____	Eye movement sideward	J.	Intensity
		K.	Information processing

THINKERS

1. Describe the differences between wave and modified wave appointment scheduling.
2. List the six LISTEN techniques used to achieve telephone effectiveness.
3. List ways to make a reception area "friendly."
4. Define the difference between a new patient and an established patient.

REFERENCES

Centers for Medicare and Medicaid Services, *MLN Matters*, www.cms.hhs.gov/MLN MattersArticles/downloads/MM5613.pdf, Accessed May 12, 2008.

Centers for Medicare and Medicaid Services, *Quarterly Updates for Providers*, www.cms.hhs.gov/QuarterlyProviderUpdates/downloads/Issuances-4Q07QPU.pdf, Accessed May 12, 2008.

Cross, M. "Doctor's fear e-mail overload." *Internet Health Care Magazine*, October 2000, pp. 34-44.

Damsey, J. *Handbook of Physician Office Letters*. Chicago, IL, AMA Press, 2000.

Hall, E., *The Hidden Dimension, Proxemic Theory*. Doubleday, 1966, New York.

LaFrance, M., Professor of Psychology and Professor or Women's and Gender Studies at Yale, Proctor & Gamble, Yale University Study, New Haven, CT, January 26, 2000.

Mancini, M., & Gale, A. *Emergency Care and the Law*. Rockville, MD: Aspen Publishers, 1987.

Matherly, S., & Hodges, S. *Telephone Nursing: The Process*. Englewood, CO, The Medical Group Management Association, 1992.

Medical Group Management Association. *MGMA Connexion*. Englewood, CO: Medical Group Management Association, November/December 2001.

Mehrabian, A.

P/S/L. "I.MD 2000—A Global Perspective of Usage and Attitudes Towards the Internet by Primary Care Physicians." Montreal, Quebec, P/S/L Research, Spring 2000.

4

WRITTEN COMMUNICATION

CHAPTER OUTLINE

CHAPTER OBJECTIVES

After completing this chapter, you will be able to do the following:

- Differentiate among the types of mail
- Understand how to handle the various types of correspondence
- Learn how to properly compose a letter
- Understand how to properly address an envelope
- Learn the importance of clear written communication
- Identify the difference between commonly confused words
- Review and comprehend grammar skills
- Understand the use of e-mail

WRITTEN COMMUNICATION

The quality of written communications leaves a lasting imprint on the reader. Written communication takes time and skill, and only a small part of the communication is actually in the words themselves. Your writing reflects your skills, work ethics, and integrity as a person. If you write in a clear and lively manner, you will be perceived as a person of high quality. Poorly written messages may cause confusion for patients or fail to achieve the purpose of the communication. Whatever your writing style, all communications should be written in clear English and in a consistent style. The vast majority of professions require some type of written communication. Effective written communication is the ability to use the conventions of the English language effectively in writing with a range of audiences in mind. Some health care professionals may be writing to patients, some to physicians, some to hospitals, and the list goes on.

The average employee receives approximately 190 communications each day as a result of voice mail, phone, letters, and e-mail.

Goals of Effective Written Communication

1. **Choose the communication medium.** A variety of media can be used for written communication, including e-mail, letters, proposals, memos, financial and technical reports, newsletters, bulletins, and business plans. E-mail is a common form of business communication and is rapidly replacing formal letters; however, it is less formal than a letter. If the person with whom you need to communicate is someone you know, e-mails work great. If you do not have a business relationship with the person, a formal letter is best to begin the business relationship.
2. **Understand the reason for the communication.** Is there something that you want or need? Do you want the person to do something? Do you need her or him to provide information to you? State the reason for the communication clearly and accurately.
3. **Clearly outline what you want accomplished with the communication.** Provide details about what you want. Do you need the person to provide you with something? Do you need something as simple as new insurance information, or is it more complex? More complex topics require more detail.
4. **Outline the benefits of a response.** Provide the benefits of responding, such as, "Once you provide the correct and current insurance information, we will submit your bill for payment of the services you received on [date]."
5. **Create credibility and acknowledge respect for the person receiving the communication.** This might include, for example, a statement about understanding the difficulties of continually changing insurances as many companies do on a yearly basis. Be sure to thank the person for the response.

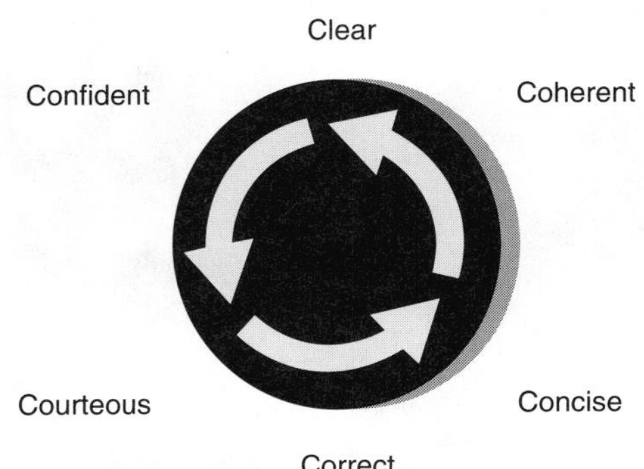

FIGURE 4-1. The "six C's" of effective communication.

The "Six C's" of Effective Writing

According to *The Business Communication Handbook* by Judith Dwyer, there are six elements to effective writing (Figure 4-1):

1. *Clear*—Be clear about your objective for the communication.
2. *Coherent*—Articulate consistent and accurate information.
3. *Concise*—Make the point, short and snappy.
4. *Correct*—Be accurate in statements.
5. *Courteous*—Give consideration to the receiver.
6. *Confident*—Be convinced and secure in what you are communicating.

Remember, whoever the audience, written communication should be in plain English.

Benefits of Written Communication

"The problem with communication is the illusion that it has been accomplished!" —GEORGE BERNARD SHAW

Written communication produces a physical document, a "hard copy" that can be kept permanently by the sender and receiver. This can then be stored for future reference. It can be easily distributed, either by hand or via e-mail. Everyone receiving the communication receives the same information—there's no miscommunication.

Understand that written communication is generally not read right away unless it is in the form of an e-mail. In the business world, people tend to read their e-mails throughout the day on a regular basis. Always prepare the communication in draft form, take a walk, and then reread it. It's almost guaranteed that you will make changes.

LETTER WRITING 101

Many situations in the business world require that letters be written. Health care is no exception. Letters are sent to patients, to other physicians, to insurance carriers, and to many other individuals and organizations. There are four main sections of a business letter: heading, opening, body, and closing. The heading comprises any printing in the letterhead portion, and the date. The letterhead will generally list the name of the practice at the top of the page, with the address and phone number either being split on each side, or located directly beneath the centered name of the practice or physician. Some letterhead designers place the address and phone number across the bottom of the page. The date should be spelled out and placed at the upper right-hand side of the paper.

Here's an example of a basic letterhead:

Lynn Marchitis, DO
100 Center Square
Suite 1A
Doctorville, PA 11111
Phone: xxx-xxx-xxxx
Fax: xxx-xxx-xxxx

The opening contains the name and address of the person or organization you are sending the letter to, which is known as the *inside address.* When sending a letter to a physician, always list the physician name, a comma, and then the appropriate designation, such as DO or MD. It is not appropriate to list the physician name as Dr. Albert Reynolds in this section of the letter. Leave two blank lines after the date. Then type the address of the person or company to whom the letter is going. An example of a correct opening is as follows:

Albert Reynolds, MD
123 Maple Avenue
Any City, Any State 11111

It also contains the salutation, such as "Dear Dr. Reynolds." End the salutation with a colon. If you don't know the name of the person, use a title instead (Dear Sir). Both the address where the letter is going and the salutation should be on the left side of the letter.

The body of the letter contains the subject, or reason for the letter. You may also use a subject line to identify the reason for the letter. Align the message on the left margin. Skip a line before starting a new paragraph, but do not indent the paragraph's first line. Make sure that each paragraph is clear and concise. For example,

Albert Reynolds, MD
123 Maple Avenue
Any City, Any State 11111
Re: Mary Smith

The reason for the letter is then typed and becomes the body of the document. The first sentence may either be indented five spaces or may be flush with the rest of the paragraph.

The closing contains the complimentary closing, signature, and typed name and title. A complimentary closing is usually one of the following:

- Respectfully
- Sincerely
- Yours truly

The type of complimentary closing used is a matter of choice of the physician. Leave two lines of space after your last body paragraph, and then use a conventional closing followed by a comma. The signature should appear below the closing. The signature should be that of the physician or other person in the office who is sending the letter and should appear below the closing. Unless you have established a personal relationship with the person to whom you are writing, use both your first name and last name. Signature stamps may be used; however, it is preferable to have an original signature on each letter. Beneath the signature should be the typed name and title of the person sending the letter. Four lines after the closing, type your full name. Do not include a title (Ms., Dr.). If you are writing on behalf of the practice, type your title on the next line. For example,

Sincerely,
Amy Grant
Amy Grant
Office Manager

The physician should sign all letters to patients that provide instructions, prognoses, or test results. Any letters to physicians or other health care professionals should also be signed by the physician. It is acceptable for the office manager to sign letters to patients involving rescheduling of appointments, asking the patient to contact the office, and overdue account balances.

If the letter contains two or more pages, a page number should be placed on all subsequent pages. The page number can be placed on the bottom right, bottom left, bottom center, top right, or top center.

The upper right-hand corner of the subsequent pages should contain the name of the person or organization to whom the letter is addressed and the date. This area can also contain the page number. For example,

Albert Reynolds, DO
December 7, 2007

Or,

Albert Reynolds, DO
Page 2
December 7, 2007

In addition to the standard sections of a business letter, there is also the return address (the address of the practice) if the letter is not printed on letterhead; the date (leave two blank lines after the return address; always spell out the month and include the day, a comma, and the year); and abbreviations at the end of the letter. If you send a copy of a letter to someone other than the person addressed, use *cc:* and the person's name. Use *Enc.* or *Enclosure* if you enclose something with the letter. If someone else types it, put the writer's initials in capitals, and then a slash and the typist's initials in lowercase: *JB/aab.* Only one abbreviation should appear on a line.

The margins of a business letter are generally 2 inches below the letterhead on the first page and 1 inch from the top of the page on all subsequent pages. This would be the place for the date to be entered. The side and bottom margins should be 1 inch from the edge of the paper. Use full block style, which is an alignment of all lines to the left, or a modified block style, which is an alignment down the middle of the page; align the return address, date, closing, and signature. There is no need to retype the information. Remember that a good business letter is brief, straightforward, and polite.

Letters are a direct reflection of you and the medical practice. They should be clear and concise with proper grammar and meaningful content. Read the following helpful hints for better letter writing and consider adopting them as your own:

- Send letters immediately after the situation or occasion; for example, a new patient welcome letter should be sent within 24 hours of the patient's appointment.
- Place the subject of the letter in the first sentence; for example, "We are sorry about the loss of your mother," or, "We saw your son's picture in the paper for the Hastings Award."
- Never use a postscript...it looks like you are in high school and can't write a letter.
- End the letter when you have accomplished the delivery of the message. Don't go on and on just to make the letter longer.
- Do not use humor in written communication; you do not know how it will be received.
- If you need to include a listing, use bullet points; this increases clarity.
- Use the tone that best matches the message.
- Keep sentences and paragraphs short.
- Try not to use negative terms; reword so that your message is positive.
- Don't use confusing words.

Sentence length is important. As a sentence gets longer, fewer people will understand what is being conveyed, and they may even stop reading. Almost 100% of all recipients understand sentences that contain 6 to 8 words. A sentence with 15 to 20 words seems to have the highest readability, whereas if your sentence has 30 words or more, you have lost half of your readers.

Word Confusion

The written word is powerful. It is a reflection of your personality and knowledge. When writing, it is important to correctly spell words that you are using. Some key words, such as homonyms, create quite a stir because they are often used incorrectly. Commonly confused words include the following:

- Accept (verb)
  To receive, or take on responsibility
  I *accept* responsibility for the broken copier.
- Except (preposition)
  If it weren't for the fact that...
  I obtained all the vital signs *except* the respirations.
- Affect (verb)
  To have influence on, to bring about a change
  Giving employees a raise based on merit can *affect* their efficiency.
- Effect (noun)
  Result
  The *effect* of the pay cut may mean a loss in personnel.
- Advice (noun)
  An opinion about an action
  The medical assistant gave *advice* on how to use the hemoccult slides.
- Advise (verb)
  To offer or to recommend
  I would *advise* you to take that medicine with food.
- Forth (adverb)
  Forward in time or place
  We went *forth* with our plans to terminate that position.
- Fourth (adjective)
  Follows third
  You are the *fourth* person who told me that.
- Its (possessive pronoun)
  Shows possession and answers the question "Whose?"
  Its tank is empty.
- It's (contraction)
  A contraction of "it is"
  It's in the examination room cabinet.
- Lose (verb)
  To misplace something
  Did you *lose* a contact lens?
- Loose (adjective)
  Not tight
  We will put a *loose* dressing on that wound.
- No (adjective)
  The negative
  There is *no* more table paper in the supply closet.
- Know (verb)
  To possess knowledge
  I *know* that you have not been taking your medication.
- New (adjective)
  The opposite of old
  I want to get a *new* stethoscope; mine is old.
- Knew (verb)
  Past tense of "know"
  I *knew* that you fell out of your chair.
- Of (preposition)
  A linking preposition
  The physician is the owner *of* the practice.
- Have (verb)
  To possess
  They *have* two children

- Principal (noun)
  Meaning important or having to do with interest
  That patient is the *principal* of the high school.
- Principle (noun)
  Basic truth, law, or policy
  It is against my *principles* to argue with that patient.
- There (adverb) (introductory word)
  Direction, introduction
  The thermometer is over *there.* OR *There* is no paper in the copier.
- Their (personal pronoun possessive)
  Possession
  This is *their* son, Mike.
- They're (contraction)
  Contraction of "they are"
  They're going to be late for the appointment.
- To (preposition)
  Linking word
  Dr. Casey went *to* the hospital.
- Too (adverb)
  Quantity; as well as
  She ate *too* much.
- Two (adjective)
  Number that follows number one
  There are *two* reasons why that could happen.
- Were (verb)
  Plural tense of "was"
  The children *were* tired.
- Where (adverb)
  Direction or place
  Where did I leave that notepad?
- Whose (adjective)
  Shows possession
  Whose purse is that?
- Who's (contraction)
  Contraction of "who is"
  Who's coming to pick you up?
- Your (pronoun)
  Shows possession
  Those are *your* prescriptions.
- You're (contraction)
  Contraction of "you are"
  You're always late for work.
- Piece (noun)
  A portion
  Can you hand me a *piece* of paper?
- Peace (noun)
  Absence of struggle
  She is at *peace.*
- Beside (preposition)
  next to; close to
  Put the chart *beside* the phone.
- Besides (preposition)
  in addition to
  Besides the medical equipment, you should move the charts.
- Can
  Physical ability
  When you have a chance, you *can* clean up the desk area.
- All ready
  Readiness of multiples
  The medical staff is *all ready* for your presentation.
- Already
  Something that previously happened
  I *already* drew the lab work on that patient.
- May
  Giving or requesting permission
  You *may* begin the prep of the patient now.
- Adapt
  Change
  She will have to *adapt* to the new office.
- Adopt
  Making your own
  We have reviewed the policies and will *adopt* them into practice.
- Adept
  Being skilled
  She is *adept* at fixing that machine.
- Adverse
  Unfavorable
  He had an *adverse* reaction to the injection.
- Averse
  Reluctant
  She was *averse* to taking the medication.
- Access
  Available
  We do not have *access* to that computer program.
- Excess
  Too much
  Please remove the *excess* plaster.

Although this list contains examples of contractions, it is *highly recommended* that they not be used in a business letter. Instead of the contraction "Who's", it is recommended that both words be written (i.e., "Who is").

Capitals

Proper nouns and adjectives derived from proper nouns should be capitalized:

- Florence Nightingale
- Paris, Parisian

General wording derived from proper nouns should be lowercase:

- Plaster of paris

Names of geographic areas and topographic features should be capitalized:

- South Pole
- Southern States
- Lake Michigan

The names of nationalities and languages should be capitalized:

- Chinese
- Russian

Names of events and important documents should be capitalized:
- Gettysburg Address
- Battle of the Bulge

The names of streets, buildings, and monuments should be capitalized:
- Fifth Avenue
- Liberty Bell
- Empire State Building

Days of the week, months of the year, and holidays should be capitalized:
- Monday
- Thanksgiving

Punctuation

Period, question mark, and exclamation point:
- Use a period after an imperative statement.
- Use a question mark after a question.
- Use an exclamation point after an exclamatory sentence.

Comma:
- To separate words in a list:

He complains of a runny nose, sore throat, and fever.
- To set off nonessential phrases and clauses:

Dr. Smith, who is board certified in cardiology, was available to lecture.
- To separate independent clauses joined by a coordinating conjunction:

He prefers to use the French technique, but others prefer the classic repair.
- To set off an introductory word or phrase:

Being so tall, Dr. Collins has to duck to enter the OR.

Colon:
- To introduce a list, or words or phrases:

Please complete the following: name, address, and insurance company.
- To separate hour and minutes:

1:00 PM
- To close a salutation:

To all my patients:

Brackets and parentheses:
- Use brackets to set off words or letters in quoted matter that have been added by someone other than the author:

He [Dr. Dunlap] is one of the leading surgeons in our area.
- Use parentheses to set off nonessential information:

He spent an hour (more or less) explaining the new regulations to the employees.

Apostrophe:
- The possessive case of singular and plural nouns, indefinite pronouns, and proper nouns:

Mary's mother is not feeling well.
She fell in front of the neighbor's house.
- The plural of numbers and letters:

There are five 7's in a row. The "six C's" of effective writing are clear, coherent, concise, correct, courteous, and confident.
- Missing letters in contractions:

I'm

Quotation Marks:
- To set off direct quotations:

The patient stated, "I felt like I was going to pass out."
- To set off titles of articles, chapters, and essays:

Chapter 10, "The Hypertensive Patient"
- To set off words and phrases that are being used out of the norm:

Charles had a "fair" day today.

Italics:
- The titles of books, newspapers, and magazines:

Newsweek
- The titles of movies, television shows, and radio shows:

Patch Adams
- The names of the plaintiff and defendant in law:

Samuel Manetti v. Robert Nelson, MD

Dashes and hyphens:
- Use a dash to indicate a sudden break in continuity or to set off an emphatic phrase:

The patient was prepped—where was the nurse?
- Use a hyphen to join the elements of a compound word:

Twenty-nine

Happy Endings

HAPPY ENDINGS: "s"

Many people just add "s" to a word to make it plural; however, there are times when one can't just add "s." Adding the letter "s" works with most words, for example, tables, wants, books, and so on.

However, if the word ends in ch, sh, s, z, or x, one must add the letters "es" to the word; for example, lunches, complexes, waxes, and so on.

If the word ends in "y" after a consonant, change the "y" to "i" and add "es"; for example, carry = carries, hurry = hurries, baby = babies.

There are also special circumstances that don't fall under any of these scenarios; for example, go and "s" is written as "goes," do and "s" is written as "does," and have and "s" is written as "has."

HAPPY ENDINGS: "ed"

Most people just add "ed" to change the tense of a word. If the word ends in "e," just add "d"; for example, rated, raked, spanked, and so on.

If the word ends in "y" after a consonant, change the "y" to an "i" and add "ed"; for example, studied, carried, hurried, and so on.

If the word is short and has a short vowel sound, double the final consonant and add "ed"; for example, capped, wrapped, mopped, and so on.

Under certain circumstances, letters are never doubled. These letters include w, x, y, and z; for example, fixed, stayed, mowed, and so on.

HAPPY ENDINGS: "ing"

To show present tense in verbs, add the ending "ing" to the word; for example, mailing, carrying, calling, and so on.

If the word ends in "e," drop the "e" and add "ing"; for example, riding, taking, hiding, and so on.

If the word is short and ends with a vowel or consonant, double the consonant and add "ing"; for example, stopping, wrapping, hopping, and so on.

Under certain circumstances, if a word has a double "e," such as *see,* don't drop the second "e," as in *seeing.* If a word ends in "ie," such as *die,* change "ie" to "y" before adding the "ing," as in *dying.*

HAPPY ENDINGS: "able/ible"

Adding the ending "able" or "ible" to a word makes it an adjective.

Add "able" to words that can stand alone, such as *return, returnable.*

Add "ible" to root words that cannot stand alone, such as *terrible* and *possible.*

A few rules: always drop the final "e," change "y" to "i," and then add "able" ending, such as adorable, available, profitable, and so on.

HAPPY ENDINGS: "ly"

Adding the letters "ly" to the end of a word changes the word to an adverb, such as quickly and timely.

If the word ends in a consonant plus "le," change the "e" to a "y," such as gently, probably, responsibly, and so on.

If the word ends in "y," change the "y" to an "i" and add "ly," such as crazily, hastily, happily, and so on.

If the word ends in "ic" or "ical," add "ly," such as logically, ethically, timely, and so on.

"i" before "e," except after "c"

Some words contain the vowels "i" and "e" in succession. The rule of thumb to remember the correct order in the "i, e" debate is *"i" before "e," except after "c" and when sounded as "a," such as neighbor and weigh.*

Exceptions to this rule are words such as seizure, either, and height.

Like/As

Use "like" or "as" as a preposition to join a noun, such as "Her temperature was as hot as a pot-bellied stove." "Her rash was like a roadmap." You *cannot* use "like" or "as" as a conjunction to introduce an adverb clause.

Incorrect: Nobody can make a diagnosis like Dr. Smith can.

Correct: Nobody can make a diagnosis as Dr. Smith can.

Misplaced Modifiers

A modifier is a word or phrase placed too far from the noun or pronoun it describes.

Incorrect: The patient was referred to a surgeon with liver disease.

Correct: The patient with liver disease was referred to a surgeon.

Misspelled Words

In our day and age, everyone uses a spell-checker. The problem is that most spell-checkers do not catch 25% of the misspelled words. For example, some spell-checkers will not find misspelled words if they are capitalized. There are occasions where the word "form" is correct but it is typed as "from" or "use" is typed as "sue." Since "from" and "sue" are words, the spell-checker will not pick them up as mistakes. Another problem with spell-checkers is that they can't tell the difference between homophones. Homophones are words that sound the same, but are spelled differently and have different meanings. Examples of homophones include the following:

rode . . . road
flower . . . flour
I . . . eye
bee . . . be
to . . . too . . . two

Because the spell-checker is not 100% foolproof, it is necessary to proofread the document before finalizing it. It is difficult to proofread your own work, but the following tips may help:

- Read what you have written out loud, if possible.
- Next, read it silently.
- Look for words that you know you commonly make mistakes with.

There are five basic rules for spelling:

1. *Rule one:* The letter "q" is always followed by a "u," with a few exceptions, such as Iraq.
2. *Rule two:* Each syllable in the word must have a vowel.
3. *Rule three:* The silent "e" rule involves dropping the "e" when adding endings beginning with a vowel, such as "have" to "having." Keep the "e" when adding endings beginning with a consonant, such as "late" to "lately."
4. *Rule four:* Make words plural. Change the "y" to "i" and add "es" when the singular form ends with a consonant plus "y", such as "baby" to "babies." When the singular form ends with a vowel plus "y," add "s," such as "boy" to "boys."

5. *Rule five:* Write "i" before "e" except after "c" or when sounded like "a" as in neighbor and "weigh." Other exceptions include codeine, Fahrenheit, neither, and either.

See the list of commonly misspelled words in Box 4-1.

BOX 4-1 Commonly Misspelled Words

Some words are commonly misspelled because of their pronunciation. The following is a list of commonly misspelled words:

Absence	Leisure
Address	Length
Advice	Library
All right	License
Alright	Maintenance
Attempt	Mathematics
Because	Mediocre
Beginning	Miniature
Believe	Miscellaneous
Besides	Mischievous
Between	Misspell
Bureau	Mysterious
Calendar	Necessary
Camaraderie	Neighbor
Ceiling	Nuclear
Cemetery	Occasion
Changeable	Occurrence
Conscientious	Odyssey
Conscious	Peculiar
Decease	Piece
Deceive	Preceded
Definite	Prejudice
Descent	Prescription
Desperate	Presence
Device	Privilege
Disastrous	Probably
Embarrass	Quantity
Environment	Receive
Equipment	Recognize
Escape	Representative
Exercise	Science
Fascinate	Scissors
February	Secretary
Fiery	Separate
Fluorescent	Sincerely
Foreign	Special
Government	Strength
Grateful	Submit
Guarantee	Suggest
Harass	Thorough
Height	Through
Humorous	Tired
Hundred	Truly
Independent	Twelfth
Jealous	Wednesday
Judgment	Weird
Knowledge	You're

WRITING LETTERS

Health care, as with any other business, requires that management prepare letters for specific occasions, such as welcome letters to new patients, sympathy, congratulations, references, job offers, terminations, and thank-you notes.

Welcome Letters

Some practices send welcome letters to all new patients within 1 week of their visit to the office. This letter will go a long way with the patient's family and friends and may generate additional new patients.

- The welcome letter should be short and to the point.
- You can provide useful information about the practice and should convey the value that you put in your patients.
- Welcome letters can also be used to welcome a new business or new doctor into the area (great marketing idea!).

Sympathy Letters

Sympathy letters are probably the most difficult letters to write. The following suggestions may help to create these heartfelt letters:

- Describe how much the deceased was respected and admired by the physician and the staff.
- Mention a few of the deceased person's (perhaps patient's) strengths, achievements, and successes.
- If appropriate, include a short personal story about the person.
- Be sure to strike a balance between the formal tone of a sympathy letter and its deeply personal nature.
- Keep in mind that the family members are emotionally drained, so keep your sympathy letter short, no more than one page.
- If this is a personal letter, you may want to offer help in some way.
- Put yourself in the family's place and imagine the kind of sympathy letter you would like to receive.

Congratulatory Letters

Congratulatory letters are happy letters to write. The following suggestions may be used when composing these letters:

- Write the letter as soon as possible after the event takes place.
- State in the beginning the specific occasion that has motivated this congratulatory letter.
- Express praise for the accomplishment.
- Keep it simple and short, no more than one page.
- Choose your words carefully so as not to exaggerate the congratulatory words or use words that seems sarcastic.

Reference Letters

There will be many times during the course of employment when the office manager may have to write reference letters for employees, temporary staff, or students. The following suggestions may be used when composing these letters:

- The letter should be favorable and should contain personal characteristics, job performance, and professional promise for the individual.
- Potential employers may accept a reference letter, instead of contacting you directly, so consider this your best shot at getting the information out.
- Many employers will keep the letter as part of the employee's personal file.
- One of the greatest advantages of a reference letter is that the employee knows what is being said about her or him.

Job-Offer Letters

When the office manager has finished the interview process and has made a decision on whom should be hired, the next step is to offer the job by way of letter. The following suggestions may be used when composing these letters:

- When extending an invitation for an interview or making a job offer, the letter should be direct and encouraging.
- All of the details that have been agreed on in the job offer should be formalized in writing. Include, for example, important information such as the agreed-on start date for employment, job title, and additional details about responsibilities, job location, and starting salary.
- A written job offer eliminates misunderstandings and clarifies important details. Use this opportunity to make the applicant feel positive about employment.
- When writing the letter, be thorough, but be as concise as possible. Stick to the facts.
- If you decide not to hire a job applicant, it is a nice gesture to write a letter informing the person of that fact. It is best to write this courtesy letter as soon as it has been decided not to hire this person.

Termination Letters

Termination letters can be hurtful to the receiver. Because of the sensitivity of this type of letter, it must be well worded to help ease the pain of the loss of position. The following suggestions may be used when composing these letters:

- The termination letter can help diminish hostility if it does not openly reproach the employee.
- It gives the employee the benefit of the doubt for facts not in evidence.
- Circumstances may change and you may decide to rehire that same employee, so choose your words well.
- Keep in mind that this letter will reflect on the physician and the medical practice as signs of courtesy and professionalism.
- As always, be careful with what you write—it can come back to haunt you!

Be Polite. . .Always Say Thank You!

One way an office manager can make patients feel special is to institute a thank-you note system. When the office treats a patient who has been referred by another patient, the office should send a thank-you note to the first patient. This can take the form of a simple handwritten message on a plain card, or the office can have preprinted thank-you cards made that the physician can simply sign. It is also appropriate for the office manager to send the note, if the physician prefers not to. Sometimes, patients will refer more than one patient to the office, so it is important to write the name of the referral on the note. This note is a great patient satisfaction tool and can generate goodwill and future referrals to the office. Some offices even send birthday cards to their patients as a personal gesture. Patients love it!

"ADDRESSING" LESSONS

The post office requires that you use the most accurate address possible. The practice is responsible for maintaining accurate addresses for all of their patients. According to the United States Postal Service (USPS), 17% of Americans change addresses annually. Forty-three million people move each year. One out of every six families move each year.

When addressing mail, it is important to use the proper format. Some commonly used formats are discussed here.

Names

When addressing letters and envelopes:

- Always use Mr., Ms., or Mrs. before the last name of the person *if* the person does not have a degree.
- Always use a comma before Jr. and Sr., but do not use a comma before a Roman numeral, for example, Robert Jones III.

Numbers

- When using numbers, the rule of thumb is to spell out the numbers if they start a sentence. Spell out numbers from one through nine, but use actual figures for number 10 and up.

- Use figures for fractions and units of measurement such as years or page numbers, for example, James is a 3-year-old, or page 1.

To Begin With . . . Salutations

Catholic nun	Dear Sister _____
Catholic priest	Dear Reverend/ Father _____
Clergyman/clergywoman	Dear Reverend _____
Rabbi	Dear Rabbi _____
Dean	Dear Dean _____
President	Dear President _____
Professor	Dear Professor _____
Assemblyman/ assemblywoman	Dear Mr./Mrs. _____
Judge	Dear Judge _____
Governor	Dear Governor _____
Mayor	Dear Mayor _____
Attorney	Dear Mr./Mrs. _____
Dentist	Dear Dr. _____
Physician	Dear Dr. _____

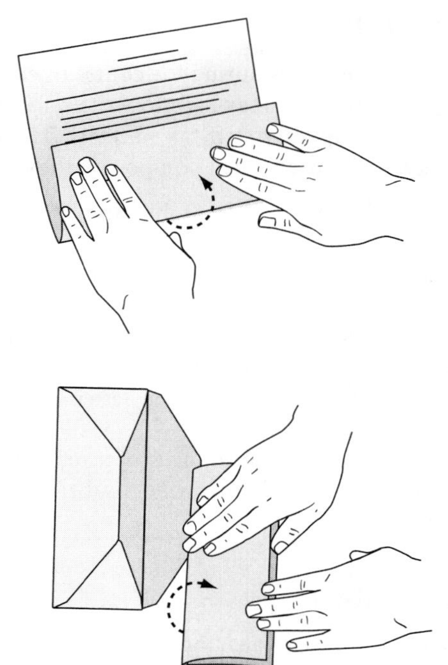

FIGURE 4-2. Folding a letter for a number 10 envelope.

THE ENVELOPE

All envelopes should have "Address Correction Requested" printed on the left-hand side of the envelope. If the mail is returned because of a bad address, the post office will place a yellow sticker on the front of the envelope with the correct address printed on it.

There are two sizes of envelopes, with the most popular business size being a number 10. This envelope measures 4½ inches × 9½ inches. The other, less commonly used envelope in the business world is a number 6, which measures 3⅝ × 6½. Office stationery uses the number 10 envelope size. When folding a letter to fit in a number 10 envelope, first fold the bottom third of the letter up with the type folding in. Next fold the top third down over the flap of the bottom third. This letter will fit perfectly into a number 10 envelope (Figure 4-2). To fold a letter to fit a number 6 envelope, first fold the letter in half with the type inside. Then fold the half into thirds and place into the envelope (Figure 4-3). When placing the address onto a number 10 envelope, place it approximately 14 lines down from the top of the envelope. For a number 6 envelope, place it approximately 12 lines down from the top of the envelope.

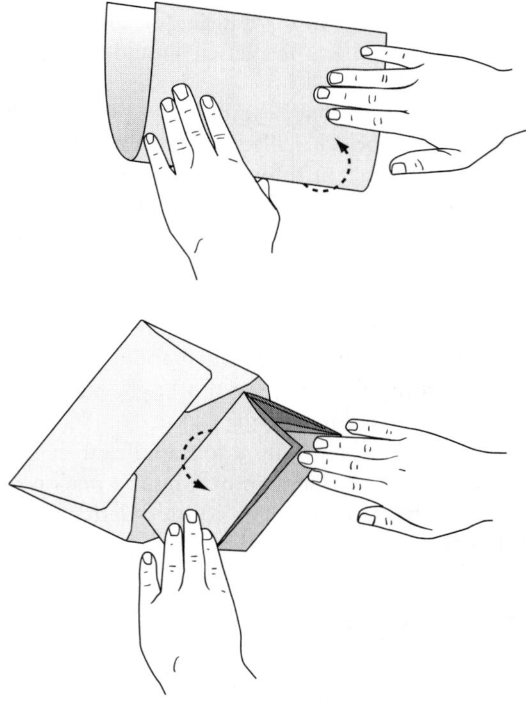

FIGURE 4-3. Folding a letter for a number 6 envelope.

TYPES OF POSTAL MAIL

Many types of mail are handled in a medical office. If you are unsure of which method to use, you can go online to the USPS Decision Tree, which will guide you to the mailing option that is best. The Web site for the Decision Tree is located at www.usps.com/businessmail101/decisiontree/decisionTree.htm. The types of mail are as follows:

- First Class
- Standard Mail

- Periodicals
- Express Mail
- Priority Mail
- Registered Mail
- Certified Mail

First Class is the most common method of mailing and is used to mail most business envelopes, postcards, note cards, flats, parcels that meet the weight requirements, and business reply mail. The maximum weight of a First Class mailing is 13 ounces. First Class mail delivery includes forwarding and return services.

Standard Mail consists of flyers, circulars, advertising, newsletters, bulletins, catalogs, and small parcels. All Standard Mail rates are bulk rates, and each mailing must meet a minimum quantity of 200 pieces or 50 pounds of mail to qualify. This is a great way to mail newsletters that the practice may want to send out to patients because it is less costly than First Class.

Periodicals are a class of mail that consists of newspapers, magazine, and other publications. This is the mode of mail transportation that may deliver office and medical supply catalogs and books. The office manager should be aware that if the office needs to send books, they can be sent inexpensively with the fourth-class or book rate.

Express Mail is the fastest mail service offered by the post office. It provides guaranteed expedited service that is offered 365 days a year, including Sundays and holidays. Express Mail must be placed into an Express Mail container (envelope, box, or tube), which can be obtained at the post office at no charge. The charge for this type of mail is based on the weight. A flat rate envelope is currently charged at $16.25.

Priority Mail consists of First Class mail that weighs over 13 ounces. If the practice wants the mail to get there fast, priority mail offers the best value. It includes forwarding and return services. Postage for Priority Mail weighing less than 1 pound is the same price, regardless of where it is going. Mail over 1 pound is priced based on its destination (based on predetermined zones).

Registered Mail is First Class or Priority Mail. Any item of value that needs to be mailed should be sent via Registered Mail. This mail route is more expensive, but it is sometimes necessary. Each piece of Registered Mail is insured for up to $25,000 against loss or damage. With Registered Mail, the office manager can track the date and time of delivery online. This type of mail can also provide the sender with a receipt for an additional charge.

Certified Mail should be used when the office requires confirmation of a letter's or package's arrival at the specified address and acknowledgment of receipt at that address. This type of mail can also be tracked online. This is more expensive than regular mail, but it is commonly used in a medical office. Certified or Registered Mail should be used for mailings of important documents, such as the following:

- Hospital and insurance company recertifications
- Letters of termination to a patient
- Documentation required by peer review organizations
- Application for staff privileges
- Requests for information from the Physician National Data Bank
- Workers' compensation and legal correspondence

Certified and Registered Mail should be sent with a delivery confirmation (slight extra charge) and a return receipt (about double the cost of the delivery confirmation).

For important and urgent mailings, the USPS offers *Priority Mail* and *Express Mail*. If you use Priority Mail, the package you send on Monday should arrive on Tuesday or Wednesday; however, this is not guaranteed. Overnight Express Mail is hand-delivered and guaranteed to arrive the following day. This delivery is guaranteed, and failure to deliver will result in a refund of your money.

Other companies also offer express mail services such as second-day delivery, standard overnight delivery, and priority overnight delivery. Standard overnight delivery is the most commonly used. It guarantees delivery by 3:00 PM the next business day and is slightly less expensive than priority overnight delivery, which guarantees delivery by 10:30 AM the next business day. Well-known and commonly used express delivery companies include the following:

- United Parcel Service (UPS)
- Federal Express (FedEx)
- DHL

METERED MAIL

Some offices with heavy mailings choose to use metered mail. Metered mail is simply mail that has been entered into a machine for the imprinting of postage, as opposed to using stamps that are purchased at the post office. Mail that is metered is delivered faster than mail with regular postage, and using the meter is faster than using postage stamps. To use metered mail, the office leases a postage meter, a piece of equipment that stamps the envelopes, and buys the postage from the USPS. Mailing costs are increased with metered mail because one must rent the postage meter. However, there is time saved by not having to affix stamps on envelopes or wait in line at the post office for accurate postage on flats and large envelopes. Whether to use metered mail is a decision that must be weighed carefully. Postage meters can be leased from companies such as Pitney Bowes and from the USPS.

OUTGOING MAIL

On any staff member's desk, at any given time, a fair number of items can be found that are waiting to be processed and mailed—laboratory work to be copied and mailed to referring doctors or patients, letters to physicians, RSVPs to various social events and workshops, membership applications to insurance companies, recertification forms for hospital privileges, and so on. The office manager might want to contact Pitney Bowes to see if it can save the office money on postage and employees' time in processing. All mail should be addressed using the zip code plus four to ensure that your mail is being handled as efficiently as possible. According to the USPS, there are currently more than 42,000 zip codes. To obtain zip codes for areas that are not local, you may search the Internet for the zip code needed or you may purchase a zip code directory from your local bookstore or office supply store. The Postmaster General prefers that everyone use the state abbreviations in mailing (Box 4-2).

BOX 4-2 Common Addressing Abbreviations

Miscellaneous Abbreviations

ALLY	Alley	EXPY	Expressway
ANX	Annex	EXTN	Extension
APT	Apartment	FLS	Falls
ASSOC	Associates	FLD	Field
ASSN	Association	FLT	Flat
AVE	Avenue	FL	Floor
BSMT	Basement	FRNT	Front
BAYOU	Bayou	FRK	Fork
BCH	Beach	FWY	Freeway
BND	Bend	GDN	Garden
BLF	Bluff	GTWY	Gateway
BLVD	Boulevard	GRN	Green
BR	Branch	GRP	Group
BRG	Bridge	GRV	Grove
BRK	Brook	HBR	Harbor
BLDG	Building	HGTS	Heights
BYP	Bypass	HWY	Highway
CP	Camp	HLS	Hills
CYN	Canyon	INLT	Inlet
CPE	Cape	IS	Island
CO	Company/County	JCT	Junction
CIR	Circle	LKS	Lakes
CORP	Corporation	LNDG	Landing
CSWY	Causeway	LN	Lane
CTR	Center	LBBY	Lobby
CIR	Circle	LDG	Lodge
CLF	Cliff	LOWR	Lower
CLB	Club	MNR	Manor
COMMON	Common	MDW	Meadow
COR	Corner	ML	Mill
CRSE	Course	MT	Mount
CT	Court	MNTN	Mountain
CV	Cove	OFC	Office
CRK	Creek	OVL	Oval
XING	Crossing	PRK	Park
DL	Dale	PH	Penthouse
DAM	Dam	PKE	Pike
DEPT	Department	PKWY	Parkway
DIR	Director	PL	Place
DIV	Division	PLZ	Plaza
DR	Drive/Doctor	REAR	Rear

BOX 4-2 Common Addressing Abbreviations—Continued

RM	Room	TER	Terrace
PT	Point	TRK	Track
PRT	Port	TR	Trail
RDG	Ridge	TRLR	Trailer
RD	Road	TPK	Turnpike
RFD	Rural Free Delivery	UNIT	Unit
SHR	Shore	UPPR	Upper
SQ	Square	VLY	Valley
STN	Station	VW	View
ST	Street	VLG	Village
STE	Suite	VL	Ville
SMT	Summit	VIS	Vista

Abbreviations for States, Commonwealths, and Districts

AL	ALABAMA	NE	NEBRASKA
AK	ALASKA	NV	NEVADA
AZ	ARIZONA	NH	NEW HAMPSHIRE
AR	ARKANSAS	NJ	NEW JERSEY
CA	CALIFORNIA	NM	NEW MEXICO
CO	COLORADO	NY	NEW YORK
CT	CONNECTICUT	NC	NORTH CAROLINA
DE	DELAWARE	ND	NORTH DAKOTA
DC	DISTRICT OF COLUMBIA	OH	OHIO
FL	FLORIDA	OK	OKLAHOMA
GA	GEORGIA	OR	OREGON
HI	HAWAII	PA	PENNSYLVANIA
ID	IDAHO	PR	PUERTO RICO
IL	ILLINOIS	RI	RHODE ISLAND
IN	INDIANA	SC	SOUTH CAROLINA
IA	IOWA	SD	SOUTH DAKOTA
KS	KANSAS	TN	TENNESSEE
KY	KENTUCKY	TX	TEXAS
LA	LOUISIANA	UT	UTAH
ME	MAINE	VT	VERMONT
MD	MARYLAND	VI	VIRGIN ISLANDS
MA	MASSACHUSETTS	VA	VIRGINIA
MI	MICHIGAN	WA	WASHINGTON
MN	MINNESOTA	WV	WEST VIRGINIA
MS	MISSISSIPPI	WI	WISCONSIN
MO	MISSOURI	WY	WYOMING
MT	MONTANA		

Other outgoing mail items may be notices to patients. They may take the form of recall notices (Figure 4-4) or notices of missed appointments. In any event, they need to be processed. The office might send a letter to a patient who did not show up for her or his last treatment and has not been heard from since (Figure 4-5).

When the office has been asked to obtain copies of records from another physician, a note from the physician may be used (Figure 4-6). The other side of the coin is when a patient wants to see another physician, and the other physician's office requests a copy of the patient's chart. If the patient has not signed a release form, it is necessary for the office to write or call the patient to request a signature permitting release of the records. A release form must be filled out completely before sending it to the patient for her or his signature. (It may not be easy to contact the patient—remember that one out of every six families moves each year.) Once permission from the patient is obtained, the records can be copied and mailed. If the office chooses to write for the patient's permission, it may send a letter such as the one shown in Figure 4-7.

Dear Mrs. Szabo:

I would like to take this opportunity to suggest that you call our office at your earliest convenience and schedule an appointment for a checkup. Our patients with chronic illnesses require periodic check-ups and reevaluations of their medications and treatment.

Sincerely,
Alexander Babinetz, M.D.

FIGURE 4-4. Sample recall notice.

Dear Mrs. Alberts:

It has been six (6) months since your last visit to our office. Your condition requires continuous medical treatments, and we are concerned about your health. If you are obtaining medical care elsewhere, we would be happy to forward copies of your medical records to your new physician. Please call our office to set up an appointment as soon as possible, or if you would like your records sent elsewhere, please call our office and the staff will be happy to assist you.

Thank you.

Sincerely,
Alexander Babinetz, M.D.

FIGURE 4-5. Sample no-show letter.

Dear Dr. Banister:

Mr. Donald Hessler, a patient of yours, has placed himself in the care of our office. He tells me that he has been a patient of yours for the last ten years. I would appreciate you forwarding to our office, copies of all his medical records up to his last visit with you. His date of birth for identification purposes is 5/14/38. A signed release from Mr. Hessler is enclosed.

Thank you.

Sincerely,
Alexander Babinetz, M.D.

FIGURE 4-6. Sample request for patient records.

Dear Mr. Carlton:

We received a request in the mail today from Dr. McDonald for a copy of your medical records. Before our office can send your records to him, we request a signed release from you that will authorize us to do so. Please sign and date the attached form and mail it back to our office.

Upon receipt of your release, we will copy and forward your medical records to your physician. Thank you for your cooperation in this matter.

Sincerely,
Alexander Babinetz, M.D.

FIGURE 4-7. Sample request for release of patient records.

Dear Mr. Keiper:

A check arrived in the mail today from Patient Health Insurance for $400 payable to our practice. The check should have been sent to you, since you have already paid for these services.

Since you obviously have insurance coverage for our services, we have deposited this check into our account. We are refunding the monies that you paid for this service.

If you have any questions, please do not hesitate to call my office. My staff will be happy to explain this further.

Sincerely,
Alexander Babinetz, M.D.

FIGURE 4-8. Sample letter regarding duplicate payment.

The office might find itself in a situation in which the insurance company pays a patient's bill and so does the patient. No, both monies cannot be kept! A simple note explaining the situation to the patient along with a refund of the monies will create goodwill. After all, how many patients receive checks from their doctors? Beyond the fact that it is illegal to keep both, the patients perceive this as an honest gesture on the part of the physician's office. With everyone aware of Medicare fraud, it is good to hear a patient saying the doctor sent a refund. A sample letter to accompany a refund can be found in Figure 4-8.

E-MAIL . . . THE NEW COMMUNICATION TOOL

E-mail stands for electronic mail. It is a way of relaying messages and has become the dominant method of communication in the business world. Most medical offices have the computer capabilities of sending e-mail. E-mail can be used by the office staff for contacting supply or pharmaceutical representatives. It can be used to correspond with the hospital; that is, the hospital can send memos (regarding staff meetings, changes, new physicians on staff, etc.) and schedules to the physician practice in place of mailing them. Physicians can even correspond with each other when taking time off by using a handheld device that has e-mail capabilities, such as a Treo or Blackberry.

E-mail can be an asset to a physician practice in many ways:

- It is invaluable when physicians are contacting their peers.
- It enables the physician and patient to communicate when they have time and are not rushed. People using e-mail tend to be more focused in their e-mails as compared to a typical phone conversation.
- Office staff can forward messages to physicians via e-mail.
- Some insurance carriers pay physicians for e-mail communications with their physicians.
- Patients can schedule their own appointments—with built-in guidelines, of course!
- Prescriptions can be refilled.
- Patients can be advised of their test results.
- Patients can be advised of new developments within the practice, for example, change in office hours, change in insurance policies, Betty the billing clerk had a baby girl, and so on.

Most physician practice management software packages contain an e-mail option. The American Medical Informatics Association has released guidelines that have been adopted by the American Medical Association. These guidelines help practices to establish e-mail policies before putting the system in place:

- Establish turnaround times for messages. E-mail should not be used for urgent matters in a physician office. A phone call is necessary for this scenario.
- Advise patients of privacy issues and who processes messages other than the doctor.
- Establish types of transactions and subject matters that can be contained in e-mail.
- Ask patients to put the purpose of the communication in the subject heading and their name or identification number (or both) in the body of the message.
- Set up an automatic reply to alert patients that their messages were received. Send a new message when their requests were completed.
- Print all messages and include them in patients' medical records.
- Maintain a mailing list of patients with their e-mail addresses, but don't send group mailings that include all recipients' e-mail addresses.
- Avoid anger, sarcasm, harsh criticism, and references to third parties in e-mail messages.
- Obtain the patient's informed consent for use of e-mail. Written forms that patients sign should itemize communication guidelines; provide instructions for when to make phone calls or office visits; describe security mechanisms that are being used; indemnify the provider

if information is lost because of technical failures; and waive the encryption requirement, if patients insist.

- Use passwords.
- Never forward patient-identifiable information without patient permission.
- Never use e-mail addresses for marketing.
- Never share professional e-mail accounts with family members.
- Use encryption for all messages when it becomes feasible.
- Double-check all e-mail addresses before sending messages.
- Back up e-mail onto long-term storage every week. A duplicate should also be made and stored off-site.
- Put policy decision both in writing and in electronic form.

Benefits of E-mail

There are many benefits to using e-mail over other mediums. They are as follows:

- E-mail can be sent and received at any time.
- It is time-effective—e-mail can be sent in a matter of seconds.
- It is cost-effective—no paper, no postage, no costs.
- E-mail allows for direct access to others.
- Messages can be saved and stored by moving them to your personal folder.
- It is easier to communicate with those who can read English, but have difficulties speaking it.
- It is an excellent mechanism for follow-up after meetings.
- It can be used to communicate with a patient's family members who live out of town.
- It can be used to communicate with colleagues from medical school.

E-MAIL AS A RESEARCH TOOL

Many physicians use e-mail to work on research projects that require collaboration. Because physicians have schedules that make it virtually impossible to collaborate, e-mail is a godsend. Manuscripts, articles, and the like can easily be e-mailed for review with comments. Once the review is completed, it is e-mailed back. E-mail eliminates a lot of phone tag for physicians. It has no geographic boundaries, so it makes research projects easy. There is no worry of time zones for calling, cost of flights for traveling, and just generally finding time to do both. E-mail can be handled at any time of the day or night and at the physician's convenience.

Drawbacks of E-mail

Even with the technology we have today, there are some drawbacks to using e-mail:

- E-mail is not confidential, which becomes a legal issue.
- E-mail does not adhere to standards—people make up their own rules.
- E-mail is too often used to distribute inappropriate material or jokes and cartoons.
- E-mail is often used to avoid confrontation and can easily be misinterpreted.
- Not everyone has access to e-mail. There are still small medical offices that do not have e-mail or Internet access.
- E-mails that are sometimes written in a very business-like manner are interpreted as rude and angry.
- E-mail is often sent without proofreading it.
- E-mails can be forwarded without the others' knowledge.
- It is assumed that all e-mails are read immediately, which could create problems.

E-mail Rules of the Road

Any business using e-mail must adopt rules regarding its use. Some e-mail rules are as follows: Only request receipt of "delivery" and "read" when absolutely necessary. Since it is possible to set your e-mail to notify you when the e-mail was delivered and when it was read, it creates three times the amount of e-mail and will clog your system. Do *not* use ALL CAPITAL LETTERS. The use of all capital letters in an e-mail denotes anger. Only "Reply to All" when "all" need to be involved. Never respond to chain e-mails, and never open spam. Both will plague you if you do. Always begin the e-mail with a salutation and the person's name, and always close the e-mail with a closing sentence and your name. Use proper grammar and spelling, just as if you were writing a letter. As with regular mail, what you write (and how you write it) is a reflection on you. E-mails should always be professional. Do not abuse the "Sent with high priority" button unless it is absolutely high priority. Always insert the subject of the e-mail in the subject line. Always consider the order of the recipients, and be sensitive to any hierarchy that may exist. E-mails with many attachments are overwhelming. Send only a few attachments at a time. Answer all e-mails in a timely fashion. The office should have a policy on the amount of time that is expected to pass before an e-mail should be answered. Always proofread the e-mail before you hit the "send" button; sometimes the fingers don't type as fast as our thought process. You will be surprised at the number of errors you may find, and you will probably change something to improve clarity. Use only accepted abbreviations; otherwise, the receiver will not understand what you are saying. Before sending the e-mail, *stop* and think...Is this the best medium to use for this type of communication?

Carefully read e-mails sent to you to be sure that you have answered all questions that were asked. If you don't answer all of the questions, there will be a "flurry" of e-mails back and forth until you do. Do not discuss confidential matters via e-mails, and never e-mail when emotional...it's just good common sense! E-mails are meant to be quick; don't go on and on. Short, clear sentences and short, clear e-mails are always best. E-mail signatures should include the sender's name, title, address, phone number, and fax number. Some practices scan signatures into the computer for a realistic e-mail signature. Don't send an e-mail that is longer than two screens; few people will read an e-mail that long. Some believe that the original message should not be sent back when replying to an e-mail. Others want the original e-mail to refer to when reading the reply.

E-mail Policy

All businesses should have an e-mail policy so that employees know the boundaries. This policy should be prepared and distributed at a staff meeting where it can be discussed. All employees should be aware of the policy and be willing to abide by it. Have all employees sign an e-mail certification form (Figure 4-9) that verifies they read the policy and understand it. Each e-mail certification form should then be placed in that employee's file. The practice e-mail policy should include the following:

- Basic rules and regulations of the practice on how to compose an e-mail
- The amount of time that should be allowed to elapse before an e-mail should be answered; some practices uses 24 hours, others use 4 hours
- When e-mails should be sent with "high priority"
- How to handle spam; there is software that can be purchased that will contain spam
- Cartoons, jokes, chain e-mails, and so on
- Personal use
- Newsletters and Listservs that are permitted by the practice

Composing The "From" and "Subject" Lines

It is important to decide what the "From" line is going to be for your e-mails. It should be consistent and change only with the change of the sender. For example, some e-mail "From" lines might look like this:

jababinetz@cardiocare.com—physician
mosimms@cardiocare.com—office manager

and so on.

The subject line in the e-mail is considered the "peep hole" to that e-mail. It shows you what the e-mail is about. Reading this subject line is a great way to "weed out" marketers.

I, ____________________________ certify that I have read the e-mail policy and understand it. I will abide by this policy.
I understand that a breach of this policy will result in termination.

Signature:____________________________

Date:______________

FIGURE 4-9. E-mail certification form.

DEALING WITH THE WHEELBARROWS OF OFFICE MAIL

The average weight of a physician's yearly mail is just less than 1 ton. The most efficient way for the physician to manage this mountain of mail is to receive it secondhand. In other words, the office staff should review the mail, handle what they can, and selectively distribute the appropriate mail to the physician. Office personnel should be able to open any mail that comes to the office (Figure 4-10). (Anything of a personal nature should, of course, be mailed to the physician's home.)

About half of a physician's mail is made up of pharmaceutical advertising. Some offices have set policies on how to handle advertisements. Many offices instruct their staff to automatically discard all junk mail that comes in. It is important that the person designated to do this job has a complete understanding of what is important and what is not. The health care professional may choose to sort the mail in an effort to obtain useful information, such as advertisements for a new copier, a less expensive long-distance service, an advertisement for the new delicatessen down the street, and so on. Some offices set advertisements aside and go through them at a later date, and then there are some who simply throw it all out!

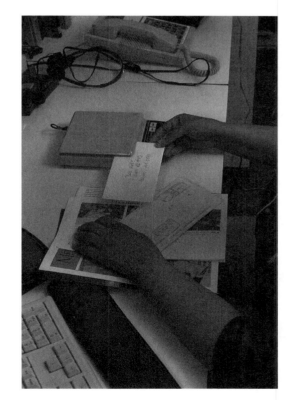

FIGURE 4-10. Receptionists are busy opening the volumes of office mail.

The staff member who will be doing the mail should be instructed to check all return addresses on envelopes to see if there is a change from the information that is currently in the office. This will save time by preventing bills from going out to the wrong address and returning 2 weeks later stamped "Forwarding Address Expired" or "No Such Address."

A properly trained office staff will save the physician volumes of time and will be appreciated by hospitals, referring doctors, insurance companies, and patients. All office staff members should be adequately trained in front-office policies and procedures, and perhaps attend workshops on streamlining the efficiency of the office. A brainstorming session involving all staff members can be helpful. Brainstorming sessions are appreciated by the staff because they give them the opportunity to provide input into the daily workings of the office. The office manager or other members of the staff can make a game out of front-office problems, asking for staff members to come up with workable solutions. The individual with the winning idea may be treated to lunch that day by the office or be able to leave early.

Incoming Mail

Each medical office should develop a policy on how the incoming mail should be handled. Sorting and processing the mail will save the physician time in the schedule each day. Some physicians want to open their own mail, whereas others want it opened and "prepared" for them. Some health care professionals are instructed to carefully review the mail and discard what they deem to be junk mail, whereas others want all mail to be reviewed by the physician. One way of preparing mail for the physician and others in the office is by using the following steps:

1. Sort the mail and place the believed junk mail in one pile, with the other letters and mail in another.
2. Slit open each letter and staple the envelope to it in the top left-hand corner.
3. Purchase a date stamp, and stamp each letter in the top right-hand corner.
4. Attach any enclosures with a paper clip or butterfly clip.
5. Purchase an "incoming mail" tray for the physician's desk. Place all opened mail in this tray.
6. If more than one person is responsible for opening the mail, have each person initial under the date.
7. If mail contains testing results on a patient, or a letter of consultation by another physician, the patient's chart should be pulled and the incoming mail should be attached with a paper clip to the front of the chart. These results must never be filed until there has been written acknowledgment that it has been reviewed. If a brochure arrives describing a conference the physician wants to attend, the dates should be written into the schedule on a tentative basis. The brochure should then be given to the physician for review.
8. General magazines such as *Golf, Newsweek, Forbes, Family Circle, Women's Day,* and so on should be placed in the waiting room. Magazines from the previous month should remain, but older magazines should be thrown out. All medical journals should be opened and placed on the physician's desk. Any medication samples that arrive in the mail should be opened and put aside. The clinical staff should be notified to see if they were specially requested by the physician for a specific patient, or if they should be placed into the sample closet.
9. Checks that arrive in the mail should be given to the person within the office who is responsible for the processing of checks and deposits.
10. Any requests for medical records should be attached to the medical record and given to the office manager for review and processing.

Patient Correspondence

When a patient writes to the physician regarding her or his medical condition, the staff should be instructed to pull the patient's chart and attach the letter to the front of it. The physician will be grateful for the time-saving effort. This is especially helpful in a group practice, where the physician may not be familiar with the patient. Even if the physician knows the patient, being human, she or he cannot possibly remember all of the details of all patients' treatments. The physician will probably never admit this to the staff, but she or he will greatly appreciate the effort and thought put into the gesture.

Some patients write short notes requesting prescription renewals. These can be handled in the same manner—by pulling the patient's chart and attaching the note to it. However, this can be delegated to the office nurse or medical assistant. The staff member can then follow previous instructions on how to handle this type of request. Any correspondence that requires a reply should be handled as soon as possible. If staff members are instructed to take care of these items on a daily basis, it will not be difficult to keep up with the mail that floods the office. Many staff members can handle a large majority of this tedious mail if properly instructed to do so. It is important to keep in mind that everything is done to streamline the workings of the medical office and the physician.

When sending important correspondence, always take the time to send it by Certified Mail and request a return receipt. This way, there is a record of the day it was received and who received it.

Suspicious Mailings

After the terrorist attacks on the United States in September 2001, it has become necessary to have procedures in place for the handling of suspicious mail or packages.

In fall 2001, the USPS was threatened with the random mailings of anthrax. Whether we like it or not, this still must be a consideration for any business (or home, for that matter). This section will help the office staff to properly respond to a suspicious package or letter. The USPS delivers 212 billion pieces of mail to over 144 million homes, businesses, and post office boxes in every state, city, and town in the country, including Puerto Rico, Guam, the American Virgin Islands, and American Samoa. The USPS handles more than 44% of the world's card and letter mail volume. It serves more than 7.5 million customers daily at more than 37,000 post offices. Since chemical or biologic warfare is a possible choice of terrorists today, businesses must be careful when accepting suspicious letters and packages.

WHAT TO LOOK FOR

The following list details some characteristics that ought to trigger suspicion:

- Excessive postage, no postage, or canceled postage
- No return address or a fictitious return address
- Improper spelling of addressee names, titles, or locations
- Unexpected envelopes from foreign countries
- Suspicious or threatening messages written on packages
- Postmark showing different location than return address
- Distorted handwriting or cut-and-paste lettering
- Unprofessionally wrapped packages or excessive use of tape, strings, or other packing materials
- Packages marked as "Fragile—Handle with Care," "Rush—Do Not Delay," "Personal," or "Confidential"
- Rigid, uneven, irregular, or lopsided packages
- Packages that are discolored, oily, or have an unusual odor or ticking sound
- Packages with soft spots, bulges, or excessive weight
- Protruding wires or aluminum foil
- Visual distractions

WHAT SHOULD I DO IF I HAVE A SUSPICIOUS PACKAGE?

If the practice receives a package that looks suspicious, an FBI Advisory tells us to follow these directions:

- Handle it with care—don't shake or bump it.
- Isolate it and look for indicators.
- Don't open it, smell it, or taste it.
- Treat it as suspect! Call 911 to be safe.

EXERCISES

MULTIPLE CHOICE

Choose the **best** *answer for each of the following questions.*

1. Which is *not* a goal of effective communication?
   a. Outline the benefits of a response
   b. Understand the reason for communication
   c. Send cartoons and jokes as a way to break the ice
   d. Choose the communication medium
2. Which of the following is *not* one of the "six C's" of communication?
   a. Confident
   b. Correct
   c. Challenge
   d. Courteous
3. E-mail can be used by which of the following?
   a. Physicians
   b. Office staff
   c. Hospitals
   d. All of the above
4. Which of the following should *not* be used when composing e-mails?
   a. All capital letters
   b. Send all attachments at one time
   c. Send all e-mails with high importance
   d. All of the above
5. Which of the following is *not* a benefit of using e-mail?
   a. Confidential
   b. Direct access to others
   c. Cost saving
   d. Faster communication
6. Which of the following is the correct use of commas?
   a. To separate words in a list
   b. To offset nonessential phrases
   c. To set off introductory words and phrases
   d. All of the above
7. Which of the following is *not* a correct use of colons?
   a. To introduce a list, words, phrases
   b. To separate hours and minutes
   c. To separate month and date
   d. To close a salutation
8. Which of the following is *not* a correct statement?
   a. "i" before "e" except after "c" and when sounded as "a"
   b. "i" before "e" except after "c" and when sounded as "u"
   c. Add "d" when the word ends in "e" to change tense
   d. Add "d" when the word ends in "ing" to change tense
9. Which of the following written communication would *not* be found in a medical practice?
   a. Newsletter
   b. Letter
   c. E-mail
   d. Bill of sale
10. Which of the following is *not* a benefit of written communication?
    a. Permanent document
    b. Nonverbal cues

c. Message is consistent
d. Easily distributed

11. What does USPS stand for?
a. United Parcel Service
b. United States Postal Service
c. United Postal Service
d. United States Parcel Service

12. What is the best length when writing a sentence?
a. 15 to 20 words
b. 25 to 30 words
c. 30 to 40 words
d. None of the above

13. Which is *not* a form of postal mail?
a. First Class
b. Registered
c. Third Class
d. Fifth Class

14. When sending an important document, the best way to send it is using
a. First Class mail
b. Certified mail
c. Fourth Class mail
d. Metered mail

15. What type of mail delivers medical journals to the office?
a. Second Class
b. Third Class
c. Fourth Class
d. Fifth Class

16. A "From" line is
a. The line in an e-mail that states the address of the recipient
b. The line in an e-mail that tells who the e-mail is from
c. The line in an e-mail that tells what the e-mail is about
d. None of the above

17. Which of the following is *not* considered a geographic abbreviation?
a. AVE
b. PKWY
c. DIV
d. CIR

18. The yearly average weight of medical office mail is
a. Under 500 pounds
b. Just under a half ton
c. Just under 1000 pounds
d. Just under 1 ton

19. Which of the following should be printed on outgoing mail envelopes?
a. Address correction requested
b. Return to sender
c. No such address
d. Forwarding address expired

20. What does the "e" in e-mail represent?
a. Electronic
b. Efficient
c. Express
d. Easy

TRUE OR FALSE

1. ______ USPS stands for United States Parcel Service.
2. ______ If a person has a degree, always use Mr., Mrs., or Ms. before the last name.
3. ______ The most popular type of postal mail is First Class.
4. ______ Most physician software packages contain an e-mail option.
5. ______ Written communication skills are not important for an office manager.
6. ______ The abbreviation ME stands for the state of Maine.
7. ______ Federal Express is less expensive than First Class mail.
8. ______ The Postmaster General prefers businesses to use abbreviations.
9. ______ Standard mail is Third Class mail.
10. ______ Certified Mail should be used to mail important documents.
11. ______ A number 10 envelope is one that is used with stationary.
12. ______ A recall notice is a form of outgoing mail.
13. ______ The words "like" and "as" are used the same way and have the same meaning.
14. ______ Never use a postscript in a business letter.
15. ______ *Adept* means "change."
16. ______ The names of geographic areas should not be capitalized.
17. ______ A salutation to a Catholic nun is "Sister."
18. ______ Congratulatory letters can be sent up to 60 days after the event.
19. ______ For efficient handling of the mail, use a zip code.
20. ______ The word "can" refers to physical ability.

MATCHING

Match the abbreviation with the word.

1. Company	A. FL
2. Freeway	B. ASSN
3. Suite	C. NE
4. Missouri	D. CO
5. Association	E. FWY
6. Nevada	F. ST
7. Nebraska	G. CT
8. Floor	H. MO
9. Court	I. STE
10. Street	J. NV

THINKERS

1. The office has develwoped an office newsletter for its patients. The newsletter must be mailed to all of the practice's patients. What class of mail should be used and why?
2. Prepare an e-mail policy for the employee handbook.
3. Describe the different types of postal mail.
4. List the "six C's" of effective writing.

REFERENCES

Cross, M., "Doctor's Fear E-mail Overload," *Internet Health Care Magazine*, October 2000, pp. 34-44.

Damsey, J. *Handbook of Physician Office Letters.* Chicago: AMA Press, 2000.

Dwyer, J. *The Business Communication Handbook* 7th edition. PrenticeHall, Australia: 2005.

5

MEDICAL RECORD

CHAPTER OUTLINE

CHAPTER OBJECTIVES

After completing this chapter, you will be able to do the following:

- Understand the medical record's importance and know the proper techniques for releasing medical records
- Compare quality and prices for electronic record software
- Recognize the benefits of dictation
- Understand the importance of proper documentation
- Differentiate among various filing systems
- Describe the life of a medical record
- Correct medical record errors properly
- Alter a medical record correctly and legally
- Properly store medical records

MEDICAL RECORD

The medical record, or patient's chart, can be the medical office manager's best friend or worst enemy. Records are an indispensable part of modern health care, yet they are not usually given the respect they deserve. Speaking physically, they are often in deplorable shape. Ragged edges and tears repaired with yards of tape are only a few indignities to which these important files are subjected.

All physicians and office managers know the importance of the medical chart. Accurate medical records are an indication that good care was delivered, whether it was a routine blood pressure check or the transfer of a patient to another doctor. Because of the medical-legal environment, the physician's office must be extremely careful about what is written in the chart, how it is written, and by whom it is written. Documentation of the entire visit is extremely important for insurance auditing and to support the practice of defensive medicine. Defensive medicine occurs when medical decisions about treatment are driven by the threat of malpractice. Under the resource-based relative value scale system (RBRVS) of reimbursement (see Chapter 8), the documentation in the patient's chart must justify the level of visit billed. If a procedure is billed with a modifier, a chart notation such as "The procedure was unusually complicated" is not sufficient documentation for the modifying code. It is necessary to document the reasons for the modifier or the procedure could be downcoded by the insurance carrier.

Putting aside for a moment the mere legal function of the medical record, accurate and neat medical records symbolize quality care and a well-informed physician. The office manager should realize the importance of the medical record and should stress to the office staff the value of neatness and clarity in every patient's chart (Figure 5-1). Well-kept medical records will result in an efficient office, and the physician will appreciate the staff's attention to detail when he or she is looking at a chart for a specific test or note. It is important to remember that the medical record is the physician's professional lifeline.

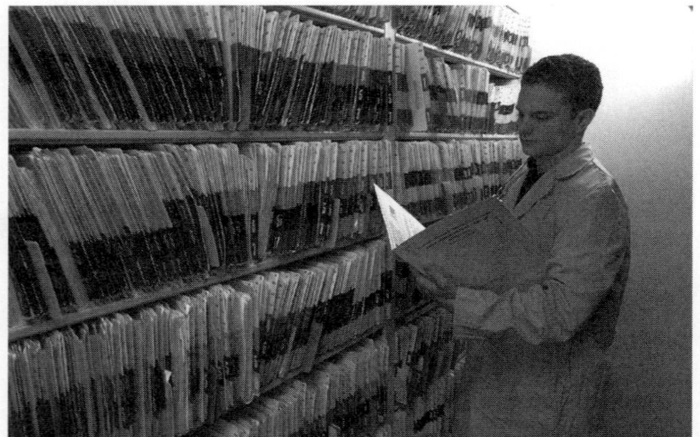

FIGURE 5-1. It is important to maintain neat and orderly medical records.

Users of the Medical Record

According to the American Medical Association, the patient's chart is used by numerous individuals. It is helpful for the office manager to understand who might have a need for the medical record. The following people are likely to consult the chart:

- Patient
- Clinical researchers
- Peer reviewers
- Reimbursement technicians
- Professional licensing and accreditation agencies

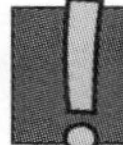

MANAGER'S ALERT

If a practice has several patients with the same name, have a label printed that says: "Warning—more than one patient has this name." This label should be placed on the cover of the charts to prevent mix-ups.

Each patient's chart should include a Patient Registration Form that provides essential demographic information such as the patient's name, address, telephone number, workplace and workplace phone number, Social Security number, date of birth, referring physician, allergies to medications, and insurance information. The Patient Registration Form is discussed in more detail later in this chapter. This form was discussed in detail in Chapter 3. Having clear and neat medical records not only helps the physician, but also aids the office staff when they must locate certain information in the chart.

For example, an organized chart will clearly identify the patient's allergies. The physician will discuss allergies with each patient; however, it is prudent to have a foolproof method of informing the office staff and reminding the physician of patients' allergies. Some offices have custom-made rubber stamps that say "ALLERGIC TO ____________." The front of the patient's chart is stamped, and the names of medications to which the patient is allergic are entered in red ink. Some practices use brightly colored stickers.

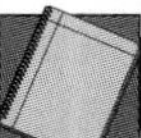

FROM THE EXPERT'S NOTEBOOK

Preprinted labels can be purchased in bright colors advising of allergies to certain medications. Because of the importance of this information, it is good practice to place these labels both on the front of and inside the patient's chart to call attention to the allergy.

Releasing Records

It is often necessary to release records to third parties. The most common releases are to courts, other physicians, and insurance companies. Documents required by a court will be requested by means of a subpoena. Subpoenas are usually served by a local constable or sheriff's office, but are often simply mailed, sometimes via certified mail with a return receipt.

A *subpoena* is a document that requires an individual to appear in court on a specified date. A *subpoena duces tecum* is a subpoena for documents to be produced at a specific time at a specific place. This subpoena is usually addressed to the *Custodian of Records.* When a medical office is issued a subpoena for a patient's medical records, the custodian of records is expected either to arrive at the designated date with the original chart, or to photocopy the records and mail them to the record copy service. A record copy service is in business to obtain records for various law offices. If the medical office does not have time to photocopy the medical records and mail them to the record copy service, the copy service will come to the office at a designated time and photocopy them. The physician should always review the records before they are released.

> **MANAGER'S ALERT**
>
> NEVER allow the original medical chart to leave the office via the mail. If the court will not accept a photocopy, someone from the office staff must go in person with the chart to the place designated.

When the office receives a request for records from another physician, the staff should be instructed to obtain a records release form signed by the patient before copying and mailing the records. (For a sample letter requesting a patient's signature on a records release form, see Chapter 3.) Once the records release form has been signed, records should be copied and mailed to the designated physician within 2 weeks. It is a good idea to send records by certified mail with a return receipt requested, so that there is no question as to whether they were received. The office should *never* refuse to send copies of a patient's medical record! The patient might sue the office on the grounds of neglect. Some states have laws applying to this situation that carry criminal penalties, so the bottom line is that once the patient has signed the records release form, send the copies of the records within 2 weeks. Records release forms (Figure 5-2) can be purchased from many different vendors and generally come in tablets of 50.

CARRIER RECORDS REQUEST

Insurance companies often request the medical records of patients applying for insurance. They generally request a recent and past medical history, along with blood pressures, weights, and copies of laboratory tests, x-ray examinations, and electrocardiograms. To expedite the release of records, the office manager should write a policy statement as to how the office handles these requests. With each request, the insurance company must send a current release from the patient. If the release is missing, the records cannot be released. Insurance companies will pay the medical office a fee to fill out the form, make copies of the test results, and send them with the release form. The office manager should have a set fee for the preparation of such requests; when insurance companies call the office, they can be told that a clerical fee for copying must accompany the request. The charge for copying medical records is usually nominal. It is always a good idea to check with the practice's lawyer to see if there is a state law that limits copying fees to a certain price. These requests should be answered in a timely fashion to avoid claim-payment delays by the insurance company. Some companies will come to the office to copy records and charge the recipient for the service. Offices that do not have sufficient personnel to make copies generally use such a service.

Name: ______________________________

Address: ______________________________

Please release any and all records on the above patient for the dates ____________ to ____________ to the office of:

Alexander Babinetz, M.D.
100 Main Street
Grand Island, NE 73604

Patient's signature: ______________________________

Witness: ______________________________

Date: ______________________________

FIGURE 5-2. Medical records release form.

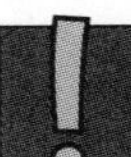

MANAGER'S ALERT

Never, under any circumstances, give patient information to insurance companies over the telephone. It must all be done in writing after the patient has signed the release form. Even with a signed release form, you can never be certain who you are talking to on the telephone. Under the Health Insurance Portability and Accountability Act, release of information over the phone is problematic from a confidentiality standpoint.

Electronic Medical Records

Most of the documents found in a medical office are actual physical documents (e.g., printed consultation reports, printed laboratory studies, printed physician letters). They arrive at the physician's office through the mail, by fax, or via hand delivery. Because of the time-consuming process of processing and delivering these physical documents, more and more practices are evaluating the benefits of computerized medical records. Most medical offices use computers for billing, accounting, and word processing. Few offices, however, use the computer to maintain their patient medical records. Maintaining medical records is the most tedious and cumbersome task in the medical office today, so it only makes sense that it should be done with the help of a computer.

Electronic medical records are referred to as EMRs or computerized patient records (CPRs). Computerization of medical records improves the quality and cost-effectiveness of medical care. For example, computerized medical records provide the following benefits:

- Increase the availability of the patient's medical history and preserve accuracy
- Facilitate clinical research by providing comprehensive views of health care delivery
- Provide diagnostic and therapeutic problem-solving support
- Increase efficiency by reducing time spent retrieving information
- Eliminate overhead and administrative costs associated with paper transfer and storage
- Maintain a comprehensive legal record of patient care
- Ensure confidentiality of patient data through the use of passwords and other security means

Not all medical offices are candidates for computerized medical records. Each office should weigh the costs against the benefits to determine whether their practice would benefit from using a computerized system of maintaining medical records. With the growth of managed care companies, computerized records are becoming more desirable. Managed care insurance companies require not only the patient's billing records, but also increasing amounts of information on the patient's care. The Institute of Medicine of the National Academy of Sciences has identified a computerized medical chart as a crucial element for improving patient care in the future. What this future holds in terms of computerized medical records can dazzle even the most high-technology physicians. As computer systems become linked together in a network throughout the country, the patient's lifetime medical records can be made available wherever the patient seeks service. Redundant tests will not have to be ordered, therefore saving money on unnecessary testing. Physicians will not have to worry about relying on patients' memories regarding historical medical events such as prior illnesses, drug allergies, and hospitalizations. All the medical information available on that particular patient will be readily accessible.

EMR systems can contain the following information:

- Laboratory results
- Radiology results
- Pharmacy information
- Respiratory therapy records
- Cardiology information
- Physical therapy records
- Physician's orders
- Medical record text consisting of the following:
  - History and physicals
  - Progress notes
  - Operative reports
  - Pathology reports
  - Discharge summaries

Electronic records can also contain nursing care information such as the following:

- Nursing assessments
- Progress notes
- Care plans
- Vital signs
- Counseling (e.g., dietary, cardiac, obstetric)
- Patient acuity levels
- Charting and clinical documentation

ADVANTAGES AND OBSTACLES

There are several advantages to a computerized patient chart system. The following is a short list of advantages as seen by one physician's office:

- The system flags patients for recall.
- Files can be retrieved faster.
- Records take up less storage space.
- Analysis reporting is easier.
- Charts are misplaced less often.

For an EMR system to be successful, it must be easy to access and use. The move from a traditional paper chart to a computerized paperless chart can, with careful planning, be a smooth transition. We have already listed the benefits to this system; now let's consider the following obstacles:

- Cost
- Downtime for training
- Lost productivity during computer conversion
- Accessibility

If you have never been involved in a computer conversion, the process will be a shock to your system, and you may find yourself holding your head every day. Let's talk about the emotions involved in a project such as this. Unfortunately, most people do not adapt well to change. Staff members who are told that the medical record is going to be changed—and that you are also taking away the tangible paper chart—will likely feel very uneasy. Telling them not to worry because it is all on the computer may sound like hollow reassurance.

Because some people are resistant to change, it is best to have them talk with others who have recently converted to a paperless system. Keep in mind that this could backfire if the other office had a difficult conversion. Planning carefully, allowing adequate time for conversion, receiving solid support from the vendor, and keeping an open mind will help to ease the change.

COST

A well-designed EMR system can save money in the following ways:

- Improves coding (the physician can search the computer master files for appropriate diagnosis codes and CPT codes for the services he or she is performing)
- Reduces labor costs (by reducing staff time to pull and refile charts)
- Lowers malpractice insurance premiums (some carriers offer a discount for the use of EMRs)
- Reduces transcription expenses (information can be entered directly into the computer by the physician)
- Dramatically reduces storage space requirements (no need for massive filing cabinets, medical records rooms, or off-site storage)
- Reduces supplies (no need to purchase charts, labels, dividers, etc.)

Although most people in health care agree that EMRs improve efficiency and quality of care, some also question the benefits based on cost. Approximately two thirds of the physicians in the United States are in solo or small group practices. The costs of an EMR, as reported by the Commonwealth Fund, which is supported by Robert Miller, PhD, and his colleagues at the University of California, is approximately $44,000 per physician for the initial setup and about $8,400 per year thereafter. Even though the costs are steep, the physicians found that the system was paid for within 2.5 years and provided the practice with a financial benefit of $33,000 per physician each year. There are two main reasons for savings from an EMR:

- More accurate coding levels
- Greater efficiency from decreased personnel costs

EMRs AND PATIENT CARE

Some physicians appreciate the ease of searching for reports with an EMR. How often does the physician spend time rifling through a chart looking for an x-ray report with no success, then call the front desk and ask them to look for it? Two employees start to look and it still cannot be located. With an EMR, the information is easily accessible. Database information can be found in seconds, which saves the physician, office staff, and patient much valuable time. An EMR streamlines patient care and any referrals needed for managed care patients. It can provide patients with health identification cards for everything from diabetes to the patient who has a titanium rod implant and needs a card when going through airport security. This system can be set up to remind the office of needed studies and can be customized with databases such as drug interactions and laboratory reference values.

Entering Data

Generally, a preprinted patient encounter slip is used for each visit. The physician checks off items and adds notations where necessary, and then a data entry clerk enters the information into the computer. If the physician dictates his or her record, the medical transcriptionist types the transcribed information directly into the computerized chart. Results of laboratory tests and x-ray examinations are typed into the patient's chart by the medical transcriptionist or data entry clerk. Letters of referral and letters from consultants are summarized and then typed into an archival storage area in the computer. Interpretations of electrocardiogram tracings are added to the patient's computerized chart. Hard-copy tracings are filed in alphabetic order in a file cabinet. It is important to keep the hard copy for comparison with other tracings the patient might have.

Some software packages will accept "scanned" text. This method reduces keystroke errors and saves time. Reports are simply placed into a scanner; handheld scanners can also be used. Once the scanning is complete, the job is done.

Vendors

The following is a list of vendors who have EMR systems:

- Misys Computer Systems
- Advanced Data Systems
- Medent
- Chart Logic
- Next Gen

Selecting a System

To ensure that you get the best system for your practice, follow these easy steps:

1. Establish the needs of the practice.
2. Prepare a budget for the purchase.
3. Establish a time line for shopping, purchase, installation, and final implementation.
4. Prepare a request for proposal (RFP) based on the information gathered above (Figure 5-3).
5. Evaluate the decision.

CORE VENDOR

When selecting a system, there are many advantages to using a core vendor that will integrate all functions into a single software package. A package from a core vendor will integrate billing, scheduling, managed care issues, and communications. With a core vendor, there is generally no need for a separate software package to help communicate within the system. An integrated system is easier to use because it requires only one phone call to get technical support, not multiple calls. One disadvantage is that core vendors are slowly becoming obsolete. Programmers writing software programs make major changes in short periods of time that require a whole system to be modified instead of just one area.

BEST-OF-BREED SOFTWARE

A best-of-breed software package integrates components from many different vendors into a single system. This approach offers opportunities for competition among vendors, with your practice coming out the winner. With

November 10, 2002

Mr. John Hamilton
Hamilton's Software Solutions
101 Center Street
Minneapolis, MN 59545

Re: Request for Proposal for Purchase of Electronic Medical Records (EMR) Software

Dear Mr. Hamilton:

Following is a request for proposal for Community Cardiology Clinic's (CCC) purchase of an electronic medical records system. Please review the information carefully and submit your bid. CCC is a cardiology practice with a staff of five physicians. The practice's primary location is 101 Center Street, with two satellite offices in nearby towns. The proposal should be for all three locations, with the understanding that other locations may be added in the future. CCC requires a system that accommodates users who have different levels of computer knowledge and varied computer skills and work styles. Some of our physicians dictate their notes, whereas others write them by hand. This system must accommodate everyone with ease and efficiency.

Scope of Service

The system provided to each office must accommodate both clinical and administrative functions within the practice. Key features that we are looking for include the following:

Must integrate with current practice management software
Must integrate with telemedical systems
Must integrate with decision support
Must contain the maximum security levels that are offered by each company
Must use either SNOCAMP or SOAP formatting
Must contain Web-based network connectivity

The vendor will provide a list and prices for all necessary hardware and computer peripherals required for running the software. The vendor will work with the office manager to coordinate installation of all equipment.

Before we select a system, we ask the vendor to provide a demonstration unit for a trial period. Once the purchasing decision is made, we request that the vendor present a timeline for installation. Following installation, we ask that the vendor provide on-site training. The vendor will provide ongoing maintenance of the program. If a new physician joins the practice, the vendor must provide full on-site training.

Proposals are requested by January 31, 2003. If no response has been received by that date, your company will be eliminated from consideration. Please provide pricing with and without financing.

If you have any questions or need clarification on any of the above, please contact me at (111) 111-1111, extension 2121.

Sincerely,
Barbara Braun
Administrator

FIGURE 5-3. Sample request for proposal (RFP).

this software, you can upgrade certain components without touching components that still satisfy your needs. You also have the benefit of access to multiple providers of expertise.

One disadvantage is that there can be a lack of organization with resulting miscommunication. A system that uses many vendors requires excellent communication and coordination. It may be necessary to hire an information specialist to help maintain this type of system.

FEATURES

The following are features to look for when investigating EMR systems:

- Pick a system that has the fewest amount of keystrokes necessary to get the job done.
- You should be able to move from screen to screen easily. You should have the option of using either a mouse or a keyboard for these functions.
- Check for inconsistencies within the program.
- The speed of the program should be something you can live with; you don't want to keep a patient standing there while the computer accesses information.
- Find a program that automatically checks for drug interactions and warns of allergies and adverse reactions.
- There should be an element of customization allowed within the system for notes, forms, appointment scheduling, and so on.

DICTATION...SINCE THE BEGINNING OF TIME

Dictation started with the Babylonians, was improved on by the Egyptians, was perfected by the Romans, and is still going strong today. Dictation, whether by manual method or more modern technology, has long been a time-saver. Reasons for dictation are generally clear to office staff and anyone else who is attempting to read the physician's writing. Dictated records can prevent having to re-file insurance claims because of poor penmanship. For compliance reasons, if the documentation in a medical record cannot be read, the service—from a legal standpoint—was not provided and any payment must be refunded. Dictated records can assist in quality care of the patient, because co-workers and colleagues cannot mistake clear, typed words.

Dictation can be handled through the physician's office or by an outside transcription service. If the office chooses to use an outside service, several things should be kept in mind:

- For correspondence, the physician must provide all mailing information. The chart is generally in the office and not available for reference.
- The physician must spell the patient's name and any other diagnostic or procedural terms that may be foreign to the transcriptionist.
- The office manager should contact references when hiring a service and ask about the service's competence and dependability.
- The office manager should discuss with the service the turnaround time of correspondence, progress notes, reports, and other transcription tasks.

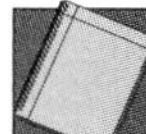

FROM THE EXPERT'S NOTEBOOK

A list of commonly used diagnoses, procedures, and medications must be given to the transcription service for reference. The office should provide the service with a list of frequently used referring physicians and their addresses, so the physician does not have to repeat this information constantly.

Today's modern technology affords much flexibility, both for the physician and for the medical transcriptionist. It is no longer necessary for the physician and the transcriptionist to be in the same country, let alone the same room! Everyone involved can work at his or her convenience from any location. If many users are tied to one system, the work may be completed with more accuracy and efficiency. Modern transcription units are very user-friendly and can be used by almost anyone. With a minimal investment in equipment and personnel, today's medical office can increase its accuracy and productivity dramatically.

It has been proven that a general business letter will take a person 10 to 30 minutes to write, depending on the technical level of the letter and the speed of the person writing it. Dictation removes those cumbersome constraints and brings us into the world of advanced technology. Most people talk five times faster than they write, which is one reason that dictation is so successful (Figure 5-4). Dictation

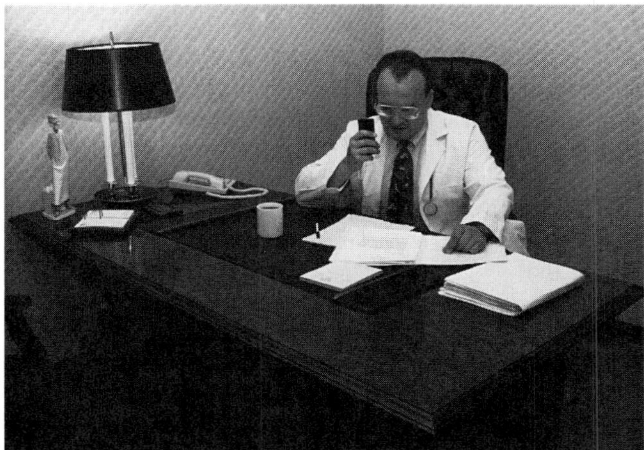

FIGURE 5-4. Physicians find that dictating medical record notes saves much-needed time.

is definitely a great time management tool and should be considered by any medical practice.

With available equipment ranging from portable units to systems serving a large medical office, the needs of any physician and his or her staff can be met. The physician can use either a handheld microcassette tape recorder or a desktop unit. A small medical practice's needs are best addressed by simple dictation units that rely on microcassette tapes, minicassette tapes, or full-size cassette tapes for information storage and retrieval. Sizes of portable dictating units vary considerably, with the smallest weighing only a few ounces.

A handheld microcassette recorder is one of the most popular units because of its versatility. This unit usually weighs a few ounces and can easily be used in a hospital setting, at home, or even in the car. Its portability increases the popularity of this method. The office manager should assess the needs of the physician so that the appropriate equipment is purchased.

Digital and analog dictation systems are available for large-volume practices. An analog system is a tape-based system in which an "endless" loop tape or cassette tape can be used. The physician either goes to a specific dictating location and dictates into a "tank" or dictates into a handheld unit. A "tank" is a unit that accepts large volumes of dictation; it provides easy access, allowing many transcriptionists to draw from it at the same time. A transcriptionist then plays the tapes on a transcriber unit and converts them into hard copy or electronic documents.

Digital dictation systems are electronic systems that are not tape based. These systems use a chip or speech board to accept the physician's voice. The voice (or, technically, its sine wave) is broken down into 1s and 0s (hence the term *digital*) and stored on a computer's hard drive. Information can be called in from any location. This system also allows information to be inserted into the body of a letter without destroying the completed sections. If a physician needs to make an addition, he or she simply inserts the material and new space is created on the disc for it without the already-dictated work being deleted. (In contrast, the portable tape units erase the previous material, and the new material is dictated over it.) In addition to this insertion feature, digital dictating technology eliminates the need to label and erase tapes on a continual basis. Digital dictation equipment is basically designed for multiple users, such as large medical groups, clinics, or hospitals.

Telephone interfacing provides similar advantages, except that there is no delay in getting tapes from the physician to the medical transcriptionist. The physician may be in another town or may be driving home from the hospital and can simply pick up the telephone to dictate progress notes reflecting work just completed. The dictated material is entered into the system at the office, where it will wait for the transcriptionist.

Voice Recognition Technology

Early voice recognition systems were clumsy, slow, and unusable in a medical office. These technologies have come a long way since their conception, and physicians have continually pushed for higher standards. There is now a voice recognition system that allows for continuous speech—the technology is able to interpret even when the speaker does not pause between words.

Voice recognition technology (VRT) used by physicians for dictation can save time and money. However, in many cases, VRT systems require that physicians create their own vocabulary by spending many hours dictating specific words and phrases commonly used by the practice. Programming VRT is like teaching a child to speak. Some specialties, such as general surgery, orthopedics, cardiology, and internal medicine, have already developed such vocabularies in a general format. Some products on the market allow for speech recognition by learning from the corrections made by the physician. It is important to judge VRTs not only by their speed, but also by their accuracy. Most VRTs have an average accuracy rate of over 95%. The office manager should check that rate against the accuracy rate of the transcriptionist before making any decisions regarding which system is best for the office. The office manager should keep in mind that VRT will not operate flawlessly; however, it does get better with age.

Dictation of Chart Entries

Dictation is the tool that keeps doctors out of trouble when others cannot read their writing. It is imperative that medical records can be read and understood. Typed progress notes are not mandatory, but they should be! One medical school in the Midwest even offers penmanship courses to physicians in an effort to improve their handwriting skills. Whether the practice is a group or solo practice, at times a staff member is called on to retrieve information from a patient record for a physician. This task becomes particularly stressful when the entries in the chart are illegible.

Dictated and transcribed case histories, initial examinations, progress notes, and medications are vital to everyone whose job brings him or her in contact with patient records. Even if the physician chooses to handwrite progress notes, dictated and transcribed case histories and initial examinations can be invaluable. Physicians who dictate their charts generally provide more information than do physicians who write them. If the physician is dictating medical records, the office manager should assign a staff member to proofread the dictation before giving it to the physician to sign. The physician must also read the dictation before signing. A physician signature acknowledges that it is correct. Remember that all chart entries must be signed by the person entering the note. It is a good idea for the office manager to check the transcription for accuracy before it is placed in the chart. It is always better to find an error in the office than in the courtroom.

In an office that uses dictated records, the physician must state the date every time he or she dictates. If the transcriptionist is given the record several days after the dictating was completed and no date is mentioned, he or she will be confused as to when the patient was in the office. The correct date is an important part of the medical record. All precautions to prevent error should be taken. It is better not to use nonmedical abbreviations when typing a medical record, because they can cause confusion at a later date. Acceptable medical abbreviations can save time and space in the medical record. A partial list of approved medical abbreviations is presented in Appendix D.

FROM THE EXPERT'S NOTEBOOK

The physician should be reminded to spell out the patient's name and any procedures or terms that might be unfamiliar to the transcriptionist. If this is not done, there will be many questions for the office manager from the transcriptionist throughout the day. It is also necessary for the physician to provide the name and address of any physician to whom he or she is dictating.

BOX 5-1 Dictation Techniques

Identification
- Doctor's name
- Date of treatment
- Patient's name
- Text to be typed
- Sequence of material
- Names and addresses of other doctors who should receive the report

Verbalization
- Speak clearly
- Speak slowly
- Enunciate properly
- Spell difficult names and diagnoses
- Do not mumble
- Avoid loud background noise at time of dictation

Grammar
- Indicate paragraph breaks
- Indicate numbering
- Indicate any special punctuation
- Indicate capitals
- Indicate indentations

If the physician does not have the time to dictate after each patient, he or she can place a sticky note on the front of the patient's chart with any pertinent information regarding the patient's visit. This will assist dictation at the end of the day. It is always best to dictate either during or immediately after the patient visit. Some physicians dictate while the patient is still in the examination room or physician's office. By using this method, the patients will again hear the instructions and can ask any questions that come to mind.

A smart office manager trains not only the transcriptionist, but also the physician. If the physician follows simple dictation techniques, the transcriptionist will save hours per week. A discussion between the physician and office manager regarding dictating techniques can increase productivity and efficiency and may prevent misunderstandings. Some physicians speak fast and low, which makes it difficult to hear them. Box 5-1 presents a simple chart on dictation techniques—share it with both the physician and the transcriptionist!

DOCUMENTATION

There isn't a single part of the medical record that isn't subject to the eyes of insurance auditors, peer reviewers, quality assurance investigators, or the law. In today's medical environment, the medical chart not only must include the diagnosis, prognosis, and plan of treatment, but also must justify the necessity of the treatment. In some cases, after insurance review, the codes may be changed before reimbursement takes place. In some states, greater than 30% of Medicare patient encounters are found to be upcoded by two to three levels of service. This is caused by insufficient documentation and translates into a lesser reimbursement than the office was expecting. More than two thirds of all Medicare evaluation and management services are found to be upcoded by one level of service. This again results in a lesser reimbursement. There is no such thing as too much documentation. Lack of documentation has always been a legal issue. Now, it is a reimbursement issue, too!

The following mnemonics are helpful for remembering the two commonly used documentation methods:

- SOAP
- SNOCAMP

Details of these documentation methods can be found in Chapter 8.

Arranging the Medical Record

There are two commonly used methods for arranging the medical record:

- Problem-oriented method
- Source-oriented method

A medical record that is arranged in a *problem-oriented* fashion contains a document with vital information regarding the patient, that is, a problem list, immunizations (if applicable), allergies, and a medications list. The patient complaints are listed on the problem list with corresponding numbers as they occur. For example, #1 may be for hypertension, #2 for diabetes, #3 for pneumonia, and so on. When the patient returns for routine blood pressure visits, #1 is used. This number is then carried throughout the chart for anything related to the patient's hypertension. Primary care physicians (family practice, internal medicine, pediatrics, obstetrics/gynecology, gerontology) generally use this method of charting for their patients. The *source-oriented* method takes like information and places it together in the medical record. For example, all laboratory results are placed together behind a tab labeled "Laboratory," all consultations are placed together behind a tab labeled "Consultations," and so on. A medical record using this type of arrangement is the most commonly used and is the one preferred by specialists. These medical records are neat and easy to access when looking for specific information about the patient. Diabetic patients, anemic patients, and other patients who undergo frequent laboratory studies should have their laboratory results layered in the chart. By layering them one on top of another, it is easy to compare the most current results with the last test. Charting is easy, as the new laboratory studies are placed on top with a single piece of tape on the top. It is easy to flip through the results to get a snapshot of the patient's blood sugars or cholesterol tests.

Liability and Documentation

Negligence is legally defined as the "failure to do what a reasonably prudent person would do under the same circumstances." *Reasonable prudence* means that a professional is required by law to act in a manner in which the average professional would act. To establish a claim for professional negligence, a patient must claim that a duty was owed to him or her, that the duty was breached, that damage was incurred, and that there was a relationship between the damages and the breach of duty. Professional negligence is discussed further in Chapter 9. Medical personnel have a duty to practice within the standards set for them by licensing or regulatory agencies. Documentation becomes a key issue when a patient claims malpractice or negligence. Having office personnel who are trained in proper documentation will reward the practice should defense in court become necessary. Most claims of this nature are filed years after the event, when most individuals no longer remember details. Proper documentation will help the physician and office staff to record specific details and the series of events that took place.

With the release of guidelines in 1995, the importance of documentation in the physician's office was not clearly defined, although it has always been a standard of practice in the hospital setting. Medical office personnel should be trained to follow the same underlying principles of documentation used by other professionals. Any information relevant to a patient's treatment and his or her response to medications or treatment should be recorded in the medical chart in a timely manner.

Documentation must be a concern for not only the physician, but also the staff. Under the legal doctrine of respondeat superior, an employer is responsible for the actions of his or her employees; thus the physician is held legally accountable for the actions of any and all personnel working in the office. All entries into the patient chart should be made in black ink or typed. Use of soft-tipped or felt-tipped marker pens can be a problem when completing two- or three-part forms, and should be avoided. A black ink ballpoint or roller-ball pen is preferable.

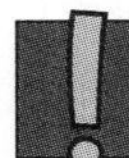

MANAGER'S ALERT

A pencil should NEVER be used. Using a pencil allows previously documented material to be altered.

LIFE OF THE MEDICAL RECORD

The length of time that a physician's office is legally required to keep a medical record varies from state to state. Each office manager should check with the practice's legal counsel or the local medical society to determine the statute of limitations for medical malpractice. This has a direct impact on the length of time the office must retain its patient records. From a strictly medical viewpoint, a medical office should retain medical records as long as the patient is active. Records should be retained indefinitely if the patient has undergone a procedure that could have an impact on him or her later in life.

In most cases, medical records should be maintained for 7 to 15 years for patients who are no longer seeing the physician. For deceased patients, records should be maintained for 5 years from the date of their last service. Pediatric and family practices that treat children must maintain medical records for 7 to 10 years past majority (the age at which full civil rights are accorded). The age of majority differs from state to state; however, it is typically age 21. The office manager should check with state authorities or legal counsel to verify this age requirement. In other words, if you treat an infant and the infant's family moves out of town, the infant's medical record may be in your office for as long as 30 years. X-ray films of inactive patients should be maintained for 5 to 10 years after the patient is no longer active. Many consulting agencies will advise a medical office to condense the patient's chart if the patient has been inactive for 3 years. This means that not every piece of paper must be kept in the chart, but only pertinent information regarding medications, certain procedures, specific treatments and tests, and so on. If a copy of the patient's chart was sent to another physician, a copy of the record release authorization should also remain in the chart.

Lost Records

Yes, it is true...medical records have been known to grow legs and walk away! Medical records become displaced and lost for a variety of different reasons. The important thing is to be able to locate them again. When looking for an entire medical record, first, don't panic. Second, use the following tips to help locate the medical record:

- Always begin by checking the charts before and after where the chart should be filed. For example, if Rachel Ragar's chart should be filed after Amanda Ragar's and before Mendy Rensinger, check to see if it was misfiled.
- Ask co-workers if they have the chart for any reason. Perhaps it was pulled for filing of x-ray results or because a prescription was waiting to be renewed. There are many reasons why the chart may have been pulled, so check with everyone.
- If the practice uses different-colored charts for different letters of the alphabet, begin by checking the charts of the same color. For example, if Amanda Ragar's chart was blue, all blue charts should be checked to see if it was accidentally misfiled.
- Check all charts within the space where it should be filed to see if the name of the label was misspelled. Some ethnic names are confusing as to which is the first and last name of the patient. Within some cultures, this is difficult to identify. There may have been some confusion between the first and last names.

COLOR ELIMINATES CHAOS

Filing Systems

Everyone has heard the old saying, "Time is money!" Time spent looking for a lost chart, or filing and pulling charts for the next day, costs the practice hundreds of dollars a month. It has been estimated that the cost of looking for and replacing one patient's chart can reach $100, and that the time spent looking for lost charts can take as much as 25% of a working day. More than half of that time is spent looking for lost or misfiled information.

Color-coded filing systems have taken the worry out of filing and pulling charts. With the help of colorful tabs located on patients' charts, the office manager can create a filing system that works for the medical office. Color-coding can shorten the length of time spent training new employees. It can also shorten the amount of time spent looking for charts that seem to have sprouted legs and walked away! Manila folders can be purchased with color-coding already on the edges, but many offices purchase plain folders and use color-coding stickers to apply the method that they prefer. This last method allows for greater flexibility in the filing system.

Color-coding schemes are based on either alphabetic or numeric systems. In alphabetic systems, 13 colors represent the first half of the alphabet, and the same colors are repeated to represent the second half, but with variations of stripes to delineate the differences. Some medical offices use the first three digits of the patient's last name, and some use the first two digits of the patient's last name along with the first digit of the patient's first name. For example, in an office that uses the last name–only method, the chart for the patient William Snyder would be labeled **SNY**. In an office that uses the other approach, William Snyder's chart would be labeled **SNW** (Figure 5-5). In either method, each letter is in a specific color.

Numeric filing (also known as *terminal digit filing*) allows for adding new files without the hassle of moving all existing files. Numeric systems use 10 colors to represent the digits 0 through 9. Each patient is assigned a number, and charts are filed according to that number. The following is a list of patients and their file or patient numbers. They may not look to be in order now, but in a minute you will see that they are.

MacKenzie Conklin **02 78 00**
Kayla Keiper **00 12 01**
Tyler Keiper **00 99 01**
Lori Curtis **02 34 02**
Kathy Miller **20 10 10**

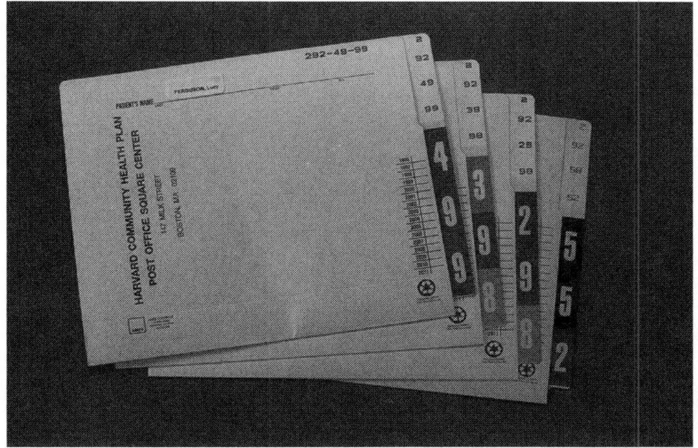

FIGURE 5-5. Numeric coding systems help offices locate medical records.

Frank Dunlap **13 64 31**
Maria Andrews **13 65 31**
Adam Barnes **00 00 65**
Joe Giononi **01 00 65**

All files ending with the same last numbers are grouped together. Then the files are grouped together according to the middle digits. Last, the files are grouped together according to the first two digits. For example, Kayla Keiper **00 12 01** comes before Tyler Keiper **00 99 01** because, although both have the same last number, Kayla's second number (12) comes before Tyler's second number (99). In the case of Adam Barnes **00 00 65** and Joe Giononi **01 00 65**, the second and third sets of digits are the same, so they are filed according to the first set. Adam's **00** comes before Joe's **01**. Each number is in a specific color.

If the office wants to use alphabetic color-coding with colored file folders, it usually assigns colors to certain letters of the alphabet. Red folders are used for last names beginning with the letters A, B, C, D, or E. Green folders are used for last names beginning with F, G, H, I, or J. Blue folders are used for last names beginning with K, L, M, N, or O. Yellow folders are used for last names beginning with P, Q, R, S, or T. Purple folders are used for last names beginning with U, V, W, X, Y, or Z.

For example, the following patients would have red folders:

Josh Bok
Jeremy Conklin
Karl Erickson

The following patients would have green folders:

Dave Fermier
Lynn Giononi
Barbara Jerkins

The following patients would have blue folders:

Kathy Keiper
Maria Lucas
Betty O'Brien

The following patients would have yellow folders:

Tom Palushok
Rachel Ragar
William Scott

The following patients would have purple folders:

Charles Whalen
Carol Vail
Lisa Zimmerman

The office manager should customize a system to meet the office's individual needs. Many companies make color-coding systems; some of the more popular companies are Colwell, Tab Products, and Smead. There are many vendors in this business, but you will find that all of them use the same colors for each system and in the same manner. This way, it allows for changing of vendors with little to no difficulty.

Other Ways Color Can Help Office Tasks

Many other tasks can be made more efficient with the use of color. Index cards in different colors can be used to designate different types of tickler files and keep the information well organized. Tickler files are set up as reminders of various types of appointments (e.g., when it is time for your yearly physical, your yearly Papanicolaou [Pap] smear, or pediatric immunizations). Color used in the appointment book helps draw attention to the most important meetings. For instance, using a red pencil to denote hospital meetings and a blue pencil to record the physician's personal appointments helps keep schedules straight and clear. Different-colored highlighters can be used for a variety of different tasks and can be very helpful in distinguishing important information.

MANAGER'S ALERT

Care should be used when choosing colored paper for office forms. Most colored paper will photocopy very poorly. Some high-end copiers have adjustments that allow for the copying of colored paper, but most do not.

WHO GETS THE RECORDS?

When a physician retires, there remains the question of who gets the records. Many physicians send their patients a letter advising them that they are retiring or leaving the practice. This letter contains instructions for the patients as to what will happen to their charts. Some physicians will have already made arrangements with other physicians to accept these new patients. The patients are given the opportunity to come to the office at certain dates and times to pick up a copy of their records to take to their new physician. Some local medical societies will act as records custodians. If the practice is being sold, arrangements should be made for the new physician to maintain the old records as a condition of the sale. If an employee wishes to take on such a task, the records can be left in his or her custody for future copying when needed. This last method should be used only as a last resort, however, because it can be a never-ending task. Off-site storage of the records is another solution, but it is a costly one. Whichever method is preferred by the physician or office manager, patients must be notified and given ample time to pick up their charts.

SIGNATURE STAMPS

Signature stamps can be the office manager's best friend or worst enemy. These stamps can save a lot of time in a medical office; however, if their use is not closely monitored they can cause serious problems. An office using a signature stamp should have a letter on file, signed by the physician, verifying the signature stamp as his or her signature. Signature stamps are helpful for the following:

- Insurance forms
- Membership applications to insurance companies
- Notes for patients to return to work or school
- Order forms for patient testing
- Letters

The downside of the signature stamp is the potential for abuse. The following suggestions will protect against misuse of signature stamps:

- Assign the stamp to one employee who will be accountable for its use.
- Have different stamps made and issue them to different employees. For example, the stamp "R. H. Hale, M.D." may be issued to one employee, the stamp "Robert H. Hale, M.D." assigned to another, and the stamp "Dr. Robert H. Hale" assigned to yet another. This way, you can track how each stamp is being used.

TROUBLESHOOTING PROBLEMS

Every office should be aware of risk-management issues associated with patients' medical charts. The office manager should instruct the staff to follow these simple guidelines:

- All laboratory results, x-ray films, and electrocardiogram tracings should be initialed by the physician before they are charted.
- All telephone calls regarding the patient's care should be noted in the chart.
- A standard procedure should be followed for missed appointments; for example, a staff member should write the date and the words "Patient missed appointment" in the patient's chart each time the patient misses an appointment (some offices have a stamp made and use red ink pads).

If the office manager delegates a specific staff member to follow through on these details, the office records will be better supported if audited or subpoenaed.

CARE AND HANDLING OF THE MEDICAL RECORD

Each chart should be well maintained and handled properly to ensure a long life. Before filing a chart, staff should verify that the proper coding, year sticker, name label, and any stickers indicating special situations (e.g., "HMO," "ALLERGIES," MEDICARE) are clearly visible. The staff member filing a chart should always check to make sure charges for the visit were entered into the computer. In the chart, all items of like nature should be filed together. All laboratory studies should be together, with the most recent on top; all progress notes should be together, with the most recent note on top; and so on. This makes filing a more pleasant task. Next, the chart is placed in its appropriate place in the file.

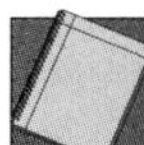

FROM THE EXPERT'S NOTEBOOK

"Out" guides can be very useful and can be purchased from a variety of vendors. They are plastic, chart-shaped guides that are inserted when a chart is pulled out. "Out" guides make it easy to return a chart to its correct place in the file without hesitation (Figure 5-6).

Correcting Errors

There is a right way and a wrong way to correct an error in a patient record. During an in-service session, the office manager should instruct the entire staff on the proper way to make corrections. To correct an error, a staff member should put a line through the mistake in ink, write in the correction near it, initial it, and date it. For legal purposes, the date is very important. It shows the date the correction was made, providing evidence that it was not made after a subpoena was served or a suit was filed. Any addenda should be acknowledged as such and dated. The appropriate time frame for inserting an addendum is generally not more than 1 week after the patient was treated. Most computer software packages have a correction function that runs a line through an error.

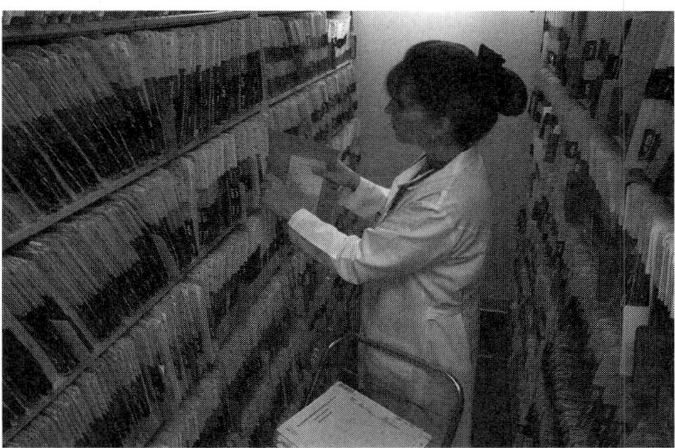

FIGURE 5-6. "Out" guides such as the ones pictured above can make refiling charts easier.

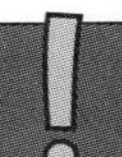

MANAGER'S ALERT

NEVER use "white-out" products for correcting errors. Government agencies and carriers performing audits will assume that you are trying to hide something.

Alterations of Medical Records

Don't even think about altering medical records! Any change made to a medical record could become a crucial part of a plaintiff's malpractice case. Many times, forgotten copies of records or portions of records will show any changes made to that record. Any missing pages or test results can and will suggest that the patient did not receive those services.

Patient Registration Form and Other Forms

The Patient Registration Form is one of the most important parts of the medical record. This form is used by every staff member. There is no such thing as too much information. A Patient Registration Form should include patient demographics, insurance and billing information, emergency information, and referring physician. Various companies provide preprinted forms for this purpose. Medical Arts Press and Colwell are two of the better-known companies. This form should be updated at each patient visit to ensure that all information is accurate. This can be done by simply asking patients when they arrive if any of the information has changed: "Is your address, phone number, and insurance still the same, Mrs. Goldenberg?" It is a good idea to have patients complete a new form yearly. Patient addresses, telephone numbers, and insurance information often change, and patients tend to assume that they have informed the office of these changes. If the office manager institutes a policy requiring that an updated form be completed every 6 months, there will be fewer problems with billing and contacting the patient. The office manager usually makes the secretary/receptionist responsible for implementing this policy, although it can also be assigned to the medical assistant or nurse, depending on the structure of the office. The important thing to remember is that someone must be held accountable for this task. A sample Patient Registration Form is presented in Figure 5-7.

Patients who receive Medicare must sign a Medicare Lifetime Signature Authorization, as shown in Figure 5-8. As a permanent part of the patient's chart, this form allows the office to bill Medicare continually. A sample Universal Authorization of Benefits Form (Figure 5-9) can be used for all patients.

Status and Purging of Medical Records

There are three types of medical records: current, inactive, and closed. *Current files* are files of patients who have been seen during the last year. *Inactive files* are of patients who have not been seen for more than a year. *Closed files* are files of patients who no longer come to the office because they have moved, are seeing another physician, or are deceased. Certain charts are generally purged from the mainstream of charts every year and filed in the inactive area of the filing system, which should be easily accessible for retrieval. The type of practice dictates the circumstances under which charts are to be purged. For instance, if a practice "recalls" patients every 3 years, charts would not be purged at the 2-year interval, but after 3 years. The charts should have year stickers on them, which can be purchased from Tab Products or any other company selling similar products. Some alphabetic color-coded stickers include the year. These color-coded year stickers help with purging and should be updated yearly as patients return to the office for treatment.

Storage of the Medical Record

Patient charts can be stored in several ways. The vertical two- or four-drawer cabinets are still in use, but in a limited fashion. They are being replaced with larger, open cabinets, which make it easier to use color-coding systems. The following four styles of file cabinets are commonly used in the medical office:

- Lateral file
- Shelf file
- Rotary file
- Vertical-drawer file

The style of file cabinet a medical office chooses depends on many factors, including cost, number of records, stage of medical practice, and space. The office manager will want to assess the office's present and future needs to determine the most appropriate type of filing cabinet.

The lateral file is generally found in the physician's or office manager's office. Lateral files use a fair amount of wall space, but they do not require as much room in front for extending drawers as vertical files do. Lateral files are made of wood, metal, or a composite; most furniture sets for offices have lateral files that match the desks and other furniture.

Because of their design, shelf files allow for more storage than do lateral files. Drawers do not pull out like conventional files. Shelves can assist the employee with the filing, because they can hold a large number of files. Files can be placed on the shelf when filing. Because of their design, more than one person at a time can use this filing system.

Rotary files are expensive and are generally used by offices with very limited space, offices with a high volume of patients, or new offices without previously existing files. They may also be used by an office that is moving. Files rotate in a circular motion and can be accessed by more than one person at a time.

PATIENT'S NAME: ______________________________

PATIENT'S ADDRESS: ______________________________

SEX: F M DATE OF BIRTH: ______________ SS#: ______________

MARITAL STATUS: S M D W

OCCUPATION: ______________________________

NAME OF EMPLOYER: ______________________________

EMPLOYER'S ADDRESS: ______________________________

EMPLOYER'S PHONE NUMBER: ______________________________

SPOUSE'S NAME: ______________________________

SPOUSE'S EMPLOYER: ______________________________

EMPLOYER'S ADDRESS: ______________________________

EMPLOYER'S PHONE NUMBER: ______________________________

REFERRED BY: ______________________________

RELATIONSHIP: ______________________________

PERSON TO NOTIFY IN CASE OF EMERGENCY: ______________________________

RELATIONSHIP: ______________ PHONE #: ______________

INSURANCE INFORMATION

PRIMARY INSURANCE COMPANY: ______________________________

ADDRESS: ______________________________

PHONE: ______________ GUARANTOR: ______________

ID #: ______________ GROUP #: ______________

SECONDARY INSURANCE COMPANY: ______________________________

ADDRESS: ______________________________

PHONE: ______________ GUARANTOR: ______________

ID #: ______________ GROUP #: ______________

FIGURE 5-7. Patient Registration Form.

______________________ ______________________

Name of beneficiary HIC number

I request that payment of authorized Medicare benefits be made to me or on my behalf to Dr. Babinetz for any services rendered by said physician. I authorize any holder of medical information about me to release to the Center For Medicare and Medicaid Services and its agents any information needed to determine these benefits or the benefits payable for related services.

I understand my signature requests that payment be made and authorizes release of medical information necessary to pay the claim. If Item 9 of the CMS 1500 claim form is completed, my signature authorizes releasing of needed information to:

Name of specific Medigap insurance company ______________________________

In Medicare assigned cases, the physician agrees to accept the charge determination of the Medicare carrier as the full charge, and the patient is responsible only for the deductible, co-insurance, and noncovered services. Co-insurance and the deductible are based upon the charge determination of the Medicare carrier.

______________________ ______________________

Beneficiary's signature Date

FIGURE 5-8. Medicare Lifetime Signature Authorization Form.

I request that payment of authorized Medicare and/or insurer benefits be made to me or on my behalf to Dr. Babinetz for services furnished to me by said physician. I authorize Dr. Babinetz to release to my insurance company any medical information needed to determine the benefits payable for related services.

I understand that if, under Medicare program guidelines, a necessary service is determined to be ineligible for benefits, I will personally be responsible for any amount denied or partially paid by the third-party payer.

_______________________ _______________________

Signature Date

I request that payment of authorized Medicare and/or insurance benefits be made either to me or on my behalf to Dr. Babinetz for any services furnished me by said physician. I authorize any holder of medical information about me to release to the Health Care Financing Administration and its agents any information needed to determine the benefits payable for related services.

_______________________ _______________________

Name of beneficiary HIC number

I request that payment of authorized Medigap benefits be made either to me or on my behalf to Dr. Babinetz. I authorize any holder of medical information about me to release to

Name of Medigap insurer _______________________

any information needed to determine benefits payable for related services.

Name of beneficiary _______________________

_______________________ _______________________

Medigap carrier Medigap policy number

Carrier's address _______________________

FIGURE 5-9. Universal Authorization of Benefits Form.

Vertical-drawer files should be used only when conditions are right. They do not take up wall space; however, they require a great amount of space in front so that each drawer can be fully extended to retrieve the files. Only one person at a time can access these files, and many filing cabinets have a safety mechanism that prevents the opening of a second drawer if one is already open.

PRESCRIPTION PADS

On October 1, 2007, legislation required that all drugs prescribed to patients with Medicaid be written on tamper-resistant prescription pads. This requirement was included in section 7002 (b) of the U.S. Troop Readiness, Veterans' Care, Katrina Recovery, and Iraq Accountability Appropriations Act of 2007.

In August 2007, the Centers for Medicare and Medicaid Services (CMS) issued a letter to the State Medicaid Directors regarding the implementation of the new requirement. The three basic requirements are as follows:

1. Prevent unauthorized copying of a completed or blank prescription form.
2. Prevent the erasure or modification of information written on the prescription by the prescriber.
3. Prevent the use of counterfeit prescription forms.

This requirement does not apply under the following circumstances:

- When the prescription is communicated by the prescriber to the pharmacy electronically, verbally, or by fax
- When a managed care entity will pay for the prescription
- When drugs are provided in certain institutional and clinical facilities

HEALTH HISTORY QUESTIONNAIRE

To avoid delay, please have all of your symptoms ready.

—ANONYMOUS

Some practices have their patients fill out a health history questionnaire (Figure 5-10) on their first visit to the office. This form can be modified for specific medical practice questions. The information provided on the completed health history questionnaire can be extremely helpful to the physician and office staff in determining the needs and problems of the patient. The questionnaire can be sent to a new patient before his or her first appointment and completed in advance of the visit to save time. Having the patient fill out the form at home improves patient flow.

Please circle the answer that seems best:

Yes No Do you need glasses to read or see far away?
Yes No Do you see better with one eye than the other?
Yes No Do you have any eye pain or blurred vision early in the morning?
Yes No Do you see haloes (circles) around lights?
Yes No Has your eyesight changed recently?
Yes No Are you having trouble with your hearing?
Yes No Have you ever had any discharge from your ear?
Yes No Have you ever had sneezing spells or frequent stuffiness of the nose?
Yes No Do you have frequent sore throats or hoarseness?
Yes No Do you have frequent nosebleeds?
Yes No Have you ever had tuberculosis or any other chest condition?
Yes No Have you ever had hay fever, asthma, hives, or any other allergic condition?
Yes No Have you ever had a close contact with a tuberculosis patient?
Yes No Do you have a cough?
Yes No If so, do you cough up phlegm?
Yes No Has your cough gotten worse in the last six months?
Yes No Have you ever had a wheeze?
Yes No Have you ever coughed up blood?
Yes No Have you ever had rheumatic fever, high blood pressure, or heart disease?
Yes No Have you ever had pain, tightness, or fullness in your chest?
Yes No Does your heart pound, skip, or miss beats?
Yes No Do you ever have distress, pain, or shortness of breath when walking?
Yes No Have your ankles ever swelled?
Yes No Do you smoke?
Yes No Have you ever smoked?
Yes No Do you need pillows or a wedge in order to sleep?
Yes No Do you suffer from severe headaches or pressure in the head?
Yes No Do you have dizzy spells or feel faint frequently?
Yes No Do you have cold hands or cold feet?
Yes No Do you have leg cramps when walking or lying in bed?
Yes No Is your appetite poor?
Yes No Do you have trouble swallowing?
Yes No Do you have indigestion, heartburn, belching, or stomach pain?
Yes No Have you ever vomited blood?
Yes No Have you ever had a stomach ulcer or duodenal ulcer?
Yes No Have your bowel movements or habits changed recently?
Yes No Do you have loose bowel movements?
Yes No Are you constipated?
Yes No Have you ever had bloody or tarry (black) bowel movements or blood on the toilet tissue?
Yes No Do you have hemorrhoids (piles)?
Yes No Were you ever anemic?
Yes No Do you bruise or bleed easily?
Yes No Do you have any pain, stiffness, or swelling in any muscles or joints?
Yes No Do you have trouble with your back?
Yes No Are you bothered by itching?
Yes No Have you had rashes or boils?
Yes No Do you have numbness, tingling, or weakness in any part of your body?
Yes No Were you ever unconscious or paralyzed?
Yes No Have you ever had fits or convulsions?
Yes No Are you passing urine more often than usual during the day or night?
Yes No Have you had bloody urine?
Yes No Have you had cloudy urine?
Yes No Have you had any pain or burning sensation while urinating?

FIGURE 5-10. Health history questionnaire. (Courtesy of Gastrointestinal Specialists, Inc.)

(*Continued*)

Yes	No	Do you sometimes lose control of your bladder, especially when coughing or sneezing?
Yes	No	Were you ever treated for syphilis, gonorrhea, or another venereal disease?
Yes	No	Do you prefer warm weather to cold weather?
Yes	No	Do you prefer cold weather to warm weather?
Yes	No	Are you ever unusually hungry or thirsty?
Yes	No	Have you ever had a goiter?
Yes	No	Have you ever had any operations, broken bones, or a serious injury?
Yes	No	Have you gained more than five pounds in the last six months?
Yes	No	Have you lost more than five pounds in the last six months?
Yes	No	Have you noticed any lumps, growths, or sores?
Yes	No	Do you take medicines, laxatives, vitamins, or other pills?
Yes	No	Do you take two or more alcoholic drinks, including beer and wine, a day?
Yes	No	Have you ever had a hernia or rupture?
Yes	No	Have you ever been turned down for life insurance, employment, or the military?
Yes	No	Do you make friends easily?
Yes	No	Are you a nervous person?
Yes	No	Is it hard for you to make up your mind?
Yes	No	Do you often feel tired?
Yes	No	Do you sleep poorly?
Yes	No	Do you often feel unhappy or depressed?
Yes	No	Have you ever had a nervous breakdown?
Yes	No	Have you ever seen a psychiatrist?
Yes	No	Have you taken hard drugs, such as heroin or cocaine?
Yes	No	Have you ever smoked marijuana?
Men Only:		
Yes	No	Has there been any change in your urinary stream in starting, strength of flow, or emptying?
Yes	No	Have you ever had any discharge or bleeding from your penis?
Women Only:		
Yes	No	Are you having hot flashes or flushes?
Date of last menstrual period? ____________		
Usual number of days of period? ________		
Usual number of days between periods? ________		
Yes	No	If your periods have stopped, have you had any vaginal bleeding since then?
Yes	No	Do you have any pain or discomfort with your periods, bleed between periods or too heavily with periods, or have irregular periods?
Yes	No	Have you ever had a vaginal discharge?
Yes	No	Have you ever noticed any lumps in your breasts or discharge from your nipples?
Yes	No	Are you now pregnant?
Yes	No	Have you ever been pregnant?
Yes	No	Have you ever had any trouble with any of your pregnancies?
Yes	No	Are you currently taking birth control pills?
(Courtesy of Gastrointestinal Specialists, Inc.)		

FIGURE 5-10 (CONTINUED). Health history questionnaire. (Courtesy of Gastrointestinal Specialists, Inc.)

In addition, by completing the form at home, the patient will take more time with it, and the information provided by the patient is much more thorough. In any event, the health history questionnaire is an integral part of the patient's chart.

FAMILY AND THE MEDICAL RECORD

Any medical receptionist will tell you that the first words the patient hears when he or she returns to the waiting room from the physician's office are, "Well, what did he say?"

A note about my patient . . . .

Alexander Babinetz, M.D.

Patient's diagnosis

____

____

Plan of treatment

____

____

____

____

____

____

FIGURE 5-11. Patient family update note.

These words are spoken by family members who have been waiting for the patient. The office manager should educate the physician to this situation so that it can be handled to everyone's satisfaction. If family members are not satisfied with the answers they are receiving from the patient, they often ask the staff to disrupt the physician's office hours and come out to speak with them. The disruption of office hours is what all good office managers need to prevent! One way to eliminate this need is to provide the patient with a note specifying a brief diagnosis and treatment plan. After reading this note, the family members would have less need to disrupt the physician's schedule and there would be no miscommunication from the patient.

Many patients bring family members into the physician's inner office to hear what the physician has to say. However, if this does not occur, using the note can save many hassles in the course of a day. The office manager can design a note (Figure 5-11) and keep a pad of them on the physician's desk for easy accessibility.

Many times patients without the company of family members need the assistance of office staff for such issues as completing forms. An example of this can be seen in Figure 5-12.

MISCELLANEOUS FILES

Hospital Records

Some offices prefer to keep their hospital records separate from their office records. This can be done by using a separate filing cabinet or by using colored folders. For example, all hospital documents could be filed in red folders, with patients in alphabetic order.

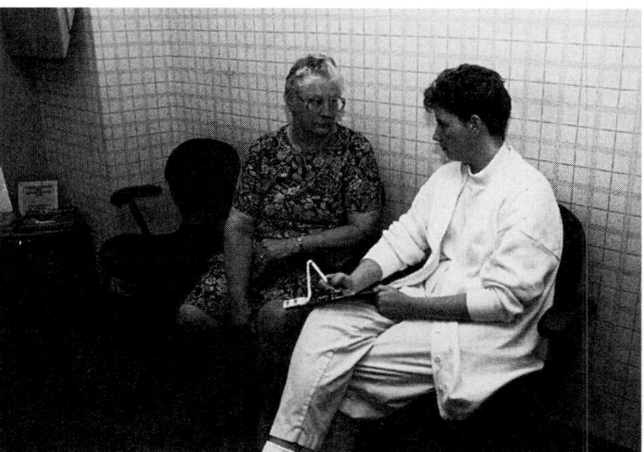

FIGURE 5-12. The secretary helps a patient fill out the patient information form.

Other Records

A separate file can be kept for miscellaneous filing, such as patient records that come into the office before the patient. These records are filed in the miscellaneous file until the patient calls or appears for an appointment. Alternatively, some offices choose to make up a patient chart as soon as records come to the office. This way, the chart is ready when the patient comes in. One problem with this approach is that many patients do not follow their referring doctor's orders and decide not to see the physician. The office is then stuck with a medical chart that will not be used. It is difficult to keep track of this type of file because of the number of patients seen in a typical physician's office. The office manager should assess the situation and institute a policy as to how these records should be handled.

SHOP AROUND

Box 5-2 lists several vendors from which the office manager can purchase the necessary supplies for the front office. Many vendors exist for every type of product. The wise office manager contacts several to check on pricing, availability, and service before deciding which company to deal with. Even though it might be easier to use the local office supply store, it is not always the most cost-effective approach. One of the office manager's main goals is to contain costs while maintaining quality care and increasing profitability. The process of contacting various vendors should be done every 6 months in order to maintain cost containment measures. Most vendors have toll-free numbers or Web sites for customers to access. Don't hesitate to call these vendors to ask for pricing. Many will offer an additional discount to secure your business. Ask them . . . you might be surprised by the answer!

BOX 5-2 Vendors/Suppliers of Office Products

Tab Products
935 Lakeview Parkway, Suite 195
Vernon Hills, IL 60061
(800) 672-3109

Veriad (Labels)
650 Columbia Street
P.O. Box 2216
Brea, CA 92622
(800) 423-4643

Colwell Systems
201 Kenyon Road
P.O. Box 9024
Champaign, IL 61820
(800) 637-1140

Medical Arts Press
8500 Wyoming Avenue North
Minneapolis, MN 55445
(800) 328-2179

Safeguard Business Systems
8585 Stemmons Freeway
Dallas, TX 75247
(800) 338-0636

Bibbero Systems, Inc.
1300 North McDowell Blvd.
Petaluma, CA 94952
(800) 242-2376

EXERCISES

MULTIPLE CHOICE

Choose the best *answer for each of the following questions.*

1. Which of the following is *not* a user of the medical record?
   a. Physician
   b. Clinical researchers
   c. Reimbursement technicians
   d. Copier repair technician
2. Which of the following would *not* be found in a medical record?
   a. Genealogic information
   b. Laboratory studies
   c. Progress notes
   d. Operative reports
3. Which of the following is an obstacle to an EMR?
   a. Cost
   b. Downtime for training
   c. Accessibility
   d. All of the above
4. Dictation was started by which group of people?
   a. Egyptians
   b. Mexicans
   c. Babylonians
   d. Romans
5. Which of the following is relevant to patient dictation?
   a. Speak slowly
   b. Speak clearly
   c. Spell unusual words or names
   d. Patient's eye color
6. Color-coding chart schemes can be based on
   a. An alphabetic system
   b. A numeric system
   c. All of the above
   d. None of the above
7. Which of the following is *not* the right way to correct a medical record error?
   a. Draw a single line through it
   b. "White" it out
   c. Place the date by the error
   d. Put your initials by the error
8. What should patients sign to ensure that they have authorized their Medicare benefits for payment for life?
   a. Medicaid Lifetime Signature Authorization Form
   b. Medicare Lifetime Signature Authorization Form
   c. Authorization of Benefits for Life
   d. None of the above
9. Types of medical records include which of the following?
   a. Current
   b. Piled
   c. Inactive
   d. Active
10. Which is *not* a style of filing cabinets?
    a. Front
    b. Vertical
    c. Lateral
    d. Rotary
11. Which is *not* a way that a subpoena is served?
    a. By the local sheriff
    b. Regular mail
    c. Certified mail
    d. FedEx overnight
12. Which of the following is an advantage of an EMR?
    a. Files are retrieved faster.
    b. Analysis reporting is easier.
    c. The chart cannot be lost.
    d. All of the above.
13. The average cost of maintaining an EMR is
    a. $575 per year
    b. $575 per month
    c. $8,500 per year
    d. $2,400 per month
14. EMRs contain such nursing information as
    a. Vital signs
    b. Nursing assessments

c. Patient acuity levels
d. All of the above

15. Which of the following is *not* a benefit of an EMR?
    a. Reduced labor costs
    b. Inexpensive
    c. Improved documentation
    d. Improved coding
16. Which of the following is asking vendors to respond with a proposal?
    a. LMP
    b. RFP
    c. CDC
    d. CMP
17. Which of the following is a technology for dictation?
    a. PSS
    b. VRT
    c. DRD
    d. DVD
18. Which of the following is a documentation format?
    a. MORE
    b. CED
    c. SOAP
    d. WASH
19. For a deceased patient, the records should be maintained for how many years after death?
    a. 5
    b. 6
    c. 7
    d. There is no set number
20. Signature stamps cannot be used on
    a. Insurance forms
    b. Membership applications
    c. Note for children to return to school
    d. Prescriptions

TRUE OR FALSE

1. ____ All laboratory and x-ray studies should be signed or initialed by the physician after review.
2. ____ Labels should never be used on the outside of a patient's chart.
3. ____ The original medical record can be mailed to the courts for review.
4. ____ One obstacle to an EMR is "downtime" for training.
5. ____ Most people are resistant to change.
6. ____ It is not necessary to include a submittal date in an RFP.
7. ____ The Egyptians were the first to use dictation.
8. ____ Illegibility is never a problem with handwritten medical records.
9. ____ Highlighters can be used to draw attention to important information in the medical record.
10. ____ Paper in dark colors should be used for office forms.
11. ____ "Out" guides are used to track employees who have left the office for lunch.
12. ____ The health history questionnaire should be completed each time the patient sees the doctor.
13. ____ The office manager should consider cost when purchasing equipment and supplies.
14. ____ The subjective part of the patient encounter is the examination.
15. ____ An authorization of benefits form does not need to be signed by Medicare patients if they signed a lifetime authorization.
16. ____ Charts are never misplaced.
17. ____ You can always change a medical record.
18. ____ You must date and sign a corrected error.
19. ____ Color can be useful in filing.
20. ____ A lateral file is a type of filing cabinet.

THINKERS

1. Define RFP and explain how it is used by the office manager.
2. A clinical assistant has entered incorrect information into a patient's chart. She has used correction fluid, written "mistake" beside it, and initialed it. Is this the correct way to handle an error? If not, how should the correction be made?
3. Signature stamps can be very useful in a medical practice. They can also be a liability. Please explain and offer examples.
4. An office manager of a pediatric practice has purged medical records on patients who have "outgrown" a pediatrician. What should be done with the records and why?

REFERENCES

Evaluation and Management Coding and Documentation Guide. Reston, VA: St. Anthony Publishing, November 2002.

Gerber, P., & Bijiefeld, M. "Medical Records: Make Sure Yours Are Trouble-Proof." *Physician's Management,* May 1993, pp. 57-76.

Gerber, P., & Bijiefeld, M. "The Medical Chart." *Physician's Management,* February 1992, pp. 42-51.

Gragg, E. "Filing Systems Evolve as Office Technology Advances." *The Office,* July 1993, pp. 12-14.

Miller, RH. "Rapid Electronic Health Record Use for Quality Improvement in Community Health Centers." *Commonwealth Fund,* University of California, 2007.

O'Donnell, W. "Your Patient Isn't the Only One Who Needs a Diagnosis." *Medical Economics,* May 18, 1992, pp. 119-123.

6

BILLING, CODING, AND COLLECTIONS

CHAPTER OUTLINE

CHAPTER OBJECTIVES

After completing this chapter, you will be able to do the following:

- Define the various types of health care insurance companies in the United States
- Identify the components of health insurance, including precertification, second opinion, advance beneficiary notice, superbills, CPT codes, insurance claims, and billing
- Use the ICD-9-CM codebook for accurate billing and reimbursement
- Understand how to use the CPT and HCPCS code books
- Comprehend the Medicare appeal process

- Know how to follow-up on claims denials
- Know how to complete the CMS 1500 form
- Determine what services should be billed "incident-to"
- Understand the life cycle of a claim and explanation of benefits
- Understand billing policy and practices for office visits, Medicare secondary payer, locum tenens, hospice care, "incident to" services, Medicare chiropractic services, credit card payments, and commercial billing services
- Identify the legal and ethical issues related to billing and collection practices
- Develop medical office forms related to billing and collection

INSURANCE

Health insurance was developed in 1694 by Hugh Chamberlen. It began as a disability insurance, because it only covered medical expenses arising from injuries that could lead to disability of the patient. In the twentieth century, traditional disability insurance as we know it evolved, and our medical insurance consists of payment for physician and hospital services, emergency department care, preventive medicine services, and, in some cases, prescription drugs.

Health insurance is a complex subject. Our past holds an unprecedented wave of mergers, acquisitions, and alliances among health care providers, insurers, managed care organizations, and patients. The reason for all of this business activity in the health care field is the growing numbers of uninsured and the increasing burden of health care costs on the federal budget. As politicians struggle to find a solution to the growing health care crisis, the media report on an almost daily basis the plight of the uninsured and the underinsured. A system that is equitable for all, as well as efficient, integrated, value driven, and accountable, is needed. This is the challenge that will be faced in the future.

The changes taking place in the health care industry are affecting medical offices in many ways. It is important for medical office managers to understand these trends so that they can make intelligent management decisions. Adapting to these changes as easily as possible will ensure the financial strength of the medical office. In the past, it was easy for physicians and their staff to be knowledgeable about the different health insurances, because there were fewer insurances than we have today. Now there are countless insurance carriers, each offering multiple plans. This has created havoc in the business office of the medical practice and has made it impossible for medical office staff to know the extent of each patient's coverage unless they call each patient's insurance company and verify the patient's insurance.

A health insurance policy is a renewable contract between the insurance company and the patient. Patients with health insurance may be required to pay some "out-of-pocket" fees. Most patients are responsible for a co-pay amount that is the responsibility of the patient to pay to the physician for each service or procedure. Some health insurance companies even offer rewards to patients for not smoking, losing weight, eating diets low in cholesterol, and other health-promoting behaviors.

According to the Census Bureau of the United States, approximately 15% of Americans do not have health insurance. Approximately 60% of individuals get their health insurance through their employer, although these plans have changed throughout the years. In the past, employee health insurance covered not only the employee, but the employee's family as well. There was little or no out-of-pocket expense that had to be picked up by the employee. Unfortunately, employers have made business decisions that cut the benefits of employees. For the most part, they no longer cover their employees' family members, and they are turning to less expensive plans such as managed care plans for their employees' coverage. Generally, medical offices (and other small businesses) with fewer than 10 employees do not offer health insurance benefits. Employers state cost as the reason for this decision.

Managed care insurance has grown from 25% to the majority of employer-based health insurance coverage. For example, in 1999, conventional insurance plans made up 10% of the insurances in the United States. Health maintenance organizations (HMOs) made up 28%, preferred provider organizations (PPOs) made up 39%, and point-of-service (POS) plans made up 24%. In 2006, conventional insurance plans went from 10% to 5%, HMOs went from 39% to 20%, PPOs went from 39% to 60%, and POS plans went from 24% to 13%.

Types of Health Insurance

Insurance companies are divided into six general categories:

1. Commercial insurance
2. Medicare

3. Medicaid
4. The Civilian Health and Medical Program for the Uniformed Services (TRICARE/CHAMPUS)
5. Managed care
   a. Health maintenance organizations (HMOs)
   b. Preferred provider organizations (PPOs)
   c. Physician-hospital organizations (PHOs)
   d. Point-of-service (POS) plans
6. Blue Cross/Blue Shield

In the past, companies covered 100% of the costs incurred from illness or injury, and individuals received this insurance coverage in the way of a benefit from their employer. This benefit usually covered employees and their families. In most practices today, third-party payers (insurance companies) are responsible for 75% to 90% of the reimbursements. However, few insurance companies today cover the entire medical costs of a patient. In addition, there are more than 42 million people in the United States with no insurance coverage, and many persons whose job provides insurance only for them, not for their families, and who must pay for insurance for their families. Understanding how the insurance system works is an important role of a medical office manager, the staff, and the physician. Many communities today have free clinics for patients who do not have any type of health care coverage.

COMMERCIAL INSURANCE

There are many different commercial insurance companies in the United States (e.g., Travelers, Prudential, Guardian, Metropolitan, and Connecticut General). These insurance companies generally write policies for groups. Some employers use commercial insurances to provide insurance for their employees. Each employee group can have different regulations, so it is always necessary to call the insurance company (the phone number should be on the member's card) to verify coverage and policies.

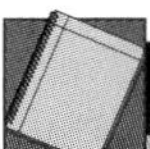

FROM THE EXPERT'S NOTEBOOK

Many commercial insurance companies offer both fee-for-service and managed care plans. Be careful to check the member's card to verify the coverage and any limitations that may apply.

MEDICARE

Medicare, a national health insurance program, was created by President Lyndon B. Johnson on July 30, 1965 (it went into effect in 1966) and covered people who are either 65 years of age or older, or who meet the criteria for a special situation. President Harry S. Truman was the first Medicare beneficiary enrolled into this newly formed health insurance plan. Medicare consists of four parts: A, B, C, and D. Medicare Part A covers the hospital expenses of the patient, some nursing facilities, hospice care, and home health. The patient pays a deductible but does not pay a premium. Any individual who receives Social Security payments is automatically enrolled in Medicare Part A. This is a benefit for senior citizens and the disabled, and is financed through the Social Security program. Part B is optional, but is selected by most because of its coverage and cost to the insured. There is a lifetime penalty of 10% per year that is imposed for not taking Medicare Part B when the beneficiary is not working. This coverage includes physician services, outpatient procedures, immunizations, laboratory and x-ray services, chemotherapy, and renal dialysis. Part B also covers durable medical equipment, such as walkers, wheelchairs, canes, and so on. This program primarily serves older patients; however, about 1 in every 10 Medicare patients is disabled and younger than 65. Some disabled and younger patients who qualify can draw on Medicare benefits. It is made up of monies provided through payroll taxes and self-employment taxes paid by all persons covered under the program. Employers are also taxed.

Medicare Part C covers the Medicare Advantage plans. The Balanced Budget Act of 1997 gave Medicare beneficiaries the option to receive their Medicare benefits through private health insurance plans, instead of through the original Medicare plans of Part A and Part B. These programs were called Medicare + Choice or Part C plans. As a result of the Medicare Prescription Drug, Improvement, and Modernization Act of 2003, the compensation and business practices changed and Medicare + Choice became known as Medicare Advantage (MA) plans. These plans offer comparable coverage to Part A and Part B, and also offer Part D coverage, which went into effect on January 1, 2006.

Medicare Part D is available through two types of private plans: the Medicare Advantage plan and the Prescription Drug plan. Annual enrollment for Medicare Part D begins November 15 of each year. Multiple prescription drug plans are available, and many beneficiaries find them confusing. Beneficiaries can be directed to an interactive tool on the Medicare Web site called "The Prescription Drug Plan Finder." This finder shows comparisons of the various different plans in each geographic area. Medicare Part D is not standardized. For beneficiaries who are dually eligible (Medicare and Medicaid), Medicaid will pay for drugs not covered by Medicare Part D, such as benzodiazepines, barbiturates, prescription vitamins, and other substances.

Medicare Part B covers 80% of outpatient and physician expenses and must be paid for by the patient in monthly premiums. This part of Medicare is financed by contributions from the federal government in addition to the monthly premium paid by the patient. This is the part of Medicare that covers physician services; therefore this is the part of Medicare that should be understood by medical office personnel.

Medicare pays for the following medical services:

- Office visits
- Hospital visits
- Therapies
- Surgeries
- Diagnostic procedures
- Consultations

To be a "covered" Medicare service, the physician or physician extender, such as a physician assistant, must either treat the patient in person or evaluate the patient's condition using technology. In other words, the physician or physician extender must actually examine the patient in a face-to-face setting or interpret a study such as an electrocardiogram (ECG) or x-ray. This is called *direct visualization* (*Medicare Carriers Manual 2020*).

Medicare Definitions

Medicare commonly calls patients *beneficiaries.* Medicare considers the following to be physicians: doctor of medicine, doctor of osteopathy, doctor of dental medicine, doctor of podiatric medicine, doctor of optometry, and doctor of chiropractic medicine.

Many patients do not understand the difference between Medicare Part A and Part B. They also do not realize that they have to pay for Part B coverage. They assume that the card that is sent to them from the Social Security Administration covers all of their medical needs. It is the office manager's responsibility to ensure that the medical biller in the office can adequately explain the difference between the two forms of coverage to these patients and advise them that they might want to carry some additional insurance to cover the 20% of expenses not covered by Medicare Part B. Many patients carry private supplemental insurance to cover the 20% balance. Medicare Part B has a yearly deductible, which generally increases each year. This deductible is the patient's responsibility and must be paid by the patient every year. It is the responsibility of the office staff to make a serious attempt to collect this deductible; failure to do so can result in fines to the physician. Most of the supplemental insurances that patients have do not cover the patient's deductible. A sample Medicare card is shown in Figure 6-1. It is important to note the difference on the card between hospital coverage (Part A) and medical coverage (Part B).

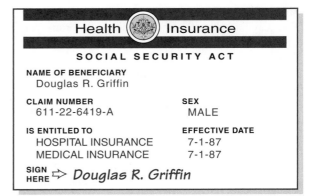

Health Insurance

SOCIAL SECURITY ACT

NAME OF BENEFICIARY
Douglas R. Griffin

CLAIM NUMBER	SEX
611-22-6419-A	MALE
IS ENTITLED TO	EFFECTIVE DATE
HOSPITAL INSURANCE	7-1-87
MEDICAL INSURANCE	7-1-87

SIGN HERE ⇨ Douglas R. Griffin

FIGURE 6-1. Sample Medicare card. (From Kinn, M.E. *The Administrative Medical Assistant,* 4th ed. Philadelphia: W.B. Saunders, 1999.)

What about Medicare HMOs?

Medicare HMOs more closely resemble HMOs than traditional Medicare contracts. The Centers for Medicare and Medicaid Services (CMS) is the largest user of managed care and offers two options:

1. Risk contract
2. Cost contract

In a *risk contract,* a calculation is based on the fee schedule and costs in the county the HMO serves and pays 95% of the average adjusted per capita cost. In a *cost contract,* the payment is based on the actual cost that is incurred by the practice and is generally the most expensive contract for CMS. The majority of the HMOs currently used are risk contract. The biggest complaint of Medicare HMOs is payment of emergency services. Patients go to the emergency department for care of what they believe is an emergency, the claim is submitted to their Medicare HMO, and then the claim is denied because the HMO rules that it was not a "true" emergency.

Who Pays?

The most common payment rules for Medicare HMOs are as follows:

- Medicare HMOs are supposed to pay for emergency services given to their patients, whether the physician is participating or not. However, the definition of an "emergency" is determined by the Medicare HMO and not the patient. What the patient believes is an emergency may not be considered an emergency by the HMO and therefore would not be covered.
- The Medicare rule against charging and accepting less from an insurer doesn't apply when it comes to managed care.
- If a patient switches from regular Medicare into an HMO and is hospitalized when the HMO plan takes effect, the carrier responsible for paying the claim depends on the type of hospital and whether or not it participates in that particular HMO.

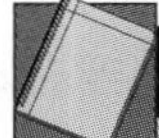

FROM THE EXPERT'S NOTEBOOK

Contact the carriers that are most commonly used for Medicare HMOs by your patients. Ask for your representative to come to the office to describe all the details of the plan with the billing staff so that claims can be submitted properly. Even though the Internet could possibly provide the office with the answers being sought, nothing beats a face-to-face meeting with the representative.

Medicare Carriers

It is sometimes necessary for physician practices to contact Medicare carriers with billing and coding questions. Appendix B contains a listing of Medicare carriers by state should you need to contact them.

MEDICAID

In 1965, the federal government, in association with the individual state governments, established a health care coverage known as Medicaid. This insurance covers some of the costs of medical care and medicines for medically indigent individuals. There are guidelines that must be met to qualify for this insurance. Individuals admitted to hospitals with no insurance benefits often qualify for this service. Applications are made through the admissions office at the hospital in an attempt to aid the individual in paying for her or his care. Medicaid is the fastest growing spending program in the United States today.

TRICARE/CHAMPUS

In 1956, CHAMPUS was created to cover the medical needs of military personnel and their families. TRICARE is the name for the health care plan formerly known as CHAMPUS. This insurance covered the fees of civilian physicians to treat any illness or injury of military dependents. Tricare consists of the following plans:

- TRICARE Prime—managed care
- TRICARE Extra—preferred provider option (PPO)
- TRICARE Standard—fee for service
- TRICARE for Life—Medicare-type product

TRICARE Prime is a managed care plan that is modeled after HMOs and is for active duty and retired uniformed services members and their families. Active duty service members are required to enroll in Prime. Others, such as retired service members and the family members of all uniformed services members, are encouraged to enroll in Prime. TRICARE prime is not offered in all areas, however, so the local TRICARE service center (TSC) should be contacted to see if it is available in your area. Enrollees have less out-of-pocket expenses with TRICARE Prime than with any of the other products.

TRICARE Extra and TRICARE Standard are available for all TRICARE-eligible beneficiaries who elect to not enroll in prime, or who are not able to enroll in prime because of geographic location. Active duty service members are not allowed to enroll in Extra or Standard. TRICARE Extra is a PPO in which beneficiaries may choose a doctor, hospital, or other medical provider within the TRICARE provider network. TRICARE Standard is a fee-for-service plan, in which members can see any provider of their choice. The out-of-pocket expenses for the Standard plan is more than for the Extra plan.

TRICARE for Life is a product that is similar to Medicare in that it can be used by military personnel over age 65, who are eligible for Medicare Part A, and who must purchase Part B. This plan acts as a secondary payer to Medicare.

MANAGED CARE (HMOs, PPOs, AND PHOs)

In 1973, the HMO was created as the first managed care insurance concept. HMOs consist of members who prepay for health insurance benefits. Most HMOs require a minimal payment at the time of service. This minimal payment ranges from $2 to $20, depending on the organization and the plan. HMOs require that their patients see a primary physician before setting up an appointment with a specialist. These primary physicians (called *gatekeepers*) must authorize any referrals for testing or specialists. Their patients must *always* obtain a referral before seeing a specialist or seeking a test. A set fee is then paid to the gatekeeper for services rendered, and any balance must be written off.

A PPO is a group of hospitals, physicians, and/or pharmacies that contracts on a discounted fee-for-service basis with employers, insurance carriers, or third-party administrators. PPOs provide services to subscribers at 10% to 20% below usual fees. A PHO is a legal entity that combines physicians and hospitals into a single organization for the purpose of obtaining payer contracts. In a PHO, the physicians remain owners of their practices, but they accept managed care patients under the terms of the contract.

Any physician's office has the right to refuse treatment to an HMO or PPO member who arrives without a referral in hand. A specialist who decides to treat a patient who does not have a referral would be wise to have the patient sign a release stating that if the patient cannot obtain a referral within 1 week, she or he will be responsible for this bill (Figure 6-2). The patient may be billed only if she or he signs this release. Otherwise, the office, as a participating HMO/PPO office, cannot bill the patient for the service.

It is important for the medical office manager to check with each individual HMO and PPO to clearly understand its rules and regulations. Some plans allow the physician's office to bill the patient if she or he does not produce a referral. Some allow the office to bill the patient only if it has obtained the aforementioned signed release from the patient. The letter shown in Figure 6-3 can be used in follow-up to the patient. In an attempt to avoid referral problems, the medical office staff can give each patient who has managed care insurance a letter explaining the office policy on payment and referrals (Figure 6-4).

One important aspect of managed care organizations for office managers to be aware of are *hold harmless clauses.* Hold harmless clauses affect the liability risks and reimbursements. Some hold harmless clauses can limit the physician reimbursement to the fee paid by the managed care organization. Physicians are not allowed to "balance bill" patients for charges that exceed the fee schedule of the carrier. *Balance billing* is defined as billing the patient for the balance after the insurance carrier has paid its portion of the bill. Other hold harmless clauses are more worrisome. They can shift the liability for damages in malpractice situations from

When an HMO or PPO member does not have a referral from his or her primary physician, the patient's signature on this release preserves the physician's right to bill the patient for the servces.

Date: ____________________

Name: ________________________________

I understand that if I am not able to obtain a referral for this visit, I will be responsible for full payment of this service.

I also understand that I have 2 weeks from this date to obtain provide this office with a referral.

Signature: ____

FIGURE 6-2. Release form for HMO or PPO patient who doesn't have a referral.

Date: ______________

Dear ______________:

Our records indicate that we have not yet received your promised referral. As you know, you must always obtain a referral from your primary physician before scheduling an appointment with our office.

According to your insurance plan, if you do not obtain a referral from your primary physician before coming to our office, it is then your responsibility to either obtain a referral within ten (10) days of your visit or pay for the visit yourself.

We have waited patiently for your referral to arrive in our mail, but, as of the date of this letter, we have not received it.

This bill is now your responsibility, and we expect payment of $___________ in the mail to our office as soon as possible. Failure to pay will result in a transfer of your account to our collection agency.

Sincerely,

Janet Casey
Office Manager

FIGURE 6-3. Letter to unreferred HMO or PPO patient requesting payment for services.

To Our HMO Patients:

Your insurance company requires that when you are seeking care from a specialist's office, such as ours, you must first obtain a referral from your primary physician. You need to have this referral with you when you arrive at the specialist's office.

These referrals are essential to facilitate our billing process, and without them we cannot complete that process. Many of our patients forget to bring their referrals with them at the time of their visit, and this presents a problem. Most insurance companies are very strict regarding their policies and procedures, and many times they will not allow referrals to be backdated or to be issued after the time of the office visit.

We request that you help us to avoid this problem by remembering that referrals are required. Regrettably, we will have to reschedule your office visit if these forms are not presented to our receptionist at your time of check-in.

We appreciate your cooperation in this matter, and if you have any questions regarding this letter, please feel free to contact our billing department located at our office at 3 Centre Street. We would also like to take this opportunity to let you know that your business is greatly appreciated, and our staff enjoys working with you on your road to recovery and superior health.

Sincerely,

Barbara Braun
Billing Manager

FIGURE 6-4. Letter explaining office policy on referrals.

the insurer to the physicians. Physicians have to assume full responsibility even if the plan was partly or wholly at fault because of utilization review decisions. There are other hold harmless clauses that give the managed care organization the right to perform background checks on its physicians. The problem with this is that the managed care organization can then release this information, without any liability, to others. It is important to have the practice attorney review all contracts before signing.

BLUE CROSS/BLUE SHIELD

Blue Cross was established in the 1930s to cover the care of the patient in the hospital setting. In 1939, its sister coverage, Blue Shield, was established to cover physician and outpatient services. These insurance companies provide medical insurance under several different plans. Some plans are designed for patients with income limits, and others make the patient responsible for a small balance. If the physician's office is a participating office in Blue Cross/Blue Shield, any balance above the approved amount must be written off. Nonparticipating physicians are allowed to bill the patient for the balance.

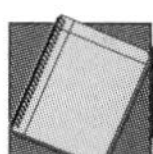

FROM THE EXPERT'S NOTEBOOK

Never attempt to guess which insurance plan a patient has. There are many regional and local plans that have different requirements. Always look at the member's card and call the carrier to verify the insurance plan and coverage.

Components of Insurance Coverage

MEDICAL

Medical insurance coverage pays the cost of services performed by a physician or an outpatient service. Outpatient services can be performed in an independent facility, the physician's office, or the hospital. These services can be office visits, x-ray examinations, laboratory tests, and physical therapy. Many plans require second opinions, and the insurance company should always be notified before further treatment is given.

SURGICAL

Surgical insurance coverage pays the surgeon's fees for any surgical procedure that the patient might require, such as an appendectomy, resetting of a fractured bone, removal of a gangrenous limb, and so on. Some plans require precertification on certain procedures. The medical office should call each insurance company to check on its rules.

HOSPITALIZATION

Hospitalization insurance coverage pays the costs incurred in a hospital setting. These are costs for room and board, pharmaceutical supplies, and medical supplies used by patients during their stay. Some plans have limitations on the number of days they cover. Each insurance plan is different and must be checked by the medical office before it admits a patient to the hospital.

MAJOR MEDICAL

Major medical coverage protects the patient from catastrophic medical bills. It is a supplement to the medical and surgical coverages and pays the balances for medical services rendered. This type of coverage keeps the patient's out-of-pocket expenses down.

Precertification/Second Opinion

Many insurance carriers require precertification of hospitalization and of certain procedures. The patient's insurance card generally indicates the type of plan the patient is carrying. The card identifies as to whether the patient is responsible for a co-pay, whether the plan calls for a second opinion, and whether the patient must obtain precertification. To save time on insurance billing, photocopy the front and back of the patient's insurance card and place the photocopy in the patient's chart or on the back of the patient's ledger card, if that is the type of system you are using. Often the physician will instruct the office to admit to the hospital a patient who is not in the office at that time. This can be done quickly and efficiently if the photocopy of the card is in the office. The office personnel can easily check on eligibility and the need for precertification without having to have the patient there. If the plan requires either precertification or a second opinion and the physician's office does not obtain this, the physician will not be paid for her or his services. When calling the insurance company to obtain precertification, have available the following information:

- Patient demographics (i.e., address, phone number, date of birth, type of insurance, etc.)
- Treatment plan
- Signs
- Symptoms
- Diagnosis

PATIENTS AND THEIR INSURANCE

Many patients are unsure of their insurance coverage. Most believe that they have coverage for everything and don't understand such things as a noncovered service or a co-pay. Even though each member of an insurance plan is provided with a manual that explains the member's specific plan, many will either not read the manual, or they will read it and not understand it. This now becomes another area where the physician's office can be of assistance.

The front desk staff members are generally well versed in the various insurance plans, and if they are dealing with a plan that they are unfamiliar with, they will either check with their colleagues in billing or call the insurance company to get answers. A letter giving patients instructions regarding insurance matters can also be helpful to some practices (Figure 6-5). Our health care system is now recognizing the needs of the patient consumer and is providing more thorough information.

Patient consumers are looking for information to help them make informed decisions about their personal health care. This new consumer can have a major impact on health care costs; the more informed that patient consumers are the more they understand the pros and cons of their insurance plans. The Blue Cross and Blue Shield Association released information from its Consumer Preferences and Usage of Healthcare Information on 2005 data, indicating that 64% of patient consumers said it was important to be able to get information about health care questions from sources other than their personal physician; 88% of these patient consumers said that if they were diagnosed with a medical condition they would search for information about treatment options, and 81% said they would search for information on their own about physicians or hospitals that could provide treatment.

This information also revealed interesting statistics regarding the use of the Internet by patients. According to this information, 8 in 10 Internet users go online for health information. The type of information accessed and the percent of patients accessing this information are listed in Table 6-1.

TABLE 6-1 Percent of Internet Users Accessing Health Information on the Web

TYPE OF INQUIRY	PERCENT OF PATIENTS IN 2006
Medicare or Medicaid Web site	13%
Health insurance	28%
Specific physician or hospital	29%
Drugs (over-the-counter and prescription)	37%
Certain medical treatments or procedures	51%
Specific diseases or medical problems	64%
Diet, nutrition, vitamins or supplements	49%

Data from Blue Cross/Blue Shield, *Medical Cost Reference Guide*, "Engaging and Empowering Consumers: Accessing Health Information," 2006.

ADVANCE BENEFICIARY NOTICE (ABN)

The advance beneficiary notice (ABN) was developed to protect Medicare patients from liability for services rendered that may or may not be medically necessary. When

To All Our Patients:
We welcome you as a new patient to our office and are happy to extend to you every possible courtesy. To avoid billing and insurance problems, we would like to acquaint you with our office procedures. Service should be paid for when rendered. If for some reason this is not possible, please discuss other arrangements with me.

If you have health insurance, please read your policy so you know your coverage. Policies vary: some cover hospital care only, and others cover both office care and hospital care. Be sure to leave the name of your insurance company and your policy number and indicate which spouse is the insured or primary holder. If you change insurance companies, please NOTIFY OUR OFFICE AT ONCE.

If you have insurance, who is responsible for your bill? Health insurance is designed to help you meet the cost of medical services. In most cases, it is not geared to pay the total fees. Your insurance contract defines your coverage. There is no contract between the company and your doctor. Therefore, the basic responsibility is yours. We would appreciate it if you pay your bill promptly, without waiting to "see what the insurance will pay," because our fees are not related to insurance coverage. Our office is interested in making you as comfortable as possible during your visits. Please feel free to call upon me for further information.

Your insurance form is prepared by both of us. Each insurance form has a "patient side," which you must complete and sign. The copy of the receipt you receive from our office is all you need to bill your insurance. Attach our form to yours and mail both to your insurance company. A check will be mailed directly to you. I suggest that you note the date of mailing, so that you are able to follow-up if necessary. Always make copies of everything you send to your insurance company. This will save everyone time and aggravation if the claim is lost.

Sincerely,

Bob MacGregor
Office Manager

FIGURE 6-5. Letter explaining the office's insurance billing policy to patients.

using this form for a specific service or procedure, it is necessary to use the modifier -GA to indicate that there is an ABN on file in the patient's medical record. This waiver only applies to services and procedures that are generally covered under the Medicare program. It would not apply to services not covered under the Medicare program, such as a hearing test. The physician's office has the responsibility of knowing Medicare's regulations.

Be sure to use the ABN correctly. It should state that coverage of the particular service or procedure has not yet been determined. It should also state that the patient accepts responsibility for the payment if Medicare does not. If patients are not notified *before* the service or procedure takes place, the patient is not responsible for paying the bill.

Below you will find various reasons for denials. These should be stated on each ABN to advise the patient as to why the practice thinks that service may not be covered. These can be customized to each patient situation and added to the notice:

- Medicare does not pay for this many services.
- Medicare does not pay for such extensive treatment.
- Medicare does not pay for this treatment.
- Medicare does not pay for this treatment because it has not been proven effective.

Any service denied by Medicare can be appealed if

- It is the initial determination of the claim
- The physician accepts assignment on the claim
- The request for the review is within 6 months of the date of the Explanation of Medicare Benefits (EOMB) or Medicare Summary Notice (MSN) denial

MANAGER'S ALERT

Patients cannot be asked to sign a blank ABN. It must meet the following criteria:

- It must be in writing.
- It must state the service or procedure that may not be covered.
- It must state why the practice believes it won't be covered.
- It must be signed by the patient.

One area of improper use of ABNs is when ordering diagnostic studies. Often, physician practices will have ABNs signed whether or not they know if the study is covered. This can place the practice at risk. It should be determined if the study is covered under the national and local carrier regulations. Once these regulations have been checked, it is necessary to identify any diagnosis restrictions that may be associated with the study.

The form from CMS (Figure 6-6) should be used by physicians to advise their Medicare patients of possible denial of services.

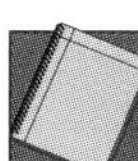

FROM THE EXPERT'S NOTEBOOK

When you are dealing with various different insurances, you might want to color-code either the patient chart or the file card. Using different colors for each insurance will help you easily keep track of all of the plans.

PATIENT ENCOUNTER FORMS

The patient encounter form is one of the most important forms found in the medical office and is used to convey the services and procedures that were provided to the patient during the encounter. It provides a great deal of information regarding the patient and the service that was provided. For example, it identifies any additional testing that may be needed, any future appointments that need to be scheduled, fees that are due by the patient, and the types of services performed for the billing staff. Because of this, it is necessary to design this form to accommodate as much information as possible. It is very important to maintain the form and update it on a yearly basis or more often if necessary.

Few medical offices use preprinted patient encounter forms that are obtained from a printer. Most computerized offices print the patient encounter form from the medical office software package.

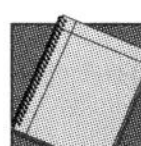

FROM THE EXPERT'S NOTEBOOK

Patient encounter forms are also known as fee slips, superbills, billing forms, service slips, charge slips, and perhaps even other names. The most common name across the country for this form is *patient encounter form.*

The CPT and ICD-9-CM codes contained on the form should be reviewed and updated semiannually. It is essential that all codes contained on the form are accurate and valid for billing purposes; failure to do so can result in claim delays or denials. A sample copy of a patient encounter form for a surgical office can be found in Appendix H.

CPT Codes

The CPT codes reflect services and procedures that can be performed during the patient encounter. These codes should be reviewed against the new CPT book that is released each November to ensure that there are no changes, deletions, or additions appropriate to the codes used within the practice. All levels within each category of evaluation and management (E&M) codes should be listed on the patient

Patient's Name ____________________ Medicare # (HICN): ____________________

ADVANCE BENEFICIARY NOTICE (ABN)

NOTE: You need to make a choice about receiving these health care items or services.

We expect that Medicare will not pay for the item(s) or service(s) that are described below. Medicare does not pay for all of your health care costs. Medicare only pays for covered items and services when Medicare rules are met. The fact that Medicare may not pay for a particular item or service does not mean that you should not receive it. There may be a good reason your doctor recommended it. Right now, in your case, **Medicare probably will not pay for –**

Items or Services:

Because:

The purpose of this form is to help you make an informed choice about whether or not you want to receive these items or services, knowing that you might have to pay for them yourself. Before you make a decision about your options, you should **read this entire notice carefully.**

- Ask us to explain, if you don't understand why Medicare probably won't pay.
- Ask us how much these items or services will cost you (**Estimated Cost: $**____________), in case you have to pay for them yourself or through other insurance.

PLEASE CHOOSE **ONE** OPTION. CHECK **ONE** BOX. **SIGN & DATE** YOUR CHOICE.

☐ **Option 1. YES. I want to receive these items or services.** I understand that Medicare will not decide whether to pay unless I receive these items or services. Please submit my claim to Medicare. I understand that you may bill me for items or services and that I mayhave to pay the bill while Medicare is making its decision. If Medicare does pay, you will refund to me any payments I made to you that are due to me. If Medicare denies payment, I agree to be personally and fully responsible for payment. That is, I will pay personally, either out of pocket or through any other insurance that I have. I understand I can appeal Medicare's decision.

☐ **Option 2. NO. I have decided not to receive these items or services.** I will not receive these items or services. I understand that you will not be able to submit a claim to Medicare and that I will not be able to appeal your opinion that Medicare won't pay.

Date **Signature of patient or person acting on patient's behalf**

NOTE: Your health information will be kept confidential. Any information that we collect about you on this form will be kept confidential in our offices. If a claim is submitted to Medicare, your health information on this form may be shared with Medicare. Your health information which Medicare sees will be kept confidential by Medicare.

OMB Approval No. 0938-0566 Form No. CMS-R-131-G (June 2002)

FIGURE 6-6. Advance beneficiary notice (ABN).

encounter form. Failure to list all levels within each category could be seen as code steering. In other words, the form is steering the physician toward *only* the codes listed and does not allow the physician to choose other levels within the category. For example, a listing on a patient encounter form may look like this *(incorrect way):*

New Patient	*Established Patient*	*Consultation*
99202	99211	99243
99203	99212	
99204	99213	
99205	99214	
	99215	

But should look like this *(correct way)*:

New Patient	*Established Patient*	*Consultation*
99201	99211	99241
99202	99212	99242
99203	99213	99243
99204	99214	99244
99205	99215	99245

If there is not enough room to list all three categories on the patient encounter form, it is acceptable to list all codes within the new and established patient categories and then print the word "Consult" with a blank line where the provider can add the appropriate level of consultation.

ICD-9-CM

ICD-9-CM codes are the diagnosis codes used in a physician office. These diagnosis codes should be reviewed every October when the new ICD-9-CM book is released. It is important to ensure that all codes are accurate, valid, and not truncated. A truncated diagnosis code is one that requires a fourth or fifth digit for specificity. For example:

Code 789.0 is the diagnosis code for abdominal pain. You can see that this is a four-digit code. This code requires a fifth digit to indicate the location of the pain. The fifth digits assigned to this code are as follows:

0	Unspecified
1	Right upper quadrant (RUQ)
2	Left upper quadrant (LUQ)
3	Right lower quadrant (RLQ)
4	Left lower quadrant (LLQ)
5	Periumbilic
6	Epigastric
7	Generalized
9	Other specified site

The best way to indicate the need for a fourth or fifth digit would be to list the code as such: **789.0__.**

When the physician sees the line following the last digit, the physician knows that she or he must indicate the location of the pain. The office staff can then assign the appropriate fifth digit to the code before submitting the claim for billing. Some physicians are familiar with fourth and fifth digits on more commonly used codes, and will be able to assign the correct number without the help of the coder.

An example of a code requiring a fourth digit would be as follows:

283.__	**Acquired hemolytic anemias**
283.0	Autoimmune hemolytic anemia
283.1	Nonautoimmune hemolytic anemia
283.2	Hemoglobinuria due to hemolysis from external causes
283.9	Acquired hemolytic anemia, unspecified

MANAGER'S ALERT

Avoid shortcuts! For example, do not print 789.00 on all patient encounter forms. This would indicate that all "abdominal pains" seen in that particular office were unspecified.

Because there is never enough space on a patient encounter form, the diagnosis codes listed should be those most commonly used by the physician. A line or two labeled "Other" should be listed for codes that are not preprinted on the form.

REMEMBER . . . BE WISE . . . PRIORITIZE

Physicians should always be reminded to prioritize their diagnosis code selections on the patient encounter form. It cannot be left up to the office staff to choose the primary diagnosis code for the visit.

The usual routine for most patients is that they pay at the time of the service. Some patients will then bill their major medical insurance provider. To make this billing easier for the patient, the office should develop a patient encounter form that lists the codes for all of the procedures and services that the practice offers, with the specific ones performed for the patient checked off. A copy of the patient encounter form is sent home with the patient. Some offices even print their most common diagnosis codes on these bills. The patient encounter form should contain all of the information required by the "Physician's Information" part of the insurance form. It should also list the following information about the practice:

- The name of the medical practice
- The address of the medical practice
- The telephone and fax numbers of the practice
- The physician's license number
- A space for the number assigned to the physician by the provider
- The practice's tax identification number
- The names of facilities where services may be performed

All patient encounter forms should be filed in the patient's chart or filed in some organized fashion where they can be accessed if necessary. Many offices choose to keep the patient encounter forms on file for just a short time, for example, 3 months, and then discard them. Each practice should check with its accountant and its attorney on this issue. Make sure the date the claim is submitted is written somewhere on the patient encounter form for easier tracking.

Computerized patient encounter forms are used in some offices and are found to be quite useful. The patient encounter form is compiled as before, with the exception of the way in which it is marked. It cannot be checked off or circled. A number 2 pencil must be used to blacken or fill in the designated circles. This form is then folded in half and fed through a scanner. The scanner is a small unit (approximately 4" × 5"). Within 4 seconds, the information is scanned into the patient charge screen of the computer and any co-pay or deductible is then printed on the screen in front of the employee. By using this software and the computerized patient encounter form, the information is in the computer and ready for billing the same day. There are no possibilities of keystroke errors because the form is being scanned. This eliminates excessive data entry workloads and delays due to the time involved in entry of the information.

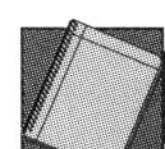

FROM THE EXPERT'S NOTEBOOK

Always remember that all codes must be supported by the documentation in the medical record.

Size Up Your Patient Encounter Form

Below is a "checklist" to allow your practice to review the currently used patient encounter form and identify any areas that may be incomplete. A space should be available for the following:

- *Aged trial balance.* Some physicians will discuss monies owed when they see a balance in the aged trial balance column of the patient encounter form. This is not generally the norm, because most physicians do not want to talk with patients about payment. By printing this information clearly in a designated area, it is easier for the discharge staff to see the balance owed and attempt to collect it.
- *Current balance.* Again, when a balance is printed in a designated area, it is easier to see, and therefore it should be easier to collect. The patient has no surprises because she or he leaves the office with the amount clearly designated.
- *Adjustments.* This space is needed for any adjustments that may be necessary.
- *Staff member initials.* If the practice has many employees, indicate which staff member handled the transaction; this makes it easier to correct errors.
- *Provider of that day's service, the appointment date, and the time of the appointment.* Printing the time of the appointment is useful in time management studies.
- *Type of appointment.* Emergency, walk-in, allergy shot only, and so on.
- *Insurance information.* Medicare, Medicaid, managed care, and so on.
- *Return visit information.* Patient's next appointment can be documented on the patient encounter form.
- *Managed care information.* Patient's deductible, co-payment, and preauthorization.
- *Office hours* (optional).

These areas should be considered for inclusion on the patient encounter form along with the previously mentioned issues of CPT codes and ICD-9-CM codes. It is helpful for office personnel to have as much information as possible.

Printing Patient Encounter Forms

Patient encounter forms can be printed either vertically or horizontally and may be any size. The normal size for patient encounter forms is 8½ by 11 inches so that they conform to other papers within the office. It is best to keep the patient encounter form short enough to fit on one printed sheet. The back of the form may also be used. In fact, many offices list their diagnosis codes on the back to allow more room for service and procedure codes on the front of the form. Many computers today have the capabilities to print patient encounter forms, and therefore printing companies are not always used. If the practice is going to print the patient encounter form "in house" it is best to keep it simple by keeping it to one page. The advantage of printing the patient encounter form in house is that changes can be made at any time and the practice does not have to wait for the stock to be "used up" before any changes can be made. Do *not* print fees on patient encounter forms. This is best left for "write-ins" when necessary. Because space is always an issue (meaning there is never enough of it on a patient encounter form), you can eliminate repetitive descriptions by listing codes and descriptions in a grid or table.

PROFESSIONAL COURTESY

The term *professional courtesy* is a "garbage can" term meaning different things to different people. True professional courtesy is defined as a physician waiving fees for service for another physician, the physician's family, or possibly professional staff at the local hospital. Others define professional courtesy as accepting "insurance only" for payment of services rendered for physicians, their family, and professional staff. Whatever you call it, the practice can't do it anymore! The letter in Figure 6-7 can be used to notify colleagues and professional staff of a new policy.

Years ago, physicians could waive payment from such patients as the local police department; the local minister, priest, and rabbi; the mailman, neighbors, and friends; and colleagues and their families. This very kind gesture can now be construed as breaking the law and, in fact, is sometimes found to be on the Office of Inspector General's (OIG's) "hit list."

In the first scenario, the physician practice may be at risk for violating the anti-kickback statute, which prohibits providing free services in order to receive patients in return. Any past or future referrals need to be considered. The letter in Figure 6-8 can be used to notify professional patients that this courtesy can no longer be offered to them.

In the second scenario, in which co-payments and deductibles are waived, the physician practice is at risk for implications of Stark and the False Claims Act through inducements to beneficiaries. It is best to check with the practice attorney and to develop and implement a policy for this situation. The Stark Law was named after United States Congreeman Pete Stark, who sponsored the bill. This bill governs physician self-referral for Medicare and Medicaid patients. Physician self-referral is when a patient is referred to a medical facility in which a physician has ownership or has an investment. For example, the physician may have ownership in an MRI center or an ophthalmologist may be invested in an eyeglass company.

Jeffrey Miller, M.D.
111 Center Avenue
Anyplace, USA

Dear Dr. Miller:
Due to the changed regulatory environment, our tradition of providing professional courtesy, regardless of referral relations, could be misinterpreted by the government agencies and other legal bodies. In light of the potential for confusion and in an effort to be as compliant as possible, this practice, based on advice of counsel, has come to the sad conclusion that we can no longer either offer professional courtesy or accept professional courtesy. Unfortunately, this also applies to the practice of accepting your insurance payment as payment in full.

We hope that you will understand the need for this decision.

Yours truly,
Alexander Babinetz, M.D.

FIGURE 6-7. Sample letter to colleague explaining discontinuation of professional courtesy services.

August 4, 2008

Dear Olivia,
In the past, we have not been charging you for our services. As you know, the cost of providing services to patients continues to rise, creating a situation whereby our paying patients are responsible for incurring all the increased costs of our practice, not to mention the legal ramifications of continuing this practice. To keep down costs and prevent an increase in our fees, we find it necessary to discontinue our courtesy policy to patients who are receiving courtesy at this time. Because we expect you to pay normal fees in the future, we are also willing to submit to your insurance company for these services. You will still be responsible for any deductible or co-pay that is not covered by your insurance.

Your understanding and cooperation are important to us. We value you and your family as patients and will continue to provide you with the very best of medical care. If you have any questions regarding this policy change, please feel free to contact me.

Sincerely,
Alexander Babinetz, M.D.

FIGURE 6-8. Sample letter to nonphysician patients explaining discontinuation of professional courtesy services.

CHARGING A PHYSICIAN'S FAMILY MEMBERS FOR SERVICES

Charging a physician's family members for services rendered is not allowed by the Medicare program. It may be allowed by other carriers; however, most carriers eventually follow Medicare regulations. Your practice should check with other carriers for their policy on this issue.

The Medicare Benefit Policy Manual, Chapter 16, Section 130 states that charges cannot be made for services by physicians that would ordinarily be furnished "gratis" because of the relationship of the physician to the patient. This refers to charges to immediate relatives or persons living in the same household. Relationships included in this Medicare regulation are as follows:

- Husband and wife
- Child, sibling, and natural or adoptive parent
- Stepparent, stepchild, stepbrother, and stepsister
- Father-in-law, mother-in-law, son-in-law, daughter-in-law, brother-in-law, and sister-in-law
- Grandparent or grandchild
- Spouse of grandparent or grandchild
- Members of the household (e.g., domestic employees or persons sharing the house as part of a family unit by blood, marriage, or adoption)

A brother-in-law or sister-in-law relationship does not exist between the physician and the spouse of his wife's or her husband's brother or sister. A father-in-law or mother-in-law relationship does not exist between a physician and his or her spouse's stepfather or stepmother. A step-relationship or in-law relationship will continue to exist even if the marriage upon which the relationship is based is terminated through divorce or death.

THE OFFICE MANAGER AND INSURANCE CLAIM SUBMISSIONS

The physician will probably expect the office manager to report insurance submissions on a weekly basis. Some offices prefer to do this on a monthly basis. The office manager should keep a record of the total number of claims, and the total dollar amount of the claims, that were submitted to each payer. It is helpful to separate these figures by the account class, in other words, by the various insurance groupings. For example:

- All Medicare claims together
- All HMO/PPO claims together
- All Blue Shield claims together

This record can be completed on a weekly basis and handed to the physician at scheduled meeting dates. This will give the physician an idea of the amount of services and billings that were generated that particular week.

Insurance submissions should be done on a daily basis. Many practices make the mistake of submitting them once a week. This causes unnecessary delays in turnaround times, and, depending on whether they are paper or paperless claims, the time required submitting a week's worth of claims together can be excessive. A medium to large practice can submit electronic claims to Medicare, Medicaid, Blue Shield, and HMOs/PPOs and paper claims to commercial insurance companies in approximately 1 hour. This can be done during the last 2 hours of the day and can be finished easily before the end-of-the-day backup has to be done. This system creates a flow of payments and shortens the turnaround time.

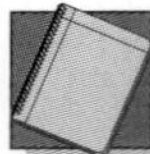

FROM THE EXPERT'S NOTEBOOK

Remember to get all the necessary insurance information from the patient during the first office visit. It will save a lot of time later.

CODING

In some offices, Medicare is the largest payer mix, may be the largest source of income, and is most probably the cause of their worst headaches. Trying to comply with all of the new Medicare rules and regulations is not only confusing, but vexing. Staff must be well acquainted with the *Physicians' Current Procedural Terminology* (CPT), *International Classification of Diseases, Ninth Revision, Clinical Modification* (ICD-9-CM), and *HCPCS Level II* codebooks. It is important to hire billing staff who have experience with insurance billing and third-party regulations. If possible, hire a certified coder who has passed the certification examination and obtained either a CPC or a CCS-P. These certifications are established for physician practice coders. Facility side coding (hospital) certifications are CPC-H and CCS. Staff may know how to fill out the forms and where to send them, but do they really understand and use the information in the explanation of benefits that they receive from Medicare and other third-party payers? Given the complexity of the new Medicare regulations and the changing codes and fee structures, staff ignorance in this area is more of a threat to the livelihood of the medical office than it has ever been.

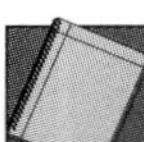

FROM THE EXPERT'S NOTEBOOK

Many courses and workshops on coding are available to medical offices. They may last anywhere from 1 to 3 days and can be very helpful in answering the everyday questions that arise. In addition, coding tips may be picked up from personnel from other offices present at the workshop.

Many publications are available to help a medical office keep informed of the various changes in the reimbursement area. *It is important for the office manager to keep up with changes as they take place.* The physician's specialty society will often send newsletters and publications that may also provide news of changes and requirements.

ICD-9-CM Codebook

The ICD-9-CM diagnosis coding system has its roots in a group of statistical studies of diseases called "The London Bills Mortality" published in England in the seventeenth century. By 1937, these statistics had evolved into the manuscript called the *International List of Causes of Death.* Many more revisions of this list were made after this point, and eventually this work became the *International Classification of Causes of Death.* The World Health Organization (WHO) used this information in 1948, when it published its morbidity and mortality lists. These lists were repeatedly revised and finally became the *International Classification of Diseases* (ICD).

In 1978, the WHO published its ninth revision of this list, and, at this point, this listing became internationally known as the ICD-9. Once the ICD-9 became recognized internationally, the U.S. National Center for Health Statistics (NCHS) addressed the need for a more precise clinical picture for its statistics. It added clinical information to the ICD-9, and thus the ICD-9-CM was born. In 1988, Congress passed the Medicare Catastrophic Coverage Act, which mandated the use of ICD-9-CM codes on all physician-submitted Part B claims. This system translates written medical terminology into numeric and alphanumeric codes. The ICD-9-CM codebook is published twice each year, in April and October, and consists of three volumes. Volume 1 contains the most specific information about diseases, symptoms, injuries, and conditions. It consists of code numbers presented in numeric order. Beside each code number is a diagnosis. In addition, each code is broken down into subcategories representing particular variations of that diagnosis. Volume 2 is an alphabetic list of the diseases, symptoms, injuries, and conditions. This volume is divided into three sections:

Section 1: Index to Diseases and Injuries
Section 2: Table of Drugs and Chemicals
Section 3: Alphabetic Index to External Causes of Injuries and Poisonings

Therefore, to code a diagnosis using the ICD-9-CM, you first use Volume 2 to find the diagnosis alphabetically. Beside the diagnosis will be a numeric code. (Never code from Volume 2; always move on to Volume 1.) Look up that numeric code in Volume 1 to see the subcategories of that code and choose the specific subcategory that represents the most specific diagnosis for the condition. Volume 3 contains procedural information reserved for hospital use.

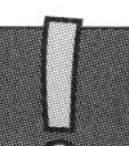

MANAGER'S ALERT

Try not to use any code in the ICD-9-CM codebook that has the acronym "NEC" after it. NEC means "not elsewhere classifiable" and indicates that the code should be used only when there is no alternative. Also, the acronym "NOS" should be avoided because it means "not otherwise specified" and is only used when there is not enough information available to assign a more specific code.

The service that was provided to the patient should correlate with the diagnosis code specified on the claim. Insurance companies reject claims in which the CPT service code specified does not match the ICD-9-CM diagnosis code specified. For instance, if a diabetic patient was seen in the office for a sore throat, it would be incorrect to use the diagnosis code of diabetes. Although the patient is a diabetic, the services she or he received on that particular day were for a sore throat and unrelated to the diabetes.

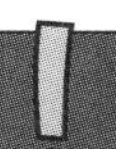

MANAGER'S ALERT

Be sure to choose the final code from Volume 1 of the ICD-9-CM codebook and not use the code found in Volume 2. Volume 2 merely directs you to the appropriate area of Volume 1 in order to choose the most specific code possible.

The ICD-9-CM disease codes are extremely precise and require some medical knowledge to understand them. Medical office staff should have some clinical background or understanding of medical terminology to be able to select the correct code for a particular claim. Regular staff meetings and explanations by the physicians will assist in the training of these staff members. It is the physician's responsibility to provide the office staff with a diagnosis for each patient. This will reduce incorrect diagnosis coding on claims.

The Centers for Medicare and Medicaid Services (CMS) provides guidelines for diagnosis coding. These guidelines can be found in the front pages of the ICD-9-CM codebook. The following is a sampling of these guidelines:

- Identify each service or procedure with a diagnosis code.
- Identify services for circumstances other than disease or injury with a V code.
- Code to the highest degree of specificity by using fourth and fifth digits.
- Code chronic diagnoses when applicable to that specific patient visit.
- For ancillary services, code the appropriate V code first, and then code the problem second.
- For surgical procedures, code the diagnosis applicable to the procedure. If the postoperative diagnosis is different from the preoperative diagnosis, code using the postoperative diagnosis.
- Do not code using "probable," "suspected," "Rule out," or "questionable."

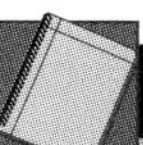

FROM THE EXPERT'S NOTEBOOK

It is the physician's responsibility to complete the patient encounter form at the time of the patient visit.

STEPS IN CODING USING THE ICD-9-CM CODEBOOK

1. Identify the main diagnosis from the physician.
2. Secure any secondary diagnoses if available.
3. Choose the appropriate modifier if needed.
4. Locate the diagnosis in Volume 2.
5. Assign the diagnosis a tentative code.
6. Cross-reference the code in Volume 1 for specificity.

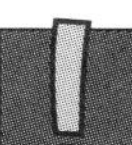

MANAGER'S ALERT

Be sure to code the diagnosis to the greatest level of specificity. Otherwise, the claim will be rejected. Be sure to note if it requires a fourth or fifth digit!

TYPES OF ICD-9-CM CODES

There are several types of diagnosis codes, including V codes, E codes, signs and symptoms codes, late effect codes, and codes used to report toxicity and poisoning, to mention a few.

V Codes

V codes are ICD-9-CM codes that are used to describe patients who are not sick but are seeking a specific health service, such as a screening, that could influence their health or have a special circumstance that could influence their health. Medicare does not recognize most V codes. Certain V codes can be used as primary diagnosis codes. Some examples of V codes that can be used as primary are as follows:

- V28: Antenatal screening
- V56: Encounter for renal dialysis
- V03-06: Need for vaccination
- V54: Orthopedic aftercare

Some examples of V codes that cannot be used as primary are as follows:

- V10: Personal history of malignant neoplasm
- V16: Family history of disease
- V09: Infection with drug-resistant organism
- V45: Other postsurgical states

There are three categories of V codes:

- *Problem oriented.* Identifies a factor that could affect the patient, but is not an injury or an illness.
  - Example: V76.11—Special screening mammogram for high-risk patient
- *Service oriented.* Identifies that the service was an examination, therapy, ancillary service, or aftercare. This diagnosis code is used to identify a patient who is not currently sick, but is seeking medical services for another purpose.
  - Example: V67.2—Follow-up examination following cancer chemotherapy
- *Fact oriented.* Simply states a fact.
  - Example: V27.2—Outcome of delivery: twins, both live born

E Codes

E codes are used to classify environmental events, circumstances, and conditions as the cause of injury, poisoning, and other adverse effects. They are used to establish medical necessity for the treatment. E codes never affect reimbursement; however, they can affect the reimbursement time by decreasing it. They can never be used as a primary diagnosis, and, if necessary, it is permissible to use more than one E code to describe a situation. When using more than one E code, the following rules must be followed:

- E codes for child and adult abuse take priority over all other E codes.
- E codes for cataclysmic events take priority over all other E codes except abuse.
- E codes for transportation accidents take priority over all other E codes except cataclysmic events and abuse.

E codes are also used to identify the place of the occurrence, as in the following example:

> *Example:* Mary accidentally burns her arm while taking cookies from the oven in her home. The E codes for this claim would be E 924.8, accident caused by hot substance, heat from heating appliance and E849.0, home.

E codes can be extremely helpful in primary care and orthopedics. The following example illustrates the medical necessity for using E codes:

> *Example:* Alex falls off of the sliding board at school, leaving him with a "goose egg" on his forehead. The school calls his mother to pick him up because he has been crying nonstop since the fall. Mom picks him up and decides that perhaps she should take him to the doctor just to be safe. At the doctor's office, Mom tells the doctor about the accident. Alex is examined and the doctor determines that he has a contusion. The doctor lists his diagnosis (Dx) as follows:
> *Dx: 1. contusion 2. E884.0, fall from playground equipment*

The E code explains how and where the injury took place. E codes can be interesting to read about in the ICD-9-CM book. There is an E code for being battered by a blender, an E code for being sucked into a jet engine, and, yes, there is an E code for decapitation by guillotine.

Signs and Symptoms

The CMS and NCHS have released instructions that if a definitive diagnosis code is not available, the codes describing signs and symptoms found in Chapter 16 of the ICD-9-CM codebook should be used. Examples of such codes are as follows:

780.4	Dizziness
780.6	Fever
784.0	Headache
786.5	Chest pain
787.0	Nausea and vomiting
788.41	Urinary frequency
790.2	Abnormal glucose tolerance test
796.2	Elevated blood pressure reading without a diagnosis of hypertension

Late Effect Codes

There are two types of late effect codes: *general* and *injury related.* A general late effect code describes a residual condition produced after the acute phase of an illness. This means generally 1 year or more after the acute illness. Examples of late effect codes are as follows:

137._	Late effects of tuberculosis (TB) (requires additional digits)
438._	Late effects of a cerebrovascular accident (CVA) (requires additional digits)

Late effects of injuries, poisonings, toxic effects, and other external causes can be used any time after the acute injury or condition. Examples of these codes are as follows:

906.3	Late effect of contusion
E929.0	Late effect of motor vehicle accident

Nonspecific/Unspecified

These can be found listed in Volume 1 of the ICD-9-CM codebook as NOS, meaning "not otherwise specified," and in Volume 2 as NEC, meaning "not elsewhere classifiable." These codes should only be used when the information is lacking and there is not a more definitive diagnosis code available. Examples of these codes are as follows:

420.90	Acute pericarditis, unspecified NOS
682.9	Cellulitis NOS
599.0	Infection, genitourinary tract NEC
533.5	Ulcer, perforating NEC

ICD-10

The NCHS and CMS have been involved in the development of the ICD-10 for the WHO. The first change that we will notice will be in the title. The new title will be *International Statistical Classification of Disease and Related Health Problems.* This new book will increase the amount of clinical detail and will address all diseases from the ICD-9-CM. The formatting of the codes will change to alphanumeric, meaning they will be one letter followed by a series of numbers. The letter "U" will not be found in the new book because it is being reserved for future use. There may be some confusion with the letters I and O, because they look very similar to the numbers 1 and 0.

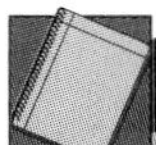

FROM THE EXPERT'S NOTEBOOK

Remember that the first character of the new diagnosis codes is always a letter. Therefore there should be no confusion between I and 1 or O and 0.

The new system will force medical practices to change claim forms and computer software and to learn an entirely new system. There are 21 chapters in the new ICD-10 as opposed to the 17 currently found in the ICD-9-CM. The new diagnosis codes will also contain a sixth digit to provide more detail of the diagnosis.

CPT CODEBOOK

The CPT codebook (Figure 6-9) is released on a semiannual basis, with updates on coding and terminology provided throughout the year. This book contains all the codes necessary to report the services performed by a physician and was created in 1966 by the American Medical Association. This book's 696 pages are broken down by body part, itemizing the different services that can be provided by a physician. There is a five-digit numeric code for each service. This numeric code is the important part of submitting a claim for insurance reimbursement. If the office does not use the correct code, the claim will be either rejected or delayed in the carrier's processing department. Either way, the claim will be delayed, and reimbursement will be late arriving at the office. This can be a problem in offices that have no claim tracking system in place. If the office does not pursue a rejected claim, the payment may never be made.

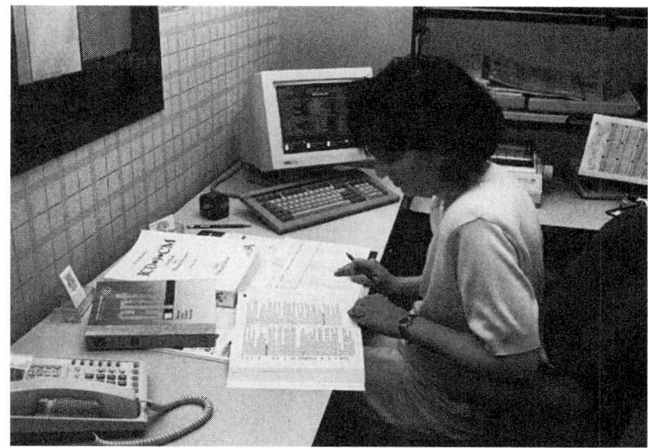

FIGURE 6-9. An employee uses coding books to prepare insurance claims.

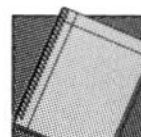

FROM THE EXPERT'S NOTEBOOK

Trying to contain costs by not buying the new CPT manual every year is a dangerous practice. Codes change and become deleted, and new codes are added every year! Make it a policy to order the new CPT manual every fall.

The specifics of the CPT codes should be carefully studied so that the physician and medical biller will recognize any changes in them from year to year. The CPT codebook is a must for the medical office and can be obtained from the American Medical Association. The address is as follows:

American Medical Association
Order Department
515 North State Street
Chicago, IL 60610

These codes may also be purchased from the American Medical Association in an electronic format.

Choosing an Evaluation and Management Code

A methodical and logical thought process should be followed when attempting to choose the correct evaluation and management (E&M) code. It is the physician's responsibility to choose the E&M codes. It is important for the office manager to have a thorough understanding of these code selections in order to ensure that the physician is correctly coding all services and procedures. Following these three simple steps will make the selection of an E&M code less painful:

Step 1: Select a group of codes by determining the following:

1. Place of service
   a. Office
   b. Hospital
   c. Emergency department
   d. Nursing home
   e. Rest home
   f. Private home
2. The type of patient
   a. Established patient
   b. New patient—haven't seen the patient for at least 3 years (for a group practice, no one in group has seen the patient in the last 3 years)
3. Whether the visit was a visit or a consultation
   a. Consultation—visit was requested by another physician
   b. Confirmatory consultation—visit provided only advice or opinion
   c. Visit—face-to-face evaluation and management of the patient

Step 2: Analyze the level of service provided by using three key components:

1. The history taking
   a. Problem focused
   b. Expanded problem focused
   c. Detailed
   d. Comprehensive
2. The examination
   a. Problem focused
   b. Expanded problem focused
   c. Detailed
   d. Comprehensive
3. The decision making
   a. Straightforward
   b. Low complexity
   c. Moderate complexity
   d. High complexity

Step 3: Choose the specific code by checking the level of service against the code listings in the CPT manual.

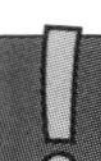

MANAGER'S ALERT

Physicians who consistently use higher codes than their colleagues will definitely hear from their carriers. Carriers have software that tracks this type of information and identifies any outliers (physicians outside the norm). This may result in an audit.

Surgery Codes

MAJOR SURGERY

The initial evaluation by a surgeon is not included in the global surgery package. The initial evaluation or consultation may be billed for separately. The "global payment" is a "package payment" that the physician receives that encompasses several services and charges, including the following:

- Preoperative visits
- Postoperative visits
- Complications after surgical procedures
- Intraoperative services
- Postoperative pain control
- Medical supplies
- Miscellaneous services

Preoperative visits include visits 1 day before surgery. Postoperative visits include all visits within 90 days of the surgery. A postoperative visit for an unrelated problem does not fall into this category. If the patient is seen for an unrelated problem that requires an additional and separate course of treatment, the visit is billed for separately. Any complication that arises from the surgery that does not require an additional trip to the operating room is included in the global package. Any additional intraoperative services that are usually necessary and part of the original procedure are included in the global fee. Postoperative pain control is included in the postoperative visits and cannot be billed for separately.

All medical supplies with the exception of tray fees are included in the original service. Surgical tray fees can be billed for separately. Any miscellaneous treatment, such as suture or staple removal, wound care, catheters, intravenous solutions, and removal of nasogastric and tracheostomy tubes, generally qualifies for the billing of a surgical tray fee.

MINOR SURGERY AND ENDOSCOPY

Minor surgeries and endoscopies are also tied into global fees. The global payment for these procedures includes the following:

- Patient visits
- Postoperative visits

- Minor surgery
- Endoscopies

Patient visits on the same day as the surgical procedure are always included in the global payment, whether they are on an outpatient or inpatient basis. For minor surgery, the postoperative days vary from 1 to 10 days, based on the procedure. The *Federal Register* contains all of the information necessary for the office manager to check the procedures that apply to the physician's specialty.

MODIFIER MANIA

A modifier is a numeric or an alphabetic character that is added to a CPT code to indicate that the service or procedure was altered for that specific circumstance. The modifier does not change the definition of the CPT code reported. Modifiers may be used to report the following:

- An unusual event
- That only part of a service was performed
- That the service was only a technical, not professional, component of a procedure (for example, the taking of an x-ray is the technical component but the interpreting of an x-ray is the professional component)
- That the service was increased
- That the service was decreased
- That the service had to be performed more than once
- That the service had to be performed by more than one physician

The following are modifiers that can be used to explain services further.

-21 Prolonged Evaluation and Management Service

The services provided were prolonged or greater than those usually required for the highest level of evaluation and management within a given category. This modifier can be used only with the highest level of care for that category. It has no effect on payment.

Example: The patient is a 76-year-old woman with Alzheimer's disease. She has been in a nursing facility for 5 years and has been basically stable. Her physician arrives for her monthly visit and discovers that she is failing physically. She is no longer able to use her wheelchair and can no longer feed herself. He reviews the complete medical record, consults by telephone with a psychiatrist regarding lowering her psychiatric drugs, and calls the family regarding the possibility of moving her to a skilled floor. Because this is above and beyond the normal nursing facility visit, the highest level of nursing home established patient visit can be billed using the -21 modifier.

-22 Unusual Procedural Service

The services provided were greater than usually required for the procedure reported. Use of this modifier may result in an increased payment if the claim has sufficient documentation attached. This can be accomplished by attaching a copy of the operative note to the claim.

Example: A child is brought to the pediatrician's office with multiple splinters in both feet. She is crying and the mother is unable to calm her down. The physician spends extensive time in an attempt to remove all of the splinters in their entirety from a noncooperative child. Some splinter areas require local anesthesia for removal. Because this is an unusual procedural service, the procedure code is billed with a -22 modifier.

-23 Unusual Anesthesia

The services required general anesthesia, as opposed to usually not requiring any anesthesia or just local anesthesia.

Example: A 3-year-old boy is brought to the hospital with a laceration involving the upper eyelid. The child is crying and the parents cannot calm him. Even with the use of the papoose board, the physician is unable to keep the child still enough to repair the laceration. It is necessary to administer general anesthesia to prevent the child from moving. Once the child is under general anesthesia, the laceration is repaired. Because this is not usually a procedure that would require general anesthesia, the modifier -23 can be attached to the procedure code.

-24 Unrelated Evaluation and Management Service

The services required an additional unrelated service by the same physician during the postoperative period. This modifier can be used only on an evaluation and management code. It has no effect on payment.

Example: A 25-year-old man comes to the surgeon's office for postoperative follow-up of removal of gallstones. While the patient is in the office, he shows the surgeon a rash that has developed on his lower right leg. The surgeon examines the rash and gives the patient a prescription for a steroid cream. Since the rash is unrelated to the removal of the gallstones, modifier -24 can be used with the appropriate level of office visit code.

-25 Significant, Separate Evaluation and Management Service

These services require a significant, separately identifiable evaluation and management service by the same physician on the same day of a procedure or other service. The E&M may be prompted by a symptom or condition for which the service or procedure was provided. Different diagnoses are not required for use of this modifier.

Example: A male patient is seen in the family practice office for his high blood pressure. It is a 6-month visit, and he needs a prescription renewal. The physician finds his blood pressure to be unacceptably high and changes his medications. At the time of the visit, he also complains of pain in his right shoulder. He has been playing softball on the weekends and thinks he might be a little out of shape. The physician examines his shoulder and diagnoses a bursitis. He explains that it will get better faster with a cortisone injection into the shoulder. He injects the shoulder and the patient is discharged for another 6 months, at which time he will return for a blood pressure check. The office visit is billed using a -25 modifier, along with the shoulder injection code. The diagnosis code for the office visit is for hypertension, and the diagnosis code for the injection is bursitis.

-26 Professional Component

Certain procedures performed are a combination of a physician component and a technical component. This modifier is used when only the physician component is being reported. Use of this modifier can affect payment. The fee schedule contains various different payment amounts for professional components.

Example: A female patient is scheduled at the hospital for an echocardiogram. The cardiologist is present for the test and interprets it immediately following the completion. He comes to the waiting room to talk with his patient before she leaves for home. He is able to bill for the interpretation of that test using the -26 modifier for professional component.

-27 Multiple Outpatient Hospital E&M Encounters on the Same Day

This modifier is used to identify multiple outpatient hospital E&M encounters on the same date. *This modifier is not used by physician practices.* It has been created for use by hospital outpatient departments.

-32 Mandated Services

The services related to a mandated consultation or related service. This has no effect on payment. This code is commonly used with workers' compensation cases when they are seeking a second opinion.

Example: A female patient is told by her orthopedist that her work-related injury will keep her out of her present job for about 6 months. The workers' compensation company requests that she see a specialist for a second opinion.

-47 Anesthesia by Surgeon

Regional or general anesthesia was provided by the surgeon. This modifier is not covered by Medicare.

Example: A male patient is examined and diagnosed as having carpal tunnel syndrome. After treating this condition conservatively, it is decided that the patient must have surgery. The surgeon provides the anesthesia for the carpal tunnel instead of an anesthesiologist. To bill for this service, the modifier -47 must be added to the procedure code to receive payment.

-50 Bilateral Procedure

Unless otherwise identified, bilateral procedures performed during the same operative session should be billed by reporting the first procedure with its five-digit code and then reporting the second procedure using the modifier. Payment on this modifier is based on 150% (200% for radiology) of the fee schedule payment amount. This modifier can be used only on certain codes.

Example: A male patient is examined by an ophthalmologist and found to have two cataracts. In follow-up, the ophthalmologist finds the cataracts to be fast growing and suggests that they both be done in the very near future. The patient is scheduled, and he has the cataracts removed with lens implants in both eyes. The modifier -50 is added to the second eye surgery.

-51 Multiple Procedures

When multiple procedures are performed on the same day or at the same session, the major procedure should be reported using the five-digit code. The second procedure is then reported using the modifier. Payment is adjusted for multiple surgeries according to standard percentages (100% for the highest fee schedule allowable, 50% for the second highest, and 25% for the third through fifth highest). Special rules apply to dermatologic, endoscopic, and anesthetic procedures. Do not use modifier -51 with add-on codes or exempt codes.

Example: A female patient is pregnant with twins. She delivers the twins, both vaginally. The second delivery is billed with a -51 modifier to indicate that the procedure was indeed performed twice.

-52 Reduced Services

The service performed was either partially reduced or eliminated at the surgeon's request. For examinations that are considered global, use of this modifier will not affect payment. For other situations, such as aborted procedures, a reduction in payment may be made. Documentation explaining the reduction should accompany the claim.

Example: A male patient comes to the urologist for a vasectomy. As he is examined, it is found that the patient is monorchid; therefore when the vasectomy code is billed, it should be billed with a -52 modifier to indicate that the service was partially reduced.

-53 Discontinued Procedure

The physician may decide to terminate a surgical or diagnostic procedure. Because of extenuating circumstances that threaten the well-being of the patient, it may be necessary to indicate that a procedure was started, but then discontinued.

Example: A male patient is scheduled to have a colonoscopy to identify and remove colon polyps. Once the scope is passed through the colon, it is determined that there is a mass associated with one of the polyps. The physician elects to discontinue the procedure and schedule the patient for a hospital procedure. To bill for the colonoscopy, it would be necessary to use the modifier -53.

-54 Surgical Care Only

One physician performed the surgery, and another provided preoperative or postoperative care. Payment is limited to the allotted time spent on preoperative and intraoperative services only.

Example: An elderly female patient arrives at the emergency department complaining of pain in the wrist after a fall out of her wheelchair. She is taken to the community hospital, where an emergency physician diagnoses and sets her wrist. She is then discharged to the nursing home, where the attending physician at the nursing home continues her care.

-55 Postoperative Management Only

One physician performed only the postoperative care, and another surgeon performed the surgery. Payment is limited to the allotted amount of postoperative care only.

Example: An elderly man requires cardiac surgery. His daughter arrives into town for the surgery and stays with her father for a while after surgery. She then returns home and discovers that her father can no longer live by himself and it is decided that her father will come to live with her in another state. He is then followed by another cardiologist for the postoperative care. These services should be billed using modifier -55.

-56 Preoperative Management Only

One physician performed only the preoperative care, and another surgeon performed the surgery. Payment is included in the payment allowed for surgery. Do not use this modifier with Medicare claims.

Example: An elderly female patient is being followed for severe knee pain by her family physician in a small town that does not have a hospital. After many different approaches, it is determined that she requires a total knee replacement. The physician phones a colleague in a larger neighboring city to perform the surgery. The patient is then transferred to the surgeon for her surgery. The visits before the surgery are billed using the modifier -56.

-57 Decision for Surgery

An E&M service that results in the decision to perform surgery is billed using a -57 modifier. The decision for surgery must be made either the day before the surgery or the day of the actual surgery.

Example: A female patient is being evaluated by a gynecologist for heavy menstrual bleeding. After the examination, the physician determines that she requires a dilation and curettage (D&C) in the morning. The D&C is scheduled for the next morning, and the consultation is billed using the -57 modifier.

-58 Staged or Related Procedure or Service by the Same Physician during the Postoperative Period

A service or procedure is planned during the postoperative period because of one of the following reasons:

- It was prospectively planned at the time of the original procedure (staged).
- It was more extensive than the original procedure.
- For therapy following the original procedure.

Failure to use this modifier may result in the denial of payment for the second procedure.

Example: A young mother is scheduled for a breast biopsy on a certain date. Once the results of the biopsy are discussed with the patient, the patient returns to the operating room for a mastectomy. Modifier -58 is used for obtaining payment for both services.

-59 Distinct Procedural Service

This modifier is used to report that a service or procedure was distinct or separate from other services performed on that same day. These services are not normally performed together. This modifier may represent any of the following:

- Different session or patient encounter
- Different procedure or service on the same day
- Different site or organ system
- Separate incision or excision
- Separate lesion
- Separate injury

Example: A female patient is scheduled for surgery for a bunion on her left foot. During the surgery, the physician identifies a suspicious lesion on her left thigh. He obtains a biopsy at this time. The biopsy is billed using modifier -59.

-62 Two Surgeons

The skills of two surgeons were required. Use this modifier when reporting both surgeons' procedures. This modifier will usually increase payment by 25%, split equally between the two surgeons. Documentation of the necessity of both surgeons must accompany the claim.

Example: A male patient is scheduled for surgery to repair a closed fracture of the spine. Two physicians are required for the surgery because one will perform the arthrodesis and the other will perform a thoracotomy. Each code would be billed with modifier -62 to indicate the use of co-surgeons.

-63 Procedure Performed on Infants less than 4 kg

Procedures (invasive) performed on neonates and infants up to a present body weight of 4 kg may involve significantly increased complexity and physician work commonly associated with these patients. This modifier may only be attached to codes in the 20000 to 69990 range.

Example: A 2-week-old infant weighing 1200 g developed abdominal distention and would not eat. The infant required intubation and radiographs, which showed a necrotizing enterocolitis. This infant required a small bowel resection. This procedure was billed using the modifier -63.

-66 Surgical Team

A team of physicians was required to perform a specific procedure. Use this modifier for each physician's procedure. Different carriers pay differently on this modifier. Documentation for the necessity of the medical team is necessary for payment on this claim.

Example: A male patient is scheduled to have a repair of a blood clot in the renal artery. Some renal calculi have also been identified by x-ray. Because two procedures are required, it is necessary for a team of surgeons to be involved in the surgery. Each surgeon would use the -66 modifier attached to the procedure that she or he performed.

-73 Discontinued Outpatient Hospital/ Ambulatory Surgery Center (ASC) Procedure before the Administration of Anesthesia

A procedure is canceled because of extenuating circumstances that may threaten the well-being of the patient. This code is used when the procedure is canceled before the administration of anesthesia.

Example: An elderly male patient is prepped for a right knee arthroscopy. Before the anesthesia is administered, there is a sudden drop in his blood pressure and the patient becomes diaphoretic. The procedure is then canceled and rescheduled for another day. The claim can be sent with the -73 modifier and the proper documentation to support it.

-74 Discontinued Outpatient Hospital/ Ambulatory Surgery Center (ASC) Procedure after Administration of Anesthesia

A procedure is canceled because of extenuating circumstances that may threaten the well-being of the patient. This code is used when the procedure is canceled after administration of the anesthesia.

Example: An elderly male patient is prepped for a right knee arthroscopy. After the anesthesia is administered, there is a sudden drop in his blood pressure and the patient becomes diaphoretic. The procedure is then canceled and rescheduled for another day. The claim can be sent with the -74 modifier and the proper documentation to support it.

-76 Repeat Procedure by the Same Physician

The physician may need to repeat the same service or procedure. This may be on the same day as the original service or procedure. Use of this modifier will help distinguish between the original and the repeat service or procedure so that the claim is not viewed as double billing.

Example: A male patient is scheduled for a thoracotomy tube placement. He has an x-ray performed before the procedure, and then again after the placement of the tube to ensure proper placement.

-77 Repeat Procedure by Another Physician

The service needed to be repeated by another physician. This modifier provides no additional payment and is used for informational purposes only.

Example: A female patient is scheduled for a thoracentesis as a result of her breast malignancy. The procedure is performed successfully; however, it needs to be repeated the following day by another physician.

-78 Return to Operating Room for Related Procedure

The physician needed to return the patient to the operating room for a related procedure during the postoperative period. Payment for use of this modifier is limited to the amount allotted for intraoperative services. Use this modifier only with surgery codes.

Example: A female patient is scheduled for a hysterectomy. The surgery is completed and the patient is returned to her hospital room. Later that evening, the patient's hemoglobin begins to drop, and it is identified that the patient is bleeding. The patient is then returned to the operating room for control of the bleeding.

-79 Unrelated Operating Room Procedure by the Same Physician

The patient required an additional unrelated procedure during the postoperative period. This modifier has no effect on payment and can be used only on surgery codes.

Example: An elderly man receives treatment for a fractured hip resulting from a fall in the backyard. Seven weeks after the surgical repair, the man falls again, sustaining a severe fracture of the right arm. This fracture requires surgical repair. The arm fracture requires the addition of the modifier to indicate that an additional surgery was required for an unrelated condition.

-80 Surgical Assistant

Surgical assistant services may be identified by adding this modifier to the surgical CPT code. During certain operations, one physician assists another physician in performing a procedure. The physician who assists the operating surgeon would report the same surgical procedure that the operating surgeon reports. However, the operating surgeon would *not* append any modifier to the procedure that she or he reports. Only the assistant surgeon would report modifier -80.

Example: An elderly female patient is scheduled for left hip replacement surgery. Because of extenuating factors with the patient, a second physician is required for this procedure. The second physician must use the -80 modifier for payment. The record must identify the medical necessity for the second physician.

-81 Minimum Assistant Surgeon

Minimum surgical assistant services are identified by adding this modifier. For example, the operating physician begins a surgical procedure alone, but during the operation, a minor problem is encountered that requires the service of an assistant surgeon for a short period of time. The services provided by the surgeon who provided this minimal assistance during the surgery would be reported with modifier -81 appended to the code for the surgical procedure.

Example: A middle-aged man is scheduled for an abdominal surgery. During the course of the surgery, the physician encounters a somewhat minor problem that requires assistance from another physician for a short period. This second physician arrives to assist and uses the modifier -81 for the billing of his or her services.

-82 Assistant Surgeon

Services required the need of an assistant surgeon. When a resident surgeon was unavailable, use this modifier. Payment is based on 16% of the fee schedule payment amount for the service rendered.

Example: A young man is brought to the emergency department with multiple injuries resulting from a motorcycle accident. He is immediately prepped for surgery and rushed to the operating room. Because the hospital is not a teaching hospital and does not have residents, it is necessary to use an assistant surgeon to help repair the multiple injuries of this patient. The second surgeon would bill for services using the -82 modifier.

-90 Reference Laboratory

A service was performed by an outside laboratory other than the treating or reporting physician. This modifier has no effect on payment.

Example: Blood is drawn for cholesterol and triglyceride testing on a patient who has a known diagnosis of high cholesterol and a cardiac condition. The blood is drawn in the office and is picked up by an outside laboratory that performs the testing and sends the results back to the physician office via phone line.

-91 Repeat Clinical Diagnostic Laboratory Test

This modifier is used when a laboratory test needs to be repeated on the same day, on the same patient, to monitor specific results.

Example: A male patient is a brittle diabetic. The physician orders a 2-hour postprandial blood sugar after breakfast, and again after lunch. The "after lunch" test would need to be reported with the -91 modifier to indicate that it is not a double billing.

-99 Multiple Modifiers

Under certain circumstances, one or more modifiers may be necessary to report a service.

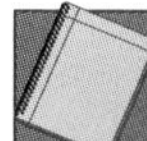

FROM THE EXPERT'S NOTEBOOK

The modifier -25 can be used to report an eligible patient visit that may have been performed on the same day as a minor surgery or endoscopic procedure.

Additional Modifiers

AH *Clinical psychologist:* Services performed by a clinical psychologist.

AJ *Clinical social worker:* Services performed by a clinical social worker and subject to Medicare fee limits of 75% of the physician fee schedule.

AS *Physician assistant, nurse practitioner, clinical nurse specialist for assistant at surgery:* Services performed by the above, in an assistant to surgery condition, must report their role using the AS modifier.

GA *Waiver of liability statement on file:* Use of this modifier indicates that the office maintains an advance beneficiary notice (ABN) on file for this claim.

GC *This service was performed in part by a resident under the direction of a teaching physician:* When a teaching physician is billing for services provided in part by a resident, the modifier GC must be attached to that service. This modifier certifies that the teaching physician was present during the key portions of service. This modifier does not affect payment.

GE *This service was performed by a resident without the presence of a teaching physician:* This modifier can only be used if the facility has acquired a primary care exception. This modifier does not affect payment.

QU *Physician providing service in a Health Professional Shortage Area (HPSA):* Use of this modifier will help to calculate the quarterly bonus payment received by the physician.

QW *Clinical Laboratory Improvement Act (CLIA)–waived test:* This modifier should be used to report any laboratory tests that are designated as waived tests.

TC *Technical component:* Use this code to bill for only the technical component of a procedure or study.

HCPCS CODEBOOK

This book contains changes and new codes for use and is available on January 1 each year. This codebook contains national codes. The following steps will assist a coder in the use of the HCPCS codebook:

1. Identify the service or procedure to be coded.
2. Look up the appropriate term in the index.
3. Assign a tentative code.
4. Locate the code or codes in the appropriate section.
5. Check for notes, symbols, or references.
6. Review the appendices for the reference definitions and any other guidelines that may exist.
7. Determine whether any modifiers should be used.
8. Assign the code.

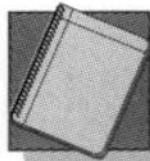

FROM THE EXPERT'S NOTEBOOK

When the CPT codebook and the HCPCS codebook both have identical code descriptions, always use the CPT code.

The HCPCS codebook is divided into the following sections:

1. Index
2. Transportation Services Including Ambulance A0000-A0999
3. Medical and Surgical Supplies A4000-A8999
4. Administrative, Miscellaneous and Investigational A9000-A9999
5. Enteral and Parenteral Therapy B4000-B9999
6. Outpatient PPS (Prospective Payment System - see chapter details in this chapter) C1000-C9999
7. Dental Procedures D0000-D9999
8. Durable Medical Equipment E0100-E9999
9. Procedures/Professional Services (Temporary) G0000-G9999
10. Alcohol and Drug Abuse Treatment Services H0001-H2037
11. Drugs Administered Other Than Oral Method J0000-J9999
12. Temporary Codes K0000-K9999
13. Orthotic Procedures and Devices L0000-L4999
14. Medical Services M0000-M0301
15. Pathology and Laboratory Services P0000-P9999
16. Q Codes (Temporary) Q0000-Q9999
17. Diagnostic Radiology Services R0000-R5999
18. Temporary National Codes (Non-Medicare) S0000-S9999
19. National T Codes Established for State Medicaid Agencies T1000-T9999
20. Vision Services V0000-V2999

It includes seven appendices:

1. Appendix 1—Table of Drugs
2. Appendix 2—Modifiers
3. Appendix 3—Abbreviations and Acronyms
4. Appendix 4—Pub 100 References
5. Appendix 5—New, Changed, Deleted, and Reinstated HCPCS Codes for 2007
6. Appendix 6—Place of Service and Type of Service
7. Appendix 7—National Average Payment

TELEPHONE MEDICINE

Many physicians spend a great deal of time with their patients on the telephone. All of these physicians want to bill for this service. Medicare will not provide reimbursement for time spent on the telephone with a patient. Medicare views this as part of the "before" and "after" work that is included in the physician's service. The office should check with other carriers, however, to see if they reimburse for this service.

THE MEDICARE CODING SYSTEM: A RATIONALE FOR CHANGE

On January 1, 1992, Medicare traded in its existing coding system for a new evaluation and management coding system. These evaluation and management codes make up approximately 45% of all Medicare Part B payments to physicians. The American Medical Association CPT Editorial Panel developed these new codes, which replaced the CPT coding system previously used. The goal in making this change was to develop a coding system that would take into consideration geographic localities and physician specialties. The previous system coded services in a uniform way that was not always appropriate for all physicians. The previous system accommodated various physician-coding practices by using a "reasonable charge" payment methodology coupled with a prevailing charge, which was calculated in each locality for each physician specialty. The resource-based relative value scale (RBRVS) payment system does not allow for any variation in physician coding.

CODING TIPS

The following tips may help the office manager and physician in dealing with these codes:

- Routinely check the patient's charts for proper documentation.
- Order the CPT and ICD-9-CM codebooks on an annual basis.
- Routinely check the CPT and ICD-9-CM codes on the patient encounter form and in the computer for accuracy.
- Have the physician take an active role in the coding process; it is the physician's responsibility to choose the correct codes.
- Read the entire Medicare special bulletins and any other bulletins from third-party payers.
- Learn when, where, and how to use modifiers.
- No distinction is made between a new and an established patient in the emergency department.
- No distinction is made between a new and an established patient for a consultation. Follow-up visits to inpatient consultations are reported using subsequent hospital visit codes.
- No distinction is made between a new and an established patient for a comprehensive nursing facility visit.
- Two office visits on the same day for the same patient may be reported if the problems were unrelated and the correct modifier is used.
- A new patient is one who has not been seen by anyone in the practice in the past 3 years.

BILLING FOR SUPPLIES

Certain services provided to patients in a physician's office require the use of a tray of supplies. Generally, the cost of those supplies is bundled into the service being provided. There are some circumstances, however, in which a "tray fee" can be billed to Medicare separately. The following procedure codes will permit the billing of a tray fee in addition to the procedure. The HCPCS code to use for billing of this fee is A4550 and can be reported with the following CPT codes:

19101	28296	43239	49080	52275	68761
19120	28297	43245	49081	52276	85095
19125	28298	43247	52005	52277	85102
19126	28299	43249	52007	52282	95028
20200	32000	43250	52010	52283	96440
20205	36533	43251	52204	52290	96445
20220	37609	43458	52214	52300	96450
20225	38500	45378	52224	52301	G0105
20240	43200	45379	52234	52305	
25111	43202	45380	52235	52310	
28290	43220	45382	52240	52315	
28292	43226	45383	52250	57522	
28293	43234	45384	52260	58120	
28294	43235	45385	52270	62270	

From *Physician's Current Procedural Terminology, CPT 2002,* Standard Edition, American Medical Association, 2002.

Occasionally, Medicare will reimburse for such items as slings (A4565), splints (A4570), casting supplies (A4580), and drugs (all "J" codes). Check with all other carriers to see if they allow for the billing of such items. Supplies such as gauze, Ace bandages, and transparent film are not reimbursable by Medicare.

PROSPECTIVE PAYMENT SYSTEM (PPS)

The PPS was implemented by the federal government in October of 1983 as a predetermined fixed amount that is paid by Medicare, which is derived based on the classification system of that service. The PPS is used to reimburse for services provided in acute inpatient hospitals, home health agencies, hospice, hospital outpatient, inpatient psychiatric facilities, inpatient rehabilitation facilities, long-term care hospitals, and skilled nursing facilities. Each patient is classified into a Diagnosis Related Group (DRG) on the basis of clinical information. The hospital is paid a flat rate for the DRG, regardless of the actual services provided. This DRG classification is a result of the following information from the patient's medical record:

- Why the patient was admitted (principal diagnosis)
- Complications and co-morbidities
- Surgical procedures
- Age

- Gender
- Discharge disposition (whether the patient was transferred, the patient expired, or it was a routine discharge)

There are over 490 DRG categories that have been defined by CMS. Each category is designed so that all patients assigned to a DRG are deemed to have a similar clinical condition. The PPS is based on paying the average cost for treating patients in the same DRG. The DRG payment for a Medicare payment is determined by multiplying the relative weight for the DRG by the hospital blended rate:

$$\text{DRG PAYMENT} = \text{WEIGHT} \times \text{RATE}$$

This hospital rate is updated annually to reflect inflation, technical adjustments, and budgetary constraints.

IS THE MEDICARE APPEAL APPEALING?

Few medical offices have ever filed an appeal to Medicare or, for that matter, have ever even thought about doing so. Most offices are intimidated by the process and are unsure how to handle such a task. A recent statistic released from Medicare shows that more than 50% of all claims sent for appeal have had their initial decisions reversed. This statistic should make the appeal process more appealing!

A few steps must be taken before starting the appeal process. First, it is best to resubmit the claim, if it hasn't already been resubmitted. This often eliminates the need for an appeal and is easier to do than an appeal. This can be done only if the claim is whole and not partial. Rejected partial claims must be submitted for an appeal. There are five steps in the appeal process:

1. Informal review
2. Fair hearing
3. Hearing by the administrative law judge
4. Review by the Appeals Council
5. Federal district court hearing

There are various time limits and monies involved in each step of the process. Every office is given a Medicare carriers' manual. Referring to the section on appeals can be very helpful during this process.

Informal Review

All requests for informal review of a claim must be made within 6 months and 5 days of the date on the Explanation of Medicare Benefits/Medicare Summary Notice. A claim for any dollar amount can be made at this point. At this point, the medical office may want to file a CMS-1964 Request for Review form; however, this is not required. All that is necessary to start this process is to write a letter asking for an informal review of the claim (Figure 6-10). This letter should include the following information:

- Patient's name
- Patient's Medicare number
- Dates of service in question
- Procedure codes

Most offices find that it is best to attach a copy of the explanation of benefits to the letter. It is also a good idea to attach any additional information that might help justify the services rendered. Remember to be specific. You have complete control over what you submit to Medicare. There is no such thing as too much information or too much documentation.

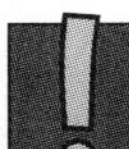

MANAGER'S ALERT

When submitting a claim for review, always send additional information to support the service rendered. If the claim is submitted just as it was initially, there is a good chance that the reviewer will pull the original claim and discuss it with the original reviewer, and the result will remain as originally decided–claim denied!

Fair Hearing

If only part of the claim was denied, the office can request a fair hearing. A fair hearing is given by an experienced reviewer designated by Medicare. It can be requested only within 6 months of the informal review decision. There is also a restriction on the amount of the claim in question. Each fair hearing must be on a claim in the amount of $100 or higher. Again, there is a form, CMS-1965, that can be used to request this hearing. The office may also request this hearing by writing a letter. The office must be aware that there are three different types of fair hearings:

1. Telephone hearing
2. On-the-record hearing
3. In-person hearing

The CMS requires that all telephone and in-person hearings be granted. When preparing for these hearings, the office must have the same information as gathered for the informal review. Any additional documentation is a must!

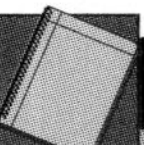

FROM THE EXPERT'S NOTEBOOK

The office may request a copy of all of the information regarding the requested appeal from the Medicare carrier. This will help in reviewing the case before the hearing. This is one of Medicare's best-kept secrets!

Medicare Part B
Department of Review
P.O. Box 890413
Camp Hill, PA 17089-0413

Dear Sir or Madam:
Please refer to the attached Medicare Explanation of Benefits form. We are challenging Medicare's denial of our daily visits, rejected as unnecessary concurrent care.

On ________________, our practice was asked to see the above-listed patient in consultation by the patient's primary care physician for a condition that required the consultative expertise of a gastroenterologist. We completed this consultation and furnished a report to the attending physician.

Due to the unique nature of this patient's condition, which related to his diagnosis of________________ , we agreed to continue to follow the patient along with the attending physician, specifically as it related to the patient's diagnosis. After a thorough evaluation, additional advice was rendered in the medical record relative to ongoing patient progress. The attending physician continued to serve as overall manager of the patient's care; however, the diagnosis was well beyond the scope of the attending physician's expertise, there by necessitating our resources.

Medicare's denial of our daily care based on too many physicians for the reported condition should in this case be overturned. The unique condition required the services of a board-certified subspecialist of internal medicine—a gastrointestinal specialist. Failure to provide these services would certainly have compromised the patient's clinical outcome.

We ask that you reconsider this claim for payment and forward the reimbursement to our office at your earliest convenience. Thank you for your attention to this matter.

Sincerely,

Betty Kelly
Billing Manager

FIGURE 6-10. Letter requesting an informal review of a rejected claim.

Hearing by the Administrative Law Judge

If the claim is denied at the fair hearing, the office may request a hearing by an administrative law judge. This hearing must be requested within 60 days of the final fair hearing decision, and the claim must be worth at least $500. At this step in the appeals process, there is no longer a Medicare employee making the decisions. A hearing officer decides at this point whether a reversal of the previous decision is warranted. If the hearing officer reverses the decision, the office wins! If the hearing officer agrees with the previous decision, the request is forwarded to an administrative law judge. These reviews take place in the Office of Hearings and Appeals at the Social Security Administration. The scheduling of this hearing can take as long as 1 year.

Review by the Appeals Council

The next step is a review by the Appeals Council. This council is also a division of the Social Security Administration. A request for a review by this council should be made through the Social Security Administration and must be made within 60 days of the administrative law judge's decision. The claim must be in the amount of $500 or more. Once the appeal process reaches this step, it is wise for the office manager to step down and enlist the help of an experienced health care attorney. An attorney is required should the appeals process go to the next step, so it is generally a good idea to engage one at this level.

Federal District Court Hearing

Should the claim be denied by the Appeals Council, a civil action must be filed in a federal district court. This claim must be filed within 60 days of the mailing date of the Appeals Council decision. To be eligible for this action, the claim in dispute must be worth $1,000 or more. Any claim under $1,000 cannot be tried at this level. The two additional requirements at this level are that the office be represented by an attorney and that the claim be filed in the federal district in which the office is located.

IDENTIFICATION NUMBERS

All carriers require that all physicians and suppliers of services maintain an identification number. The main numbers required by carriers used to be as follows:

- Unique provider identification number (UPIN)
- Provider identification number (PIN)
- National Supplier Clearinghouse (NSC) numbers

These numbers are now called legacy numbers or legacy identifiers. Providers are now required to obtain a National Provider Identifier (NPI), which will be used on all billing. For a certain period of time, legacy numbers may also be included. When applying for an NPI number, it is important to include the legacy numbers of the provider in order to be properly identified. Under the Health Insurance Portability and Accountability Act (HIPAA), all providers must apply for and submit an NPI number. Because of the creation of this number, it has been necessary to make changes to the CMS 1500 form in order to allow for reporting space.

THE NEW CMS 1500 FORM

Any "paper" claims submitted to commercial companies, Medicare, Medicaid, and others require the completion of a CMS 1500 form (Figure 6-11). This form was developed by CMS originally for billing to Medicare and was updated in 2006, and the older version was discontinued on February 1, 2007. This form was changed to accommodate the reporting of the NPI. Now, this form is widely used by most third-party carriers and contains 33 information fields that need to be completed when submitting a claim. The following information is a step-by-step guide to completion of and changes to this form.

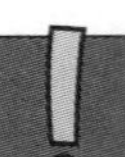

MANAGER'S ALERT

If you check FECA Black Lung Program, it is then necessary to complete Items 11a through 11d.

Item 1: Type of Insurance. The insurance selections for this line are Medicare, Medicaid, TRICARE/CHAMPUS, CHAMPVA, Group Health Plan, FECA Black Lung Program, and Other. Simply identify the type of insurance the patient carries and place a checkmark in the appropriate box. Under CHAMPVA, the box titled "VA File #" has been changed to "Member ID #."

Item 1a: Insured's Identification Number. The patient's health insurance claim (HIC) number for that specific carrier is placed in this block.

Item 2: Patient's Name. The patient's name, last name first, is entered into this block. Use Jr. or Sr. if applicable. Leave a space between the suffix and the last name, then enter the first name, for example, *Nordmark Jr. Albert.* For hyphenated names, capitalize both last names and separate by a hyphen, for example, *Miller-Andrews.* Do not leave a space between a prefix and the last name, for example, *McCarter.*

Item 3: Patient's Date of Birth and Sex. Place the patient's date of birth in month, day, and year formatting. Use eight numbers to enter, for example, 08041954 for a date of birth August 4, 1954. The patient age must correspond to the diagnosis code; for example, an age of 17 or less must be listed when the diagnosis code in Item 21 is a pediatric diagnosis code. An age of 0 must be listed when the diagnosis code in Item 21 is a newborn diagnosis code. If the date of birth does not correspond, the claim will be denied. The gender of the patient is simply checked in the appropriate box labeled "M" for male and "F" for female. Occasionally, an incorrect patient sex is entered and the claim is denied for "this diagnosis for this patient sex."

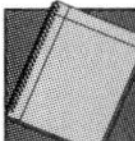

FROM THE EXPERT'S NOTEBOOK

Enter the patient's name exactly as it appears on her or his insurance card; otherwise there is a chance for error or misidentification.

Item 4: Insured's Name. Place the name of the insured person in this block. When entering the name, enter the last name first. If Medicare is the primary insurance, this block must remain blank. If the insured is also the patient, simply enter "same" in this block.

Item 5: Patient's Address (and telephone number). Place the patient's mailing address and telephone number using the first line for the street address, the second line for the city and state and the zip code, and the third line for the telephone number.

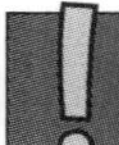

MANAGER'S ALERT

If there is punctuation in the name of the city, do not use it. For example, enter St Paul Minnesota.

Item 6: Patient Relationship to Insured. This block identifies the relationship of the patient to the insured, that is, "self," "spouse," "child," and "other."

Item 7: Insured's Address (and telephone number). Enter the address and telephone number of the insured as before on this form. If the insured and the patient are the same, indicate "same" in this area.

Item 8: Patient Status. This block is used to identify the marital status of the patient and the employment or

1500

HEALTH INSURANCE CLAIM FORM

APPROVED BY NATIONAL UNIFORM CLAIM COMMITTEE 08/05

PICA | PICA

CARRIER

1. MEDICARE (Medicare #) | MEDICAID (Medicaid #) | TRICARE CHAMPUS (Sponsor's SSN) | CHAMPVA (Member ID#) | GROUP HEALTH PLAN (SSN or ID) | FECA BLK LUNG (SSN) | OTHER (ID)

1a. INSURED'S I.D. NUMBER (For Program in Item 1)

2. PATIENT'S NAME (Last Name, First Name, Middle Initial)

3. PATIENT'S BIRTH DATE MM DD YY SEX M F

4. INSURED'S NAME (Last Name, First Name, Middle Initial)

5. PATIENT'S ADDRESS (No., Street)

6. PATIENT RELATIONSHIP TO INSURED Self Spouse Child Other

7. INSURED'S ADDRESS (No., Street)

CITY STATE

8. PATIENT STATUS Single Married Other

CITY STATE

ZIP CODE TELEPHONE (Include Area Code) ( )

Employed Full-Time Student Part-Time Student

ZIP CODE TELEPHONE (Include Area Code) ( )

9. OTHER INSURED'S NAME (Last Name, First Name, Middle Initial)

10. IS PATIENT'S CONDITION RELATED TO:

11. INSURED'S POLICY GROUP OR FECA NUMBER

a. OTHER INSURED'S POLICY OR GROUP NUMBER

a. EMPLOYMENT? (Current or Previous) YES NO

a. INSURED'S DATE OF BIRTH MM DD YY SEX M F

b. OTHER INSURED'S DATE OF BIRTH MM DD YY SEX M F

b. AUTO ACCIDENT? YES NO PLACE (State)

b. EMPLOYER'S NAME OR SCHOOL NAME

c. EMPLOYER'S NAME OR SCHOOL NAME

c. OTHER ACCIDENT? YES NO

c. INSURANCE PLAN NAME OR PROGRAM NAME

d. INSURANCE PLAN NAME OR PROGRAM NAME

10d. RESERVED FOR LOCAL USE

d. IS THERE ANOTHER HEALTH BENEFIT PLAN? YES NO ***If yes***, return to and complete item 9 a-d.

READ BACK OF FORM BEFORE COMPLETING & SIGNING THIS FORM.

12. PATIENT'S OR AUTHORIZED PERSON'S SIGNATURE I authorize the release of any medical or other information necessary to process this claim. I also request payment of government benefits either to myself or to the party who accepts assignment below.

SIGNED ________ DATE ________

13. INSURED'S OR AUTHORIZED PERSON'S SIGNATURE I authorize payment of medical benefits to the undersigned physician or supplier for services described below.

SIGNED ________

PATIENT AND INSURED INFORMATION

14. DATE OF CURRENT: MM DD YY ◄ ILLNESS (First symptom) OR INJURY (Accident) OR PREGNANCY(LMP)

15. IF PATIENT HAS HAD SAME OR SIMILAR ILLNESS. GIVE FIRST DATE MM DD YY

16. DATES PATIENT UNABLE TO WORK IN CURRENT OCCUPATION FROM MM DD YY TO MM DD YY

17. NAME OF REFERRING PROVIDER OR OTHER SOURCE 17a. 17b. NPI

18. HOSPITALIZATION DATES RELATED TO CURRENT SERVICES FROM MM DD YY TO MM DD YY

19. RESERVED FOR LOCAL USE

20. OUTSIDE LAB? YES NO $ CHARGES

21. DIAGNOSIS OR NATURE OF ILLNESS OR INJURY (Relate Items 1, 2, 3 or 4 to Item 24E by Line)

1. ___ . ___ 3. ___ . ___

2. ___ . ___ 4. ___ . ___

22. MEDICAID RESUBMISSION CODE ORIGINAL REF. NO.

23. PRIOR AUTHORIZATION NUMBER

	24. A. DATE(S) OF SERVICE From MM DD YY	To MM DD YY	B. PLACE OF SERVICE	C. EMG	D. PROCEDURES, SERVICES, OR SUPPLIES (Explain Unusual Circumstances) CPT/HCPCS	MODIFIER	E. DIAGNOSIS POINTER	F. $ CHARGES	G. DAYS OR UNITS	H. EPSDT Family Plan	I. ID. QUAL.	J. RENDERING PROVIDER ID. #
1												
2												
3												
4												
5												
6												

PHYSICIAN OR SUPPLIER INFORMATION

25. FEDERAL TAX I.D. NUMBER SSN EIN

26. PATIENT'S ACCOUNT NO.

27. ACCEPT ASSIGNMENT? (For govt. claims, see back) YES NO

28. TOTAL CHARGE $

29. AMOUNT PAID $

30. BALANCE DUE $

31. SIGNATURE OF PHYSICIAN OR SUPPLIER INCLUDING DEGREES OR CREDENTIALS (I certify that the statements on the reverse apply to this bill and are made a part thereof.)

SIGNED DATE

32. SERVICE FACILITY LOCATION INFORMATION

a. b.

33. BILLING PROVIDER INFO & PH # ( )

a. b.

NUCC Instruction Manual available at: www.nucc.org

OMB APPROVAL PENDING

FIGURE 6-11. The new CMS 1500 claim form.

student status. The marital status blocks are "single," "married," and "other." The employment status blocks are "employed," "full-time student," and "part-time student."

Item 9: Other Insured's Name. Place the name of the person responsible for the Medigap policy in this block. If the insured is also the patient, the word "same" can be entered. If there are no Medigap benefits, this block would be left empty. Again, when entering the name, use last name first.

FROM THE EXPERT'S NOTEBOOK

If the physician is not participating in the Medicare program, it is not necessary to fill in Item 9.

Item 9a: Other Insured's Policy/Group Number. Place the Medigap number in this block.

Item 9b: Other Insured's Date of Birth and Sex. Enter date of birth using eight digits, for example, 08/01/1950. Enter the sex of the insured in this block.

Item 9c: Employer's Name or School Name. Place the address of the Medigap insurer in this blank. Ignore the title that is printed on the form (Employer's Name or School Name).

Item 9d: Insurance Plan Name, Program Name, or PAYERID. Place the name of the other insured's health insurance plan or program.

Item 10: Is Patient's Condition Related. This block identifies if the patient's condition is related to employment, motor vehicle accident, or other accident.

Item 10a: Employment. If the condition is employment related, place an "X" in the block to identify if it is current or previous employment.

Item 10b: Auto Accident. Place an "X" in the box to identify that the condition is related to an auto accident. Be sure to enter the date of the accident in Item 14. Enter the name of the state in which the accident occurred using standard post office abbreviations.

Item 10c: Other Accident. This identifies whether the patient's condition is related to an accident other than employment or auto related. If the accident is "other," place an "X" in the "YES" box. Enter the date of the accident in Item 14.

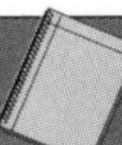

FROM THE EXPERT'S NOTEBOOK

Any items checked "yes" in blocks 10a, 10b, or 10c will require a completed Medicare secondary payer (MSP) form.

Item 10d: Reserved for Local Use. This block is reserved for Medicaid information only.

Item 11: Insured's Policy/Group/Federal Employees Comp. Act (FECA) Number. Enter the policy, group, or FECA number of any insurer that is primary to Medicare.

Item 11a: Insured's Date of Birth and Sex. Enter the date of birth and sex of the insured if not the patient.

Item 11b: Employer's Name or School Name. Place the employer's name in this block. If the insured is retired, enter the retirement date followed by the word "retired."

Item 11: Insurance Plan Name or Program Name. Place the name of the insurance company that is primary to Medicare in this block. The ID number must also be added.

Item 11d: Is There Another Health Benefit Plan? If the patient has Medicare, leave this block empty.

Item 12: Patient's or Authorized Person's Signature. The patient's signature, or a representative of the patient, must be placed in this block. If the patient has signed a "lifetime authorization form," the letters "SOF" can be placed in this block. This signifies that there is a "signature on file." The form must then be maintained in the patient's file.

Item 13: Medigap Benefits Authorization. The patient, or patient representative, must sign separately for the Medigap benefits. A "lifetime assignment on file" may be used; however, it is carrier specific.

Item 14: Date of Current Illness, Injury, or Pregnancy. Place the date of the first symptom or the date the accident occurred in this block. For chiropractic services, enter the date of the initiation of the course of treatment.

Item 15: If Patient Has Had Same or Similar Illness, Give First Date. This is not a required block for Medicare. If the patient has not had a same or similar illness, leave this block empty.

Item 16: Dates Patient Unable to Work. This block is especially important for workers' compensation patients. Enter the dates that the patient was gainfully employed but unable to work because of illness or injury.

Item 17: Name of Referring Physician or Other Source. This block is used to enter the name of the referring physician or other referral source.

Item 17a: ID Number of Referring Physician. The qualifying number should be listed to the left of the other ID number for the referring or ordering provider. The qualifying numbers are as follows:

OB	State license number
1B	Blue Shield provider number
1C	Medicare provider number
1D	Medicaid provider number
1G	Provider UPIN
1H	CHAMPUS ID number
E1	Employer's ID number
G2	Provider commercial number
LU	Location number

N5	Provider plan network ID number
SY	Social Security Number
X5	State industrial accident provider number
ZZ	Provider taxonomy

Item 17b: NPI Number. Place the NPI number of the referring physician or ordering physician.

Item 18: Hospitalization Dates Related to Current Services. This block is used only when the patient is hospitalized. Place the date of admission and the date of discharge in this block.

Item 19: Reserved for Local Use. This block is used for many different messages. For example, if a patient refuses to assign benefits, that is written in this block; if the patient is in hospice care, the block must state that this is the attending physician, not a hospice employee.

Item 20: Outside Diagnostic Services. This block is used to identify diagnostic tests that may be performed outside the physician's office. Place an "X" in the "YES" box when the test is being performed by another provider. Place an "X" in the "NO" box when the tests are performed in the physician's office (not a purchased test).

Item 21: Diagnosis or Nature of Illness or Injury. Place the appropriate ICD-9-CM code for the services rendered in this block. A maximum of eight may be listed. This block must be completed for the claim to be paid. Codes should be listed in order of priority. Medicare claims do not use the description of the ICD-9-CM.

Item 22: Medicaid Resubmission. This block is used when resubmitting a claim to Medicaid. If billing the claim to Medicare, this block would remain empty.

Item 23: Prior Authorization Number. If the service performed required preauthorization, that number would be entered in this block. It is generally a 10-digit number. This block is also used for the Home Health Agency (HHA) number or hospice number when billing for care plan oversight services. It is also used for the Clinical Laboratory Improvement Act (CLIA) identification number when billing for tests performed in the physician office laboratory.

Item 24a: Dates of Service. Place the dates of service involved in the procedure code. If the service is performed on a single day, the "from" and "to" would be the same date. If services carry over into another month, list each month separately.

Item 24b: Place of Service. Place the two-digit place of service code in this block. Place of service codes are as follows:

11	Physician's Office (O)
12	Patient's Home (H)
21	Inpatient Hospital (IH)
22	Outpatient Hospital (OH)
23	Department—Hospital (OH)
24	Ambulatory Surgery Center (ASC)
25	Birthing Center (OL)
26	Military Treatment Facility (OL)
31	Skilled Nursing Facility (SNF)
32	Nursing Facility (NH)
33	Custodial Care Facility (OL)
34	Hospice (OL)
41	Ambulance—land
42	Ambulance—air or water
50	Federally Qualified Health Center (FQHC)
51	Inpatient Psychiatric Facility (OL)
52	Psychiatric Facility Partial Hospitalization
53	Community Mental Health Care (CMHC)
54	Intermediate Care Facility/Mentally Retarded (STF)
55	Residential Substance Abuse Treatment Facility (RTC)
56	Psychiatric Residential Treatment Center (RTC)
60	Mass Immunization Center
61	Comprehensive Inpatient Rehabilitation Facility (OL)
62	Comprehensive Outpatient Rehabilitation Facility (CORF) (COR)
65	End-Stage Renal Disease Treatment Facility (KDC)
71	State or Local Public Health Clinic (OL)
72	Rural Health Clinic (RHC) (OL)
81	Independent Laboratory (IL)
99	Other Unlisted Facility (OL)

Item 24c: EMG. This block identifies a service performed in a hospital department. This block does not have to be completed for Medicare billing.

Item 24d: Procedures, Services, or Supplies. Place the appropriate HCPCS/CPT code for the service rendered. Enter any modifiers that are appropriate in the modifier block.

Item 24e: Diagnosis Pointer. Place the appropriate reference number (pointer) of the diagnosis code for the service performed.

Item 24f: Dollar ($) Charges. Place the amount charged for the procedure or service performed.

Item 24 g: Days or Units. List the number of days or units for the procedures described in block 24d. When billing for drugs, it is important to list the quantity of the drug administered.

Item 24h: EPSDT (Family Plan). This block identifies that early and periodic screening, diagnosis, and treatment services were provided. This block does not have to be completed for Medicare billing.

Item 24i: ID Qualifier. The qualifying number should be listed to the left of the other ID number for the referring or ordering provider. The qualifying numbers are as follows:

OB	State license number
1B	Blue Shield provider number
1C	Medicare provider number
1D	Medicaid provider number
1G	Provider UPIN
1H	CHAMPUS ID number
E1	Employer's ID number

G2	Provider commercial number
LU	Location number
N5	Provider plan network ID number
SY	SSI number
X5	State industrial accident provider number
ZZ	Provider taxonomy

Item 24j: Rendering Provider ID #. Enter the NPI number of the rendering physician.

Item 25: Federal Tax ID Number. This block is used for the federal tax identification number of the physician. The number can be either a Social Security number or a federal tax ID number. The federal tax ID number must be present to submit a claim to Medigap.

Item 26: Patient's Account Number. The patient's account number assigned by the physician's office should be placed in this block.

Item 27: Accept Assignment. This block identifies if the physician is willing to accept assignment on the claim. If the physician accepts, place an "X" in the "YES" block.

Item 28: Total Charge. This is a total of the charges on the claim form. Do not use a dollar sign ($) in this block.

Item 29: Amount Paid. The block identifies the amount paid by the patient toward this claim.

Item 30: Balance Due. This block identifies the amount due after calculating from the amount charged and the amount paid.

Item 31: Signature of Physician or Supplier Including Degrees or Credentials. Place the signature of the provider of the service in this block along with the date the form was signed. An authorized representative of the physician may sign the physician's name.

Item 32: Name and Address of Facility Where Services Were Rendered. Place the name and address of the facility where the services were performed other than the physician's office or the patient's home (hospital, clinic, nursing facility, etc.).

Item 32a: NPI Number. Enter the NPI number of the service facility location.

Item 32b: Other ID Number. The qualifying number should be listed to the left of the other ID number for the referring or ordering provider. The qualifying numbers are as follows:

OB	State license number
1B	Blue Shield provider number
1C	Medicare provider number
1D	Medicaid provider number
1G	Provider UPIN
1H	CHAMPUS ID number
E1	Employer's ID number
G2	Provider commercial number
LU	Location number
N5	Provider plan network ID number
SY	SSI number
X5	State industrial accident provider number
ZZ	Provider taxonomy

Item 33: Physician's, Supplier's Billing Name, Address, Zip Code, and Phone Number. Place the name, address, and phone number of the provider of the service.

Item 33a: NPI Number. Enter the NPI number of the service facility location.

Item 33b: Other ID Number. The qualifying number should be listed to the left of the other ID number for the referring or ordering provider. The qualifying numbers are as follows:

OB	State license number
1B	Blue Shield provider number
1C	Medicare provider number
1D	Medicaid provider number
1G	Provider UPIN
1H	CHAMPUS ID number
E1	Employer's ID number
G2	Provider commercial number
LU	Location number
N5	Provider plan network ID number
SY	SSI number
X5	State industrial accident provider number
ZZ	Provider taxonomy

THE LIFE CYCLE OF A CLAIM

A claim to a third-party carrier takes on a life of its own as it travels through the cycle (Figure 6-12). In Stage 1, the information obtained by the front office is of paramount importance in submitting a "clean claim." If information is either incomplete or incorrect at this stage, the claim will most probably be denied; it will then have to be corrected and resubmitted. At this point, the practice has lost valuable time because instead of having the claim paid in about 2 to 3 weeks, it has now been 6 weeks.

In Stage 2, the information documented by the physician, physician extender, or clinical staff in the office plays the most important role in getting paid. The documentation must be present and complete to support the level of service or procedure being billed.

In Stage 3, the billing information, that is, the patient encounter form, is often sent to a coder for verification and completeness before being submitted to the carrier.

In Stage 4, the accurate information is entered into the computer and the claim is submitted to the appropriate carrier.

In Stage 5, if the claim is incomplete, it is denied.

In Stage 6, if the claim is "clean," it is paid.

EXPLANATION OF BENEFITS/ REMITTANCE ADVICE

Both the terms *explanation of benefits* (EOB) and *remittance advice* (RA) are used to describe the explanation of

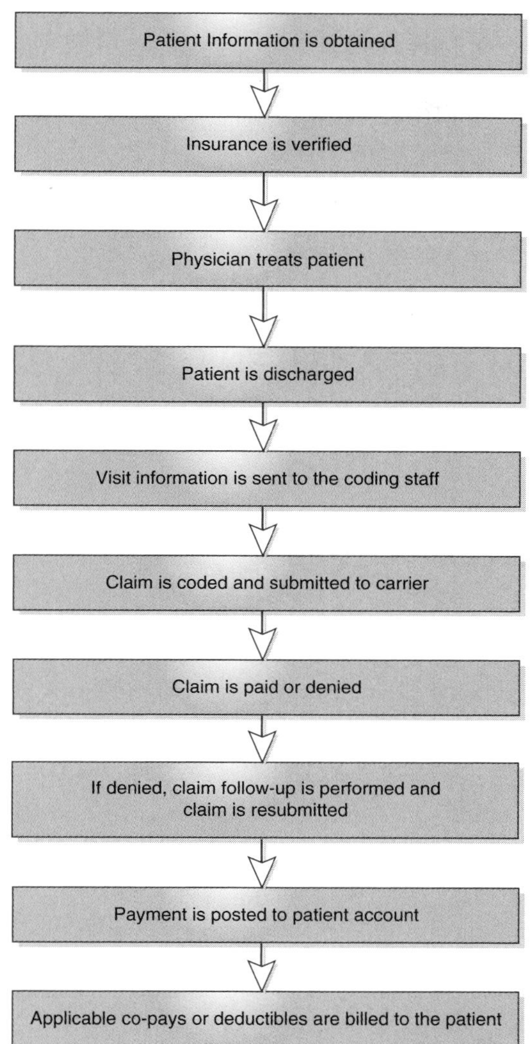

FIGURE 6-12. Flow chart showing what happens to third-party carrier claims.

payment or denial that is issued for every claim processed by a third-party carrier. This form (EOB/RA) is invaluable to a medical practice because it contains the following important billing information:

- What has been approved for payment
- What has actually been paid
- What has been denied
- Why it may have been denied
- What errors were identified on the claim
- What adjustments may have been made

The Anatomy of an EOB/RA

The information contained on an EOB/RA is as follows:

- Patient name
- Health insurance claim (HIC) number
- Patient account number (assigned by the practice)
- Provider name (physician, physician assistant [PA], nurse practitioner [NP], etc.)
- Claim number
- The amount billed
- The amount allowed (by contract)
- The amount applied to deductible/co-pay
- The amount payable from secondary insurance
- The amount paid
- The amount of interest paid, if applicable
- The amount paid to the patient, if applicable
- Codes billed
- Date of service
- Balance owed by the patient
- Claim total
- Explanations or messages regarding the claim

The EOB/RA should be used to identify errors and specific carrier requirements for more accurate coding in the future. Occasionally the carrier may make a mistake and deny a valid service. This error could be immediately identified and rectified. Denials can be addressed and possibly corrected based on the reason for the denial (see later in this chapter under "Reference Remark Codes" for specific descriptions of denial codes). If it is a medical necessity issue, which is the largest reason for denial across the country, there may be additional information available in the medical record that could be submitted to support the medical necessity for the service or procedure.

If your physician does not accept assignment, an EOB or RA would be sent as informational only. The example in Figure 6-13 illustrates a medical necessity scenario. In this scenario, the justification for the biopsy was documented in the progress note from 8/1/02. This note should be forwarded to the carrier to support the reason for the biopsy.

DENIED CLAIMS

An incomplete claim will be denied if certain information is missing for the insurance submission. According to CMS, the most common billing errors are as follows:

- The patient cannot be identified as a Medicare patient. *Always use the HIC number and name as it appears on the patient's Medicare card.*
- The referring/ordering physician's name and UPIN/NPI were not present on the claim. *Remember that this information is required in Items 17 and 17a for all diagnostic services, including consultations.*
- Evaluation and management procedure codes and the place of service do not match. *An incorrect place of service has been submitted with the E&M procedure code.*
- Diagnosis codes being used are either invalid or truncated. Diagnosis codes are considered invalid

Nordmark, Albert
000-11-2222

8/1/02 BP-136/84 P-84

cc- pt in for BP check. No other complaints. Denies chest pain, shortness of breath, cough, vision problems. No GI or GU problems. Pt states no problems with current medications. No changes in family or social history since last visit.

Exam- Pt is a well-developed, well nourished male in no acute distress. Heart-RRR, no murmurs. Resp-clear to auscultation, no bruits, Abd- soft, non-tender, no masses, no hepatomegaly. No swelling of legs or ankles, pedal pulses. Skin-suspicious lesion on R temple. Pt has very tanned skin. He states it is a "retirement tan."

Imp: Well-controlled hypertension
Possible malignant lesion R temple

Tx: 1) Continue Lotensin 10 mgs. 1 BID
2) Return for bx of lesion

Alexander Babinetz, M.D.

8/14/02 B.P. 154/86 P-88

cc- pt here for bx of lesion R temple

The patient was given 0.5 cc of Xylocaine to anesthetize the area around the lesion. Punch biopsy of lesion R temple taken. Pt tolerated bx well, was given a band-aid and discharged. Was told to take Tylenol for any discomfort. Pt instructed to call the office in 1 week for results of bx.

Alexander Babinetz, M.D.

FIGURE 6-13. Sample of progress notes sent to justify medical necessity.

usually because an extra digit is being added to make it five digits. *Remember that not all diagnosis codes are five digits. Check the ICD-9-CM codebook for the correct diagnosis code.*

- Procedure code/modifier was invalid on the date of service. *CMS no longer provides a grace period for discontinued CPT/HCPCS codes.*
- Claims are being submitted with deleted procedure codes. *This information can also be found in the CPT book.*

Claims Lacking Necessity

There are a few common reasons for claims to be denied due to lack of necessity. Because diagnosis coding is so important these days, many practices are seeing denials because the *diagnosis not payable for service billed.* Simply put, this means that the procedure code submitted is only payable with certain diagnosis codes and the one that was submitted was not one of those codes. Another commonly used denial is *allowance included in payment made for the surgery or procedure.* This type of denial occurs when an E&M service is provided during the postoperative period of a procedure. In this situation, it may be necessary to bill for the E&M code using a modifier. Modifier -24 can be used in this case when the E&M service is unrelated to the procedure.

Use of the diagnosis code reference number in Item 24e can be another reason for denial. This must be present for all claims submitted to the carrier. Last but not least, the physician (UPIN) who orders the procedure or service should be listed in Item 17a.

Duplicate Claims (Double Billing)

Duplicate claims will be denied if received by the carrier once the payment has been released to the practice. Many practices automatically resubmit claims that have not been paid within 60 days. Some computer software can be set to automatically resubmit these claims, whereas others require manual resubmission. This is not a good idea. Federal carriers can view this as a fraudulent billing issue. It is important to understand the status of a claim before resubmitting it.

Reference Remark Codes

These codes can be found on the EOB/RA form and describe the reason for the rejection of the claim. These codes are Medicare codes only. The following list can be referenced if the practice receives Medicare rejections:

MA36	Incomplete/invalid name of patient
MA51	Incomplete/invalid procedure code
MA52	Incomplete/invalid date of service
MA53	Incomplete or missing number of days or units of service
MA58	Incomplete release of information indicator
MA60	Incomplete/invalid relationship of patient to the insured
MA61	Missing or incomplete HIC number or Social Security number
MA75	Missing patient (or patient representative) signature
MA76	Incomplete/invalid diagnosis
MA77	Incomplete/invalid place of service
MA78	Missing appropriate HCPCS modifier(s)

MA79 Missing charge for service listed
MA81 Missing physician signature
MA82 Missing Medicare number or billing name, address, and phone number
MA83 No indication of Medicare as primary or secondary (see Item 11on the CMS form)
MA 84 Records indicate that a primary payer (not Medicare) exists, but missing employer's name or date of retirement
MA85 Records indicate that a primary payer (not Medicare) exists, but missing insurance plan or group name
MA86 Records indicate that there is an insurance primary to Medicare, but missing group number of primary insurer
MA87 Records indicate that a primary payer (not Medicare) exists, but missing insured's name
MA88 Records indicate that a primary payer (not Medicare) exists, but missing insurance address or telephone number
MA89 Records indicate that a primary payer (not Medicare) exists, but missing patient relationship to insured
MA91 Records indicate that there is insurance primary to Medicare, but missing or incomplete employer location
MA92 Records indicate that there is insurance primary to Medicare, but the information is either missing or incomplete
MA93 Records indicate that there is insurance primary to Medicare, but missing a copy of the EOB
MA99 Records indicate that a Medigap policy exits, but missing the required information
MA100 Missing or incorrect date of current illness, injury, or pregnancy
MA102 Missing or incorrect referring/ordering/supervising physician's name or UPIN
MA104 Missing or incorrect date the patient was last seen and the UPIN of the attending physician
MA110 Records indicate that a diagnostic test was billed, but not clarified if performed by an outside entity or if no purchased tests are included on the claim
MA111 Records indicate that a diagnostic test was billed; claim indicated it was performed by an outside entity, but missing purchase price of test or performing laboratory's name and address
MA112 Records indicate that the performing physician is a member of a group practice but missing or incomplete carrier-assigned provider number
MA114 Missing or incomplete name and address, or carrier-assigned provider number of the entity where services were furnished
MA115 Records indicate services were billed for in a Health Professional Shortage Area, but no physical location was supplied
MA116 Missing the statement "Homebound" on the claim to validate whether the laboratory services were performed at home or in an institution

MEDICARE SECONDARY PAYER

In 1966, Medicare was established under the Social Security Act for payment of health expenses for the elderly (age 65 and over). After the birth of Medicare, Congress recognized that some Medicare patients may also be covered under another insurance carrier. This led to the birth of the Medicare secondary payer (MSP) program. Once the primary insurance has paid, Medicare picks up the balance as the secondary payer.

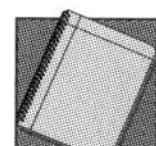

FROM THE EXPERT'S NOTEBOOK

Medicare will not pay if the primary insurance is accepted as payment in full by the provider.

It is important to understand when and when not to bill Medicare as primary. If the physician practice does not follow the rules of billing for an MSP, the practice can be subject to penalties of up to $2,000 for each incorrect billing. This can be made clear to the carriers by completion of Item 11c on the CMS 1500 form. The following list identifies scenarios where Medicare is primary:

- Patients with no additional insurance who are 65 or over
- Patients who have TRICARE/CHAMPUS
- Patients who are younger than 65 and are disabled
- Patients whose income qualifies them for the Medicaid program

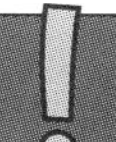

MANAGER'S ALERT

If the claim is denied by the primary insurer, submit the claim to Medicare. Primary carrier rejection does not necessarily mean automatic rejection by a secondary carrier, such as Medicare. Medicare will process the claim according to Medicare rules, which may result in acceptance of the claim.

Calculating the MSP payment

Follow these easy steps to understanding how to calculate the MSP payment:

1. Establish the Medicare payment.
2. Establish the Medicare reasonable and customary charge or the primary's allowable charge.
3. Subtract the amount paid by the primary from Item 2.
4. Payment will be the lowest amount of either Item 1 or Item 3.

For example: A patient is billed $200. The patient deductible has been paid. The primary insurer pays $125.00 of an allowable of $150.00. Medicare's reasonable charge is $125.00.

1. $125.00 × 80% = $100.00 (Medicare payment)
2. Primary allowable is $150.00, which is higher than Medicare's at $125.00.
3. The primary allowable charge of $150.00 − payment of $120.00 = $30.00
4. Payment is based on whichever is lower, Item 1 or Item 3. Since Item 1 is $100 and Item 3 is $30, payment would be $30.00, the lowest amount.

RENT-A-DOC (LOCUM TENENS)

There are times in the life of a medical practice when the practice must retain a substitute physician. Indications for such a situation are

- Physician illness
- Physician vacation
- Physician pregnancy/maternity leave

The practice of a substitute physician is referred to as *locum tenens.* The physician hired generally does not have an established practice and has the flexibility to move from one area to another. In some of these situations, physicians will often have established a reciprocal billing arrangement with other physicians in town. When this is not possible, a locum tenens physician is hired to fill the gap. Congress passed legislation through the Social Security Amendments of 1994 that made this type of arrangement legal.

Billing Arrangements

The following scenarios must be in place for a locum tenens billing to take place:

- The regular physician must *not* be available to treat patients.
- The regular physician must pay the locum tenens physician for services on a per diem or similar fee-for-time basis.
- The locum tenens physician cannot provide Medicare services for more than 60 continuous days.
- All services billed by the regular physician for locum tenens services must be submitted with a Q6 modifier to identify that the service was performed by a locum tenens physician.
- The locum tenens NPI number must be listed in Item 23 of the CMS 1500 form. The billing or regular physician number should still be reported in Item 33 for solo physician and Item 24k for group practice.
- "Incident to" services by the regular physician's staff may still be performed with the locum tenens physician if they meet the requirements for "incident to" billing.

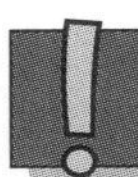

MANAGER'S ALERT

The Office of Inspector General (OIG) has issued a fraud alert for potential billing violations of locum tenens situations. Be careful to follow the guidelines for this billing.

HOSPICE CARE

Medicare patients who are terminally ill and have a life expectancy of less than 6 months can use "hospice benefits" instead of standard Medicare coverage. When Medicare patients choose hospice coverage, they waive their right to curative treatment and realize that they are only allowed palliative care. In other words, they cannot seek any additional treatments or services under Medicare Part B. Hospice care is available for two 90-day periods and one 30-day period. If the patient needs an additional period, a fourth period can be added.

Billing

When billing for physician services for hospice care, a statement must be entered in Item 19 explaining that the physician is the patient's attending physician and not a physician who is employed by the hospice. If this statement is not entered in Item 19, there is a strong possibility that the physician will not be paid. An example of such a statement would be, "Dr. George Casey is the attending physician of hospice patient, Eileen Brostowicz, and is not an employee of the hospice."

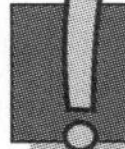

MANAGER'S ALERT

Hospice services are also being scrutinized by the OIG, and a fraud alert has been issued.

THE RETURN ENVELOPE

The return envelope is a very important tool of the billing office, but it is often dismissed as an unneeded expense.

It is a proven fact, however, that individuals will pay bills that include a return envelope before they pay bills for which they have to provide their own envelope. Whether the reason is that it is convenient for them or they feel they are getting something for free, customers pay a bill faster when it is accompanied by a return envelope. It works for the utility companies; why not for the doctor? Some offices prefer to use a colored envelope for their return envelope, so they can detect it easily in the mail. Colored or plain white, the return envelope is well worth the few pennies it costs to enclose it.

SUBMITTING CLEAN CLAIMS

A clean claim is one that has been submitted with no errors. It contains the necessary information regarding the patient's coverage and diagnosis and the services rendered. It contains all of the necessary information regarding the treating and referring physician. A clean claim is one that can be processed electronically; it has no error that requires the services of an individual. Claims that arrive at an insurance processing center with errors must be transferred to an individual for processing. This delays the claim processing and therefore payment to the physician. It is critical for the office manager to stress the importance of a clean claim and to ensure that the billing process in the office promotes clean claims. The errors most commonly made on the CMS 1500 form are listed in Box 6-1.

ELECTRONIC CLAIMS

By using electronic claims submission, the office spends less time preparing the claim for submission and receives reimbursement sooner than if a paper claim was submitted. This paperless processing of claims goes by several names: *electronic media claims, electronic data interchange,* and *electronic claims processing.* Medicare and Blue Cross/Blue Shield have had electronic claim submission systems in place for many years. Larger HMOs, Medicaid, and commercial insurance company clearinghouses are now also going electronic. There are several reasons why electronic claims submission is preferable to paper claims submission:

- Payment is faster.
- Paperwork is reduced.
- Staff time and costs are reduced.

Submitting claims electronically makes payment dramatically faster. The checks are automatically deposited into the practice's bank account, and the explanation of benefits is either printed out on the office's printer or mailed to the office. In any case, the turnaround time for a claim is much faster. Faster claim turnaround times translate into improved cash flow. The average physician's office submits approximately 80% of its gross earnings to third-party insurances; therefore the cash flow improvement can mean substantial increases in revenue. There is no need for postage, and thus there is a reduction in paperwork costs and staff time. It has been estimated that by using an electronic claims submission system, a medical office saves between $1 and $4 on each claim submitted. There is no need for an employee to print the claim form, fold it, place it in an envelope, and stamp and finally mail it.

Electronic claims are submitted to the insurance carrier from the computer via the telephone lines and take only a short time to transmit. The software of the computer translates, edits, and formats the data according to the rules of each insurance carrier. When considering whether to purchase electronic claims submission software, you should do the following:

- Ask neighboring practices if they have any experience with electronic claims. Ask if you can visit their office and see their system in operation.
- Contact the carriers whom you bill and ask for the names of qualified software vendors.
- Consider attending the next professional meeting to speak with software vendors and look at their displays.
- Ask your office's health care consultant, if you have one, to recommend a qualified vendor.
- Ask the vendor how long it has been involved with electronic claims submissions.
- Ask the vendor for references, that is, the names of offices for whom the vendor has installed systems.
- Ask the references about the vendor's service and support.
- Ask the vendor about charges associated with electronic claims packages.
- Ask the vendor about the cost of service contracts.
- Ask the vendor about updates on the software.
- Ask the vendor whether training for the staff and physicians is available and included.

BOX 6-1 Errors Commonly Made on the CMS 1500 Form

- Health insurance number is missing or incorrect.
- Provider number is missing or incorrect.
- Unique provider identification number (UPIN) is missing or incorrect.
- Place of service is missing or incorrect.
- Guarantor information is incomplete.
- Date of service is incorrect.
- Form is addressed to incorrect carrier.
- Modifiers are missing or incorrect.
- Diagnosis codes are truncated or not appropriate for service billed.
- Number of units billed is incorrect.

MEDICARE AUDITS

There is a simple way to avoid Medicare audits—learn exactly what the auditors are looking for when they review a practice's claims. Every insurance carrier has a manual on payment procedures. This manual contains guidelines as to how many records each carrier should select for a comprehensive medical review. Reviewers will look for patterns and abnormal practices. The CMS manual includes a section titled "Post Payment Alert List," which describes types of abuse that have been detected across the nation. If records are requested, it is imperative that they are copied and sent in a timely fashion.

PATIENT TRANSFERS

When a patient is transferred from one hospital to another, selecting the proper billing codes can be tricky. When a patient is in Hospital A and is transferred to Hospital B, Medicare will pay for discharge-day management from Hospital A and for hospital admission to Hospital B. Generally, the hospital admission service is a lower-level code, because the patient is already an established patient of the physician.

"INCIDENT TO" SERVICES

"Incident to" billing is defined as billing for services furnished to patients as an integral, although incidental, part of the physician's personal professional services in the course of diagnosis or treatment of an illness or injury. Medical personnel performing these services must be employed by the physician. The personnel must be full-time employees, part-time employees, or employees leased by the physician. A leased employee is one who is a non-physician working under a written employee leasing agreement that provides services as a leased employee of the physician with the physician controlling all actions of the employee.

In a medical office, this refers to "incident to" the professional services of a physician in private practice and is limited to scenarios where there is direct physician supervision. This applies to the following groups of people:

- Nurses
- Anesthetists
- Psychologists
- Technicians
- Therapists
- Nurse practitioners
- Physician assistants
- Clinical social workers
- Clinical nurse specialists

The services of a nurse practitioner (NP) and physician assistant (PA) cannot be billed "incident to" in a hospital setting. In other words, NP or PA services cannot be billed for using the following codes:

- Inpatient consultations (99251 to 99255)
- Initial hospital services (99221 to 99223)
- Subsequent hospital services (99231 to 99233)

Even though NPs and PAs are licensed under state law to perform certain medical procedures without physician supervision, if service is billed as "incident to," the NP or PA must perform the service under the direct personal supervision of a physician. NPs and PAs can bill using their own individual UPIN for such services.

DIRECT SUPERVISION

In a medical office, direct supervision doesn't mean the physician must be in the examination room when the service is being performed, but it does mean that the physician must be present in the office suite and immediately available to provide assistance and direction. Being available by phone does not count!

Here is another scenario that doesn't count. A physician's office is on the second floor of the hospital, in the west wing. He is on the second floor of the hospital, east wing, making rounds on inpatients. Yes, he is close, but not close enough. This scenario would not meet the requirements.

MEDICAL OFFICE REGISTRATION AND BILLING

The following is the core of information needed from each patient, regardless of her or his financial status, at the time of registration:

- Insurance information—photocopy both sides of the insurance card
- Driver's license number
- All demographic and financial information
- Employment information
- Consent/authorization signatures

All patients should be reminded of their financial responsibility, be it a $10 co-pay or a $100 deductible. Each individual payer requires different information, as the following lists indicate:

- Medicare:
  - Policy number
  - Spouse's employment
  - Patient's retirement date
  - Whether the patient has been in the hospital in the last 60 days

- Medicare questionnaire
- Secondary insurance information, if any, and card copy, if applicable
- Medicaid:
  - Current monthly card
  - Address
  - Birth date
  - Card holder's name
  - Secondary insurance information, if any, and card copies
- Workers' compensation:
  - Date of injury
  - Address of place of injury
  - Letter from employer
  - Workers' compensation form
  - Workers' compensation number of previous injury
  - Secondary insurance information and card copy
- Health maintenance organization (HMO)/preferred provider organization (PPO):
  - Name of primary care physician
  - Referral number for visit
  - Commercial/Blue Cross
  - Plan code
  - Correct policy number
  - Correct group number
  - Name as written on card

Billing and Statement Types

Two main categories of billing and statement types are commonly used by medical practices:

1. Computerized
2. Manual

COMPUTERIZED BILLING

Most offices today are computerized and run their billings from their computer system. This can be done in two ways: data mailers and statements.

Data mailers are composed of several sheets of paper that are arranged in such a way that when the computer prints, it imprints the patient bill and the mailing envelope at the same time. Some data mailers may also contain a return envelope for the patient's convenience. This is an efficient way to bill patients; however, it can be costly. The office manager should evaluate the time it takes employees to fold, stuff, and address these bills. This can be weighed against the cost of the data mailer to determine the most cost-effective way in which to bill patients.

Statement billing is a computer printout of a patient's statement. These statements are continuous and must be separated, folded, and stuffed into envelopes to be mailed. This bill may contain such information as

- Service rendered
- Charge for service
- Date submitted to insurance company
- Date paid
- Balance due

Most computers will print specific notes on these bills, such as the following:

- "This bill is now 30 days past due. Please send payment."
- "This bill is now 60 days past due. Please remit!"
- "This bill is now 90 days past due. Avoid collection proceedings by remitting today!"

There might be a limitation as to the number of characters the computer can print in such a note, so some abbreviations might need to be used.

MANUAL BILLING

Some offices are not computerized and use manual billing systems. For instance, large offices may use a ledger system, in which a ledger card is kept for each patient or family. This card is photocopied at the end of each month, placed into a window envelope, and mailed to the patient. These cards are generally used with a pegboard system, which is a "one-write" system.

As discussed in the beginning of this chapter, many medical offices use a "patient encounter form," a form that serves as a charge slip, patient receipt, patient billing statement, and insurance reporting form. Patient encounter forms are imprinted with the physician's name, office address, and phone number. They also contain the space necessary for the information required by the various different insurance companies. Today's patient encounter form may look quite different from patient encounter forms of the past. There are companies today that offer a computerized patient encounter form that can be used with a scanner to input the charges and diagnoses directly into the patient's computerized account. The patient encounter form is fed through a scanner that immediately prints the information on the computer screen. This saves the office valuable time and is less likely to contain errors because no keystrokes are involved in the data entry process.

Offices using noncomputerized billing systems can apply brightly colored pressure-sensitive labels with collection warnings on them to the front of patient statements. Box 6-2 shows some warnings that may be printed on the labels.

Payment at the Time of Service

Another part of patient education is alerting patients that payment is expected at the time of the visit. The front-desk staff should be trained to ask for payment at this time. When patients schedule office visits, they should be informed of the office's payment and collection policy

BOX 6-2 Collection Warning Labels

- Please remit promptly to avoid collection agency action.
- PAST DUE.
- Please contact our office immediately if there is a problem.
- We accept VISA and MasterCard. Do you wish to pay for your overdue balance using your credit card?
- YOUR ACCOUNT IS 90 DAYS PAST DUE! PLEASE PAY NOW!
- No payment has been received from your insurance company. This bill is now payable by you!
- This bill is your RESPONSIBILITY!!
- SERIOUSLY OVERDUE ACCOUNT!!
- Your insurance company has paid its share of this bill. The balance is now your responsibility!
- *FINAL NOTICE:* If we do not hear from you within 10 days, this account will be turned over to our collection agency.
- *FINAL NOTICE:* This is the last statement you will receive from this office. The next notification will be from our collection agency!

and told that payment is expected at the time of service. Staff should be trained to expect the common responses: "I forgot my checkbook," "I always get billed," "I just wrote my last check before coming here," "I'll mail the check to you," "They always bill my insurance." Instruct the staff to be firm but courteous when dealing with patients who delay in paying.

The Billing Cycle

It is critical to have a billing policy in place. Patient statements should be mailed in a timely manner. If the number of statements to be mailed each month is large, it might be easier to mail them in a cycle. In cycle billing, patient statements are split into quarters of the alphabet and billed on a weekly rotation. The first week of the month, all patients with last names that begin with the letters A through F are billed. The second week of the month, all patients with last names that begin with the letters G through L are billed. The third week of the month, all patients with last names that begin with the letters M through R are billed. The fourth week of the month, all patients with last names that begin with the letters S through Z are billed. Use of a system such as this will allow for better cash flow in the practice. This type of billing is also referred to as "batch" billing.

Step 1: The patient calls to schedule an appointment with the physician and is reminded to bring her or his insurance card to the office at the time of the appointment. While the patient is on the phone, her or his demographic and insurance information is obtained. If the patient has a managed care plan, she or he is reminded to bring a referral for the visit from a primary physician.

In addition, it is important that patients know exactly what is expected of them in the office before they schedule an appointment. The informed patients of today often call and ask a series of questions regarding procedures of the office before they will schedule an appointment. If they do not like what the office is telling them, they will simply call another. The office should not be concerned about turning down patients who do not seem willing to pay its fees and follow its payment guidelines. This policy should be discussed with the physician before it is instituted.

Some physicians still believe that a medical practice is not a business. However, more and more physicians are changing their view on this issue. For example, when prospective patients without insurance call to schedule an appointment, they should be instructed that the fee for a new patient office visit can be anywhere from $55 to $170. They should also be told that follow-up visits can be anywhere from $38 to $125. *These amounts listed are for explanation purposes only and do not represent actual fees. Your office fees would be substituted.* It is best to explain that this fee does not cover any diagnostic workup that they might also have to have done, if the physician deems it necessary. Most offices submit these diagnostic tests to the patient's insurance company for payment. This is a courtesy and should not be abused. There will always be the patient who refuses to pay for an office visit before submitting the claim to her or his insurance company. Train the staff to explain to the patient that this is not the policy of the office and that payment for the visit must be made at the time of service. Some patients do not have insurance coverage for office visits. The staff should give these patients a copy of their patient encounter form or a CMS 1500 form that they can send to the insurance company for reimbursement from major medical. Patients with insurance coverage would only have to pay for co-payments or deductibles, because the balance of the charges would be submitted to their insurance carrier.

Step 2: The patient arrives at the office for the appointment. Her or his demographic information is obtained, if it was not obtained on the phone. The patient is asked for her or his insurance card, and the front and back of the card are photocopied. If the patient is a Medicare patient, a Medicare authorization is signed. If the patient has insurance other than Medicare, a general medical authorization is signed. If the patient is a managed care patient, in a specialty office, a valid referral is collected. If the patient is responsible for a co-pay, it is best to try to collect the co-pay at this time.

All patients who belong to an HMO must be told that they cannot be seen without a referral from their primary physician. Physicians will not backdate a referral, so it is extremely important that patients have the referral at the time of their visit. The physician who treats the patient without a referral runs an excellent chance of not getting paid. It is the front-desk person's responsibility to establish whether the patient has a referral for her or his visit. It is also important to check the referral to see what services have been approved for your office to do at that visit. Any service performed without the primary physician's permission will not be paid for by the HMO.

If the physician for whom you work has established a policy that she or he will not participate in any insurance, it is important for the office staff to make this policy clear to patients. The staff can be helpful in assisting patients with their insurance forms. Financial arrangements can be made with the office manager regarding payment plans. Some offices hand out financial arrangement sheets to all new patients. This financial agreement sheet can be tailored to fit any practice and its policies. When patients are given this sheet, they will have a full understanding of the policy of your office, and payment should be smoother.

Step 3: The patient receives care and exits the examination room. The patient then goes to the front desk, where a follow-up appointment and testing are scheduled, if appropriate. Payment, if not covered by insurance, is collected for the physician's service at this point. If the visit is covered by insurance, this information should be confirmed now.

Step 4: Services are billed to the appropriate insurance companies.

Step 5: The patient statement is mailed to the patient on the normal monthly billing cycle.

Overpayments

Occasionally, patients and carriers overpay on patient accounts. For patient overpayments, the check should be returned to the patient with VOID written across the front of it. However, because of the system used in some offices, it is difficult to intercept the check before it is entered into the computer as a credit. When this occurs, an office check is written for the amount paid and is sent to the patient. The adjustment is made in the computer on the day the office check is mailed to the patient.

Carrier overpayments, however, are an entirely different issue. If an overpayment is received from a carrier, specifically Medicare, the carrier should be notified and the payment should be returned. If the practice does not refund the overpayment, the physician could be accused of fraud. Since all physicians need and want to abide by Medicare regulations, it is their responsibility to follow the rules and refund promptly.

Overpayments can result from a variety of incidents:

- A computer "glitch"
- An error in calculation of the deductible
- Payment when another carrier is primary
- Data entry errors
- Payment being sent to the patient instead of the physician

Medicare can request a refund of an overpayment for up to 3 years after the date the payment was made to the practice. This is a great argument for retaining the practice's copies of EOBs/RAs. Actually, by law, the Data Match Project, which is collaboration by the Internal Revenue Service (IRS), Social Security Administration (SSA), and CMS, can request a refund at any time within 1 year after it is discovered. If you think that the refund notice is an error, it can be appealed. Written notice must be made to the carrier with supporting evidence that this is indeed an error. Check with the local Medicare carrier to identify the time frame in which the refund must be made. This time period is generally about 30 days.

SIMPLE STEPS TO CORRECT AN OVERPAYMENT

1. Immediately notify the carrier in writing and explain how the overpayment occurred.
2. Send notification by certified mail with a return receipt requested.
3. If the check is for the services of only one patient, return the actual Medicare check with VOID written across the front and back. Keep a copy of the check you refund.
4. Most checks are for the services of more than one patient. In this case, the check should be deposited and a check from the practice should be issued for the refund amount. Always make two copies of the check; keep one on file and send one copy with the refund.
5. Attach a copy of the EOB/RA to the letter.
6. Include the patient's Social Security number; this identifies the patient and eliminates confusion and errors.

It is wise to keep a log of overpayments for tracking purposes. This can be done simply by writing them in a notebook. The entry should contain the following information:

- The patient's name
- The number of the patient's check or the carrier's check
- The number of the returned check
- The amount of the returned check
- The date the check was received
- The date the check was refunded
- The reason for the refund
- The initials of the employee requesting the refund

The staff member requesting a refund check should fill out a patient refund form (Figure 6-14) and submit it to the bookkeeper or office manager for reimbursement. The form should have a copy of the patient's check attached to it.

Mistakes in Billing

Always admit any mistakes the office may have made in billing. Patients often tell the office that they think there

Date: ______________________

Refund check payable to: ______________________________________
Address:

Reason for refund:

Name of person requesting refund: ______________________________
____

Approved by: ______________________________

Date of refund: ______________________

FIGURE 6-14. Patient refund form.

is a mistake on their bill. This is sometimes a stall tactic so that they do not have to pay their bill. However, if the office did make a mistake, it should be admitted and rectified immediately. This shows the patient the integrity of the office and the staff members.

FROM THE EXPERT'S NOTEBOOK

When the office has made an error in billing to an insurance company, it is important to notify the insurance company immediately and ask how to go about correcting the situation. Some insurance companies ask that you wait to send a reimbursement check to them until they send you the necessary paperwork. Others will ask for a check in the amount they paid, accompanied by a copy of the EOB/RA.

FINANCIAL DISCLOSURE LETTERS

It is important to realize that not everyone will pay her or his bills. It is impossible to collect certain accounts, not because the collection system in place is faulty or the staff are not doing their job, but because some patients suffer from true economic hardship. However, there should be a policy in place for these occasions. A copy of the patient's first complete tax return (Form 1099) should be requested in every case of hardship. The poverty guidelines released by the Department of Health and Human Services each year are used for these types of determinations. In 2008, according to the *Federal Register*, the poverty level for one individual was $10,400 for the 48 contiguous states. Alaska was $13,000, and Hawaii was $11,960. For a family of four, this figure increased to $22,200 for the 48 contiguous states, $26,500 for Alaska, and $24,380 for Hawaii. This level refers to all income sources before taxes. The financial disclosure form shown in Figure 6-15 can be used to determine the financial stability of a patient. Any patient who claims hardship should be asked to fill out this form. It is sent to the patient with a cover letter and is followed by either an acceptance letter or a rejection letter, as shown in the figure.

UNDELIVERED PATIENT STATEMENTS

The U.S. Postal Service (USPS) offers a service whereby any mail sent from a professional office can be located by the use of "Address Correction Requested." All of the medical office's envelopes should have these words printed on them. If these words are either printed or stamped on the envelope sent to the patient who has moved, the Post Office will automatically research and locate the new address of that patient. It will send the office a form with the new address stamped on it. (However, if the patient did not arrange to have her or his mail forwarded, it will not be possible to obtain the new address.) This tool is very helpful when offices are attempting to send statements to patients who no longer live in the area.

Some mail will be returned with various phrases handwritten on the front of the envelope. This is usually the work of patients attempting to avoid paying their bills. Such phrases as "Not here" or "Refused" are generally written by the patient, a family member, or a friend. The USPS uses a stamp to explain the undelivered mail.

If the mail is returned and the USPS cannot help, there are a few other methods to locate lost patients. The following is a list of possible means of obtaining patients' addresses or phone numbers:

- Call the patients' employers for updated information.
- Check the telephone book—it can come in handy sometimes.
- Call the emergency contact or relative of the patient.
- The hospital billing department may have the information.
- A referring physician may have updated information on a mutual patient.

Date:
Re:
Amount:

Dear: ______________________________

Per our telephone conversation, you stated that you could not afford to pay the above balance.

Enclosed you will find a **Financial Disclosure Form** for you to fill out. Please return this form to my attention at the address above, and a determination regarding your financial situation will be made.

If you fail to return this form, we will have no choice but to start legal collection proceedings for this account. If you have any questions, please feel free to contact our office at (222) 222-4444.

Sincerely,

Sue Malloy
Billing Manager

FIGURE 6-15. A, Financial disclosure form cover letter.

Patient name: ______________________
Social Security #: ______________________
Guarantor: ______________________
Relationship: ______________________
Address: ______________________
____
____
Phone#: ______________________
Are you currently employed? Y N
Disabled? Y N
Employer, if applicable: ______________________

Employer's address:
____
____
____
Other sources of income:
____
Spouse's name: ______________________
Employed? Y N
Total monthly income: ______________________
Number of dependents: ______________________
Total monthly expenses: ______________________
Rent: ______________________

Mortgage: ______________________

List other significant monthly expenses (car loans, medical, personal, etc.)
1. $
2. $
3. $

Please attach a copy of the following:
_____Prior year's income tax form _____Payroll stubs
_____Prior year's W-2 form

I understand that if my request for waiver of co-insurance charges is approved, it will apply as long as my primary insurance carrier's reimbursement is as stated above. I also understand that I am responsible for all deductibles and denial charges.

I, ______________________, certify that the facts set forth in this Financial Disclosure Form are true and correct to the best of my knowledge.

Patient's signature: ______________________

Date: ______________________

FIGURE 6-15. B, Financial disclosure form.

Date:
Re: *Sussex County Internal Medicine Associates Serious Past Due Balance of:* $ ___________

Dear Mr. ______________:
I am in receipt of your **Financial Disclosure Form** regarding your financial situation pertinent to the above outstanding balance. After thoroughly researching your form, I have determined that you are financially capable of paying the above balance of $ ___________ .

I am willing to set you up on a payment plan of at least $___________ per month. You will receive a monthly statement showing your payments.

If this account goes 60 days with no payment, it will be necessary to turn it over for legal collection proceedings. Thank you in advance for your cooperation. I'm looking forward to the resolution of this situation.

Sincerely,

Peg Knowles
Billing Manager

FIGURE 6-15. **C,** Letter to establish payment plan.

Date:

RE: *Sussex County Internal Medicine Associates Serious Past Due Balance of:* $ ________________

Dear Mr. ________________:
We have received your **Financial Disclosure Form** regarding your financial situation pertinent to the above balance. After thoroughly researching your form, I have decided to waive your portion of the bill.

If you have any questions, please feel free to contact our office at (222) 222-4444.

Sincerely,

Sharon Fuller
Billing Manager

FIGURE 6-15. **D,** Letter approving patient's request to waive balance due.

CREDIT CARDS—FRIEND OR FOE?

Health care providers are constantly looking for more effective ways to collect patient fees. If the medical office accepts credit cards, patients can pay for services even if they do not have the cash to do so. VISA, MasterCard, American Express, and Discover are busily visiting medical offices in an attempt to get them to accept credit card payments. Many medical offices offer patients more flexible and convenient payment terms by the use of these cards, because patients simply do not have the funds available for payment at the time of the office visit. If the office itself has a cash flow problem, the accountant may urge the office to accept credit card payment. This payment method decreases the office's billing expenses and increases its cash flow.

Patients who have major medical insurance find that using a credit card gives them the flexibility to pay for medical services at the time of the visit and then submit the bill to their major medical payers. In most cases, by the time the patient receives the credit card statement, the payer has issued a check to the patient for reimbursement of services. Medical practices that accept credit cards decrease their accounts receivable and reduce the average time for overdue accounts by 9 days. One of the most common reasons credit cards are accepted by medical practices is so that accounts receivable can be collected over the telephone. This decreases the number of accounts that need to be placed with outside collection agencies.

The credit card option gives patients an alternative way to clear their balances. Patients who always have an excuse as to why they cannot pay for their visit at the time of service now have the option of putting it on their credit card. If a practice chooses to accept credit cards, it is best to advertise this, so that the patients are aware that this is now an option available to them. This can be done by installing a sign that is provided by the credit card company (which is tastefully done with a caduceus on it, for those physicians who still cringe at the thought of patients using credit cards), by having the credit card insignias printed on the patient statements, and by placing the insignias on collection notices as an option for payment. Some practices have great success with the credit card option of payment, and can honestly report that their collections have improved since the implementation of credit cards.

Even though credit card acceptance is high in the medical field, the percentage of patient payments made with credit cards or debit cards is only 31%. Most patients still prefer to write a check for the medical service they received. It has been found that practices that are frequently paid with credit cards receive payment in full from their patients 2.5 times more often than practices that are only occasionally paid with credit cards.

There are drawbacks to this system, however. Credit card companies charge anywhere from 2% to 10% on each transaction. This fee can be kept to a minimum, depending on the volume of use and the size of the bill. There are application fees to pay and equipment fees to consider. Some offices purchase the equipment outright, whereas others lease it. Some offices use electronic "point of service" machines, whereas others use the less expensive manual imprinting units. The office should understand that it is responsible for the verification of each card on charges over $50 or more. In addition to these costs, some banks will also bill the practice for the charge slips used in the imprinters. It is necessary to evaluate the type of clientele the practice has. Are they generally older patients who would not use credit cards? Are they young and middle-aged professionals who live in a world of credit? The type of clientele the practice serves is an important consideration when deciding whether to accept credit cards.

Credit cards are becoming increasingly accepted by physicians, such as dermatologists and plastic surgeons, whose services are not always covered by insurance plans. When this happens, many patients choose to use their credit cards as a form of payment. The 24-hour care center, or "Doc-in-a-Box," as some people call it, also often encourages patients to pay by credit card, so that it is ensured payment by these walk-in patients it will likely not see again.

Debit cards have become more popular over the past 5 years, and are constantly used by patients for medical services and medications. It is simply more convenient to use a debit card than to write a check. With a debit card the patient has two options for payment, credit or debit. Credit will take a few days to catch up with your bank account, whereas when using a debit card, the amount is subtracted from your checking or savings account immediately upon use. These cards are also referred to as check cards.

BILLING SERVICES

Many offices have difficulty maintaining an efficient billing department. The billing process is sloppy, and the rules and regulations of the insurance companies boggle the mind. Is an outside billing service the answer?

A billing service is just what it says it is: a service that contracts with you to provide you with insurance billing. It will handle all bookkeeping and patient billing for the practice. It is the billing service's job to be up to date on the latest in Medicare and insurance company regulations. If you have decided the office could use the help of a billing service, contact several such services and obtain information regarding their services and fees. Inquire about the frequency of insurance claim submissions and whether or not they submit claims electronically.

One area to research when considering a billing service is the way it collects the claims from your office. Some billing services have representatives who arrive at the office at certain intervals to collect the claims. Other services use a courier or ask that the claims be sent via overnight mail. Some sophisticated services have their computer dial into your office computer to retrieve the information. When and how often the claims are sent is also valuable information for the office to have before signing a contract with a billing service.

Their fees are generally negotiable, and the fee should be a major factor in hiring the right billing service for your practice. Some billing services charge the practice by selling it vouchers and charging a certain amount per voucher. Others take a percentage of what they collect.

It is also important to discuss patient confidentiality with the billing service, ask how it maintains privacy when working with these claims, and ask for references.

COLLECTIONS

One in every five debt collectors works for a collection agency. The rest work for stores, banks, hospitals, and physician offices. These collectors keep track of accounts that are overdue and attempt to collect payment on them. Although some are employed by third-party agencies, many work in house and are direct employees of hospitals and physician practices. In larger physician practices, there may be one person whose only job is to provide in-house collections for the practice. The duties of collectors are the same whether they are collecting for a hospital or physician practice, and whether they are third-party collectors or in-house collectors, because they are all used to locate patients and notify them of delinquent accounts. Their process is as follows:

- When patients move without leaving a forwarding address, collectors may check with the post office, telephone companies, credit bureaus, or former neighbors to obtain the new address. This is called "skip-tracing." Collectors may spend a great deal of time on the telephone or the Internet during this process.
- Once the patient is located, the collector informs the patient of the overdue account and attempts to obtain payment. The collector may ask the patient why there was a delay in paying the bill.
- If the patient agrees to pay the overdue account, the collector will record this commitment and check later to verify that the payment was made. If the patient does not pay, the collector will prepare a statement indicating the conversation and action or nonaction

that took place. This account may then be turned over to an attorney for legal collections. This decision, however, needs to be made by the physician or the office manager at the direction of the physician. Patients should not be sent for legal collection without the physician's approval.

As cash flow is becoming increasingly important to practices, there is greater emphasis on collecting overdue or unpaid accounts. Hospitals and physicians' offices are two of the fastest growing industries requiring collectors. With insurance reimbursements steadily decreasing and costs steadily increasing, physicians and hospitals are seeking to recover even the smallest of balances. Because of the economy, employment of collectors is expected to grow faster than the average for all occupations through 2014.

Collection Policy

The words "prompt payment" are not often heard in a medical office. Many offices have accounts that are seriously overdue, thus creating a large accounts receivable balance that negatively affects the practice.

It is extremely important for the medical office to have a collection policy in place. Many offices are lax in the organization of their overdue accounts. However, the smart office has a specific process for collecting overdue accounts. It is a good idea to include this policy in the patient handbook that is given to patients at the time of their first visit. If the office does not provide a patient handbook, a written explanation of billing and collection procedures should be given to all patients as they register at the office. This "patient education" is a necessary part of the collection process.

Develop an In-Office Collections System

The office should determine the action it will take on delinquent accounts and when to take them. Many offices do not have a policy in place and therefore have a large percentage of their accounts receivable sitting unattended. The collection process described previously will be beneficial in setting up this system. Having a plan in place helps educate the patient to the fact that the office expects to be paid.

Once you have a plan in place, you must stick to it and not let emotions guide actions. Sometimes, staff members will let a bill "slide" because they feel the patient will eventually pay it. In all but a few of these cases, these employees have been deceived, and no payment is ever received. All this does is delay the collection process. Many patients pay their doctor last, feeling that the doctor has a lot of money and doesn't need it. Figure 6-16 shows a sample billing status report that can be used to document follow-up actions taken regarding delayed payment.

Stay within the Law: Collection Do's and Don'ts

There are two governing bodies that the medical office should be aware of when doing collections: the federal government and the state government. In some states, the physician's office must follow the same guidelines that the collection agencies in that state follow. Negligence of the rules can inadvertently negate the debt. Serious repercussions can result from not following these guidelines, so it is imperative that they are strictly followed. Be wise—stay within the law! The following are some guidelines to help you do so:

- Most state collection laws allow telephone collections only between 8:00 AM and 9:00 PM. Do not call at any other time of the day or night. Call the state bureau of collections and ask for information regarding collection laws.
- Do not call a patient's place of employment unless it is absolutely necessary, because some employers prohibit personal phone calls at work. Check your state's law. The number of calls that can be made to a patient's place of employment varies from state to state.
- Do not use a postcard as a collection tool.
- Do not misrepresent your identity.
- Do not misrepresent the office by using a form designed to create a false belief.
- Do not use a misleading letterhead.
- Do not accuse the patient of fraudulent behavior.
- Do not engage in continuous or repeated phone calls, "continuous" meaning making a series of phone calls, one right after another, and "repeated" meaning calling with excessive frequency under the circumstances.
- Do not shame a patient into payment.
- Do not speak to anyone *except* the patient.
- Do not leave a message that states the purpose of the call.

Develop an in-office collections procedure. The billing department, along with the office manager, should develop a system for handling overdue accounts. An example of such a system is as follows. At 30 days, the patient receives a phone call from a staff member, who says that she or he is following up to make sure that the statement arrived at the patient's home. At 60 days, the statement is sent printed or stamped with a message advising the patient that the account is now 60 days past due and remittance should be immediate to avoid collection proceedings. A "Final Notice" is sent at 90 days, a week after the billing statement. This "Final Notice" advises the patient that if payment is not received within 7 days of the receipt of the notice, legal collection proceedings will be started. It is advisable to make one last call to the patient before sending her or his account off to the collection agency. Have the

Patient Name/ Account Number	Date	Issue	Action Taken

FIGURE 6-16. Billing status report.

staff state that the patient's account has been pulled for legal collection proceedings and that they are making a courtesy call before the account is sent.

Telephone Calls

Patients do not like to be reminded of their outstanding debts. A series of telephone calls to them regarding these debts can be very beneficial to the collections process. However, as already mentioned, telephoning must be done within the hours designated by state law. In addition, staff should be trained to be professional at all times and not to respond to anger with anger.

Some patients are easily reached at dinnertime. Staff should be instructed that when a phone call fails to find the patient at home, they should note the time the call was made and should do this after subsequent unsuccessful attempts to contact the patient. A pattern in the patient's absence will often appear. For instance, if the office staff are calling at dinnertime, late afternoon, or early evening and finding no one at home, it might be concluded that the patient works evenings. By placing that account on the morning calls list, staff might catch the patient at home.

Instruct staff to *always* be certain that the person they are speaking to is the patient. If it's not the patient, they should leave a message, but not the reason for the call. A patient's outstanding debt can be discussed only with the patient in some states; the patient's debt cannot be discussed even with her or his spouse. The office must obtain the state regulations regarding this before making calls.

Thus a collections call should take place as follows. When someone picks up, staff should say, "Hello, Mrs. Brenner?" If the person identifies herself as Mrs. Brenner, it is permissible to discuss the outstanding debt. If the person says, "No, this is her daughter. Can I help you?" staff must simply give their own name and the name of the physician's office and leave a message for Mrs. Brenner to call the office at her earliest convenience. Staff must be trained to never state to anyone except the patient that they are calling in reference to an overdue account.

A "pregnant pause" placed at the right time in the conversation will sometimes evoke a response from patients regarding their nonpayment. For instance, after identifying themselves and stating the name of the physician's office, staff can say, "I'm calling about your overdue account balance of $45.00." A pause at this point in the conversation generally works! In most cases, it is best for staff to take a positive stand and say that they know the patient intends to pay this overdue account, but that perhaps she or he needs some type of payment arrangement. The patient should be given a time frame in which to work; for example, "Can we expect your monthly payment of $20.00 by the end of the week?" If the payment does not reach the office by that date, a reminder call should be made. Failure to follow up on these situations will result in nonpayment and a lackadaisical attitude on the part of the patient. Follow-up is extremely important when making collection calls.

MANAGER'S ALERT

Never threaten a patient with a debt collection action that you have no intention of pursuing. Under the Fair Debt Collection Practices Act, it is a violation to threaten to take action that is not intended to be taken. The office that makes such idle threats can be sued for harassment.

Collection Letters

Some offices have found the use of collection letters to be helpful. You can design a series of collection notices and letters for the office similar to that shown in Figure 6-17. Many offices buy brightly colored paper and, with the use of the computer and photocopier, print professional-looking notices. The use of a letter format as opposed to a form for the first contact with the patient has been found to be beneficial. It exudes a more personal touch and many times the effect is positive. A form is interpreted as being cold and ruthless.

The Collection Agency

The best way for medical services to collect fees is through in-office collection processes, which is the way some offices handle their severely overdue accounts. Most offices, however, do not have the resources and personnel to handle these accounts past a certain point. They focus their efforts on collecting overdue accounts up to and including 90 days and at that point refer overdue accounts to collection agencies, the "pros." If the patient hasn't paid in 90 days, it is clear that the patient does not intend to pay this bill. The likelihood that in-office collection methods will succeed greatly decreases after the 90-day period. According to the Commercial Collection Agency Section of the Commercial Law League of America, 25% of the accounts that are delinquent for 3 months are not recovered (Box 6-3 shows the death of the value of a dollar after time). At 6 months, there is a 40% account mortality rate, and at 12 months, 75% of the accounts must be written off and forgotten.

To choose a competent and efficient collection agency, the office manager might want to call other offices to see which agencies they use. It is wise to hire a collection agency on the basis of a solid referral. Some offices choose to request a list of collection agencies from the local medical society or hospital.

Once information is secured from the prospective agencies, it is very important to analyze their collection methods and find out the fees they charge for the accounts collected. The collection agency chosen should be ethical and provide services in a manner with which the office feels comfortable. After all, the collection agency is a reflection of the office. Collection agencies charge for their services in a variety of ways. Some take a percentage, between 30% and 50% on average, and some collect a flat fee for each account handed over to them. These fees are negotiable. There are two advantages to flat rates:

- The agency gives every account equal treatment and does not "pick off" the larger-balance accounts that come with a bigger payoff.
- There is more comfort in turning over large accounts because the charge is the same. Some practices that are charged on a percentage basis will tend to keep these accounts in house longer to try to collect.

Many collection agencies use vouchers to obtain information regarding the account being placed. Some agencies charge for these vouchers and some include it in the price of the collection service. Investigate all methods to ascertain which is best for your practice.

Fees can always be negotiated based on the following:

- The volume of accounts being referred or the total dollars associated with these accounts.
- If you promise to use them and only them.
- The age of the accounts deem them to be more collectible. In other words, the accounts referred for collections may be 90 days old as opposed to 2 years old.

March 24, 2008

Name: Eugenia Safin
Amount Due: $ ______________
Account #: 101625

The above amount of $___________ has been applied to your Medicare deductible. This charge results from your visit with the doctor on ________________.

We would appreciate it if you could forward a check in the amount of $___________ to our office as soon as possible. A self-addressed envelope is enclosed for your convenience.

Thank you for your cooperation in this matter.

Sincerely,

William Scott
Billing Manager

FIGURE 6-17. A, Collection notice for Medicare deductible.

November 10, 2008

Brenda Lingle
P.O. Any Box
Anytown, USA

Dear Mrs. Lingle:
Our records indicate that you have a seriously overdue account balance of $_________ and that **no** payment has been made. We would appreciate **immediate payment** to avoid any further collection proceedings. If you have any questions, please feel free to call our office.

Thank you for your cooperation in this matter.

Sincerely,

Kathleen McWilliams
Billing Manager

FIGURE 6-17. B, Overdue account letter.

September 18, 2008

Brian Brostowicz
270 Wendell Street
Big City, USA

Dear Mr. Brostowicz:
Our records indicate that your account balance is 60 days past due. We have submitted this balance of $ ___________ to your insurance company, but we have not received any payment as of this date.

Your insurance policy is a contract between you and your insurance company. Unfortunately, we do not have the personnel to continue to pursue this matter. This unpaid balance of $___________ is now your responsibility. Please mail a check to our office in this amount and contact your insurance company for payment to reimburse you. Thank you for your prompt attention to this matter.

Sincerely,

Lisa Gatto
Administrator

FIGURE 6-17. C, Sixty-day collection letter.

FINAL NOTICE

DATE: August 4, 2008
ACCOUNT NUMBER: 000007640

NAME: Rita Palit

YOUR ACCOUNT IS NOW SERIOUSLY PAST DUE—FAR BEYOND OUR USUAL LIMITS. UNLESS YOU MAKE IMMEDIATE ARRANGEMENTS TO PAY YOUR ACCOUNT, WE WILL HAVE NO CHOICE BUT TO REFER IT TO OUR COLLECTION AGENCY.

REMIT PAYMENT WITHIN 10 DAYS TO ABOVE ADDRESS.

BALANCE DUE $ ________.

Maryanne Dunlap
Billing Supervisor

FIGURE 6-17. **D,** Ninety-day collection notice.

October 30, 2008

Ann Colantonio
1600 Park Hill Street, Apt. 3
Any City, USA

Dear Mrs. Colantonio:
Your account with our office is long past due, but I don't believe in sending collection letters to receive payment for my services. I believe most people are fair, and want to pay their bills as soon as possible. So, instead of harassing you with dunning letters, may I appeal to your sense of fairness:

If money is tight for you right now, please pay any other bills that are older than ours. We will wait for any patient who makes an effort to meet his obligations. But, if it's our turn, please send a check to us soon.

If you want more time to pay your bill or want to set up a payment plan, just call us and tell us how we can help you. We will appreciate this courtesy, and it will save both of us a lot of worry.

Sincerely,

Danelle Kelly
Accounts Supervisor

FIGURE 6-17. **E,** Soft collection letter.

September 9, 2008

Cecelia Alberts
10 Down Street
Any Town, USA

Dear Mrs. Alberts:
After two reminders, we still haven't received your check for the balance of your overdue account. Perhaps there is some question in your mind about this balance. If so, please contact us at once; I am certain we can straighten the matter out immediately.

However, if you have no questions, and our figures agree, why delay payment any longer? Even partial payment will be greatly appreciated. We shall expect a prompt reply. Thank you.

Amount Due: $ ___________

Sincerely,

Bill Snyder
Billing Department

FIGURE 6-17. **F,** Soft reminder letter.

August 1, 2008

A Friendly Reminder . . .

It is entirely possible, Mrs. Miller, that you have already settled this account and that our letters have crossed in the mail. If so, please disregard this notice.

If, however, you have not yet paid your account balance of $________________, will you please do so today? We appreciate your attention to this matter.

Thank you.

Sincerely,

Gail Reinhart
Billing Manager

FIGURE 6-17. **G,** Friendly reminder letter.

November 6, 2008

John Anthony
RD 2
Lake Town, USA

Dear Mr. Anthony:
Our accountant has brought to our attention that you have an overdue account balance of $100.00. We are sure that this is just an oversight on your part, and that payment will be made within the week. However, if there is a problem, we are sincerely interested in helping. If you require us to set up a payment plan for you, please call our office and our billing clerk, Ann, will be happy to help you.

If there is a problem that needs special attention, we invite you to come to our office to discuss this problem. Should you wish to do so, please call our office to set up an appointment with Donna. We would like to help with any special arrangements that might be necessary.

If this has just been an oversight on your part, please drop a check in the mail so that we may credit your account as soon as possible. We thank you for your cooperation in this matter, and look forward to hearing from you.

Sincerely,

Laurie Bass
Office Manager

FIGURE 6-17. **H,** Oversight collection letter.

COLLECTION DEPARTMENT FINAL NOTICE
DATE: ______________
ACCOUNT NUMBER: ______________
NAME: ______________________________
BALANCE DUE: ______________

WE HAVE CORRESPONDED WITH YOU ON SEVERAL OCCASIONS REGARDING YOUR CHARGES FOR SERVICES PERFORMED BY OUR PHYSICIANS. BECAUSE OF YOUR FAILURE TO PAY THIS ACCOUNT OR TO MAKE SATISFACTORY PAYMENT ARRANGEMENTS, WE MUST TAKE FURTHER ACTIONS.

WE DO NOT DESIRE TO INITIATE ANY ACTIONS THAT WOULD HARM YOUR CREDIT RATING. HOWEVER, WE MUST INSIST THAT THE BALANCE DUE ON YOUR ACCOUNT BE PAID WITHOUT FURTHER DELAY. IF WE DO NOT RECEIVE YOUR CHECK WITHIN *10 DAYS*, THE NEXT COMMUNICATION YOU RECEIVE WILL BE FROM OUR COLLECTION AGENCY.

SINCERELY,

Kim Hamilton
Billing Supervisor

FIGURE 6-17. **I,** Collection Department Final Notice.

BOX 6-3 Time Marches On . . .

How many times have you heard that the value of the dollar decreases rapidly? In looking at accounts receivables, the value of the dollar decreases at the following rate:

Current value	$1.00
After 2 months	$0.90
After 6 months	$0.66
After 1 year	$0.45
After 2 years	$0.23
After 3 years	$0.16

This is an important factor to keep in mind when collecting overdue account balances in a medical office. Calculate the cost of collecting accounts when they are severely overdue. In many cases, it is simply more cost-effective to write them off than to pay office staff to collect them.

MANAGER'S ALERT

Have the practice attorney review any contract with a collection agency *before* you sign it.

The office manager should always have the last say regarding whether an account should be turned over to the collection agency. There may be extenuating circumstances regarding one or two of the patients that the biller might not be aware of. *No* accounts should be placed into collections before they are reviewed. Review helps to prevent any counterallegation that could come up. The normal period of time an account should remain in collections is 6 months. After that time, the account should be returned to the office and a decision should be made as to the next course of action. At this point, many offices simply write off these accounts and place a sticker on the patient's chart regarding this action.

Some offices cease to provide care for patients who have neglected to pay for their services. They send termination letters to the patients after the collection agency returns the account. This action eliminates any liability that might arise in the future with these patients. A few offices have either the billing manager or the office manager file in small-claims court for the balance on the bill. This is costly and often is just throwing good money after bad. If patients get to this point, experience says cut your losses and go forward! Patients who are covered under the Americans with Disabilities Act cannot be terminated because of lack of payment.

All accounts should be logged into a loose-leaf book or into a spreadsheet for tracking purposes. This creates a paper trail of these accounts and allows the success of the collection agency to be tracked. The monthly reports sent by the collection agency should be compared with the book in the office for evaluation of the collection agency's services. Many collection agencies want the patients to pay the monies directly to them and not to the medical office. This is also a negotiable point. If the agency wants the business, it will do anything to satisfy the customer—you!

Looking for a collection agency for patients is a bit trickier than if the collections were for a retail store. The following questions should be asked of all collection agencies that are being interviewed:

- How does the agency pay collectors?
- Does it regularly monitor telephone calls?
- Will it allow a review of its collector's code of professional conduct?
- Can you contact clients as references—especially other medical offices?

Collection Percentages

Statistics show that new physicians have a lower collection rate than established practices. Type of communities, geographic location, and age of physician are also important statistics in collections.

Collecting from an Estate

Collecting payment for service to the deceased requires great tact, because the family of the deceased is already on an emotional roller coaster. This is not the time to offend the family by sending threatening letters and collection notices. The best way to start collections on a deceased patient is to be sure to collect all that is appropriate from the third-party payers involved. Once these payers have reimbursed their share, the balance must be treated with care. A simple call to the family to obtain the name and address of the executor who will be handling the estate is the next step. Estates usually close within 12 months of the date of death, so it is imperative to follow through in a timely manner. Contact the executor involved and provide the proper documentation to support the outstanding debt. The executor will then add you to the list of creditors for payment. The executor of the estate can be a lawyer, family member, or friend. It is necessary to keep in constant contact with that person to check on the status of the claim.

MANAGER'S ALERT

Do not "write off" a bill for a deceased patient without first attempting to collect your fees. An automatic write-off may look like the office is trying to cover up a problem.

A claim can also be filed at the local courthouse with the registrar of wills. This claim is filed against the estate, and if the estate is solvent at the time of probate, the bill is paid. Should the estate not be solvent, the state establishes a priority system to determine who is paid and in what order. The first three bills to be paid from an estate are

1. Funeral costs
2. Expenses of settling the estate
3. Claims due for the deceased person's last illness

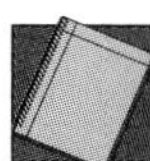

FROM THE EXPERT'S NOTEBOOK

The claims submitted by the billing service are only as good as the information that is provided by the office. The office is responsible for all claims and actions by the billing service, so check the billing service out before hiring it!

Laws vary from state to state, so be certain to check with your practice's attorney on policy. Some offices have their attorney collect this fee for them; however, it is best to pay office personnel rather than an attorney for this service.

Educating the Staff and Patients about Payment for Services

No matter how successful a practice is, if it is not making a profit, no one wins. It is as important to the office staff as it is to the physician that all monies owed are paid in a timely fashion. The factors in successful collection are simple:

- Listen carefully to the patient's explanation for nonpayment. Sometimes, the staff must interpret what the patient is saying.
- Communicate clearly.
- Show consideration for the patient.
- Develop a policy.

If a medical practice has a difficult time with overdue accounts it is often because the office has not established a payment policy that the patient must follow. Much success can be attributed to proper education of the patient about your billing procedures and policies.

It is better for patients to be aware of your payment policies before they come to the office; however, many physicians think it is unprofessional to have their office speak of fees before the visit. This is slowly changing, and the future will bring more and more office policy changes as cutbacks in reimbursement from insurance carriers and government agencies hit each individual physician's office. Of particular importance is that the employees know the rules and regulations of each insurance company. It is better to know ahead of time what is and is not covered by the insurance company than to provide a specific service and later find out that the office will not be paid for this service. The office staff must understand that there are three entities involved in patients' care: the physician, the patient, and the patient's insurance company.

Both the physician and the staff must be aware of the collection rules. It is essential for office personnel to be aware of the internal workings of all insurance companies. Medicare, Blue Shield, and many major HMOs and PPOs are now sending bulletins on a regular basis to keep physicians' offices aware of changes in regulations. It is important that not only the insurance clerk, but also the receptionist/secretary, is aware of all the regulations and changes taking place with insurances. It is the office manager's duty to oversee these rules and regulations and to conduct office meetings on a regular basis to explain and answer any questions the office personnel might have.

Many collection seminars are given throughout the United States at various times of the year. It is always a good practice to send the collection staff to one or two of these seminars. They can be costly, but the money can come back to the office in efficient collections. Some offices send copies of Medicare bulletins to their patients to show that the office is harassed just as much as, if not more than, patients. This also points out to patients that it is not the office's rule, it is the insurance companies.

EXERCISES

MULTIPLE CHOICE

Choose the best *answer for each of the following questions.*

1. What is the first bill paid from a patient's estate?
   a. Electric bill
   b. Physician's bill
   c. Funeral bill
   d. Hospital bill
2. The value of $1.00 at 6 months is
   a. $0.66
   b. $0.20
   c. $0.45
   d. $0.75
3. Which of the following is *not* a necessary part of the letter requesting an informal hearing?
   a. Patient's name
   b. Patient's address
   c. Patient's Medicare number
   d. Procedure codes
4. The average percentage paid to collection agencies is
   a. 45%
   b. 20% to 60%
   c. 30% to 50%
   d. None of the above
5. Signs and symptoms codes can be found in what chapter of the ICD-9-CM codebook?
   a. Not in a chapter, in Appendix A
   b. Chapter 1
   c. Not in a chapter, in Appendix C
   d. Chapter 16

6. E&M codes are selected based on which of the following?
   a. Place of service
   b. Type of service
   c. None of the above
   d. All of the above
7. Which of the following is *not* a key component used to choose an E&M code?
   a. Examination
   b. Medical decision making
   c. Insurance
   d. History
8. Which of the following is *not* a category of V code?
   a. Insurance oriented
   b. Problem oriented
   c. Service oriented
   d. Fact oriented
9. Medicare Part A pays for which of the following services?
   a. Physician visits
   b. Outpatient x-rays
   c. Outpatient laboratory tests
   d. None of the above
10. Which of the following insurances was established in 1965 by the federal government with the state governments?
    a. Medicare
    b. Medicaid
    c. CHAMPUS
    d. CHAMPVA
11. In addition to procedure and diagnosis codes, office patient encounter forms should contain what categories of E&M codes?
    a. New patient codes
    b. Established patient codes
    c. Outpatient consultations
    d. All of the above
12. An inpatient consultation code is
    a. 99255
    b. 99233
    c. 99215
    d. 99245
13. A moderate complexity level is part of which key component of an E&M service?
    a. Medical decision making
    b. Examination
    c. History
    d. Medical necessity
14. The global fee package does *not* contain which service?
    a. Preoperative visits
    b. Office visits 1 year after the procedure
    c. Postoperative visits
    d. Intraoperative services
15. Which of the following is *not* a coding system?
    a. CDC
    b. ICD-9-CM
    c. CPT
    d. HCPCS
16. Which of the following is *not* a type of Medicare hearing?
    a. Telephone hearing
    b. On-the-record hearing
    c. Hearing by proxy
    d. In-person hearing
17. One of the blocks on the CMS form that is affected by the NPI number is
    a. Block 2
    b. Block 9
    c. Block 21
    d. Block 33
18. The place of service code for physician office is
    a. 22
    b. 11
    c. 21
    d. 12
19. Which document provides information about the payment of the claim?
    a. EOB
    b. RFP
    c. OIG
    d. MSP
20. Which of the following modifiers is used to bill for a covering physician for a short-term absence of the staff physician?
    a. Q9
    b. W4
    c. W2
    d. Q6

MATCHING

Match the following items.

1. Established patient level 3	A. OL
2. New patient level 3	B. 22
3. Place of service for hospice	C. 53
4. Modifier for unrelated E&M service	D. PC
5. Modifier for reduced service	E. 99243
6. Modifier for discontinued service	F. 99213
7. Modifier indicating professional component	G. 24
8. Outpatient consultation code	H. GA
9. Place of service for outpatient hospital	I. 52
10. Modifier indicating the office maintains an ABN	J. 99203

TRUE OR FALSE

1. _____ There are advantages to collection agencies that charge flat rates.
2. _____ Many commercial insurance companies have HMOs and PPOs.
3. _____ Part A Medicare covers the hospital expenses.
4. _____ ICD-9 codes are used to describe the diagnosis of the patient.
5. _____ Code 99203 is used to submit for an established patient office visit.
6. _____ A V code establishes medical necessity.
7. _____ Use a "signs and symptoms" code when a definitive diagnosis code is not available.

8. ______ Modifier -53 is used to report a discontinued procedure.
9. ______ You do not need an NPI number to bill for services.
10. ______ "Incident to" services can be billed in a hospital setting.
11. ______ Only four diagnosis codes can be submitted per claim.
12. ______ Always use postcards as a collection tool.
13. ______ A reference remark code identifies why the service was rejected.
14. ______ The place of service is not important when sending in a claim.
15. ______ The form used to bill for physician services on paper is the UB92.
16. ______ Modifier -91 is used for Repeat of a Clinical Diagnostic Laboratory Test.
17. ______ Always use Volume 1 before Volume 2 when assigning a diagnosis code.
18. ______ *Patient encounter form* is another term for a *superbill.*
19. ______ It is necessary to prioritize all diagnosis codes for billing.
20. ______ TRICARE is a military insurance.

THINKERS

1. An overpayment has been made by Medicare for patient Josh Bok. Determine whether a refund should be made. If not, explain the reasoning behind your decision. If so, what steps should be taken to refund the overpayment?
2. Why is the reference remark important to a medical practice?
3. Develop a policy regarding ABNs and how they would be used in your medical practice.
4. Design a patient encounter form for a medical practice. (Do not include ICD-9-CM or CPT codes.)
5. A long-time patient of the practice has recently fallen on "hard times" and cannot pay the "patient balance due" after his surgery. How should the office manager handle this patient?

REFERENCES

American Medical Association. *CPT 2008.* Chicago, 2008.

American Medical Association. *ICD-9-CM 2008.* Chicago, 2008.

Association of Credit and Collection Professionals, Debt Collection, www.acainternational.org.

Blue Cross/Blue Shield Association, Health Insurance Basics 2000-2008, www.bcbs.com.

Centers for Medicare and Medicaid, *Medicare Special Bulletin,* June 25, 1993.

Comeau, J.F. "Collection Systems That Deter Lawsuits." *Physician's Management,* February 1992, pp. 113–118.

"Federal poverty guidelines." *Federal Register,* Vol. 72, No. 15, January 24, 2007, pp. 3147–3148.

Fox, S. "Online Health Search 2006." American Life Project, 2006. Accessed 05/31/08.

Ingenix. *HCPCS Level II, 2008.* Eden Prairie, MN, 2007.

Lewin, R. "The Touchiest Billing Situation You'll Ever Face." *Medical Economics,* August 23, 1993, pp. 117–123.

Medicare Carriers Manual. www.cms.hhs.gov.

Medicare National Coverage Determination Manual, Chapter 1, Part 1, Coverage Determinations, (Section 10-80.12), revised 4-4-08, www.cms.hhs.gov.

Tricare Management Activity, Military Health System, Medical, www.tricare.mil.

U.S. Census Bureau. Washington, DC, Issued August 2007.

U.S. Department of Labor, Bureau of Statistics, Health Diagnosis and Treating Occupations, www.bls.gov/OCO/.

7

FRAUD, ABUSE, AND COMPLIANCE

CHAPTER OUTLINE

CHAPTER OBJECTIVES

After completing this chapter, you will be able to do the following:

- Define *fraud* and *abuse* and understand how they affect a medical practice
- Use fraud alerts and special advisory bulletins
- Know the function of the Office of Inspector General (OIG) and how it can affect a medical practice
- Identify OIG risk areas and their implications
- Recognize the ramifications of exclusion from Medicare and Medicaid
- Recognize the ramifications of civil and criminal penalties
- Understand the Beneficiary Incentive Program and its effect on a medical practice
- Identify the various fraud and abuse legislative acts and their implications
- Draw conclusions from fraud statistics
- Understand why a compliance plan for a physician practice is important

WHAT IS FRAUD?

Fraud is an intentional deception or misrepresentation made by an individual who knows that the false information reported could result in a benefit to herself or himself or another person. There are many ways in which a medical practice can be guilty of fraud, including the following:

- Billing for services or supplies that were not provided
- Unbundling (i.e., coding components of a procedure separately when only a single code is necessary)
- Upcoding (i.e., coding and billing for a level of service that is not supported by the medical record documentation)
- Falsifying a diagnosis in order to obtain payment for services
- Altering claims to obtain more money
- Submitting duplicate claims to receive additional money
- Completing Certificate of Medical Necessity forms when necessity is not supported by the medical record
- Soliciting, offering, or receiving kickbacks, bribes, or rebates
- Submitting claims involving collusion between a provider and a patient
- Overusing services
- Billing for noncovered services
- Signing blank prescriptions
- Making excessive referrals to an ancillary facility

The Federal Bureau of Investigation (FBI) can investigate federal and private payer cases of fraud, but has no jurisdiction to impose sanctions on providers. Any time there is a question regarding a service performed or a diagnosis given, it is best to clarify it with the physician before keying information into the computer (Figure 7-1).

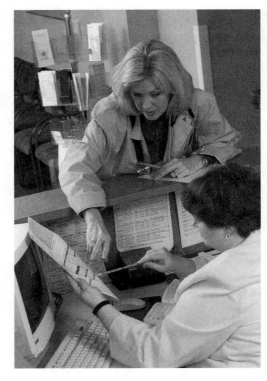

FIGURE 7-1. To prevent fraudulent billing, the physician should always be consulted on anything questionable before entering billing information.

WHAT IS ABUSE?

Abuse is an incident or a practice that is not consistent with sound medical, business, or fiscal practices. Examples include providing medically unnecessary care or care that does not meet the standards of care. It is considered abuse when Medicare reimburses for services or items for which the provider is not entitled to compensation. Abuse is similar to fraud except that it cannot be proven that the abusive acts were committed knowingly, willingly, and intentionally. To determine whether a practice is guilty of abuse, answer the following questions:

1. Is the service or supply necessary?
2. Is the service or supply appropriate according to professionally recognized standards?
3. Has a fair price been charged?

Answering "no" to any of these questions confirms that abuse has occurred in the practice.

SOME CRIMINAL STATUTES RELATING TO FRAUD AND ABUSE

False Statements Relating to Health Care Matters

ITEM 18 U.S.C.1035

It is a crime to knowingly and willfully falsify or conceal a material fact, or to make any false statement or use any false writing or document in connection with the delivery of health care or relating to health care payment for items or services. For example, billing for any service that wasn't performed is considered fraud. Penalties could include fines and imprisonment for up to 5 years. This law applies to claims filed with most third-party carriers.

Obstruction of Criminal Investigations of Health Care Offenses

ITEM 18 U.S.C. 1518

It is a crime to willfully prevent, obstruct, mislead, or delay or to attempt to prevent, obstruct, mislead, or delay the communication of records relating to a federal health care offense. For example, if the Office of Inspector General (OIG) requests copies of records, the request cannot be ignored by the physician's office manager. Penalties for this obstruction could result in fines and imprisonment for up to 5 years. This law applies to claims filed with most third-party carriers.

Mail and Wire Fraud

ITEM 18 U.S.C. 1341 AND 1343

It is a crime to use a mail, courier, or wire service to conduct a scheme to defraud another of money or property. The term *wire services* includes the use of a telephone, fax machine, or computer. Every time one of these services is used, it is considered a separate violation punishable by fines and imprisonment for up to 5 years. Consider a gerontologist who bills for services to nursing home patients but did not perform the services. If these claims were submitted to Medicare and Medicaid electronically, the physician is guilty of mail and wire fraud.

Theft or Embezzlement in Connection with Health Care

ITEM 18 U.S.C. 1035

It is a crime to knowingly and willfully embezzle, steal, or intentionally misapply any of the assets of a health care benefit program. For example, an office manager embezzled some Medicare checks and "doctored" the books so that they would not be missed. Because he deposited the monies from the federal government into his own account, he can now be punished by fines and imprisonment for up to 10 years if the amount embezzled was $100 or more, or fines and imprisonment for up to 1 year if less than $100. This law applies to claims filed with most third-party carriers.

FRAUD AND ABUSE CONTROL PROGRAM

The Fraud and Abuse Control Program was established by the federal government under subtitle A of HR 3103. The Office of Inspector General (OIG), Federal Bureau of Investigation (FBI), and Department of Justice (DOJ) share in the prosecution and investigation of suspected fraud and abuse. The OIG investigates fraud cases that involve federal programs such as Medicare, Medicaid, and Child Health Grant programs. The OIG can impose civil monetary penalties and program exclusions on providers guilty of fraud. The FBI investigates federal and private payer cases of suspected fraud, but does not have the authority to impose sanctions on providers. Both the OIG and the FBI refer cases to the DOJ, which prosecutes fraudulent providers for violations of any criminal laws.

The responsibilities of this fraud and abuse control program are as follows:

- To investigate and audit the delivery of medical services and payments associated with those services
- To facilitate enforcement of statutes
- To provide education to providers through fraud alerts and advisory opinions
- To share information with public and private third-party payers

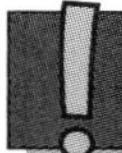

MANAGER'S ALERT

The Fraud and Abuse Control Program is applicable to any plan or program that provides medical benefits to patients; it is not restricted to Medicare or Medicaid.

This program is funded by civil monetary penalties, fines, forfeitures, and damages assessed in health care cases, along with monetary gifts and bequests. A Health Care Fraud and Abuse Control Account was established to maintain these funds and was created within the Federal Hospital Insurance Fund. The FBI also uses these funds for health care prosecution, audits, and educational efforts.

Fraud Alerts

The OIG and the Centers for Medicare and Medicaid Services (CMS) warn physicians of suspected fraudulent practices by issuing fraud alerts. These alerts notify physicians of practices that are currently being investigated so that they can examine their practices for any possible issues or oversights that must be corrected. The first alert was issued in 1988. Since that time, alerts have been issued for the following areas:

- Prescription drug marketing practices
- Routine waiver of Medicare deductibles and co-payments
- Joint venture arrangements
- Hospital incentives to referring physicians
- Clinical laboratory arrangements
- Home health fraud
- Nursing home services
- Physician liability for certifications with medical equipment and home health services
- Rentals in physician offices by persons or entities to which physicians refer
- Hospice arrangements with nursing homes

Special Advisory Bulletins

The OIG also issues Special Advisory Bulletins, such as the bulletins issued on the following subjects:

- Patient Anti-dumping Statue
- The effect of exclusion from participation in federal health care programs
- Gain-sharing arrangements and civil monetary penalties (CMPs) for hospital payments to physicians to reduce or limit services to beneficiaries

Operation Restore Trust

In 1995, Operation Restore Trust (ORT) was developed with many new antifraud approaches. In its original form, it covered the states of California, Florida, Illinois, New York, and Texas, whose populations include more than one third of Medicare and Medicaid beneficiaries. In its first 2 years, this program recouped $187.5 million in restitution, fines, and settlements. This program was expanded in 1997. It now includes sophisticated methods for identifying providers for investigation, increasing investigations in conjunction with the DOJ, training local aging organizations to detect and report nursing home fraud, monitoring home health agencies to identify inappropriate billing, and developing teams to identify system problems.

Medicare Integrity Program

The Medicare Integrity Program (MIP) allows the U.S. Department of Health and Human Services (DHHS) to partner with private companies to audit cost reports, develop lists of durable medical equipment that requires authorization, educate providers and beneficiaries on quality assurance, review provider services, and determine appropriate payment under Medicare Part B.

Office of Inspector General

The OIG investigates suspected fraud and abuse, and audits and inspects CMS programs and contractors. The OIG has access to CMS's files and data, as well as the files of CMS contractors who assist as a case develops. The OIG conducts investigations of specific providers that may be suspected of fraud, waste, or abuse to determine whether criminal, civil, or administrative actions are warranted. It conducts audits and analyses that identify Medicare and Medicaid policy weaknesses, and makes recommendations for any corrections that should take place. It conducts reviews and special projects to identify performance in health provider fraud and abuse control. It participates in program communications, which keeps the OIG in touch with the health care community, Congress, and others. Last, it participates with other governmental agencies and private health insurers in special programs to share knowledge on preventing fraud and abuse.

Providers are encouraged to report any situations involving fraud and abuse. A confidential hotline has been established at 1-800-HHS-TIPS (1-800-447-8477) for reporting fraud and abuse. Concerns may also be e-mailed to Htips@os.dhhs.gov or faxed to 1-800-223-8164. You can mail information to the following address:

Office of Inspector General
U.S. Department of Health and Human Services
Attn: HOTLINE
330 Independence Ave., SW
Washington, DC 20201

When filing a complaint, the following information should be provided if possible:

1. Type of carrier
   a. Medicare Part A
   b. Medicare Part B
   c. Child Support Enforcement
   d. National Institutes of Health (NIH)
   e. Indian Health Service (IHS)
   f. Food and Drug Administration (FDA)
   g. Centers for Disease Control and Prevention (CDC)
   h. Substance Abuse and Mental Health Services Administration (SAMHSA)
   i. Health Resources and Services Administration (HRSA)
   j. Aid to Children and Families
   k. All other DHHS agencies or related programs
2. Name of department or program being affected by your allegation of fraud
   a. Administration for Children and Families
   b. Child Support Enforcement (CSE)
   c. Centers for Medicare and Medicaid Services (CMS)
   d. Food and Drug Administration (FDA)
   e. National Institutes of Health (NIH)
   f. Centers for Disease Control and Prevention (CDC)
   g. Indian Health Service (IHS)
   h. Office of Inspector General (OIG)
   i. Office of the Secretary of DHHS
   j. Health Resources and Services Administration (HRSA)
   k. Substance Abuse and Mental Health Services Administration (SAMHSA)
   l. Administration on Aging (AOA)
   m. Agency for Health Care Policy and Research
   n. Other
3. Your name and address (confidentiality will be maintained)
4. E-mail address, if applicable
5. Alleged fraudulent act and the person committing the fraud
   a. The name of the subject/person/practice
   b. Title of subject/person/practice
   c. Address of the subject/person/practice
6. Brief summary of the facts relating to the allegation

Self-Disclosure

If you are aware of any potential fraud or abuse that may exist within your practice, you may want to discuss self-disclosure with the practice attorney. The self-disclosure program encourages anyone believing that there are irregularities within her or his practice to disclose them using the self-disclosure protocol. Self-disclosure allows providers to reduce their costs, minimize the extent of the audit, negotiate settlements, and often avoid exclusion from governmental programs. There are times when the practice may be required to enter into an integrity agreement. A corporate *integrity agreement* is a corrective plan of action that is negotiated between carriers and medical practices. These contracts are used as part of a settlement to resolve violations of the civil false claims act and whistleblower suits. In this agreement, the physician practice does not accept liability or admit fault. Complete details of the self-disclosure protocol can be found on the OIG's Web site at www.hhs.gov/oig. Details can also be found in the *Federal Register,* Vol. 63, No. 210, p. 58399.

Whistleblowers

Many fraudulent activities are discovered through whistleblowers. Whistleblowers are employees who report illegal or wrongful activities of the employer or fellow employees. For reporting such activities, whistleblowers can receive a percentage of the recovered monies. Employees cannot be terminated for this action. Many whistleblower suits have been prevented through exit interviews. These interviews are discussed in Chapter 2.

OIG Work Plan

Each year, the OIG releases what the agency has planned for health care for the coming year. It identifies areas of suspected fraud and abuse within the health care system. This work plan can be obtained from their Web site at www.os.dhhs.gov/oig. It is a good idea for the practice to obtain a copy and review what's on the "hit list" for the coming year. By reviewing this list, the office manager can identify areas of risk within the practice and implement a corrective action.

OIG-Identified Risk Areas

The following is a list of risk areas for medical practices, as determined by the OIG. The office manager should review this list carefully to determine any risk that the practice might face.

- Billing for services not documented
- Duplicate billing
- Upcoding
- Unbundling
- Improper use of provider numbers
- Misuse of billing and coding software
- Billing companies with questionable practices
- Focus on certain evaluation and management (E&M) codes (e.g., 99214, 99233, 99244, 99254, 99245, 99255)
- Credit balances
- Waiver of co-pays and deductibles
- Professional courtesy, discounted services
- Code steering

BILLING FOR SERVICES NOT DOCUMENTED

There are times when services or procedures are billed and not documented. These instances can arise from the following situations:

1. The service or procedure was checked off on the superbill, but for some reason was not performed. Perhaps the patient did not want to have that procedure done that day, and asked if it could be done on the next visit.
2. The service or procedure was checked off on the superbill, was actually performed, but was not documented in the medical record. Perhaps the physician ordered a flu shot, checked it on the superbill, but forgot to document it in the medical record. The nurse who administered the shot also forgot to document it.
3. The hospital billing form was completed and given to the office staff for billing. For example, the physician mistakenly checked off that he or she had seen the patient and provided a level two subsequent inpatient service (99232), when actually the patient was in x-ray and was never seen.

DUPLICATE BILLING

There are situations in which a practice may bill for the same service twice. This can occur either as a simple error or as a malicious attempt to collect a double payment from insurers. Some offices automatically resubmit claims that have not been paid after a predetermined period but without any investigation into why it has not been paid. This is a bad habit to get into. All claims should be thoroughly investigated before they are resubmitted. If you do not have the staff to follow up on these claims, hire them! It is much better than the alternative. Participating in this type of rebilling could expose the practice to violations of the False Claims Act.

UPCODING

Upcoding is the practice of choosing a level of service that is higher than the documentation in the medical record supports. For example, the physician chooses a level three, 99213 office visit for an established patient. When documenting the patient encounter in the medical record, the physician omits the documentation of the review of systems and the level of medical decision making is only straightforward. This level now becomes a level two, 99212. Billing at the higher level of 99213 constitutes upcoding.

UNBUNDLING

A bundled service is one whose payment is already included in another service code. Unbundling is the fragmenting of one service into its component parts and coding each component part as if it was a separate service. Unbundling can be either unintentional or intentional. For example, an obstetrics/gynecology practice performs ultrasound examinations in their office. They own the equipment and the physician personally performs the ultrasound. They bill the appropriate ultrasound code with a professional courtesy (PC) modifier and then bill that code again with a technical component (TC) modifier. They should instead bill the global code that includes the component parts.

The National Correct Coding Primer, which is continually updated and has been released by the CMS under its National Correct Coding Policy, is an effective tool to help medical practices avoid claim denials for component part combinations. A practice can investigate codes to identify whether there is a correct coding edit for that code. These edits were implemented in 1996 by the Correct Coding Initiative (CCI) of the National Correct Coding Council under CMS. By using this manual, inappropriate billing such as unbundling can be prevented.

IMPROPER USE OF PROVIDER NUMBERS

Under the law, payment cannot be made to someone other than the patient or the provider who rendered services. For example, if a physician group hires a new physician, it is the responsibility of the office manager to obtain the necessary credentialing and provider numbers for the new physician. It is improper for the office to use the provider number of another physician within the group for services provided by the new physician. This is why it is important to file for these numbers as soon as you are aware that a new physician will be joining the group. There are only a few instances in which reassignment of benefits is allowed. You may read more detailed information in the *Federal Register,* Code 42, Section 424.70.

BILLING AND CODING SOFTWARE

The practice should be cautious when using billing and coding software, because its use is under the watchful eye of the OIG. Errors that may arise from billing software are usually not with the software itself, but how it is used. The OIG is concerned that medical practices will allow the software to choose the levels of service. The OIG is examining the use of such software as it relates to physician service encoding to determine whether it is the cause of error. Encoding software packages can be invaluable to a medical practice if used correctly. These packages combine codes from the ICD-9-CM, CPT, HCPCS, and CCI manuals; they can save valuable time when coding, because all codes can be found in the same place. These packages can also assist the practice in coding accurately by identifying bundled procedures, truncated diagnosis codes, and mutually exclusive CPT codes.

Coding software, such as Flashcode by Medical Coding and Compliance Solutions, LLC, can be a big advantage for the billing staff. This software allows you to easily determine the proper ICD-9-CM code by typing the diagnosis in description form. It will then guide you through the diagnoses and will identify any additional digits that may be required. The CPT portion of the software will work in the same manner by assisting you in correctly identifying the most accurate procedure or service code possible. This software also has built-in CCI edits, so that the risk for unbundling is reduced. (For more details on this software, see Chapter 10.) Some software packages, however, suggest billing combinations that may be a bit "creative." This is not what you are looking for. Use software packages that assist you only in accurate coding and therefore don't put you at risk for fraud! Carefully investigate any software before purchasing it.

BILLING COMPANIES

When hiring a billing company for your practice, be sure to find one that does not offer a percentage or an incentive. This could be misconstrued as a violation of the anti-kickback statute (see the *Federal Register,* Code 42, U.S.C., Section 1320a and 59, p. 65372).

FOCUS ON CERTAIN E&M CODES

The OIG is focusing on certain codes that it believes are subject to abusive practices. These codes are as follows:

- 99214, established patient office visit level four
- 99233, subsequent hospital visit level three
- 99244, outpatient consultation level four
- 99245, outpatient consultation level five
- 99254, inpatient consultation level four
- 99255, inpatient consultation level five

The office manager must be certain that the physician, clinical staff, physician extenders (i.e., nurse practitioners, physician assistants, and clinical nurse specialists), and billing staff thoroughly understand the documentation guidelines for these services. Ideally, they should understand the guidelines for all E&M services, but in practice they must be aware of the codes that are subject to particular OIG scrutiny.

CREDIT BALANCES

Credit balances arise when two separate entities make payment for the same service. For example, Medicare reimburses for a service that is also covered by another insurer. Sometimes these balances are allowed to sit as "credits" on the patient's accounts and the payments are deposited by the practice. This practice can be viewed as fraudulent. If your practice is currently handling overpayments in this way, it is imperative to stop. Any and all credit balances sitting on patient accounts should be refunded to the appropriate entities. There should be a policy in the billing manual regarding proper handling of overpayments. If the practice is implementing a compliance plan, this policy definitely needs to be included.

WAIVER OF CO-PAYS AND DEDUCTIBLES

The OIG has issued a Special Fraud Alert identifying the risk of waiving co-pays and deductibles. It is each practice's responsibility to attempt collection of all co-payments and deductibles that are due the physician. Failure to do so can result in violations of the False Claims Act and the anti-kickback statute. This alert also applies to discounting services that many offices refer to as insurance only. Check out the Special Fraud Alert issued by the OIG in May 1991, "Routine Waiver of Part B Co-payments and Deductibles." This can be found on the OIG Web site at www.oig.hhs.gov.

PROFESSIONAL COURTESY/DISCOUNTED SERVICES

Extending professional courtesy can land a practice in big trouble. This practice is under the ever-watchful eye of the OIG. Professional courtesy is the practice of either not charging or "accepting insurance payment only" for other physicians, their families, hospital personnel, and other medical professionals. This is discussed in detail in Chapter 6 with sample letters that can be used to advise patients and colleagues of your new policy.

Whether your professional courtesy falls into a risk area depends on how professional courtesy is extended. When extended to someone who has referred patients in the past or still refers to your practice, either directly or indirectly, the practice could face a problem involving the anti-kickback statute. If professional courtesy is extended by "accepting insurance only," it could violate the Civil False Claims Act, and perhaps even the prohibition of inducements to beneficiaries (see *Federal Register*, Code 42, U.S.C., Section 1320a).

CODE STEERING

Code steering can be an issue if all levels of E&M codes are not listed on the superbill or patient encounter form. Not listing all levels could be a very dangerous practice. For example, when looking at a superbill, the practice may list all the levels within the category of established patient office visits (99211, 99212, 99213, 99214, 99215) on the superbill. When it comes to new office patients, however, it lists only the top three levels (99203, 99204, 99205) and excludes levels 99201 and 99202. The usual justification for this practice is that "the physician hardly ever uses those levels, so why list them?" You must list all levels within each category of E&M codes listed on the superbill. Space is always a problem, but it can be done and must be done! With proper formatting of codes (Table 7-1), the practice can save space on the superbill and still list all levels within the E&M categories.

TABLE 7-1 Example of How to List Complete Set of Office Visit Codes on the Superbill

CORRECT WAY			INCORRECT WAY
New		*Established*	*Established Patient*
99201	Level 1	99211	Level 1- 99211
99202	Level 2	99212	Level 2- 99212
99203	Level 3	99213	Level 3- 99213
99204	Level 4	99214	Level 4- 99214
99205	Level 5	99215	Level 5- 99215
			New Patient
			Level 3- 99213
			Level 4- 99214
			Level 5- 99215

Exclusion from Medicare and Medicaid

Physicians guilty of fraud and abuse can be excluded from participation in the Medicare and Medicaid programs. A mandatory exclusion, which requires that a provider cannot bill Medicare or Medicaid for at least 5 years, is initiated when the provider is convicted of criminal offenses. Any provider who has been convicted on two or more previous occasions of health care–related crimes will be permanently excluded. Providers will receive no payment from Medicare or Medicaid once they are excluded. All applications for reinstatement must be made to the OIG. A permissive exclusion is initiated by the OIG for criminal violations, including filing a false claim, failing to respond to the CMS or the OIG for an investigation, and failing to provide all necessary information requested by the CMS or the OIG.

Civil Monetary Penalties

Any fraudulent claim submitted to Medicare or Medicaid is subject to civil monetary penalties. This penalty is $10,000 for each service or item. Penalties of up to $10,000 may be imposed for each instance of medically unnecessary services.

Criminal Penalties

Any provider convicted of a federal health care offense may be ordered to forfeit all real estate and personal property derived from proceeds that are directly or indirectly traceable back to the offense.

Administrative Remedies

Administrative remedies may be enforced to correct abuse practices within a medical practice. Such remedies include the following:

- Education
- Recovery of overpayments
- Withheld payments

The carrier (in this case, Medicare or Medicaid) may require that physicians attend educational sessions to learn the documentation guidelines. It can recover any overpayments made to the practice by requesting by letter that a refund be made. The carrier may also withhold the overpayment from future reimbursements until paid in full.

Beneficiary Incentive Program (HR 3103)

The Beneficiary Incentive Program (HR 3103) was established to encourage patients to report fraud and abuse against the Medicare program. Each time a patient reports fraud and abuse, a monetary reward of at least $100 is sent to the patient. On January 1, 1999, Medicare beneficiaries were granted the right to request copies of itemized statements from their health care providers, including physicians and physician extenders, home health agencies, nursing facilities, durable medical equipment suppliers, and hospitals. The provider is allowed 30 days to respond to the beneficiary by sending the requested statement. This request must be made in writing by the beneficiary, and failure of the medical office to comply with this request may result in civil monetary penalties of approximately $100 for each offense. If the practice does not respond within 30 days, the carrier will assist the beneficiary in this request. If the carrier is not successful, the case will then be referred to the Program Integrity Group at CMS's central office. At this point, civil monetary penalties may be imposed. Bottom line: If the practice gets this type of request from a patient, respond within 30 days!

All beneficiary notices include statements that provide the Medicare fraud hotline telephone number. The toll-free number provided for these Medicare patients is 1-800-447-8477.

Incentive Reward Program

The Incentive Reward Program was established to encourage individuals to report known cases of fraud and abuse against the Medicare program. Individuals will be rewarded for leads that recover at least $100 from the offending entity. Any cases already under investigation will not fall under the Incentive Reward Program, and therefore no remuneration will be made. The cap on the reward is $1,000, or 10% of the recovered funds, whichever is less. Fines and penalties are not included in the calculation of the reward, and others that may be involved in the same case will share the reward equally.

FRAUD AND ABUSE LEGISLATION

The following sections describe legislation directed at fraud and abuse in health care.

Fraud and Abuse Amendments of 1972

The Fraud and Abuse Amendments of 1972 enforce exclusion from the Medicare program for health care providers who knowingly and willfully submit false claims.

Anti-kickback Statute of 1974

The Anti-kickback Statute of 1974 permits criminal penalties of up to $25,000 and/or imprisonment for up to 5 years for every offense. These penalties are in addition to exclusion from Medicare and Medicaid. In 1980, the phrase "knowingly and willingly" was added as the criteria of intent to the kickback provision.

Antifraud and Abuse Amendments of 1977

These amendments increased the penalty provisions for health care providers to not more than $25,000 and/or imprisonment for up to 5 years for each offense, in addition to exclusion from the Medicare and Medicaid programs. For the same crime on the patient side, a patient could face a fine of up to $10,000 and/or imprisonment of up to 1 year.

Civil Monetary Penalties Act of 1981

The Civil Monetary Penalties Act of 1981 provides for the imposition of civil monetary penalties and assessments on any individual who submits a claim for services or supplies that were not provided as claimed. It also covers any charges that exceed the standards. In 1987, the scope of this legislation was expanded to make employers accountable for staff billing errors.

Medicare and Medicaid Patient and Program Protection Act of 1987

This act allows health care providers, individuals, and businesses to be excluded from receiving payment for services rendered under Medicare, Medicaid, and other federal programs because of abuse to those systems. Every sanction calls for assessments of up to double the violation amount, civil monetary penalties of up to $2,000 per violation, and exclusion from the Medicare program for up to 5 years.

Safe Harbor Regulations of 1991–1993

The "safe harbor" regulations, first implemented in 1991, specified 11 safe payment practices that were exempt from the Anti-kickback Statute. The interim safe harbor rules were published in 1992, and were known as the "Managed Care Safe Harbors." Seven additional safe harbors were proposed in 1993. In 1996, guidelines for the safe harbor provisions to protect specific health care plans such as health maintenance organizations (HMOs) and preferred provider organizations (PPOs) were published. In 1997, the Negotiated Rulemaking Committee developed the interim final rule for shared risk exception. This rule established exception from liability under the Anti-kickback Statute for remuneration between an eligible organization under section 1876 of the Social Security Act and an individual or entity providing services in accordance with a written agreement between these parties.

Self-referral Prohibitions (Stark Law) of 1989–1996

The Omnibus Budget Reconciliation Act (OBRA) of 1989 included Stark I provisions, which banned physicians from referring laboratory specimens to any entity with which the physician has a financial relationship. Stark I became effective on January 1, 1992, and was amended by OBRA 1990 to exclude financial relationships between hospitals and physicians if the relationships were unrelated to clinical laboratory services. Final regulations were issued in 1995. Stark I was expanded by OBRA 1993 to include 10 other designated health care services. This expanded version is now referred to as Stark II and became effective on January 1, 1995.

Health Insurance Portability and Accountability Act of 1996 (HIPAA) (HR3103)

The Health Insurance Portability and Accountability Act of 1996 (HIPAA) was responsible for establishing the Fraud and Abuse Control Program, which was a combined effort by the DHHS and the U.S. Attorney General. It imposes civil monetary penalties for improper coding practices and for seeking reimbursement for services that do not meet the medical necessity standards. This act enforces criminal penalties for "knowingly and willingly" defrauding any health care benefit program.

Three amendments have been added to the HIPAA:

1. The Women's Health and Cancer Rights Act of 1998 (WHCRA). This law was enacted in October 1998 and mandates coverage for breast reconstruction surgery by all insurance plans when performed at the time of a mastectomy.
2. The Newborns' and Mothers' Health Protection Act (NMHPA). This law was enacted in September 1999 and provides insurance coverage to all mothers and newborns for the first few days after birth. It prevents insurance carriers from limiting hospital stays to less than 48 hours after a vaginal birth and 96 hours after a cesarean section.
3. The Mental Health Parity Act (MHPA). This law prohibits imposing aggregate lifetime or annual dollar limits for mental health services that are less than the limits of the medical and surgical benefits.

The Balanced Budget Act of 1997

The Balanced Budget Act includes antifraud provisions that allow the government access to records that may document fraud and abuse. Part of the act prohibits participation in programs because of noncompliance with Medicare regulations. It requires a raised beneficiary awareness of fraud and abuse. The act established penalties for anti-kickback violations of $50,000 and up to three times the total amount of the remuneration offered, paid, or received. It established a new penalty of $25,000 for health plans that do not report information on adverse actions against them as required under the fraud and abuse data collection program. It requires that all nonphysician providers of patient care choose diagnosis codes, just as physicians do, and removes the place of service restriction for nonphysician practitioners.

Publication of the OIG's Provider Self-disclosure Protocol of 1998

The self-disclosure protocol provides specific guidelines for self-policing and self-auditing by providers and for self-disclosure to the OIG of any practices that violate federal criminal, civil, or administrative laws. It provides detailed audit methodology and guidelines with respect to reporting improper practices identified through internal investigations.

Publication of the OIG's "Rulemaking 1999"

"Rulemaking 1999" was a revision of the OIG's exclusion and civil monetary penalty authorities and increased OIG's authority to exclude individuals not only from Medicare and Medicaid, but also from all other federal health care programs. These regulations also provide for permanent exclusion of individuals who are convicted of three or more offenses, and for a 10-year exclusion for individuals who are convicted of two offenses.

Safe Harbor Regulations of 1999

This 1999 final rule contained eight new safe harbor regulations and clarified six existing regulations. The new rules address provisions such as the following:

- Investments in ambulatory surgery centers
- Group practice issues
- Recruiting of physicians
- Sale of physician practices to hospitals
- Malpractice insurance subsidies for obstetricians
- Specialty referral arrangements between providers

Final Rule: HIPAA Privacy Regulations of 2000 (Health Insurance Portability and Accountability Act)

On December 28, 2000, final regulations were released for national standards to protect the privacy of personal health information maintained by health care providers, hospitals, health plans, and health insurers. The regulations became effective April 14, 2003, for most plans, and later in 2003 for small health plans. These regulations will have an enormous impact on the health care industry because they require the implementation of national standards for the electronic submission of specific medical information. It is expected that because of this law, all carriers will convert to automation for electronic transmissions within the next 5 years. The regulations will also ensure privacy for all electronic transactions, security for information systems, and unique health identification numbers for all providers, employers, individuals, and carriers.

The following are the most important computer-related requirements of HIPAA:

- Software that can handle unique identifiers and new formats
- Coding and security standards for electronic record-keeping software
- Policies and procedures for electronic storage of information
- Filing systems for submission of claims
- Compliance policies for information security processes

Violations of these privacy standards are punishable by fines, civil monetary penalties, and imprisonment. Punishment depends on the severity of the violation. Civil monetary penalties can range from $100 per violation to $25,000 for noncriminal violations. Violations that are committed knowingly are subject to higher penalties. For disclosing or procuring protected medical information, the fine could be as high as $50,000 and 1 year of imprisonment. If the information is obtained under false pretenses, the fines rise to $100,000 with up to 5 years of imprisonment. The worst offense is obtaining information with the intent to sell it, transfer it to others, or use it for malicious activities, which can lead to fines up to $250,000 and imprisonment for up to 10 years.

HIPAA Risk Assessment and Gap Analysis

Because the office computer vendor should handle the transactions part of HIPAA, the main concern of the office manager should be the issues associated with privacy.

A meeting with the staff can prove beneficial for identifying the areas of risk within the office. During a staff meeting, implement a brainstorming session by asking employees to perform a mock "patient walk-through" of the office. This exercise will identify what is heard and what is seen by patients in the office. Follow these steps and discover the eye-opening areas of risk identified along the way:

- Walking into the reception area and proceeding to the front desk to register
- Sitting in the reception area
- Walking back to the examination room
- Sitting in the examination room
- Proceeding to a testing area or scheduling area
- During discharge, including payment for services, next appointment, scheduling of testing, and so on

What areas of privacy infringement can be identified during this process?

COMMON RISK AREAS

A listing of some commonly identified areas of HIPAA risk are as follows:

- Reception desk in reception area is "open." This area should be in a secure location and not in an open space of the reception area.
- Receptionist sits behind window, but window is open. Conversations about patients with co-workers and physicians can be overheard. Receptionist's phone conversations can be overheard. The window should be closed, voices should be low, and music should be playing to create "white noise" in the office suite. Employees should discuss patients in an area of the office that is off-limits to patients.
- A sign-in sheet is used for patients to register their presence using their full names and the physicians they are scheduled to see. Patients signing in can see who else has an appointment and what physician they are seeing. This is especially important for multispecialty groups. Vendors (pharmaceutical representatives, cleaning staff, computer vendors, copy machine repairpersons, laundry crew, shredding company personnel, etc.) can also read the sign-in sheet as they stand at the front window. Ask patients to sign only their first names on the sign-in sheet along with their appointment time.
- Computer monitor on front desk can be seen and read by patients or vendors standing at the window. Reposition the monitor so that it cannot be seen by anyone standing at the window. Set the screen saver to come on quickly if the computer is not in use.
- Receptionist discusses patients' insurance with them standing at the window. Patients should be directed to a secure area within the office before discussing patient demographics, insurance, and other confidential matters.
- A message book is open on the front desk allowing patients at the window to view messages. The message book should be closed unless in use.
- Patient is escorted to an examination room. Patient walks past charts hanging outside of examination rooms and can read the patients' names. Frequently, diagnostic studies are paper-clipped to the outside of the chart, where patients walking by can read the results. Charts should be placed in chart holders backwards.
- Patient walks past a daily appointment schedule that has been taped to the wall in the hallway. Anything

with patient information on it should be protected. These schedules should be kept in a folder at a nursing station.

- A message from a patient is taped to the wall outside of an examination room so that the physician can see it when returning to the hallway. Any message containing patient information should not be in an open area allowing other patients, vendors, or visitors to read it.
- While in the examination room, patient overhears staff talking about another patient outside of the examination room door. Voices should be low, music should be playing throughout the office to create "white noise," and conversations should take place in a nonpatient area.
- Employee or physician takes a phone call while in the examination room with a patient. During the call, another patient, who has been identified during the call, is discussed. All calls should be handled in a secure area of the office.
- Another patient's test result is left on the counter in the examination room. Be certain that room is cleaned properly before using it for a new patient. Always file patients' information in their chart to avoid loss.
- The physician's operating room schedule is open at the scheduling desk and can be viewed by anyone standing or sitting there. All schedules containing patient information must be covered or closed.
- Patients' charts are piled on the scheduling desk awaiting employees to call patients to schedule procedures. Charts should be placed in a more secure area until scheduling is completed.
- While employees are away from their desks, charts are left out on their desks, patient information is left on computer screens, the message book is left open, and so on. Clutter and work papers should be organized and secured before leaving workstations or desks.
- When patient is standing at the discharge desk, other patient charts are piled there awaiting input into the computer. Find a more secure area for the placement of charts for the day.
- The patient charts for the day are piled onto the counter next to the desk where the patient names can be seen. Find a more secure area for the placement of charts for the day.

What about identification of risk that is not face-to-face?

- Faxing protected information to the wrong number. Use speed-dial whenever possible to avoid incorrect entering of a phone number.
- Faxing protected information to a number where it sits for a while before it is retrieved. Call ahead to alert the recipient that the fax is coming.
- Calling and leaving a message (either on an answering machine or with another family member) for a patient to remind him or her of an appointment or to inform him or her of test results. Can be a breach of confidentiality; leave a message for the patient to call the office phone number without stating it is a medical office (for example, "This is a message for Mrs. Rita Jones, please call 555-111-2222 at your earliest convenience. Thank you").
- Sending a postcard to the patient reminding him or her of an appointment or informing him or her of test results. Anyone can read what is written on a postcard. Reminders can be sent in sealed envelopes. Test results should be sent in a sealed envelope or should be handled with the patient on the telephone.
- Talking with the physician on a cell phone regarding a patient. Because of security and cell phones, protected patient information should not be discussed on cell phones.

It is the office manager's responsibility to identify and correct any areas where there may be infringement of patient privacy.

Stark II Regulations of 2001

Phase I of the final regulations regarding physician self-referral was issued on January 4, 2001. Phase I includes self-referrals, statutory definitions, in-office ancillary service exceptions, and compensation arrangement exceptions. New exceptions were added to include risk-sharing arrangements, fair market value compensation, payments to physician members of faculty practice plans, and non-cash compensation from a hospital to a medical staff member.

The Stark Law states that a physician cannot have a financial relationship with an entity that provides health care services. A good office manager will ask two questions to determine whether the practice is in violation of the Stark Law:

1. Does the practice make referrals (Medicare or Medicaid patients only) for laboratory, x-ray, and physical therapy services, for example, or for durable medical equipment, outpatient drugs, and so on?
2. Does a financial relationship exist between the practice and the referral entities?

If the answer to both of these questions is yes, it is necessary to speak with the physician about the possibility of a violation under Stark.

FRAUD STATISTICS

Fighting health care fraud is a great source of income for the government. Through the False Claims Act alone, the DOJ reclaimed $1.68 billion from 1997 to 2000. With the cost of those recoveries at $202 million, the return on the dollar is

$8 for all False Claims Act violations. CMS (formerly the Health Care Financing Administration [HCFA]) was allocated $630 million for fraud control for 2000 and $680 million for 2001. Efforts to prevent wasteful spending and improper payments have saved an estimated $60 billion.

Taxpayers Against Fraud (TAF) reported the following results:

- From 1986 through 2001, almost $3 billion in civil penalties was recovered.
- In the year 2000 alone, $732 million was recovered in health care cases. It is estimated that the current antifraud statutes are generating billions in additional savings because of their deterrent effect.
- Whistleblower cases have been responsible for the recovery of $2.3 billion since 1986.

MEDICARE FRAUD UNITS

Medicare fraud units have been established across the United States to handle Medicare fraud and abuse. They are responsible for collection of overpayments and exclusions from the Medicare program, among other things.

Medicare-Specific Fraud

- Billing Medicare or another insurer for services or items that were never delivered
- Billing Medicare for services or items of equipment that are different from what was expected
- Use of another person's Medicare card to obtain medical care, supplies, or equipment
- Billing Medicare for home medical equipment after it has been returned

MEDICAID-SPECIFIC FRAUD

- Billing for services not rendered
- Billing separately for services in lieu of an available combination code
- Misrepresentation of the service/supplies rendered
- Altering claims
- Submission of any false data on claims
- Duplicate billing for the same service
- Billing for services provided by unlicensed or unqualified persons
- Billing for used items as new
- Falsifying credentials
- Fraudulent enrollment practices
- Offering free services in exchange for a recipient's MA ID number
- Overuse of services
- Providing unnecessary services
- Kickbacks—accepting or making payments for referrals
- Concealing ownership of related companies
- Forging or altering prescriptions or orders
- Using multiple ID cards
- Loaning ID cards to others
- Reselling items received through the program

COMPLIANCE PLANS

In September 2000, the OIG released the "Compliance Program Guidance for Individual and Small Group Physician Practices." This program was developed to help physicians adhere to federal guidelines and take proactive and protective measures to ensure proper conduct. An effective plan reduces the risk of civil and criminal action and provides a safety net in the event of an audit.

A compliance plan requires the practice to accomplish the following:

- Review all billing procedures
- Correct any weaknesses or errors
- Establish controls

This plan is not mandatory; however, by implementing a strong system of controls and checks, it allows medical practices to prevent future problems.

Seven Basic Components of a Compliance Plan

The OIG provides seven basic components that provide practices with a solid base on which to practice medicine. The seven components are as follows:

1. Monitor compliance by conducting periodic audits.
2. Implement compliance and practice standards by developing written standards and procedures.
3. Designate a compliance officer or contact to monitor compliance efforts and enforce practice standards.
4. Conduct appropriate training and education on practice standards and procedures.
5. Respond appropriately to detected violations by investigating allegations and disclosing incidents to appropriate government entities.
6. Develop open lines of communication, such as (a) discussion at staff meetings regarding how to avoid erroneous or fraudulent conduct, and (b) community bulletin boards, to keep employees updated regarding compliance activities.
7. Enforce disciplinary standards by adhering to well-publicized guidelines.

ONE: AUDITING AND MONITORING

By performing an audit, the practice is able to identify any areas of noncompliance and the risks associated with their findings. This step will also determine whether the compliance plan is working, because the auditing and monitoring process is ongoing. This review consists of two parts: the standards and procedures audit and the claims submission audit.

The standards and procedures audit should be performed (either in house or by contract) periodically to determine the effectiveness and completeness of the plan. Any issues identified during this audit should be corrected using the standards released by the government and the CPT and ICD-9-CM codebooks.

The claims submission audit should be performed initially as a baseline and then at least yearly afterward. This audit will identify coding, billing, and documentation issues that may not be in compliance. These audits will provide information on medical necessity, incomplete documentation for services billed, and inaccurate and accurate coding of services, procedures, and diagnoses. The recommended number of records for the audit is either 5 for each federal payer, or 5 to 10 for each physician.

TWO: ESTABLISHING PRACTICE STANDARDS AND PROCEDURES

After the audit has been completed, the practice will have an understanding of its exposure. It now becomes necessary to develop written standards and procedures to address any risk areas. The risk areas that physicians need to monitor are as follows:

Coding and Billing

The most common issues investigated by the OIG are as follows:

- Billing for items or services not rendered or not provided as claimed
- Submitting claims for equipment, medical supplies, and services that are not reasonable and necessary
- Double billing resulting in duplicate payment
- Billing for noncovered services as if they were covered
- Misuse of provider identification numbers, which results in improper billing
- Unbundling
- Failure to properly use coding modifiers
- Clustering
- Upcoding

Reasonable and Necessary

A physician may bill Medicare only for services that meet the standard of being reasonable and necessary for the diagnosis and treatment of a patient.

Documentation

One of the most important compliance issues is timely, accurate, and complete documentation. Documentation is not only important for compliance issues, but also for legal issues and continuity of care. (Detailed documentation guidelines can be found in Chapter 8.) The documentation in the medical record may be used to validate the following:

- Site of service
- Appropriateness of the services provided
- Accuracy of the billing
- Identity of the provider

Another area where problems arise is in the completion of the CMS 1500 form. To avoid problems with claims submissions, the office manager should be aware of the following:

- Link the diagnosis codes with the appropriate service or procedure
- Use modifiers when necessary
- Provide all insurance coverage information, including Medicare secondary payer coverage

Improper Inducements, Kickbacks, and Self-Referrals

The practice should have policies regarding compliance with anti-kickback regulations and the self-referral law. Possible risk areas relating to these subjects are as follows:

- Financial arrangements with outside entities to whom the practice may refer federal health care program business
- Joint ventures with entities supplying goods or services to the practice or its patients
- Consulting contracts or medical directorships
- Office and equipment leases with entities to which the physician refers
- Soliciting, accepting, or offering any gift or gratuity of more than nominal value to or from those who may benefit from a practice's referral of federal health care program business

Record Retention

This section of the compliance plan should contain a policy regarding the retention of the practice's medical, financial, and compliance records. The following guidelines are suggested by the OIG in its compliance plan guidelines:

- Length of time that a practice's records are to be retained can be specified in the medical practice's standards and procedures.
- Medical records need to be secured against loss, destruction, unauthorized access, unauthorized reproduction, corruption, and damage.
- Standards and procedures need to stipulate the disposition of medical records in the event the practice is sold or closed.

THREE: DESIGNATING A COMPLIANCE OFFICER

In a large practice or hospital setting, the appointment of a compliance officer is the norm. However, in a practice with limited resources, a physician within the group, the office manager, or a small committee may perform the following duties of the compliance officer:

- Overseeing and monitoring the implementation of the compliance program.
- Establishing methods, such as periodic audits, to improve the practice's efficiency and quality of services and to reduce the practice's vulnerability to fraud and abuse.
- Periodically revising the compliance program in light of changes in the needs of the practice or changes in the law, standards, and procedures of government and private payer health plans.
- Developing, coordinating, and participating in a training program that focuses on the components of the compliance program and seeks to ensure that training materials are appropriate.
- Ensuring that the DHHS-OIG's "List of Excluded Individuals and Entities" and the General Services Administration's "List of Parties Debarred from Federal Programs" have been checked with respect to all employees, medical staff, and independent contractors.
- Investigating any report or allegation concerning possible unethical or improper business practices and monitoring subsequent corrective action and compliance.

FOUR: CONDUCTING APPROPRIATE TRAINING AND EDUCATION

Educational sessions are an important part of the compliance plan and should be tailored to the practice's needs. The three basic steps for setting up educational sessions are as follows:

1. Determine who needs training in coding, billing, or compliance.
2. Determine the type of training that best suits the practice's needs (e.g., seminars, one-on-one sessions with physicians, self-study, in-service training).
3. Determine when and how often education is needed and how much each person should receive.

Because training is a key factor in a successful compliance plan, medical practices should ensure that all necessary information is communicated to the physicians and staff.

Compliance Training

The operation and importance of the compliance plan should be a high priority. The consequences of violating the standards and procedures of the program and the role of each employee in the operation of the program should be discussed and understood.

Coding and Billing Training

Some physicians are not versed in the documentation requirements for coding and billing in accordance with federal health care programs. Some items of importance for billing and coding education are as follows:

- Coding requirements
- Claim development and submission processes
- Signing a form for a physician without the physician's authorization
- Proper documentation of services rendered
- Proper billing standards and procedures and submission of accurate bills for services or items rendered to federal health care program beneficiaries
- Legal sanctions for submitting deliberately false billings

Format of the Training Program

Training can be conducted by office staff or by outside sources. Consultants can provide on-site educational sessions and will do so at the convenience of the practice (e.g., early mornings, evenings, Saturdays). Training is also offered in 1-day workshops and seminars by coding and billing organizations. Some carriers also offer compliance training programs.

Continuing Education on Compliance Issues

Compliance guidelines do not specify a set number of training sessions that should occur. They do suggest, however, that educational sessions be performed at least annually. Newly hired billing and coding staff should be trained soon after they start work. All educational sessions should be documented with "sign-in" sheets that are maintained by the office manager or compliance officer if the practice has one.

FIVE: RESPONDING TO DETECTED OFFENSES AND DEVELOPING CORRECTIVE ACTION INITIATIVES

Once the practice has identified a possible violation, it becomes necessary to correct the problem. A corrective action plan will aid in this. Develop a set of indicators such as the following that will alert the practice of possible exposure:

- Significant changes in the number or types of claim rejections or reductions
- Correspondence from carriers and insurers challenging medical necessity or validity of claims
- Illogical patterns or unusual changes in the pattern of CPT, HCPCS, or ICD-9-CM code utilization
- Unusually high volumes of charge or payment adjustment transactions

SIX: DEVELOPING OPEN LINES OF COMMUNICATION

Compliance training communication is an integral part of any compliance plan. Good communication does not necessarily require costly methods and processes. It can be as simple as an "open door" policy that allows for a free flow of information between physicians, staff, compliance personnel, and employees. An open communication policy should include the following elements:

- The requirement that employees report conduct that a reasonable person would, in good faith, believe to be erroneous or fraudulent

- The creation of a user-friendly process (such as an anonymous drop box for larger practices) for effectively reporting erroneous or fraudulent conduct
- Provisions in the standards and procedures that define failure to report erroneous or fraudulent conduct as a violation of the compliance program
- The development of a simple procedure to process reports of erroneous or fraudulent conduct
- A process that maintains the anonymity of the persons involved in the possible erroneous or fraudulent conduct and the person reporting the concern
- Provisions in standards and procedures that prohibit retribution for reporting conduct that a reasonable person acting in good faith would believe to be erroneous or fraudulent

If a billing company is used, there must be regular communication between the practice's compliance officer and the billing company's compliance officer or other responsible staff to coordinate billing and compliance activities. Communication can include, as appropriate, lists of reported or identified concerns, initiation of internal assessments and the results of those assessments, training needs, regulatory changes, and other operational and compliance matters.

SEVEN: ENFORCING DISCIPLINARY STANDARDS BY ADHERING TO WELL-PUBLICIZED GUIDELINES

An effective compliance plan must include a procedure for enforcing its provisions and disciplining individuals who violate those provisions. Disciplinary actions should include the following:

- Warnings (verbal)
- Reprimands (written)
- Probation
- Demotion
- Temporary suspension
- Termination
- Restitution of damages
- Referral for criminal prosecution

If it becomes necessary to invoke these actions, it is of utmost importance to document them in a compliance file. This documentation must include the following:

- Date of the incident
- Name of the reporting party
- Name of the person responsible for taking action
- Follow-up action taken

HOTLINES

One of the seven basic components of an effective compliance plan is a "hotline" for reporting fraudulent activities. A hotline can be managed in house or by an outside agency. The actual intake of information should be handled in a manner comfortable to the practice. Confidentiality must be maintained or the hotline will fail. The intake process should be structured with the proper gathering of information, the caller's concern, and documentation of the call.

Be sure that the existence of the hotline is well publicized within the office. It should also be explained in the compliance plan. When advertising the hotline, be certain to emphasize that all information is held strictly confidential.

The office manager should routinely monitor the hotline for effectiveness by implementing the following steps:

1. Document the number of calls monthly.
2. Evaluate and improve, if necessary, the level of trust between the compliance officer and employees.
3. Maintain a response time of 24 hours for all investigations.

HOTLINE AUDITING AND MONITORING

An in-house hotline should be maintained by the office manager or another designated employee. In some offices a compliance officer maintains the hotline. Box 7-1 provides policies and procedures for auditing, maintaining, and monitoring a hotline.

Hotlines are becoming more common as compliance is continually emphasized. Box 7-2 lists the top issues reported on hotlines.

BACKGROUND CHECKS

Some job candidates have less-than-desirable backgrounds. The physician you interview may seem perfect for the job, but a background check may reveal a problem in another state. As discussed in Chapter 2, background checks help us select the best and most trusted employees.

The OIG released a Special Advisory Bulletin regarding the "Effect of Exclusion from Participation in Federal Health Care Programs." This bulletin clarified that services provided by an excluded provider are not reimbursable. Because of this, it is extremely important for medical practices to be aware of any employees or prospective employees who are on the exclusion lists. One source of information about problems in an employee's background is the Internet. Another way to obtain a background check is to use a company that specializes in such services. One company, Government Management Services, Inc., identifies sanctioned individuals in health care by using its proprietary Fraud and Abuse Control Information System. This company conducts searches of sanctioned information gathered by the Office of Inspector General (OIG), General Services Administration (GSA), and other federal agencies. It will search for disciplinary actions taken by federal agencies and licensing and certification agencies in all 50 states.

BOX 7-1 Sample Hotline Policy and Procedure

Parties Necessary for Development and Implementation

Corporate compliance officer

Compliance committee (management)

Issues to Consider

Must be relatively easy to implement once the hotline is established

Can help define the annual compliance auditing and monitoring plan

Purpose

One of the primary responsibilities of the compliance team is to ensure that the hotline operates in conformance with its objectives. Periodic audits of the hotline operation will ensure that the hotline is operating efficiently.

Policy

Hotline operations will be audited periodically.

ABC Medical Practice will take necessary steps to ensure continued integrity and effectiveness of the hotline.

Rita Peters is the primary person responsible for the hotline operations.

Procedures

Rita Peters will conduct or oversee periodic audits of all aspects of the hotline operation. Rita's audits will focus on the following:

Receiving Calls

Accessibility—Calls should be answered promptly during established hotline hours.

Continuity—Callers should hear a recorded message.

Uniformity and completeness—Callers should be asked a set of uniform questions, be treated professionally, and be encouraged by the operator to elaborate on all important information.

Closure—Callers should be provided an appropriate report identification number and thanked for calling the hotline.

Logistics and Operations

Confidentiality—The practice's telephone system should be structured to ensure that the origin of the call is not identified and cannot be traced.

Operations security—Monitor calls and report preparation areas (in-house areas) to ensure that all information is kept confidential and cannot be overheard or seen by others.

Records management—Examine files and record retention policies to ensure that documents are maintained in a secure area.

Follow-up—Review follow-up and investigative activities to confirm that issues are handled promptly and appropriately.

Effectiveness

Employee awareness and understanding—Solicit feedback from employees to ensure that the hotline continues to be viewed as a viable method of communication.

Rita will provide reports on the results of any hotline audits to the appropriately designated people, who in turn will report to the compliance committee.

Rita will recommend to the compliance committee any necessary changes to the hotline.

Adapted from Joseph, A., & Kusserow, R. *Corporate Compliance Policies and Procedures.* Boston: Opus Communications, 2000.

PHYSICIANS AT TEACHING HOSPITALS (PATH)

Medicare's rule for physicians at teaching hospitals (PATH) became effective on July 1, 1996. This rule covers services provided by physicians and residents in teaching facilities such as hospitals and clinics, and replaces the I.L. 372 rule. This first rule, Intermediary Letter 372 (I.L. 372), was titled "Part B Payments for Services of Supervising Physicians in a Teaching Setting" and was effective in April 1969.

A notorious case of teaching physician fraud occurred at the University of Pennsylvania. After the investigation was completed, charges of upcoding were levied on that health system and it received a settlement figure of $30 million. The $30 million consisted of $10 million in actual false claims and $20 million in fines and penalties. In addition, the settlement included the implementation of a corporate compliance plan and centralization of billing services. This case was the beginning of a major initiative against teaching hospitals that continues across the country today. Details on regulations affecting teaching hospitals can be found in Chapter 8.

ORGANIZATIONS

It can be very helpful for the office manager to join compliance organizations. These organizations can provide guidance, education, and networking opportunities. Two organizations

BOX 7-2 Top 14 Reported Hotline Issues

1. Billing and coding
2. Conflict of interest
3. Fraud
4. Health violation
5. Human resources
6. Medical staff
7. Patient care
8. Policy violation
9. Prejudice
10. Sexual harassment
11. Substance abuse
12. Theft
13. Time/attendance
14. Workplace violence

From *Compliance Hot Line Benchmarking Report.* Boston: Opus Communications, 2000.

that might warrant further investigation are the Health Care Compliance Association (www.hcca.org) and the National Health Care Anti-Fraud Association (www.nhcaa.org).

EXERCISES

MULTIPLE CHOICE

Choose the best *answer for each of the following questions.*

1. Which of the following is an example of fraud?
   a. Upcoding
   b. Unbundling
   c. Altering a claim
   d. All of the above
2. What is defined as an incident or practice that is not consistent with sound medical, business, or fiscal practices?
   a. Fraud
   b. Abuse
   c. Compliance
   d. Falsification
3. Billing for a service that wasn't performed is an example of
   a. Wire fraud
   b. Embezzlement in connection to health care
   c. False statements relating to health care matters
   d. None of the above
4. Who refers cases to the DOJ?
   a. OIG
   b. FBI
   c. Both the FBI and OIG
   d. None of the above
5. The first fraud alert was issued in what year?
   a. 1993
   b. 1997
   c. 1988
   d. 1980
6. Operation Restore Trust was developed in what year?
   a. 1995
   b. 1997
   c. 1993
   d. 2000
7. The program in which the DHHS partners with private companies to audit cost reports is
   a. OIG
   b. MIP
   c. ORT
   d. None of the above
8. Which one of the following do you not need when you call the OIG hotline?
   a. Carrier name
   b. Patient name and address
   c. Name of person alleged fraudulent
   d. Name of emergency contact
9. What is one way to deter a whistleblower suit?
   a. Call the carrier
   b. Hire well-trained employees
   c. Perform exit interviews
   d. None of the above
10. Which of the following is a risk area identified by the OIG?
    a. Duplicate billing
    b. Credit balances
    c. Professional courtesy
    d. All of the above
11. What is the term for a service whose payment is included in another service code?
    a. Downcoding
    b. Upcoding
    c. Unbundling
    d. Code steering
12. To avoid claim denials, a medical practice should use
    a. CCI
    b. CCP
    c. CSS
    d. None of the above
13. Which of the following is an overpayment that is left on the books?
    a. Code steering
    b. Debit
    c. Credit
    d. Credit balance
14. When only certain codes are listed on the patient encounter form, it is known as
    a. Bundling
    b. Code steering
    c. Ping-ponging
    d. None of the above
15. Which of the following is an administrative remedy?
    a. Education
    b. Recovery of overpayments
    c. Withheld payments
    d. All of the above

TRUE OR FALSE

Determine whether the following issues have been listed by the OIG as risk areas for physicians.

1. ______ Code steering
2. ______ Upcoding
3. ______ Preventive medicine codes for Medicare patients
4. ______ Critical care time calculations
5. ______ Waiver of co-pays
6. ______ Collection agencies
7. ______ Waiver of deductibles
8. ______ Billing companies
9. ______ Duplicate billing
10. ______ Compliance plans

THINKERS

1. An office manager is new to a practice. She discovers that there are several credit balances on the books for a patient. Is it necessary for her to do anything about this discrepancy, or can she allow them to stay there until the patient returns to the office (to use up the credit)?
2. A good friend of the physician arrives for an office visit. The physician instructs the receptionist not to charge this individual. The receptionist comes to the office manager for guidance. How should the office manager handle this situation?
3. Describe the self-disclosure program and how it may be used by a medical practice.
4. Dr. Martin submits claims electronically for services that were not performed. What criminal statute(s) could this practice involve?

REFERENCES

Compliance Hotline Benchmarking Report. Boston: Opus Communications Publications, 2000.

Joseph, A., & Kusserow, R. *Corporate Compliance Policies and Procedures.* Boston: Opus Communications Publications, 2000.

Federal Fraud Enforcement. "Physician Compliance." Available at www.ama.assn.org/ama/pub/category/4598.html.

Physicians Fraud and Abuse Prevention. Salt Lake City, UT: Ingenix Publishing, 2000.

8

DOCUMENTATION AND RISK ASSESSMENT

CHAPTER OUTLINE

Introduction
Documentation
Audits

CHAPTER OBJECTIVES

After completing this chapter, you will be able to do the following:

- Understand the principles of documentation
- Recognize the key components of evaluation and management services
- Recognize the various components of history, examination, and medical decision making
- Understand the importance of medical necessity
- Differentiate between new and established patients
- Know the various types of office and hospital services
- Identify consultation requirements
- Know the documentation requirements for operative reports
- Recognize the importance of a medical record audit and be able to perform one

INTRODUCTION

After finishing Chapters 6 and 7, perhaps you are asking yourself, "Why do office managers need to know coding, billing, and documentation?" Office managers need to know everything about how to run a medical office. They must understand each job within the practice, what purpose it serves, how important it is to the practice, and how it is performed. Most office managers at some point in their careers have found themselves scheduling appointments and surgeries, checking in patients, discharging patients, and filing charts, and yes, some have even performed clinical duties. It is often necessary for the office manager to pitch in when staff is short-handed.

Billing, coding, and documentation are the lifeline of the practice. Documentation is a major issue for physicians; it has had a major impact on medical practices since the release of documentation guidelines in 1995. An office manager must be able to assist the physician in this task by understanding all aspects of documentation. The responsibility of medical office operations ultimately falls into the lap of the office manager.

DOCUMENTATION

Proper documentation can mean the difference between receiving and not receiving reimbursement for services the physician performs. Communication between the office staff and the physician plays an invaluable role in this process. The quality of current documentation can have significant consequences. Many managed care organizations require documentation of quality medical care and consequent outcomes before executing or renewing contracts. Their goal is to obtain quality medical care for their members at reasonable costs while controlling the increase in those costs. This type of "purchaser" is growing in number each year.

On the Medicare side, because of the increasing number of health care fraud and abuse cases, Medicare requires random prepayment audits on their beneficiaries. In a prepayment audit, the practice submits the Medicare claim; Medicare then requests a copy of the record before making payment. Medicare audits the record and reimburses the amount that it determines is correct for that patient encounter. In the event of an audit, the office manager and the physician will soon realize the critical importance of proper documentation. Proper documentation also reduces liability. When coding and billing, each visit should be carefully examined to establish the proper code for the visit. The office manager must fully explain to the physician the evaluation and management (E&M) coding system. If the physician constantly uses the same codes for every office visit, this bad habit will raise a red flag during processing and can automatically trigger an audit.

We are all looking for value in our daily lives. Health care is no exception. Optimal medical record documentation has significant present and future value, but physicians must "buy in" to the importance of proper documentation because it affects their personal, professional, and financial success. You as the office manager play a key role in helping the physician to accomplish this!

Principles of Documentation

In 1995, a list of documentation principles for physicians and physician extenders was released. These guidelines were a combined effort between the Centers for Medicare and Medicaid Services (CMS) and the American Medical Association (AMA) to standardize the documentation of patient services. The guidelines are as follows:

1. The medical record should be complete and legible.
2. The documentation of each patient encounter should include the date; the reason for the encounter; appropriate history and physical examination; review of laboratory results, x-ray data, and other ancillary services, where appropriate; assessment; and plan for care (including discharge service, if appropriate).
3. Past and present diagnoses should be accessible to the treating and/or consulting physician.
4. The reasons for and results of x-rays, laboratory tests, and other ancillary services should be documented or included in the medical record.
5. Relevant health risk factors should be identified.
6. The patient's progress, including response to treatment, change in treatment, change in diagnosis, and patient noncompliance, should be documented.
7. The written plan for care should include, when appropriate, treatments and medications, specifying frequency and dosage; any referrals and consultation; patient/family education; and specific instructions for follow-up.
8. Documentation should support the intensity of the patient's evaluation and treatment, including thought processes and the complexity of medical decision making.
9. All entries must be dated and contain the identification of the provider of the service.
10. Reported *Physicians' Current Procedural Terminology* (CPT) and *International Classification of Diseases, Ninth Revision, Clinical Modification* (ICD-9-CM) codes must be supported by the documentation in the medical record.

Evaluation and Management Documentation Basics

Ignorance of the law excuses no man; not that all men know the law, but because it is an excuse every man will plead, and no man can tell how to confute him.

—JOHN SELDEN (1584–1654), ENGLISH LAWYER AND SCHOLAR

In 1992, the Resource-Based Relative Value Scale (RBRVS) system was introduced. At that time, the seven factors driving the selection of an E&M code were as follows:

1. History
2. Examination
3. Medical decision making
4. Counseling
5. Coordination of care
6. Presentation of the problem
7. Time

We now use the first three items—history, examination, and medical decision making—as the key components in selecting a level of E&M service. The final four items—counseling, coordination of care, presentation of the problem, and time—are no longer driving forces for choosing these E&M levels.

"THREE OUT OF THREE" RULE

All three key components of history, examination, and medical decision making must be documented for the following categories of E&M codes:

- All consultations (except follow-up)
- Initial hospital care
- Comprehensive nursing facility care
- Emergency department services
- Observation services
- Observation services/inpatient hospital
- Domiciliary care, new
- Home, new patient
- Office visit, new patient

"TWO OUT OF THREE" RULE

Only two out of three key components of history, examination, and medical decision making need to be documented for the following categories of E&M codes (any two of the three components can be used):

- Subsequent hospital care
- Subsequent nursing facility care
- Domiciliary care, established
- Home services, established
- Office visit, established patient

HISTORY LEVELS

There are four levels of history: problem focused, expanded problem focused, detailed, and comprehensive. There are four components within these history levels: chief complaint; history of present illness (HPI); review of systems (ROS); and past, family, and/or social history that need to be documented based on the level of service.

1. *Problem focused*: This level must contain a chief complaint and a brief HPI that consists of one to three elements.
2. *Expanded problem focused*: This level must contain a chief complaint, a brief HPI that consists of one to three elements, and a problem-pertinent ROS, which documents at least one system.
3. *Detailed*: This level must contain a chief complaint; an extended HPI that consists of four or more elements or the status of three chronic conditions; an extended ROS that consists of two to nine systems; and a pertinent past, family, or social history that consists of documentation of one history area (i.e., past, family, or social history).
4. *Comprehensive*: This level must contain a chief complaint; an extended HPI that consists of four or more elements or three chronic conditions; a complete ROS that consists of 10 or more systems; and a complete past, family, and social history. Depending on the category of E&M service, this will be either two out of three or three out of three areas of past, family, and social history.

Chief Complaint

The chief complaint, or reason for the visit, is generally a brief phrase about why the patient is seeking care. It is usually in the patient's own words and should not consist of vague language. Examples of vague language would be as follows:

- cc—routine
- cc—follow-up visit
- cc—checkup

Examples of correct documentation of the chief complaint are as follows:

- cc—routine visit for high blood pressure
- cc—follow-up visit for sciatica
- cc—checkup on left knee pain

The simple language of "routine," "follow-up," and "checkup" does not state why the patient sought care (i.e., check up on what?).

History of Present Illness

The history of present illness is a description of the present illness from the beginning of symptoms to the time of the patient encounter. There are eight elements in the history of present illness:

1. **Duration**—How long do the symptoms last? How long have you been in pain? *I have had the paid since yesterday.* OR *The pain usually lasts about an hour.*
2. **Location**—Where is the pain? *The pain is in my ankle.*
3. **Severity**—On a scale of 1 to 10, how bad is the pain? OR Using descriptive wording, how bad is the pain? *The pain is about at a level 5 now.* OR *I had severe pain all night.*
4. **Timing**—When did the pain start? *It started last week.*
5. **Quality**—What type of pain is it? *It is a burning sensation.* OR *It is a sharp pain.*
6. **Modifying factors**—What helps or doesn't help the pain? *When I lay down, it gets better.* OR *I took over-the-counter pain pills but it didn't help.*
7. **Context**—What were you doing when this occurred? *I was riding my exercise bike when the pain started.*
8. **Associated signs and symptoms**—What else bothers you when this occurs? *Well, when I got the chest pain, I also got pain down my left arm.*

There are two levels of history of present illness: brief and extended. A brief history focuses on the patient's problem, whereas the extended history of present illness goes beyond that to elicit information that may support multiple diagnoses.

1. *Brief:* One to three of the eight elements
2. *Extended:* Four or more of the eight elements or the status of three chronic conditions of the patient

Review of Systems

The review of systems is a series of questions regarding the signs and symptoms of various organ systems. Fourteen systems are included in the review of systems:

1. Constitutional
2. Eyes
3. Ears, nose, mouth, throat
4. Cardiovascular
5. Respiratory
6. Gastrointestinal
7. Genitourinary
8. Musculoskeletal
9. Integumentary
10. Neurologic
11. Psychiatric
12. Endocrine
13. Hematologic/lymphatic
14. Allergic/immunologic

There are three levels of review of systems:

1. Problem pertinent, which includes questions about one system
2. Extended, which includes questions about two to nine systems
3. Complete, which includes questions about 10 or more systems

A problem-pertinent review of systems involves a review of system(s) that can be affected by, play a role in, or are likely to be involved in the patient's problem. An extended review includes a more in-depth review of systems. A complete review includes 10 of the 14 systems. This type of review is considered comprehensive in nature.

Past, Family, and Social History

A past history contains information about the patient's past experiences with illnesses, injuries, and treatments. A family history contains information about the patient's family, and a social history contains information about past or current activities and conditions.

There are two levels of past, family, and social history:

1. *Pertinent:* One area.
2. *Complete:* There are two levels of a complete past, family, and social history. These levels depend on the category of E&M code. There is the "three out of three" rule and the "two out of three" rule.
   a. "Three out of three" rule: All "initial contact" levels require all three areas to be documented. Examples of these levels are as follows:
      (1) All consultations
      (2) Initial hospital care
      (3) Comprehensive nursing facility care
      (4) Emergency department services
      (5) New office patient
   b. "Two out of three" rule: All "follow-up" levels require only two out of three areas to be documented. Examples of these levels are as follows:
      (1) Subsequent hospital care
      (2) Subsequent nursing facility care
      (3) Established office patient

PAST HISTORY

The elements of a past history include such documentation as the following:

- Medications
- Hospitalizations
- Surgeries
- Allergies
- Age-appropriate immunization status

FAMILY HISTORY

The elements of a family history include such documentation as the following:

- Health status or cause of death of parents, siblings, and children

- Specific diseases related to problems identified in the chief complaint, history of present illness, and/or review of systems
- Any diseases of family members that may be hereditary or place the patient at risk

SOCIAL HISTORY

The elements of a social history include such documentation as the following:

- Smoking
- Alcohol
- Controlled substance use
- Type of employment and occupational history
- Type of living conditions
- Sexual history
- Marital status
- Level of education

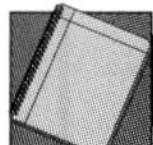

FROM THE EXPERT'S NOTEBOOK

If the history is unobtainable because of such conditions as dementia, loss of consciousness, or confusion, you must document that it was unobtainable and why. If documented properly, it will be considered at a comprehensive level. If left blank, it will be assumed that this portion of the visit was not performed.

EXAMINATION

The examination portion of the visit contains documentation of the objective findings of the provider of the service. Because the revised guidelines for E&M services have not yet been released, CMS allows physicians to choose either the 1995 or 1997 guidelines for documentation of the examination portion of the visit.

1995 Guidelines

The 1995 guidelines are much more subjective than the 1997 guidelines, because they are based on what the clinician feels is a "limited examination" or an "extended examination." The level of examination under the 1995 guidelines can consist of body areas and/or organ systems for the problem-focused, expanded problem-focused, and detailed levels. The comprehensive level of 1995 examination consists only of the documentation of organ systems. Documentation of body areas does not count toward a comprehensive level of examination.

The body areas are as follows:

- Chest
- Abdomen
- Back (including spine)
- Neck
- Genitalia, groin, and buttocks
- Head (including the face)
- Extremities; each one is an area

The organ systems are as follows:

- Constitutional
- Eyes
- Ears/nose/mouth/throat
- Cardiovascular
- Respiratory
- Gastrointestinal
- Genitourinary
- Musculoskeletal
- Integumentary
- Neurologic
- Psychiatric
- Hematologic/lymphatic/immunologic

There are four levels of examination under the 1995 guidelines:

1. *Problem focused*: Examination that is limited to the affected body area or organ system (generally one system is examined).
2. *Expanded problem focused*: Examination of the affected body areas or organ systems and any other symptomatic or related organ systems (generally five to seven systems are examined).
3. *Detailed*: Extended examination of the affected body areas or organ systems and any other symptomatic or related organ systems (generally five to seven systems are examined).
4. *Comprehensive*: Complete single-system specialty examination or complete multisystem examination (generally eight or more systems are examined). Documentation of body areas cannot be counted toward a comprehensive examination.

1997 Guidelines

The 1997 examination guidelines consist of a multispecialty examination and 10 single-specialty examinations. As stated previously, a physician can use either set of guidelines, and the guidelines can be changed from patient to patient. For example, Dr. Babinetz may examine Frank Dunlap using the 1997 guidelines for documentation and then examine Steve White using the 1995 guidelines. The 1997 single-specialty guidelines consist of "shaded" areas where each bullet point must be examined and documented. These single-specialty examinations consist of the following systems:

- Cardiovascular
- Ears/nose/mouth/throat
- Eye
- Genitourinary
- Hematologic/lymphatic/immunologic

- Musculoskeletal
- Neurologic
- Psychiatric
- Respiratory
- Integumentary

The multispecialty examination does not contain "mandated" areas. The details of these guidelines can be found on the CMS Web site at www.hcfa.gov or any state Medicare carrier Web site.

There are four levels of examination under the 1997 guidelines:

1. *Problem focused*: One to five of the elements identified by a bullet point.
2. *Expanded problem focused*: At least six of the elements identified by a bullet point.
3. *Detailed*: At least two of the elements identified by a bullet point from each of six areas/systems, or at least 12 of the elements identified by a bullet point in two or more areas/systems.
4. *Comprehensive*: For a multisystem examination, perform all elements identified by a bullet point in at least nine organ systems or body areas and document at least two elements identified by a bullet point from each of nine areas/systems. For a single-specialty examination, perform all elements identified by a bullet point and document each element in each shaded box and at least one bullet point in each unshaded box.

MEDICAL DECISION MAKING

The medical decision-making portion of the visit consists of the complexity of establishing the diagnosis and/or management option(s). The complexity of medical decision making is measured by two of the following three elements:

1. The number of possible diagnoses and/or the number of management options that must be considered
2. The amount and/or complexity of medical records, diagnostic tests, or other information that must be obtained, reviewed, and analyzed
3. The risk of significant complications and/or morbidity associated with the presented problems, diagnostic procedures, and possible management options

There are four types of medical decision making:

1. Straightforward
2. Low complexity
3. Moderate complexity
4. High complexity

The matrix in Table 8-1 illustrates the various components and levels of medical decision making. This matrix will help you choose the proper type of decision making for each situation.

TABLE 8-1 Medical Decision-Making Matrix

TYPE OF MEDICAL DECISION MAKING	NUMBER OF DIAGNOSIS/ MANAGEMENT OPTIONS	AMOUNT AND/OR COMPLEXITY OF DATA	RISK OF COMPLICATIONS AND/OR MORBIDITY OR MORTALITY
Straightforward	Minimal	Minimal/ none	Minimal
Low complexity	Limited	Limited/ low	Low
Moderate complexity	Multiple	Moderate	Moderate
High complexity	Extensive	Extensive	High

If a patient has multiple diagnoses and multiple management options, the complexity of the visit would be increased. The data that are collected and analyzed during the patient encounter must be clear and concise. For test results, document thought processes, analysis, and evaluation of both positive and negative findings. Their impact on treatment should be documented. Review of the patient medical record, past and present, should be documented with comments. Note the extent of the records and data reviewed. The potential risk to the patient is an important element in assessing the complexity of this key component of medical decision making.

COUNSELING

Counseling consists of any conversation or discussion with a patient or family concerning one or more of the following areas:

- Diagnostic results or studies
- Prognosis
- Risks and benefits of management options
- Instructions for management or follow-up
- Importance of compliance with management option
- Risk factor reduction
- Education of patient and family

Presentation of the Problem

The presenting problem is the disease, condition, injury, symptom, sign, illness, complaint, or any other reason for the patient visit, with or without the diagnosis being established at the time of the visit. There are five types of presenting problems:

1. *Minimal*: A problem that may not require the presence of a physician but is treated under his or her supervision
2. *Self-limited or minor*: A problem that runs a definite course, is transient, and is not likely to change the patient's general health permanently, or has a good prognosis with management

3. *Low severity*: A problem with a low risk of morbidity without treatment, little or no risk of mortality without treatment, and full recovery without physical impairment
4. *Moderate severity*: A problem with moderate risk of morbidity without treatment, moderate risk of mortality without treatment, and a prognosis of increased probability of physical impairment
5. *High severity:* A problem with a high risk of morbidity without treatment, a moderate to high risk of mortality without treatment, and a high probability of severe physical impairment

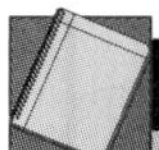

FROM THE EXPERT'S NOTEBOOK

When physicians are covering hospital rounds for other physicians, or if they are seeing a patient in the office setting, they must code their visits as if the patient was already an established patient.

Time

The specific times expressed in the visit codes are averages and represent a range of times that vary with each clinical situation. Unless it is a time-based code, time can only be used when counseling is 50% or more of the visit. Documentation must include the total amount of time spent with the patient, the amount of time spent counseling the patient, and the subject matter of the counseling. Sample documentation might look something like Figure 8-1.

MEDICAL NECESSITY

Insufficient documentation of medical necessity is the number one reason for denial of Medicare claims nationwide. In the policies and regulations section of the Physician Center at CMS, the medical necessity exclusion is described as follows:

No payment may be made under Part A or Part B for any expenses incurred for items or services which are not reasonable and necessary for the diagnosis or treatment of illness or injury or to improve the functioning of a malformed body member.

The AMA document entitled *Prepare that Claim, 2008*, identifies the definition as :

Health care services or products that a prudent physician would provide to a patient for the purpose of preventing, diagnosing, or treating an illness, injury, disease, or its symptoms in a manner that is:

1. In accordance with generally accepted standards of medical practice;

2. Clinically appropriate in terms of type, frequency, extent, site, and duration;

3. Not primarily for the convenience of the patient, physician, or other health care provider.

11/10/2003

Braun, Robert

I spent 50 minutes with Bob Braun today. Of that time, 30 minutes were spent counseling Bob and his wife in the results of his cardiac testing. Bob's prognosis and treatment options of ________________ were explained. Bob and his wife had the concern of ________________, but were satisfied with my recommendation of ______________.

Bob will go home and discuss our meeting today with his daughters. He will call me on Monday to let me know how he wishes to proceed.

Dr. Alexander Babinetz

FIGURE 8-1. Sample documentation.

NEW VERSUS ESTABLISHED PATIENTS

The CPT E&M codes were designed to classify the work of physicians and require far more clinical documentation than the previous visit codes. This documentation must indicate that a service was actually performed at the level that was reported and was medically necessary. In the E&M system of coding, a *new patient* is defined as any patient who has not been seen by the physician or anyone in his or her group in the past 3 years. The three key components (history, examination, and medical decision making) and the nature of the presenting problem must be documented in the new patient's record. An *established patient* is a patient who has been seen by the physician or one of the members of his or her group during the past 3 years. Two of the three key components and the nature of the presenting problem must be documented in the established patient's medical record.

CONSULTATIONS

One area of serious misunderstanding is the consultation. When assigning an E&M code to a service, one must be careful to differentiate between a consultation and a visit. The medical record documentation for a consultation must contain the following:

- The name of the requesting physician
- The reason for the consultation
- Date the consultation was requested
- Date and time the consultation was completed
- History
- Evidence of a physical examination and system review of the affected body areas or organ systems
- The consultant's written opinion sent back to the requesting physician
- The services that were ordered or performed
- Signature of the consultant

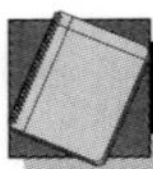

FROM THE EXPERT'S NOTEBOOK

Medicare reserves the right to downcode the service if the consultation does not read as an opinion. Thus the wording the physician uses when writing the consultation report is extremely important. He or she must write, "I recommend that an MRI be done," instead of simply writing an order for the test. When the consultant *orders* the MRI, he or she is no longer considered a consultant, and the reimbursement may be lowered.

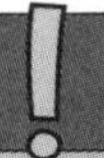

MANAGER'S ALERT

A referral from another physician is not the same thing as a consultation. A visit is not a consultation unless the office sends a written report back to the requesting physician. The words used in the documentation of a consultation must not include any form of the word "referral." CMS uses the managed care definition of this word, which indicates a "transfer of care." If the documentation uses the word "referral," the visit would not be a consultation and payment for these services would have to be refunded.

From a professional liability standpoint, clear and concise medical records will often prevent an attorney, a third-party carrier, or a governmental agency from filing a claim. Every complication and unusual occurrence should be documented. Any issues that arise from a patient's family members should be documented. Noncompliance, informed consent, telephone calls, prescription renewals, and all other relevant issues should be documented. In this era of cost-conscious health care, there is an increasing emphasis on documentation and quality of care. Keep this in mind: If you don't document it, you didn't do it! Failure to document services provided may affect the practice in a way in which other practices have been affected: seeing themselves in the headlines (Figure 8-2). Physicians often ask one another questions about what needs to be documented (Figure 8-3). Box 8-1 describes commonly overlooked aspects of thorough medical documentation. **Remember: If you didn't document it, you didn't do it!**

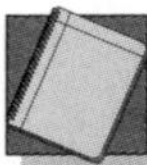

FROM THE EXPERT'S NOTEBOOK

Type the various categories of office codes and their descriptions on a 3 × 5 card and have it laminated for durability. The card will easily fit into the physician's coat pocket so that he or she can refer to it if needed when coding patient visits.

Office Services

This section explains the documentation necessary for new and established office visits. A new patient is one who has never been seen by the physician or group, or who is an established patient who has not been seen by a physician within the group in the last 3 years. An established patient is already recognized as a patient of the practice and is returning for a visit. All examination guidelines illustrated with the CPT codes are based on the 1995 guidelines for examination. The office manager should have a thorough understanding of these components.

NEW PATIENT, OFFICE

"Office patient, new" codes are used to report patient encounters in a physician office or other outpatient facility. These codes are used to report services on patients who are new to the physician. They have chosen this physician on their own and were not sent by another physician. If the visit was at the request of another physician, the service type would be one of a consultation.

New Patient 99201

History: Problem Focused

Chief complaint, brief history of present illness (one to three elements).

Examination: Problem Focused

Limited examination of the affected body area or organ system.

Medical Decision Making: Straightforward

Number of diagnoses or management options: minimal
Amount of or complexity of data: minimal or none
Risk of complications and/or morbidity or mortality: minimal

New Patient 99202

History: Expanded Problem Focused

Chief complaint, brief history of present illness (one to three elements), problem-pertinent review of systems.

Examination: Expanded Problem Focused

Limited examination of the affected body area or organ system and other symptomatic or related organ systems.

Medical Decision Making: Straightforward

Number of diagnoses or management options: minimal
Amount of or complexity of data: minimal or none
Risk of complications and/or morbidity or mortality: minimal

New Patient 99203

History: Detailed

Chief complaint; extended history of present illness (one to three elements); extended review of systems (two

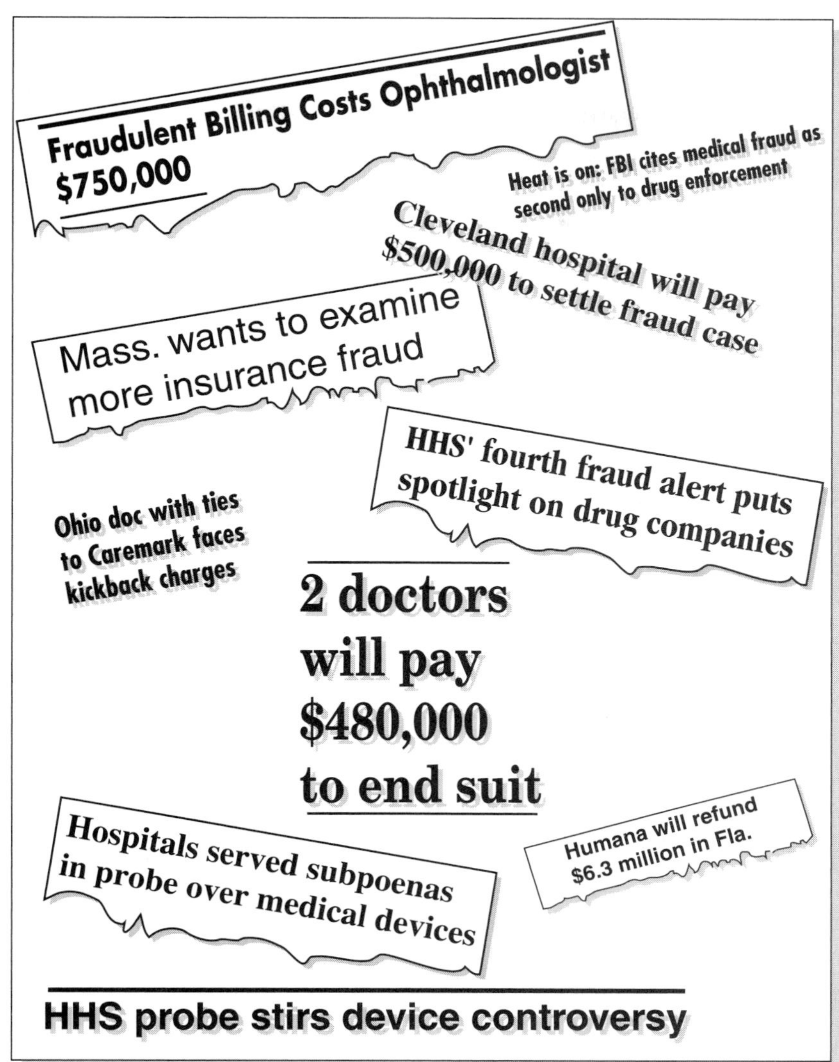

Fraudulent Billing Costs Ophthalmologist $750,000

Heat is on: FBI cites medical fraud as second only to drug enforcement

Cleveland hospital will pay $500,000 to settle fraud case

Mass. wants to examine more insurance fraud

HHS' fourth fraud alert puts spotlight on drug companies

Ohio doc with ties to Caremark faces kickback charges

2 doctors will pay $480,000 to end suit

Hospitals served subpoenas in probe over medical devices

Humana will refund $6.3 million in Fla.

HHS probe stirs device controversy

FIGURE 8-2. News headlines reflect the importance of documentation of services.

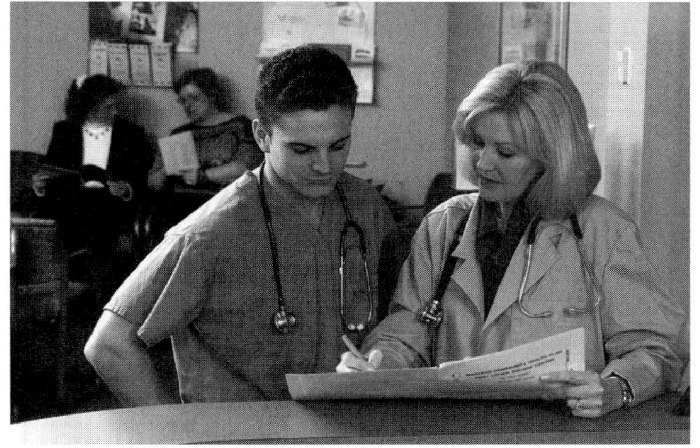

FIGURE 8-3. Physicians discuss proper documentation.

to nine systems); pertinent past, family, or social history (one area).

Examination: Detailed

Extended examination of the affected body area and other symptomatic or related organ systems.

Medical Decision Making: Low

Number of diagnoses or management options: limited

Amount of or complexity of data: limited

Risk of complications and/or morbidity or mortality: low

New Patient 99204

History: Comprehensive

Chief complaint; extended history of present illness

BOX 8-1 Commonly Overlooked Elements of Thorough Medical Documentation

Relevant Diagnoses, Symptoms, and Conditions
When diagnoses, symptoms, and conditions affect the medical decision making, document them! The guidelines relate to possible diagnoses. For example, a patient with chest pain could have a number of possible diagnoses (e.g., myocardial infarction, angina, pneumonia, rib fracture). It often helps to list some of the things you have to rule out, even if the final diagnosis is indigestion.

Treatment Options
If a patient has shoulder pain, for example, document the treatments you considered (e.g., medications, hot packs, exercise, joint injections).

Test Results Reviewed (or To Be Reviewed)
Document all test results you reviewed (e.g., laboratory tests, x-rays, electrocardiograms). It is a good idea to initial each result after reviewing it. If you order additional studies based on the results that you reviewed, write them down on the chart.

Consulting the *Physician's Desk Reference* (PDR)
Document when you look up medications in the PDR or search a database for information.

If Another Physician Is Called
Document all calls to other physicians (e.g., radiologist, cardiologist, gastroenterologist).

Past Medical Records
If you reviewed past medical records from a hospital or another physician, document this review. It is also important to convey through language the extent of the records reviewed. Use statements such as, "Reviewed last two hospitalizations," "Extensive review of old records from nursing home," or "Spent an hour reviewing the patient's medical record." The physician must convey in the medical record the complexity and amount of the review.

Communication with Family
Document any conversations with nursing home personnel or family members regarding the care and medical decision making for the patient. Document the extent of the conversation by the subject matter and time involved.

Risk Factors
Document any risk factors or multiple symptoms that justify a more complex medical decision-making process.

Statements to Avoid
Do not use statements or phrases such as "Patient feels fine," "Patient has no complaints today," and "No change." Statements that are vague do not identify details of the patient encounter that are necessary for medical record documentation.

Medical Necessity
Medical necessity for all diagnostic tests should be clear. Medical necessity includes symptoms, monitoring of drug therapy, follow-up of abnormal test results, and toxicity of certain medications. Remember, insufficient documentation of medical necessity is the number one reason nationwide for denial from Medicare.

Family and Social History
Both the family history and the social history must be included in notes to support a level 4 or 5 visit in certain categories of E&M service.

Review of Systems
Document the review of systems thoroughly. Document even normal findings.

(four or more elements); complete review of systems (at least 10 systems); complete past, family, and social history (all three history areas).

Examination: Comprehensive

General multisystem examination or a complete examination of a single organ system.

Medical Decision Making: Moderate

Number of diagnoses or management options: multiple
Amount of or complexity of data: moderate
Risk of complications and/or morbidity or mortality: moderate

New Patient 99205

History: Comprehensive

Chief complaint; extended history of present illness (four or more elements); complete review of systems (at least 10 systems); complete past, family, and social history (all three history areas).

Examination: Comprehensive
General multisystem examination or a complete examination of a single organ system.

Medical Decision Making: High
Number of diagnoses or management options: extensive
Amount of or complexity of data: extensive
Risk of complications and/or morbidity or mortality: high

New patient office visit codes require that all three key components be documented and in the same level to determine the code. If either the history, examination, or medical decision making is documented in the level below, the correct level for billing would be the lower level.

ESTABLISHED PATIENT, OFFICE

"Office patient, established" codes are used to report patient encounters in a physician office or other outpatient facility. These codes are used to report services on patients who are established and are not new to the physician.

Established Patient 99211

Minimal (generally 5 minutes) E&M service for an established patient that does not require a physician. It can be billed only when the physician is in the office suite; not down the hall and around the corner, but in the office suite! Box 8-2 lists ways in which this code should not be used.

Established Patient 99212

History: Problem Focused
Chief complaint, brief history of present illness (one to three elements).

Examination: Problem Focused
Limited examination of the affected body area or organ system.

Medical Decision Making: Straightforward
Number of diagnoses or management options: minimal
Amount of or complexity of data: minimal or none
Risk of complications and/or morbidity or mortality: minimal

BOX 8-2 When *Not* to Use Code 99211

1. When administering a flu shot
2. When calling in a prescription
3. When faxing tests to another physician
4. When talking with a patient on the telephone
5. When performing a venipuncture
6. When copying a patient's records for another physician
7. When changing a dressing that is still in the global fee period

Established Patient 99213

History: Expanded Problem Focused
Chief complaint, brief history of present illness (one to three elements), problem-pertinent review of systems.

Examination: Expanded Problem Focused
Limited examination of the affected body area or organ system and other symptomatic or related organ systems.

Medical Decision Making: Low
Number of diagnoses or management options: limited
Amount of or complexity of data: limited
Risk of complications and/or morbidity or mortality: low

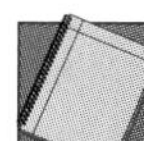

FROM THE EXPERT'S NOTEBOOK

Code 99213 is the most commonly used E&M code in the nation. More than half of all E&M services billed across the country are 99213.

Established Patient 99214

History: Detailed
Chief complaint; extended history of present illness (one to three elements); extended review of systems (two to nine systems); pertinent past, family, or social history (one area).

Examination: Detailed
Extended examination of the affected body area and other symptomatic or related organ systems.

Medical Decision Making: Moderate
Number of diagnoses or management options: multiple
Amount of or complexity of data: moderate
Risk of complications and/or morbidity or mortality: moderate

Established Patient 99215

History: Comprehensive
Chief complaint; extended history of present illness (four or more elements); complete review of systems (at least 10 systems); complete past, family, and social history (all three history areas).

Examination: Comprehensive
General multisystem examination or a complete examination of a single organ system.

Medical Decision Making: High
Number of diagnoses or management options: extensive
Amount of or complexity of data: extensive
Risk of complications and/or morbidity or mortality: high

Established office visit codes require at least two of the three components to be present to determine the level of care. The code selection is based on the level that contains two of the key components.

Outpatient Consultation Codes

This section describes the components of an outpatient consultation. A consultation occurs when a physician is asked to provide an opinion or advice regarding a specific problem. This E&M service must be requested by another physician or appropriate party. These codes have a defined use such as in a physician's office, home service, an emergency department, custodial care, or other ambulatory setting.

OFFICE CONSULTATION 99241

History: Problem Focused

Chief complaint, brief history of present illness (one to three elements).

Examination: Problem Focused

Limited examination of the affected body area or organ system.

Medical Decision Making: Straightforward

Number of diagnoses or management options: minimal
Amount of or complexity of data: minimal or none
Risk of complications and/or morbidity or mortality: minimal

OFFICE CONSULTATION 99242

History: Expanded Problem Focused

Chief complaint, brief history of present illness (one to three elements), problem-pertinent review of systems.

Examination: Expanded Problem Focused

Limited examination of the affected body area or organ system and other symptomatic or related organ systems.

Medical Decision Making: Straightforward

Number of diagnoses or management options: minimal
Amount of or complexity of data: minimal or none
Risk of complications and/or morbidity or mortality: minimal

OFFICE CONSULTATION 99243

History: Detailed

Chief complaint; extended history of present illness (one to three elements); extended review of systems (two to nine systems); pertinent past, family, or social history (one area).

Examination: Detailed

Extended examination of the affected body area and other symptomatic or related organ systems.

Medical Decision Making: Low

Number of diagnoses or management options: limited
Amount of or complexity of data: limited
Risk of complications and/or morbidity or mortality: low

OFFICE CONSULTATION 99244

History: Comprehensive

Chief complaint; extended history of present illness (four or more elements); complete review of systems (at least 10 systems); complete past, family, and social history (all three history areas).

Examination: Comprehensive

General multisystem examination or a complete examination of a single organ system.

Medical Decision Making: Moderate

Number of diagnoses or management options: multiple
Amount of or complexity of data: moderate
Risk of complications and/or morbidity or mortality: moderate

OFFICE CONSULTATION 99245

History: Comprehensive

Chief complaint; extended history of present illness (four or more elements); complete review of systems (at least 10 systems); complete past, family, and social history (all three history areas).

Examination: Comprehensive

General multisystem examination or a complete examination of a single organ system.

Medical Decision Making: High

Number of diagnoses or management options: extensive
Amount of or complexity of data: extensive
Risk of complications and/or morbidity or mortality: high

Office consultation codes require that all three key components be present and in the same level to determine the code.

Hospital Services

Hospital services are performed in the hospital setting. They consist of initial hospital services, subsequent hospital services, and inpatient consultations.

INITIAL HOSPITAL SERVICES

The following codes are used to report initial hospital E&M services (H&Ps) that take place in a hospital setting. They are reported by the admitting physician and are also used in partial hospitalization programs. They include all services provided in conjunction with the admission of the patient.

Initial Hospital Care 99221

History: Detailed or Comprehensive

Detailed: Chief complaint; extended history of present illness (one to three elements); extended review of systems (two to nine systems); pertinent past, family, or social history (one area).

Comprehensive: Chief complaint; extended history of present illness (four or more elements); complete review of systems (at least 10 systems); complete past, family, and social history (all three history areas).

Examination: Detailed or Comprehensive

Detailed: Extended examination of the affected body area and other symptomatic or related organ systems.

Comprehensive: General multisystem examination or a complete examination of a single organ system.

Medical Decision Making: Straightforward or Low

Straightforward:

Number of diagnoses or management options: minimal
Amount of or complexity of data: minimal or none
Risk of complications and/or morbidity or mortality: minimal

Low:

Number of diagnoses or management options: limited
Amount of or complexity of data: limited
Risk of complications and/or morbidity or mortality: low

Initial Hospital Care 99222

History: Comprehensive

Chief complaint; extended history of present illness (four or more elements); complete review of systems (at least 10 systems); complete past, family, and social history (all three history areas).

Examination: Comprehensive

General multisystem examination or a complete examination of a single organ system.

Medical Decision Making: Moderate

Number of diagnoses or management options: multiple
Amount of or complexity of data: moderate
Risk of complications and/or morbidity or mortality: moderate

Initial Hospital Care 99223

History: Comprehensive

Chief complaint; extended history of present illness (four or more elements); complete review of systems (at least 10 systems); complete past, family, and social history (all three history areas).

Examination: Comprehensive

General multisystem examination or a complete examination of a single organ system.

Medical Decision Making: High

Number of diagnoses or management options: extensive
Amount of or complexity of data: extensive
Risk of complications and/or morbidity or mortality: high

Initial hospital care codes require that all three key components be present and in the same level to determine the code.

SUBSEQUENT HOSPITAL CARE

Subsequent hospital care codes are used to report services provided after the initial hospital service or the inpatient consultation. These codes report services for each day following and include such services as review of the medical record, review of test results, review of nurses' notes, and review of changes in the patient's status.

Subsequent Hospital Care 99231

History: Problem Focused

Chief complaint, brief history of present illness (one to three elements).

Examination: Problem Focused

Limited examination of the affected body area or organ system.

Medical Decision Making: Straightforward or Low

Straightforward:

Number of diagnoses or management options: minimal
Amount of or complexity of data: minimal or none
Risk of complications and/or morbidity or mortality: minimal

Low:

Number of diagnoses or management options: limited
Amount of or complexity of data: limited
Risk of complications and/or morbidity or mortality: low

Subsequent Hospital Care 99232

History: Expanded Problem Focused

Chief complaint, brief history of present illness (one to three elements), problem-pertinent review of systems.

Examination: Expanded Problem Focused

Limited examination of the affected body area or organ system and other symptomatic or related organ systems.

Medical Decision Making: Moderate

Number of diagnoses or management options: multiple
Amount of or complexity of data: moderate
Risk of complications and/or morbidity or mortality: moderate

Subsequent Hospital Care 99233

History: Detailed

Chief complaint; extended history of present illness (one to three elements); extended review of systems (two to nine systems); pertinent past, family, or social history (one area).

Examination: Detailed

Extended examination of the affected body area and other symptomatic or related organ systems.

Medical Decision Making: High

Number of diagnoses or management options: extensive
Amount of or complexity of data: extensive
Risk of complications and/or morbidity or mortality: high

Subsequent hospital care codes require that at least two of the three components be present to determine the level of care. The code selection is based on the level that contains two of the key components.

HOSPITAL DISCHARGE SERVICE 99238

This service requires a discharge time of 30 minutes or less and includes the following components:

- Final examination of the patient
- Discussion of the hospital course
- Instructions for continuing care
- Preparation of discharge records
- Prescriptions, if needed
- Completion of referral forms, if needed

HOSPITAL DISCHARGE SERVICE 99239

This service requires a discharge time of more than 30 minutes and includes the following components:

- Final examination of the patient
- Discussion of the hospital course
- Instructions for continuing care
- Preparation of discharge records
- Prescriptions, if needed
- Completion of referral forms, if needed

If the higher level of discharge is chosen for billing, it is important to document the time spent discharging the patient and why the discharge took that amount of time.

Inpatient Consultation Codes

The following codes are used to report consultations to inpatients, nursing facility patients, and patients in a partial hospital setting. Physicians can bill for only one inpatient consultation per admission. The consultant may evaluate and initiate treatment during a consultation. A consultation requested by a patient or patient's family does not constitute an inpatient consultation.

INPATIENT CONSULTATION 99251

History: Problem Focused

Chief complaint, brief history of present illness (one to three elements).

Examination: Problem Focused

Limited examination of the affected body area or organ system.

Medical Decision Making: Straightforward

Number of diagnoses or management options: minimal
Amount of or complexity of data: minimal or none
Risk of complications and/or morbidity or mortality: minimal

INPATIENT CONSULTATION 99252

History: Expanded Problem Focused

Chief complaint, brief history of present illness (one to three elements), problem-pertinent review of systems.

Examination: Expanded Problem Focused

Limited examination of the affected body area or organ system and other symptomatic or related organ systems.

Medical Decision Making: Straightforward

Number of diagnoses or management options: minimal
Amount of or complexity of data: minimal or none
Risk of complications and/or morbidity or mortality: minimal

INPATIENT CONSULTATION 99253

History: Detailed

Chief complaint; extended history of present illness (one to three elements); extended review of systems (two to nine systems); pertinent past, family, or social history (one area).

Examination: Detailed

Extended examination of the affected body area and other symptomatic or related organ systems.

Medical Decision Making: Low

Number of diagnoses or management options: limited
Amount of or complexity of data: limited
Risk of complications and/or morbidity or mortality: low

INPATIENT CONSULTATION 99254

History: Comprehensive

Chief complaint; extended history of present illness (four or more elements); complete review of systems (at least 10 systems); complete past, family, and social history (all three history areas).

Examination: Comprehensive

General multisystem examination or a complete examination of a single organ system.

Medical Decision Making: Moderate

Number of diagnoses or management options: multiple
Amount of or complexity of data: moderate
Risk of complications and/or morbidity or mortality: moderate

INPATIENT CONSULTATION 99255

History: Comprehensive

Chief complaint; extended history of present illness (four or more elements); complete review of systems (at least 10 systems); complete past, family, and social history (all three history areas).

Examination: Comprehensive

General multisystem examination or a complete examination of a single organ system.

Medical Decision Making: High

Number of diagnoses or management options: extensive
Amount of or complexity of data: extensive
Risk of complications and/or morbidity or mortality: high

Inpatient consultation codes require that all three key components be present and in the same level to determine the code.

DOMICILIARY CARE

Domiciliary care codes are used to report E&M services provided to patients who reside in personal care facilities, any facility that provides room and board and personal assistance, or facilities that are assisted living. These facilities do not provide medical care to the residents living there.

DOMICILIARY CARE, NEW PATIENTS 99324

History: Problem Focused

Chief complaint, brief history of present illness (one to three elements).

Examination: Problem Focused

Limited examination of the affected body area or organ system.

Medical Decision Making: Straightforward

Number of diagnoses or management options: minimal
Amount of or complexity of data: minimal or none
Risk of complications and/or morbidity or mortality: minimal

DOMICILIARY CARE, NEW PATIENTS 99325

History: Expanded Problem Focused

Chief complaint, brief history of present illness (one to three elements), problem-pertinent review of systems.

Examination: Expanded Problem Focused

Limited examination of the affected body area or organ system and other symptomatic or related organ systems.

Medical Decision Making: Low

Number of diagnoses or management options: limited
Amount of or complexity of data: limited
Risk of complications and/or morbidity or mortality: low

DOMICILIARY CARE, NEW PATIENTS 99326

History: Detailed

Chief complaint; extended history of present illness (one to three elements); extended review of systems (two to nine systems); pertinent past, family, or social history (one area).

Examination: Detailed

Extended examination of the affected body area and other symptomatic or related organ systems.

Medical Decision Making: Moderate

Number of diagnoses or management options: multiple
Amount of or complexity of data: moderate
Risk of complications and/or morbidity or mortality: moderate

DOMICILIARY CARE, NEW PATIENTS 99327

History: Comprehensive

Chief complaint; extended history of present illness (four or more elements); complete review of systems (at least 10 systems); complete past, family, and social history (all three history areas).

Examination: Comprehensive

General multisystem examination or a complete examination of a single organ system.

Medical Decision Making: Moderate

Number of diagnoses or management options: multiple
Amount of or complexity of data: moderate
Risk of complications and/or morbidity or mortality: moderate

DOMICILIARY CARE, NEW PATIENTS 99328

History: Comprehensive

Chief complaint; extended history of present illness (four or more elements); complete review of systems (at least 10 systems); complete past, family, and social history (all three history areas).

Examination: Comprehensive

General multisystem examination or a complete examination of a single organ system.

Medical Decision Making: High

Number of diagnoses or management options: extensive
Amount of or complexity of data: extensive
Risk of complications and/or morbidity or mortality: high

All three key components are necessary to choose the level of service.

DOMICILIARY CARE, ESTABLISHED PATIENTS 99334

History: Problem Focused

Chief complaint, brief history of present illness (one to three elements).

Examination: Problem Focused

Limited examination of the affected body area or organ system.

Medical Decision Making: Straightforward

Number of diagnoses or management options: minimal
Amount of or complexity of data: minimal or none
Risk of complications and/or morbidity or mortality: minimal

DOMICILIARY CARE, ESTABLISHED PATIENTS 99335

History: Expanded Problem Focused

Chief complaint, brief history of present illness (one to three elements), problem-pertinent review of systems.

Examination: Expanded Problem Focused

Limited examination of the affected body area or organ system and other symptomatic or related organ systems.

Medical Decision Making: Low

Number of diagnoses or management options: limited
Amount of or complexity of data: limited
Risk of complications and/or morbidity or mortality: low

DOMICILIARY CARE, ESTABLISHED PATIENTS 99336

History: Detailed

Chief complaint; extended history of present illness (one to three elements); extended review of systems (two to nine systems); pertinent past, family, or social history (one area).

Examination: Detailed

Extended examination of the affected body area and other symptomatic or related organ systems.

Medical Decision Making: Moderate

Number of diagnoses or management options: multiple
Amount of or complexity of data: moderate
Risk of complications and/or morbidity or mortality: moderate

DOMICILIARY CARE, ESTABLISHED PATIENTS 99337

History: Comprehensive

Chief complaint; extended history of present illness (four or more elements); complete review of systems (at least 10 systems); complete past, family, and social history (all three history areas).

Examination: Comprehensive

General multisystem examination or a complete examination of a single organ system.

Medical Decision Making: Moderate

Number of diagnoses or management options: multiple
Amount of or complexity of data: moderate
Risk of complications and/or morbidity or mortality: moderate

Medical Decision Making: High

Number of diagnoses or management options: extensive
Amount of or complexity of data: extensive
Risk of complications and/or morbidity or mortality: high

Requires two of the three key components to determine the level of service.

HOME SERVICES

These codes are used to report E&M services that are provided in the home setting. These patients can be either new or established.

HOME SERVICES, NEW PATIENTS 99341

History: Problem Focused

Chief complaint, brief history of present illness (one to three elements).

Examination: Problem Focused

Limited examination of the affected body area or organ system.

Medical Decision Making: Straightforward

Number of diagnoses or management options: minimal
Amount of or complexity of data: minimal or none
Risk of complications and/or morbidity or mortality: minimal

HOME SERVICES, NEW PATIENTS 99342

History: Expanded Problem Focused

Chief complaint, brief history of present illness (one to three elements), problem-pertinent review of systems.

Examination: Expanded Problem Focused

Limited examination of the affected body area or organ system and other symptomatic or related organ systems.

Medical Decision Making: Low

Number of diagnoses or management options: limited
Amount of or complexity of data: limited
Risk of complications and/or morbidity or mortality: low

HOME SERVICES, NEW PATIENTS 99343

History: Detailed

Chief complaint; extended history of present illness (one to three elements); extended review of systems (two to nine systems); pertinent past, family, or social history (one area).

Examination: Detailed

Extended examination of the affected body area and other symptomatic or related organ systems.

Medical Decision Making: Moderate

Number of diagnoses or management options: multiple
Amount of or complexity of data: moderate
Risk of complications and/or morbidity or mortality: moderate

HOME SERVICES, NEW PATIENTS 99344

History: Comprehensive

Chief complaint; extended history of present illness (four or more elements); complete review of systems (at least 10 systems); complete past, family, and social history (all three history areas).

Examination: Comprehensive

General multisystem examination or a complete examination of a single organ system.

Medical Decision Making: Moderate

Number of diagnoses or management options: multiple
Amount of or complexity of data: moderate
Risk of complications and/or morbidity or mortality: moderate

HOME SERVICES, NEW PATIENTS 99345

History: Comprehensive

Chief complaint; extended history of present illness (four or more elements); complete review of systems (at least 10 systems); complete past, family, and social history (all three history areas).

Examination: Comprehensive

General multisystem examination or a complete examination of a single organ system.

Medical Decision Making: High

Number of diagnoses or management options: extensive
Amount of or complexity of data: extensive
Risk of complications and/or morbidity or mortality: high

All three key components are necessary to choose the level of service.

HOME SERVICES, ESTABLISHED PATIENTS 99347

History: Problem Focused

Chief complaint, brief history of present illness (one to three elements).

Examination: Problem Focused

Limited examination of the affected body area or organ system.

Medical Decision Making: Straightforward

Number of diagnoses or management options: minimal
Amount of or complexity of data: minimal or none
Risk of complications and/or morbidity or mortality: minimal

HOME SERVICES, ESTABLISHED PATIENTS 99348

History: Expanded Problem Focused

Chief complaint, brief history of present illness (one to three elements), problem-pertinent review of systems.

Examination: Expanded Problem Focused

Limited examination of the affected body area or organ system and other symptomatic or related organ systems.

Medical Decision Making: Low

Number of diagnoses or management options: limited
Amount of or complexity of data: limited
Risk of complications and/or morbidity or mortality: low

HOME SERVICES, ESTABLISHED PATIENTS 99349

History: Detailed

Chief complaint; extended history of present illness (one to three elements); extended review of systems (two to nine systems); pertinent past, family, or social history (one area).

Examination: Detailed

Extended examination of the affected body area and other symptomatic or related organ systems.

Medical Decision Making: Moderate

Number of diagnoses or management options: multiple
Amount of or complexity of data: moderate
Risk of complications and/or morbidity or mortality: moderate

HOME SERVICES, ESTABLISHED PATIENTS 99350

History: Comprehensive

Chief complaint; extended history of present illness (four or more elements); complete review of systems (at least 10 systems); complete past, family, and social history (all three history areas).

Examination: Comprehensive

General multisystem examination or a complete examination of a single organ system.

Medical Decision Making: Moderate

Number of diagnoses or management options: multiple
Amount of or complexity of data: moderate
Risk of complications and/or morbidity or mortality: moderate

Medical Decision Making: High

Number of diagnoses or management options: extensive
Amount of or complexity of data: extensive
Risk of complications and/or morbidity or mortality: high

Emergency Department Services

These codes are used to report patient encounters that take place in the emergency department. There is no difference between a new and an established patient. Patients arriving for care may require care for a stroke or may require care for an earache. Many hospital emergency departments now have a "fast track" system in which patients with non–life-threatening conditions are treated (e.g., a patient who cut her finger with a kitchen knife, a patient who sprained an ankle playing volleyball, or a child with an earache). All services, whether "fast track" or regular emergency department services, should use the codes 99281 to 99285.

EMERGENCY DEPARTMENT SERVICES, 99281

History: Problem Focused

Chief complaint, brief history of present illness (one to three elements).

Examination: Problem Focused

Limited examination of the affected body area or organ system.

Medical Decision Making: Straightforward

Number of diagnoses or management options: minimal
Amount of or complexity of data: minimal or none
Risk of complications and/or morbidity or mortality: minimal

EMERGENCY DEPARTMENT SERVICES, 99282

History: Expanded Problem Focused

Chief complaint, brief history of present illness (one to three elements), problem-pertinent review of systems.

Examination: Expanded Problem Focused

Limited examination of the affected body area or organ system and other symptomatic or related organ systems.

Medical Decision Making: Low

Number of diagnoses or management options: limited
Amount of or complexity of data: limited
Risk of complications and/or morbidity or mortality: low

EMERGENCY DEPARTMENT SERVICES, 99283

History: Expanded Problem Focused

Chief complaint, brief history of present illness (one to three elements), problem-pertinent review of systems.

Examination: Expanded Problem Focused

Limited examination of the affected body area or organ system and other symptomatic or related organ systems.

Medical Decision Making: Moderate

Number of diagnoses or management options: multiple
Amount of or complexity of data: moderate
Risk of complications and/or morbidity or mortality: moderate

EMERGENCY DEPARTMENT SERVICES, 99284

History: Detailed

Chief complaint; extended history of present illness (one to three elements); extended review of systems (two to nine systems); pertinent past, family, or social history (one area).

Examination: Detailed

Extended examination of the affected body area and other symptomatic or related organ systems.

History: Comprehensive

Chief complaint; extended history of present illness (four or more elements); complete review of systems (at least 10 systems); complete past, family, and social history (all three history areas).

Examination: Comprehensive

General multisystem examination or a complete examination of a single organ system.

EMERGENCY DEPARTMENT SERVICES, 99285

History: Comprehensive

Chief complaint; extended history of present illness (four or more elements); complete review of systems (at least 10 systems); complete past, family, and social history (all three history areas).

Examination: Comprehensive

General multisystem examination or a complete examination of a single organ system.

Medical Decision Making: High

Number of diagnoses or management options: extensive
Amount of or complexity of data: extensive
Risk of complications and/or morbidity or mortality: high

Prolonged Care Services

Prolonged care services are reported when the care of the patient requires direct (face-to-face) patient involvement beyond the usual service. These services can be either inpatient or outpatient. The reporting of these codes can be tricky. Before using them, the section on prolonged care in the CPT book should be studied so that the time is calculated correctly.

PROLONGED CARE SERVICES, 99354

Prolonged physician services in the office or outpatient setting requiring direct (face-to-face) patient contact beyond the usual service. First hour.

PROLONGED CARE SERVICES, 99355

Each additional 30 minutes.

PROLONGED CARE SERVICES, 99356

Prolonged physician services in an inpatient setting requiring direct (face-to-face) patient contact beyond the usual service. First hour.

PROLONGED CARE SERVICES, 99357

Each additional 30 minutes.

PROLONGED CARE SERVICES, WITHOUT DIRECT PATIENT CONTACT 99358

Prolonged physician service before and/or after direct (face-to-face) patient care. First hour.

PROLONGED CARE SERVICES, WITHOUT DIRECT PATIENT CONTACT 99359

Each additional 30 minutes.

Care Plan Oversight Services

These codes are used to manage a patient who is in hospice, is homebound, or is in a nursing facility or domiciliary care. These codes consist of documentation of development and revision of care plans; review of tests and reports; review of patient status reports; decisions regarding patient care discussed with other health care professionals, family members, and caregivers; and integration of new information into the medical treatment plan. The physician must track time spent on each aspect of care plan oversight. If, at the end of the calendar month, there are 15 to 29 minutes accumulated, the physician may bill for the appropriate codes for this time frame, that is, 99374, 99377, and 99379. For time spent over 30 minutes in care plan oversight, the codes 99375, 99378, and 99380 should be used.

CARE PLAN OVERSIGHT SERVICES 99374

Physician supervision of a patient under care of a home health agency in home, domiciliary, or equivalent environment requiring complex and multidisciplinary care modalities involving the following:

- Regular physician development and/or revisions of care plans
- Review of subsequent reports of patient status
- Communication (including phone calls) for purposes of assessment of care decisions with other health care professionals, family members, surrogate decision makers, and/or key caregivers
- Integration of new information into the medical treatment plan and/or adjustment of medical therapy
- Within a calendar month: 15 to 29 minutes

CARE PLAN OVERSIGHT SERVICES 99375

Within a calendar month: 30 minutes or more

CARE PLAN OVERSIGHT SERVICES 99377

Physician supervision of a patient under care of hospice requiring complex and multidisciplinary care modalities involving the following:

- Regular physician development and/or revisions of care plans
- Review of subsequent reports of patient status
- Communication (including phone calls) for purposes of assessment of care decisions with other health care professionals, family members, surrogate decision makers, and/or key caregivers
- Integration of new information into the medical treatment plan and/or adjustment of medical therapy
- Within a calendar month: 15 to 29 minutes

CARE PLAN OVERSIGHT SERVICES 99378

Within a calendar month: 30 minutes or more

CARE PLAN OVERSIGHT SERVICES 99379

Physician supervision of a patient under care of a nursing facility requiring complex and multidisciplinary care modalities involving the following:

- Regular physician development and/or revisions of care plans
- Review of subsequent reports of patient status
- Communication (including phone calls) for purposes of assessment of care decisions with other health care professionals, family members, surrogate decision makers, and/or key caregivers
- Integration of new information into the medical treatment plan and/or adjustment of medical therapy
- Within a calendar month: 15 to 29 minutes

CARE PLAN OVERSIGHT SERVICES 99380

Within a calendar month: 30 minutes or more

Preventive Medicine Services

Preventive medicine service codes are used to report a "well visit" for a patient who is healthy and has no complaints. These codes are based on the age of the patient and whether the patient is new or established. The extent and the focus of these services depend on the age of the patient. A minor problem that is identified during a preventive medicine service that does not require additional workups or treatment should not be reported separately. If a problem is identified or a preexisting problem is addressed during the preventive medicine visit and these problems require significant additional workup or treatment, a separate E&M service should be billed using the -25 modifier.

PREVENTIVE MEDICINE SERVICES, NEW PATIENT

99381 Initial preventive medicine E&M of an individual, including an age-appropriate history, examination, counseling/anticipatory guidance/risk factor reduction interventions, and the ordering of appropriate laboratory/diagnostic procedures, infants (age under 1 year)
99382 Early childhood (age 1 to 4 years)
99383 Late childhood (age 5 to 11 years)
99384 Adolescent (age 12 to 17 years)
99385 Age 18 to 39 years
99386 Age 40 to 64 years
99387 Age 65 years and over

PREVENTIVE MEDICINE SERVICES, ESTABLISHED PATIENT

99391 Initial preventive medicine evaluation and management of an individual, including an age-appropriate history, examination, counseling/anticipatory guidance/risk factor reduction interventions, and the ordering of appropriate laboratory/diagnostic procedures, infants (age under 1 year)
99392 Early childhood (age 1 to 4 years)
99393 Late childhood (age 5 to 11 years)
99394 Adolescent (age 12 to 17 years)
99395 Age 18 to 39 years
99396 Age 40 to 64 years
99397 Age 65 years and over

If a new condition or injury or a preexisting problem is addressed and is significant enough for additional work, a separate E&M code my be used to report this service. The modifier -25 should be attached to the problem E&M service to indicate that this was a separately identifiable service.

Observation Services

Observation service codes are used to report patient encounters for patients who do not have a documented illnesses serious enough to meet the requirements for hospital admission. These services are not site specific; the patient does not have to be in an "observation unit."

OBSERVATION SERVICES 99218

History: Detailed

Chief complaint; extended history of present illness (one to three elements); extended review of systems (two to nine systems); pertinent past, family, or social history (one area).

Examination: Detailed

Extended examination of the affected body area and other symptomatic or related organ systems.

Medical Decision Making: Straightforward

Number of diagnoses or management options: minimal
Amount of or complexity of data: minimal or none
Risk of complications and/or morbidity or mortality: minimal

History: Comprehensive

Chief complaint; extended history of present illness (four or more elements); complete review of systems (at least 10 systems); complete past, family, and social history (all three history areas).

Examination: Comprehensive

General multisystem examination or a complete examination of a single organ system.

Medical Decision Making: Low

Number of diagnoses or management options: limited
Amount of or complexity of data: limited
Risk of complications and/or morbidity or mortality: low

OBSERVATION SERVICES 99219

History: Comprehensive

Chief complaint; extended history of present illness (four or more elements); complete review of systems (at least 10 systems); complete past, family, and social history (all three history areas).

Examination: Comprehensive

General multisystem examination or a complete examination of a single organ system.

Medical Decision Making: Moderate

Number of diagnoses or management options: multiple
Amount of or complexity of data: moderate
Risk of complications and/or morbidity or mortality: moderate

OBSERVATION SERVICES 99220

History: Comprehensive

Chief complaint; extended history of present illness (four or more elements); complete review of systems (at least 10 systems); complete past, family, and social history (all three history areas).

Examination: Comprehensive

General multisystem examination or a complete examination of a single organ system.

Medical Decision Making: High

Number of diagnoses or management options: extensive
Amount of or complexity of data: extensive
Risk of complications and/or morbidity or mortality: high

Requires all three key components to determine the level of service.

OBSERVATION DISCHARGE SERVICES 99217

This code is used to report discharge services provided to a patient on discharge from "observation status" if the discharge is on other than the initial date of "observation status." It includes such services as the following:

- Final examination of the patient
- Discussion of the hospital stay
- Instructions for continuing care
- Preparation of discharge summary and other relevant records

Hospital Observation or Inpatient Care Services

These codes are used to report observation or inpatient hospital care services provided to patients admitted and discharged on the same date of service. When a patient is admitted to the hospital from observation status on the same date, the physician should report only the initial hospital care code. The initial hospital care code reported by the admitting physician should include the services related to the observation status services he or she provided on the same day of the inpatient admission. If the patient is admitted from observation status, the observation code becomes bundled into the initial hospital visit and cannot be billed for separately.

HOSPITAL OBSERVATION OR INPATIENT CARE SERVICES 99234

History: Detailed

Chief complaint; extended history of present illness (one to three elements); extended review of systems (two to nine systems); pertinent past, family, or social history (one area).

Examination: Detailed

Extended examination of the affected body area and other symptomatic or related organ systems.

Medical Decision Making: Straightforward

Number of diagnoses or management options: minimal
Amount of or complexity of data: minimal or none
Risk of complications and/or morbidity or mortality: minimal

History: Comprehensive

Chief complaint; extended history of present illness (four or more elements); complete review of systems (at least 10 systems); complete past, family, and social history (all three history areas).

Examination: Comprehensive

General multisystem examination or a complete examination of a single organ system.

Medical Decision Making: Low

Number of diagnoses or management options: limited
Amount of or complexity of data: limited
Risk of complications and/or morbidity or mortality: low

HOSPITAL OBSERVATION OR INPATIENT CARE SERVICES 99235

History: Comprehensive

Chief complaint; extended history of present illness (four or more elements); complete review of systems (at least 10 systems); complete past, family, and social history (all three history areas).

Examination: Comprehensive

General multisystem examination or a complete examination of a single organ system.

Medical Decision Making: Moderate

Number of diagnoses or management options: multiple
Amount of or complexity of data: moderate
Risk of complications and/or morbidity or mortality: moderate

HOSPITAL OBSERVATION OR INPATIENT CARE SERVICES 99236

History: Comprehensive

Chief complaint; extended history of present illness (four or more elements); complete review of systems (at least 10 systems); complete past, family, and social history (all three history areas).

Examination: Comprehensive

General multisystem examination or a complete examination of a single organ system.

Medical Decision Making: High

Number of diagnoses or management options: extensive
Amount of or complexity of data: extensive

Risk of complications and/or morbidity or mortality: high

Requires all three key components to determine level of service.

Comprehensive Nursing Facility Services

The following codes are used to report professional services to patients in a skilled nursing facility or nursing facility. No distinction is made between a new patient or an established patient in a nursing facility. There are two levels of nursing facility E&M services: *comprehensive nursing facility assessment* and *subsequent nursing facility care.* A discharge from the hospital and admission to a nursing facility may both be billed.

COMPREHENSIVE INITIAL NURSING FACILITY 99304

History: Detailed/Comprehensive

Chief complaint; extended history of present illness (one to three elements); extended review of systems (two to nine systems); pertinent past, family, or social history (one area).

Examination: Detailed/Comprehensive

General multisystem examination or a complete examination of a single organ system.

Medical Decision Making: Straightforward or Low

Straightforward:

Number of diagnoses or management options: minimal
Amount of or complexity of data: minimal or none
Risk of complications and/or morbidity or mortality: minimal

Low:

Number of diagnoses or management options: limited
Amount of or complexity of data: limited
Risk of complications and/or morbidity or mortality: low

COMPREHENSIVE INITIAL NURSING FACILITY 99305

History: Comprehensive

Chief complaint; extended history of present illness (one to three elements); extended review of systems (two to nine systems); pertinent past, family, or social history (one area).

Examination: Comprehensive

General multisystem examination or a complete examination of a single organ system.

Medical Decision Making: Moderate

Number of diagnoses or management options: multiple
Amount of or complexity of data: moderate
Risk of complications and/or morbidity or mortality: moderate

COMPREHENSIVE INITIAL NURSING FACILITY 99306

History: Comprehensive

Chief complaint; extended history of present illness (four or more elements); complete review of systems (at least 10 systems); complete past, family, and social history (all three history areas).

Examination: Comprehensive

General multisystem examination or a complete examination of a single organ system.

Medical Decision Making: High

Number of diagnoses or management options: extensive
Amount of or complexity of data: extensive
Risk of complications and/or morbidity or mortality: high

Comprehensive initial nursing facility codes require that all three key components be present and in the same level to determine the code.

Subsequent Nursing Facility Codes

As with established patients in an office setting, subsequent nursing facility codes require that only two of the three key components be performed and documented. These codes are used for all follow-up visits after the initial service is performed in the nursing facility.

SUBSEQUENT NURSING FACILITY 99307

History: Problem Focused Interval

Chief complaint, brief history of present illness (one to three elements).

Examination: Problem Focused

Limited examination of the affected body area or organ system.

Medical Decision Making: Straightforward

Number of diagnoses or management options: minimal
Amount of or complexity of data: minimal or none
Risk of complications and/or morbidity or mortality: minimal

SUBSEQUENT NURSING FACILITY 99308

History: Expanded Problem Focused Interval

Chief complaint, brief history of present illness (one to three elements), problem-pertinent review of systems.

Examination: Expanded Problem Focused

Limited examination of the affected body area or organ system and other symptomatic or related organ systems.

Medical Decision Making: Low

Number of diagnoses or management options: limited
Amount of or complexity of data: limited
Risk of complications and/or morbidity or mortality: low

SUBSEQUENT NURSING FACILITY 99309

History: Detailed Interval

Chief complaint; extended history of present illness (one to three elements); extended review of systems (two to nine systems); pertinent past, family, or social history (one area).

Examination: Detailed

Extended examination of the affected body area and other symptomatic or related organ systems.

Medical Decision Making: Moderate

Number of diagnoses or management options: multiple
Amount of or complexity of data: moderate
Risk of complications and/or morbidity or mortality: moderate

SUBSEQUENT NURSING FACILITY 99310

History: Comprehensive Interval

Chief complaint; extended history of present illness (one to three elements); extended review of systems (two to nine systems); pertinent past, family, or social history (one area).

Examination: Comprehensive

Extended examination of the affected body area and other symptomatic or related organ systems.

Medical Decision Making: High

Number of diagnoses or management options: extensive
Amount of or complexity of data: high
Risk of complications and/or morbidity or mortality: high

Subsequent nursing facility codes require that at least two of the three components be present to determine the level of care. The code selection is based on the level that contains two of the key components.

COMPREHENSIVE ANNUAL ASSESSMENT 99318

This code is used to report an annual nursing facility assessment. This assessment must be made on a yearly basis to all residents in a nursing facility.

History: Detailed Interval

Chief complaint; extended history of present illness (one to three elements); extended review of systems (two to nine systems); pertinent past, family, or social history (one area).

Examination: Comprehensive

Extended examination of the affected body area and other symptomatic or related organ systems.

Medical Decision Making

Low:

Number of diagnoses or management options: limited
Amount of or complexity of data: limited
Risk of complications and/or morbidity or mortality: low

Moderate:

Number of diagnoses or management options: multiple
Amount of or complexity of data: moderate
Risk of complications and/or morbidity or mortality: moderate

There is no time associated with this code.

NURSING FACILITY DISCHARGE DAY MANAGEMENT 99315

This service requires a discharge time of 30 minutes or less and includes the following components:

- Final examination of the patient
- Discussion of the hospital course
- Instructions for continuing care
- Preparation of discharge records
- Prescriptions, if needed
- Completion of referral forms, if needed

NURSING FACILITY DISCHARGE DAY MANAGEMENT 99316

This service requires a discharge time of more than 30 minutes and includes the following components:

- Final examination of the patient
- Discussion of the hospital course
- Instructions for continuing care
- Preparation of discharge records
- Prescriptions, if needed
- Completion of referral forms, if needed

When choosing the higher-level code, 99316, it is necessary to document the time spent performing the discharge service and the reason why the discharge took that long.

ADDITIONAL EVALUATION AND MANAGEMENT CODES

Details regarding the additional E&M codes listed below can be found in the CPT. Some of these codes, such as prolonged care, are time-based codes and require documentation of the time spent with the patient.

- Domiciliary care: new patient (99324 to 99328)
- Domiciliary care: established patient (99334 to 99337)
- Home services: new patient (99341 to 99345)

- Home services: established patient (99347 to 99350)
- Emergency services (99281 to 99285)
- Prolonged services: office (99354 and 99355)
- Prolonged services: hospital (99356 and 99357)
- Prolonged services: without patient contact (99358 and 99359)
- Physician standby services (99360)
- Team conferences (99361 and 99362)
- Telephone calls (99371 to 99373)
- Care plan oversight services (99374 to 99380)
- Preventive medicine services: new patient (99381 to 99387)
- Preventive medicine services: established patient (99391 to 99397)
- Preventive medicine counseling: individual (99401 to 99404)
- Preventive medicine counseling: group (99411 and 99412)
- Newborn care (99431 to 99440)
- Neonatal intensive care: initial (99295 and 99296)
- Neonatal intensive care: subsequent (99297 and 99298)
- Critical care services (99291 and 99292)
- Observation or inpatient care (99234 to 99236)
- Observation care (99217 to 99220)

Documenting by Specialty

When documenting for certain specialty services, it is important to remember specifics that need to be included in the documentation. Most of this information is common sense. For example, tips for documenting urology services may include the following:

- The final diagnosis must reflect the underlying cause of the patient's symptoms. For example, "cancer: prostate" is much more specific than "urinary retention," or "hematuria."
- If the patient's "cystitis" is due to a specific cause, such as radiation therapy, it must be documented as such.
- If there are calculi, the location must be documented (e.g., ureter, kidney, bladder).
- If there is an "incontinence" problem, specify the type (i.e., stress, urge, or mixed).
- If the patient has a cystocele, document whether the patient has undergone a hysterectomy.
- If lithotripsy was performed, specify the type used.

When documenting services of an orthopedist, documentation should include the following:

- If a patient has had a spinal fusion and returns for additional treatment, document the level of the previous fusion, whether it failed, and whether the spine needs to be fused again at the same level.
- If a patient complains of a joint condition, document whether it was due to trauma, is chronic, or is spontaneous.
- For procedures involving joints, specify whether the joint space was entered.
- If a debridement is performed on a patient with an open fracture, it must be documented.
- Document all injuries by anatomic site.

These examples help illustrate the types of documentation assigned to physicians by specialty. These guidelines apply mostly to hospital services and are not all-inclusive.

Documenting the Operative Report

The role of the operative report is crucial for payment of services to physicians and hospitals. A well-documented operative report can provide accurate coding and, therefore, reimbursement of services. For the most part, it is not necessary that physicians change what they are doing; they just need to document what they are doing. Figure 8-4 describes the "four C's" of documenting an operative report properly.

"FOUR C'S" OF AN OPERATIVE REPORT

- *Complete*: The documentation tells the whole story, thus providing the necessary information for reporting the services performed and for reimbursement.
- *Communicative*: The documentation tells what was done and why. It describes the how and where of services, and each element supports the others.

  What: the steps in the procedure that were performed

  How: the way the steps were taken, instruments used, preparation of the patient

  Where: the organs and/or tissues involved in the procedure

  Why: the reason for the surgery (e.g., the diagnosis, condition, problem) and the medical necessity for the procedure

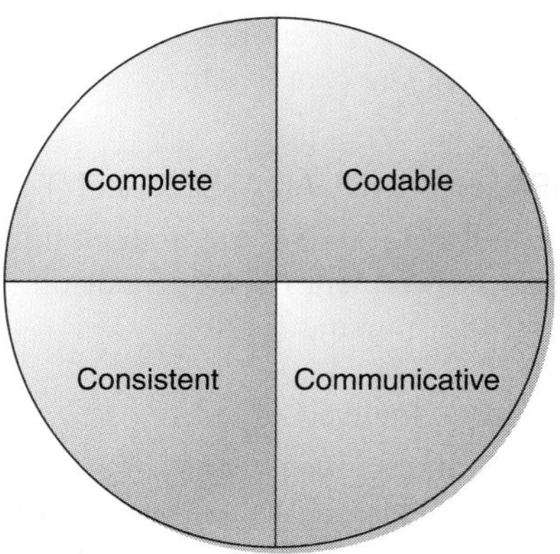

FIGURE 8-4. The "four C's" of documenting an operative report.

- *Consistent*: All documentation must be complementary and paint a big picture. There should be no unanswered questions.
- *Codable*: All procedures and their respective diagnoses must be accurately translated into procedural (CPT) and diagnostic (ICD-9-CM) codes.

"CANNED" REPORTS

A "canned" report is one that uses a template. In other words, the same general wording is used for the dictation of all patient reports. In only a few exceptions is the report personalized. CMS refers to these reports as cookie-cutter reports. Many physicians look to the easy solution of canned reports because they save time and are practical. However, this is not a practice that physicians should consider. As the office manager, it is important to point out the drawbacks of this system.

- Each patient is an individual. No two patients are the same.
- Occasionally, after a procedure is started, a different approach or an entirely different procedure may need to be performed.
- A canned procedure report is often generated by a master list of what is on the operating room schedule for that day. If the procedure changes, the physician would have to dictate a note, which could result in two operative reports for the same patient on the same day.
- Canned reports can be a legal liability, should the record find its way to a courtroom.

Yes, shortcuts are good when they can be used in an efficient and effective manner. This, however, is not the case with canned reports.

GUIDELINES FOR DICTATING OPERATIVE REPORTS

Very few physician services involve as much detail as surgery. Many surgical techniques can often be performed on almost any body part; however, the method can be quite different. Proper documentation provides the specific information necessary regarding a surgical procedure. The operative report should read like the instructions on how to build a birdhouse, only in much more detail. It must provide procedure details such as where, what, who, when, and how, down to the most minute of details. It should describe any complications, loss of blood, types of instruments used, history of the condition, type of anesthesia, who administered it, and the condition of the patient after the surgery. The following list illustrates key areas that should be addressed when dictating an operative report. If the physician follows this list, there should be no documentation problems!

1. Patient name, medical record number, age, sex
2. Date of operation
3. Primary surgeon and co-surgeons
4. Team surgeons and assistant surgeons
5. Preoperative, postoperative, and surgical diagnoses
6. Anatomic location
7. Unilateral or bilateral
8. History of diagnosis
9. Trauma
10. Type of anesthesia
11. Anesthesiologist
12. Procedure performed
13. Clinical indications
14. Findings during surgery
15. Complications
16. Estimated blood loss
17. Blood administered
18. Drains and tubes
19. Specimens
20. Postoperative condition of patient

Teaching Physician Services

TERMS YOU SHOULD KNOW

When talking about teaching physician services, it is important to understand the differences between a teaching physician, resident, and moonlighting fellow.

Teaching physician: A teaching physician is a physician who involves residents in the care of patients. This new term has replaced the term *attending physician*.

Resident: A resident is someone who is approved as part of a graduate medical education (GME) program. This person can be a resident, a fellow, or an intern. Medical students do not fall into this category.

Moonlighting fellow: Moonlighting fellows provide services outside the scope of the graduate medical education program. Such situations are generally found in emergency departments and office settings.

Billing for E&M Services in a Teaching Setting

Services that are paid by Medicare and are furnished in a teaching hospital must be personally furnished by a physician who is not a resident, furnished by a resident when a teaching physician is physically present during the critical or key portions of the service, or furnished by residents under a primary care exception within an approved GME program. A *teaching setting* is defined as a hospital-based or nonprovider setting that receives payment for resident services from the fiscal intermediary through the GME program. A teaching hospital is a GME-approved hospital with a residency program in medicine, osteopathy, or dentistry. This includes services in hospitals, clinics, and nursing facilities where there are teaching programs.

Both residents and teaching physicians may document in the medical record. The documentation must be dated and contain a legible signature or identity of the person who performed the service or procedure. The documentation may be either dictated and transcribed, typed, handwritten, or computer generated. If an electronic medical record is being used, it may generate a predetermined note. It is the responsibility of the teaching physician to personalize the information and to provide documentation to support the medical necessity of the service or procedure. If only the computerized documentation is used, it will not be sufficient for billing.

When teaching physicians bill for services, they must personally document that they performed the service or were physically present during the key or critical portions of the service furnished by the resident, and the teaching physician must document his or her participation in the management of the patient.

Moonlighting Fellows

Moonlighting services are those services that are furnished by an intern or a resident that are not related to the training program and are outside the teaching setting. The following criteria must be met:

- The services are identifiable physician services, which require treatment by a physician in person and contribute to the diagnosis or treatment of the patient.
- The intern or resident is fully licensed to practice medicine, osteopathy, dentistry, or podiatry by the state in which the services are performed.
- The services furnished can be separately identified from those services that are required as part of the training program.

Medical Students

Medical students may document in the medical record; however, only the review of systems and past, family, and social history can be used by the teaching physician. None of the additional documentation by medical students can be used and must be redocumented by the teaching physician. For example, the teaching physician must verify and redocument the balance of the history portion (chief complaint and history of present illness), must perform and document the examination, and must perform and document the medical decision making.

GUIDELINES FOR INITIAL HOSPITAL SERVICES, EMERGENCY SERVICES, NEW PATIENT OFFICE SERVICES, AND CONSULTATIONS

Scenario 1: All elements are obtained personally by the teaching physician without a resident present. If a resident was not involved in the service, the physician bills for services as if the patient was a private patient.

Scenario 2: All elements are obtained by the resident in the presence of, or jointly with, the teaching physician and documented by the resident. Documentation of the teaching physician's participation in the service does not meet the teaching physician requirements. The teaching physician must personally document this information. The documentation by the teaching physician is minimal, but must contain confirmation of the key components that have been documented by the resident in the presence of the teaching physician. The combination of both forms of documentation should be used to choose the appropriate level of E&M service.

GUIDELINES FOR SUBSEQUENT HOSPITAL SERVICES AND ESTABLISHED PATIENT OFFICE VISITS

A personal note by the teaching physician must document two out of three key elements of history, examination, and medical decision making. The "primary care exception rule" applies for patient services furnished by residents without the presence of a teaching physician. The facility must request in writing that all of the elements below have been met to qualify. Residents can bill for services using the following codes:

- 99201 to 99203
- 99211 to 99213

Under this "exception" arrangement, they are not permitted to use higher-level codes such as 99204 and 99205 or 99214 and 99215. They can also bill for the initial preventive physical examination (the "Welcome to Medicare Physical"), code G3044. This code, which became effective in January 2005, covers face-to-face visits that are limited to new beneficiaries during the first 6 months of their Medicare enrollment.

For a facility to meet the exception rule, the following must apply:

- Services must be furnished in a center located in the outpatient department of a hospital or clinic run by the teaching hospital.
- The resident must have completed more than 6 months of the residency program.
- Patients must consider the center to be the primary source of their health care.
- Residents generally follow the same patients throughout their course of study.

The supervising (teaching) physician

- Cannot supervise more than four residents at a given time and must be immediately available.
- Must have no other responsibilities at the time the service is being rendered.
- Must accept responsibility for all patients seen by residents.
- Must ensure that all services are appropriate and necessary.
- Must document the extent of his or her participation in the direction of the services furnished.

- Must review with the resident (either during or immediately after each visit) the history, examination, diagnosis, and record of tests and therapies.
- Must maintain daily clinic schedules of residents assigned to a teaching physician or preceptor.

The types of facilities that may qualify for the primary care exception rule are as follows:

1. Family practice
2. Internal medicine
3. Pediatrics
4. Obstetrics/gynecology
5. Geriatrics
6. Rural health clinic
7. Preventive medicine

In some circumstances, psychiatric programs may qualify.

TEACHING PHYSICIAN SURGEON

Special rules apply to surgeons in teaching physician programs. The teaching physician must be present for the critical and key portions of the procedure and must be immediately available to furnish services during the entire length of the procedure. The following are the key conditions that must be met for teaching physician surgeons:

- The teaching physician must be responsible for the preoperative, operative, and postoperative care of the patient.
- If the teaching physician leaves the operating room during the procedure, he or she must be immediately available to return, if needed.
- If the teaching physician becomes involved in another surgery, he or she must appoint another surgeon who can be immediately available to intervene in the original case.
- The teaching physician is not required to be present for all postoperative visits with the patient. The teaching physician can determine which visits are important and require his or her presence.

Single Surgery

The teaching physician must document his or her presence for the entire period of time between the opening and closing of the patient by the teaching physician, the resident, or an operating room nurse. The notes must be specific and must be signed and dated by the individual making the entry. No other documentation guidelines are necessary for single surgery. An example of documentation for surgery can be found in Box 8-3.

Two Overlapping Surgeries

To bill for two overlapping surgeries, the teaching physician must be present for the key portions of both surgeries. Obviously, this means that these surgeries cannot take place at the same time! Once the key portion of the first surgery has been completed, the surgeon can then go to the second surgery. The teaching physician must personally document the key portion of both procedures so that the documentation clearly reflects to auditors and reviewers that the physician was immediately available to return to either case if need be. Immediate availability is not defined in terms of geographic location from the operating room.

BOX 8-3 Example of Documentation for Surgery

- "The key portions of this surgery were the removal of foreign body from pharynx and the pharyngoesophageal repair. I directly supervised the removal of foreign body from pharynx and personally performed the pharyngoesophageal repair."
- "I directly supervised the exploration of the abdomen, which was the key portion of the procedure."
- "The key portions of this procedure were the removal of the aneurysm and the bypass graft of the splenic artery. I was physically present for both procedures."

Three Surgeries

When three simultaneous or overlapping surgeries are performed, the teaching surgeon's role is considered supervisory rather than a physician service. Services are not recognized under Medicare Part B.

Assistants at Surgery

Services for an assistant at surgery will not be covered if they are performed in a teaching institution and a qualified resident is available to perform the service. If a resident is not available, a written statement must be attached to each claim for which payment is sought. An example of such a statement is illustrated in Box 8-4.

Minor Surgery

Examples of minor surgery are simple sutures and incision and drainage. The teaching physician must be present for the entire procedure in order to bill for the procedure or surgery. A minor procedure or surgery usually takes 3 to 5 minutes to perform.

BOX 8-4 Example of Assistants-at-Surgery Statement

"I understand that Section 1842(b) of the Social Security Act generally prohibits Medicare payments to physicians for the services of assistants at surgery in teaching hospitals when qualified residents are available. I certify that the services for which payment is claimed were medically necessary, and that no qualified resident was available to perform the services. I further understand that these services are subject to postpayment review by the carrier."

Endoscopic Procedures

The teaching physician must be present during the entire viewing portion of the endoscopy or similar procedure conducted by the resident. The viewing portion includes insertion and removal of the scope. If a teaching physician views the entire procedure through a monitor in another room, this does not meet the requirement for teaching physicians. The documentation must clearly state that the teaching physician was present during the entire viewing or that he or she performed the actual viewing portion of the procedure. A simple "time-in" or "time-out" statement of the teaching physician's presence will not satisfy the requirements.

Complex and High-Risk Procedures

The teaching physician must be present with the resident for all complex or high-risk procedures or must personally perform the service. Documentation should include a statement that the teaching physician was personally present during the procedure. Examples of high-risk procedures include the following:

- Cardiac catheterization
- Cardiovascular stress tests
- Interventional radiology
- Transesophageal echocardiography

ANESTHESIA

The teaching anesthesiologist's presence is not required during preoperative or postoperative visits. The teaching anesthesiologist must be present for critical or key portions of the procedure or surgery, including induction and emergence. The teaching anesthesiologist must be immediately available to furnish services during the entire procedure. If the teaching anesthesiologist is involved in concurrent procedures with more than one resident or a resident and a nonphysician anesthetist, the services are paid as "medical direction."

PSYCHIATRY

Some psychiatry residency programs may qualify under the primary care exception rule, but it is important to check before performing any services. The requirement that the teaching physician be present may be met by observing the resident and patient through a one-way mirror or video equipment; however, audio equipment alone is not sufficient. These observations must be concurrent. The teaching physician must document in the medical record that he or she observed the session via video or a one-way mirror and the actual time it was observed. The teaching physician supervising the resident must be a physician; psychologists who supervise residents do not meet the requirements for billing these services. The teaching physician must meet with the patient after the visit and discuss relevant issues concerning the patient.

For the following time-based codes, the teaching physician must be present for the entire period of time:

- Individual therapy (90842 to 90844)
- Psychologic testing (96100)

The following codes are not time based:

- Psychologic diagnostic interviews (90801)
- Family/group psychotherapy (90846 to 90853)
- Pharmacologic management (90862)

The teaching physician can bill for only the actual time spent observing the session. Review of videotape following the actual psychotherapy session does not meet the requirement. The teaching physician must document the amount of time spent "face-to-face" in video or one-way mirror contact.

MATERNITY SERVICES

The teaching physician presence requirement must also be met for both types of delivery. When the teaching physician is involved only in the delivery, the code for the delivery is the only code that can be billed. To bill for a global procedure, the teaching physician must be present for the minimum number of visits, as defined by the procedure code.

INTERPRETATION OF DIAGNOSTIC RADIOLOGY AND OTHER DIAGNOSTIC TESTS

A physician other than a resident must perform the interpretation. If a resident prepares and signs the interpretation, the teaching physician must indicate that he or she personally reviewed the image, slide, or strip, and the resident's interpretation. A note should be included stating whether the teaching physician agrees with or modifies the resident's findings. If a resident was not involved in the interpretation, the carrier will assume that the teaching physician personally performed the service if only his or her signature is on the interpretation. A teaching physician may no longer simply countersign or initial the resident's interpretation.

TIME-BASED CODES

Teaching physicians must be present for the period of time for which payment is sought for time-based procedures. Time spent with a patient by the resident in the absence of the teaching physician cannot be added to the time spent by the resident and teaching physician or the teaching physician alone. For example, if a code specifically describes a service of 20 to 30 minutes, it should be billed only if the teaching physician is present for that time period. Examples of such codes are as follows:

- Individual psychotherapy
- Critical care services
- E&M services where counseling was greater than 50% of the total visit time

- Prolonged services
- Care plan oversight services

TEACHING PHYSICIAN MODIFIERS

Services provided in whole or in part by a resident must be identified by adding one of the following modifiers:

- -GC: This service is performed in part by a resident under the direction of a teaching physician. This modifier is to be used with all services provided by a teaching physician except where modifier -GE is appropriate. Use of this modifier acknowledges the presence of the teaching physician during the key portion of the service.
- -GE: This service is performed by a resident without the presence of a teaching physician under the primary care exception. This modifier is used to indicate that the teaching physician was not present during the E&M service under the primary care exception being billed, but that the requirements for billing have been met.

Documentation Formats

There are two commonly used formats for documenting E&M services:

1. SOAP
2. SNOCAMP

SOAP METHOD

SOAP is a mnemonic used to recall a method of organized and comprehensive documentation. Documentation compiled under this method covers the following areas:

- *Subjective view of the case*: Documentation includes patient complaints; history of injury or illness; answers to questions about organ systems; and past, family, and/or social history.
- *Objective data*: Documentation includes findings on examination of the patient.
- *Assessment*: Documentation includes prognosis and/or differential diagnosis of the patient and diagnostic studies.
- *Plan for treatment*: Documentation includes patient instructions, prescriptions, testing to be performed, and next appointment.

By faithfully following this method of documentation, the physician imposes organization on the information he or she compiles about a patient, and reduces the chance of omitting information. Some physicians are reluctant to use this method because they think it is not comprehensive enough. This method does, however, serve as a basic system for preparing a medical record. Figure 8-5 provides the practice with a template for documentation using this method.

SNOCAMP METHOD

The SNOCAMP method was developed by a physician in Florida named Walter Larimore, MD. This method is more defined than the SOAP method and follows the E&M guidelines closely.

- *Subjective:* Documentation includes patient complaints; history of injury or illness; answers to questions about organ systems; and past, family, and/or social history.
- *Nature of presenting problem:* A disease, illness, injury, symptom, or finding that relates to the chief complaint or reason for the visit.
- *Objective:* Documentation includes findings on examination of the patient.
- *Counseling and/or coordination of care:* Documentation includes patient encounters for which counseling and/or coordination of care constitute more than 50% of the visit.

Patient name: ____________________

Date: ____________ Patient account #: (optional) ____________________

Subjective Review:

Objective Review:

Assessment:

Plan for Treatment:

FIGURE 8-5. Method for documenting patient encounters.

- *Assessment:* Documentation includes prognosis and/or differential diagnosis of the patient and diagnostic studies.
- *Medical decision making:* Documentation includes complexity of the visit and the physician's thought process. This component is somewhat subjective and is based on the following three components:
  1. Number of diagnoses or management options
  2. Amount and/or complexity of data
  3. Risk of mortality/morbidity
- *Plan:* Documentation includes the treatment plan being considered for managing the patient's case. It should also include the rationale for ordering additional studies and/or procedures.

AUDITS

When physicians are in residency, they understand and comply with documentation requirements. In many cases, however, once a physician is out in private practice, things change. Managed care pressure to see more and more patients to meet expenses often causes documentation to suffer. To make matters worse, documentation requirements have become more cumbersome. Over the last 10 years, the government and other third-party payers have increased their auditing efforts in an attempt to recover possible overpayments. Box 8-5 provides a list of actual documentation retrieved from various medical records.

Internal medical record audits can identify areas of risk in a medical record. They can also identify uncaptured charges and lost revenue. Audits can be performed by an outside individual such as a consultant, or by a member of the physician's staff. The first step is to choose a person who has the knowledge and understanding of documentation and coding guidelines. This may be another job for the office manager! The individual chosen to perform an audit must have a working knowledge of medical terminology and a thorough understanding of the principles of documentation. Candidates for this role include the following:

- Office manager/administrator
- Medical records technician
- Compliance specialist
- Nurse
- Coding specialist

The audit schedule must be determined by the office manager and the physician. Some offices prefer to audit records every quarter, whereas others audit only once or twice a year. The number of medical records audited per provider must also be determined by the office manager and the physician. The average number of records chosen for audit is 6 to 10 per provider. A provider is anyone providing services to patients (e.g., nurse practitioners, physician assistants, or physicians). These records should be chosen randomly and should contain a sample of the various types of E&M services that the provider performs. For instance, if the physician has hospital patients, nursing home patients, and office patients, a sample from each category should be reviewed.

There are two types of audits: retrospective and prospective. A retrospective audit is an audit performed on services that have already been billed to the carrier. Should this audit identify overpayments made to the practice, the practice must issue a refund to the insurance carrier. A prospective audit is an audit performed on services that have not yet been billed, and is designed to reduce liability. A claim isn't fraudulent if it has not been billed.

BOX 8-5 It's All in the Charts: Excerpts from Actual Charts

- The laboratory tests indicated abnormal lover function
- The skin was moist and dry
- Rectal exam revealed a normal size thyroid
- The patient had waffles for breakfast and anorexia for lunch
- She stated that she had been constipated for most of her life until 1989, when she got a divorce
- I saw your patient today, who is still under our car for physical therapy
- Patient was alert and unresponsive
- When she fainted, her eyes rolled around the room
- Bleeding started in the rectal area and continued all the way to Los Angeles
- She is numb from her toes down
- Coming from Detroit, this man has no children
- While in the Emergency Room, she was examined, x-rated, and sent home
- Between you and me, we ought to be able to get this lady pregnant
- The patient suffers from occasional, constant, infrequent headaches
- Both breasts are equal and reactive to light and accommodation
- Exam of genitalia was completely negative except for the right foot
- The patient was to have a bowel resection, however, he took a job as a stockbroker instead
- The patient lives at home with his mother, father, and pet turtle, who is presently enrolled in adult day care three times a week

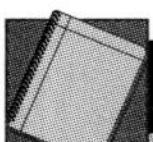

FROM THE EXPERT'S NOTEBOOK

It is a good idea to audit services that have not yet been billed. If the review uncovers an error in the level of service, it can be corrected before the claim is submitted. It is not fraudulent if it has not been billed!

How to Audit a Medical Record

Once a sample has been chosen and the records are obtained, the following steps should be followed to properly audit an E&M service:

1. Open the medical record to the date of service that you chose to review.
2. Look at the patient encounter form for that date of service.
3. By reviewing the documentation, determine the category of service provided (e.g., new office patient, subsequent hospital visit, consultation).
4. Using the documentation guidelines, carefully review the history portion of the visit.
   a. Is there a chief complaint or reason for the visit?
   b. Is there a history of present illness? How many elements of the history of present illness are documented?
   c. Is there a review of systems? How many systems?
   d. Is there a past, family, and/or social history?
5. Carefully review the examination portion of the note. Using the guidelines listed previously, what level of examination is documented?
6. Carefully review the medical decision-making portion of the note.
   a. How many diagnoses or management options are there?
   b. What quantity of data were reviewed?
   c. What was the complexity of the data that were reviewed?
   d. What is the risk of morbidity and mortality?
7. After identifying the medical decision-making elements, determine the level of medical decision making. Two out of three areas will determine the level of medical decision making.
8. After you have determined the levels of all three key components of E&M services, according to the guidelines, what level of service should be billed?
9. Compare the reviewer's level and category with the level and category checked on the patient encounter form. Does it match?
   a. If the level of documentation supports the level checked on the form, it is correctly coded.
   b. If the level of documentation supports a higher level of code than the one checked, the original code was downcoded.
   c. If the level of documentation does not support the level of service checked, the original code was upcoded.
10. Next, verify the medical necessity for the visit and any ancillary services that were performed.
    a. Is the medical necessity for that level supported?
    b. Is the medical necessity documented for any additional services performed during that visit?
11. Do the diagnosis codes checked on the patient encounter form match the codes listed in the medical record for that date of service?
    a. Are they correct? Are they in the same order? Are any diagnosis codes missing?
    b. Are any diagnosis codes listed that are not supported in the medical record?
12. Were any services performed that were not captured for billing?
13. Did the provider of the service (e.g., physician, nurse practitioner, physician assistant) sign the note?
14. Does the note contain the same date of service as the patient encounter form?
15. Is the patient's name or identifying number on each page (front and back) of the medical record?
16. Is the service part of a teaching physician service?
    a. Did this service involve a resident?
    b. If so, were the teaching physician regulations followed?
    c. Is it legible?
    d. Are modifiers used correctly?
17. Once you have determined all of the above, you have finished your first audit of a medical record.

An audit sheet (Figure 8-6) can be developed by the practice to successfully capture all of the information necessary for the audit; however, manual audits are labor intensive. An easier way to perform an audit is to use medical record compliance software. One such software package is auditXpress by Parente Healthware, Inc. This software can guide the auditor through all steps of a medical record audit. After information is entered into the computer, the click of a button will generate a printed text report describing any issues found during the audit and their relative percentage ranking. With this software, all the details of each medical record audited can be transferred into an Excel spreadsheet. This tool can be used to educate the physician by showing the areas within the medical record that were not in compliance with the level of service chosen.

In the sample auditXpress screen shown in Figure 8-7, the physician, provider of the service, or clinic/hospital name is entered. Entering by physician or provider allows for easy tracking of noncompliant physicians. This screen provides preliminary results of the audit performed. These results can then be printed in a text-formatted report and an Excel spreadsheet illustrating the detailed findings of each medical record audited.

Figure 8-8 shows the actual audit screen. By completing elements within the history, examination, and medical decision-making fields, the appropriate level of service is depicted in the derived documentation screen. Users of the program are asked to complete additional patient demographics for each service audited, such as the following:

Patient ID ____________________ Date of birth ________________________

Date of service ________________________ Physician level ____________________

Provider _____________________ Auditor level ____________________

History:

CC: _________ Present _________ Missing

HPI: _________ Location _________ Duration _________ Quality _________ Severity

_________ Timing_________ Modifying factors _________ Signs and symptoms

_________ Context

ROS: _________ Constitutional _________ Eyes _________ ENMT _________ Cardiac

____ Resp____GI ____ GU ____ Musculo ____Skin ____Neuro ____Psych ____ Endo ____ Hem/Lymph ____ All/Immuno

PFSH:

____ Past ____

____ Family ____

____ Social ________________________________ ______________________________

Examination:

____**Problem focused:** a limited exam of the affected body area or organ system (one system).

____**Expanded problem focused:** a limited exam of the affected body area or organ system and other symptomatic or related organ systems (2-4 systems).

____**Detailed:** an extended exam of the affected body areas and other symptomatic related organ systems (5-7 systems).

____**Comprehensive:** a general multisystem exam or a complete exam of a single organ system (8 or more systems).

Medical decision making:

Number of diagnoses and/or number of management options: ________________________________

____

Amount and complexity of medical records, diagnostic tests, and other information obtained, reviewed, analyzed:

____

____

Risk of significant complications, morbidity, and/or mortality: ____________________________

____

____ Medical necessity issues: ____

____ Signature issues: ____

____ Diagnosis issues: ____

____ Uncaptured services: ____

____ Other: ____

____

FIGURE 8-6. Audit sheet.

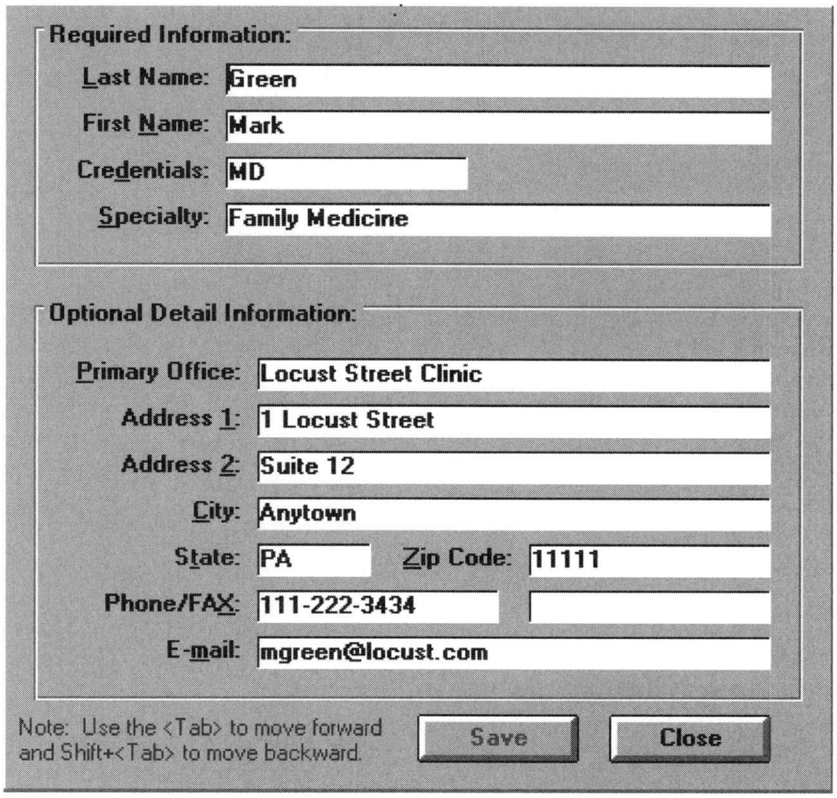

Required Information:
Last Name: Green
First Name: Mark
Credentials: MD
Specialty: Family Medicine

Optional Detail Information:
Primary Office: Locust Street Clinic
Address 1: 1 Locust Street
Address 2: Suite 12
City: Anytown
State: PA Zip Code: 11111
Phone/FAX: 111-222-3434
E-mail: mgreen@locust.com

Note: Use the <Tab> to move forward and Shift+<Tab> to move backward.
Save Close

FIGURE 8-7. Physician/provider information screen. (Courtesy of Parente Healthware, Inc.)

Patient Chart Documentation Audit
File View Help
Patient: Conklin, Betty
Insurance: General Insurance
Date: 7/19/2002 DOB: 1/1/1950
Payor Class: Commercial Gender: Female Visit Type: New
Date of Service: 12/2/2002 Age: 52
Select: History = Missing
Select: Examination = Missing
Select: Medical Decision Making = Missing
Derived Documentation Level: Invalid Code
Select Charge Level Used: 99204
Documentation Result: Invalid Code
Select Items of Documentation:

	On/Off	Chart Documentation Items
1.		Missing Documentation
2.		Missing Language for Chief Complaint
3.		Missing Documentation of Review of Systems
4.		Missing Past, Family, Social History
5.		Missing Medical Necessity

Save Close
Enter Other Pertinent Information:
Copyright PARENTE HEALTHWARE, INC.

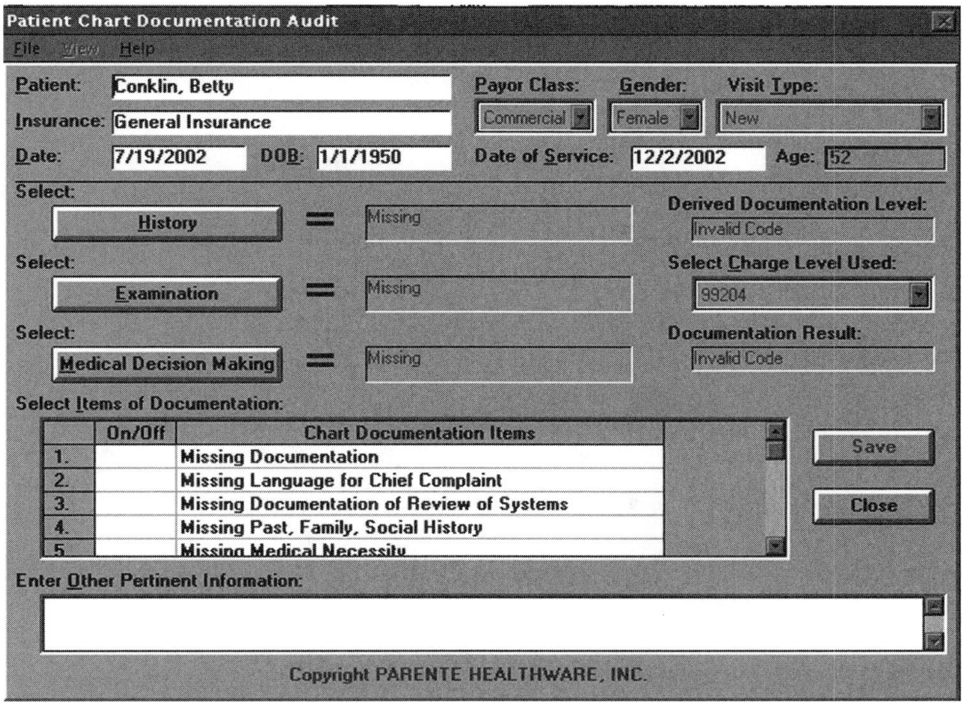

FIGURE 8-8. Audit screen. (Courtesy of Parente Healthware, Inc.)

- Patient name
- Insurance company
- Payer class
- Gender
- Visit type
- Date of service
- Date of birth
- Age (calculated by the software once the date of birth field is completed)

Once the user clicks on the history button, the history screen will appear. This screen will help the auditor capture the elements of history that are documented in the patient medical record. The screen shown in Figure 8-9 illustrates that the auditor found the chief complaint to be documented. The history of present illness elements that were documented in the medical record were as follows:

- Location
- Severity
- Modifying factors
- Signs and symptoms

Ten systems were reviewed and documented in the medical record. These systems are "checked" to document the review of systems. The last element of the history portion of the patient visit is the documentation of a past, family, and social history. The audit shows there was complete documentation of all three histories. Once these items are "checked," the next button is clicked and the program returns to the audit screen with the level of history appearing in the history field.

The examination portion of the visit is completed in the same manner and allows for the use of either 1995 or 1997 examination guidelines. The medical decision-making screen (Figure 8-10) is also completed and "drives" the level of medical decision making that is documented in the patient record.

Figure 8-11 shows an example of upcoding. In this example, a new patient was seen and examined. The physician chose level 99204 for the visit. Once the documentation information found in the medical record was entered, the software chose level 99203. The software then indicates that this service had been upcoded. This discovery demonstrates to the office manager that the practice is at risk. It is necessary to schedule a one-on-one meeting with the physician or a group meeting with all physicians to clear this up quickly. Proper documentation guidelines should be stressed.

A patient received a flu shot, but the flu shot was not marked on the billing form. This results in an uncaptured service, which is a loss of revenue if not discovered. This service was not checked on the billing form, resulting in a loss of revenue. This finding will print out in a report because the auditor checked Item 17 (Uncaptured Service) in the "Chart Documentation Items" list. There is a space to make notes regarding these findings.

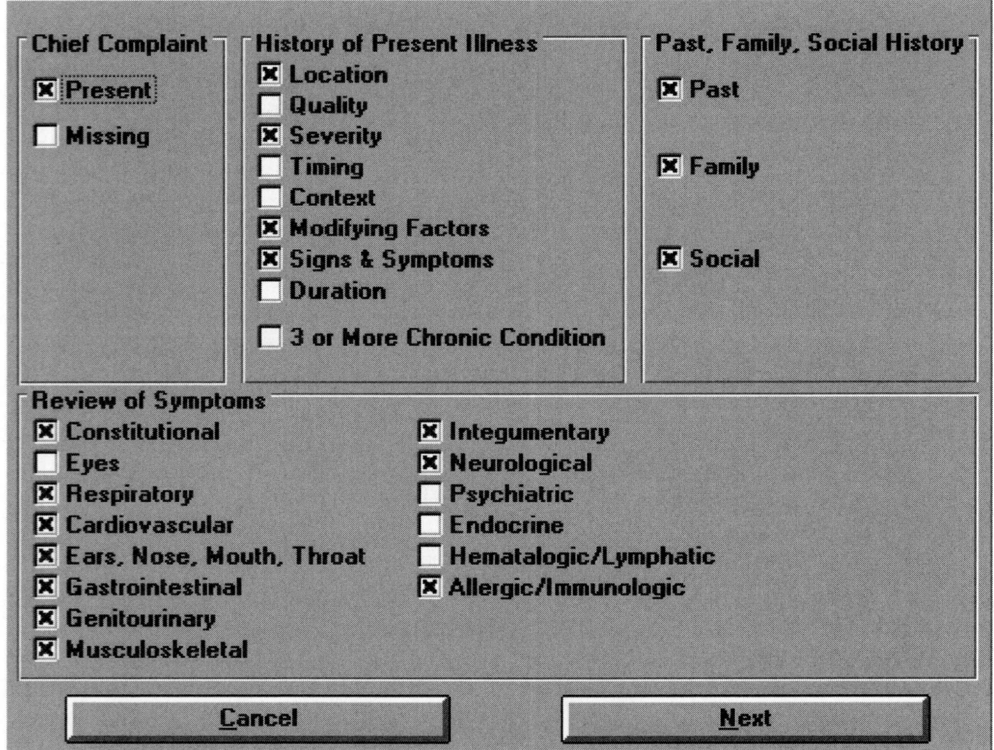

FIGURE 8-9. History screen. (Courtesy of Parente Healthware, Inc.)

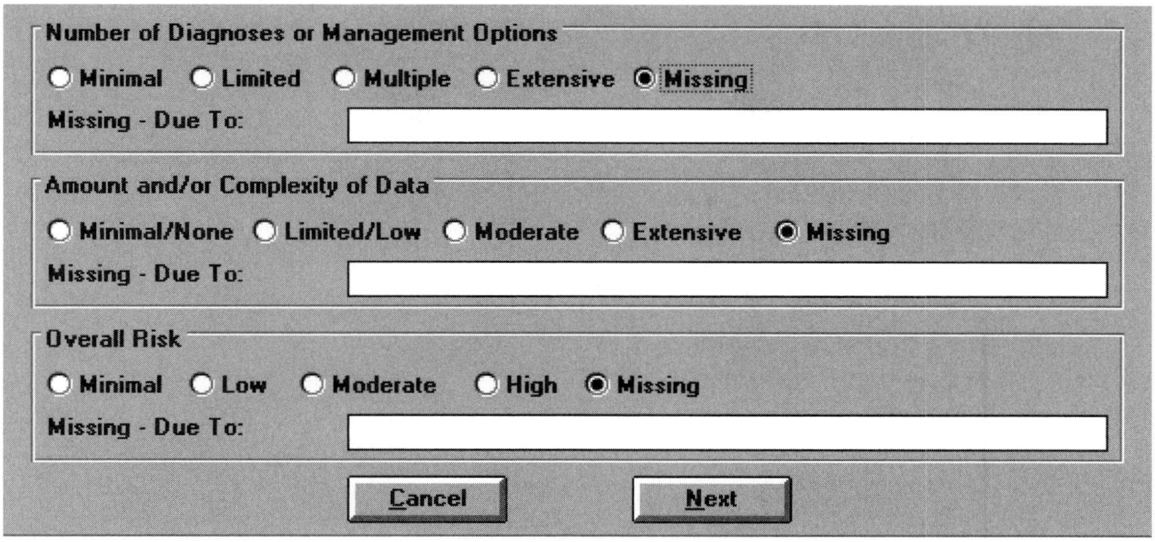

Number of Diagnoses or Management Options
○ Minimal ○ Limited ○ Multiple ○ Extensive ◉ Missing
Missing - Due To:

Amount and/or Complexity of Data
○ Minimal/None ○ Limited/Low ○ Moderate ○ Extensive ◉ Missing
Missing - Due To:

Overall Risk
○ Minimal ○ Low ○ Moderate ○ High ◉ Missing
Missing - Due To:

Cancel Next

FIGURE 8-10. Medical decision-making screen. (Courtesy of Parente Healthware, Inc.)

Patient Chart Documentation Audit
File View Help
Patient: Black, Rachel Payor Class: Medicare Gender: Female Visit Type: New
Insurance: Medicare
Date: 7/19/2002 DOB: 1/1/1925 Date of Service: 10/30/1923 Age: 77
Select: History = Detailed
Select: Examination = Comprehensive
Select: Medical Decision Making = Moderate Complexity
Derived Documentation Level: 99203
Select Charge Level Used: 99204
Documentation Result: Upcoded
Select Items of Documentation:

	On/Off	Chart Documentation Items
1.		Missing Documentation
2.		Missing Language for Chief Complaint
3.		Missing Documentation of Review of Systems
4.		Missing Past, Family, Social History
5		Missing Medical Necessity

Save Close
Enter Other Pertinent Information:
Missed billing for flu shot and admin code

Copyright PARENTE HEALTHWARE, INC.

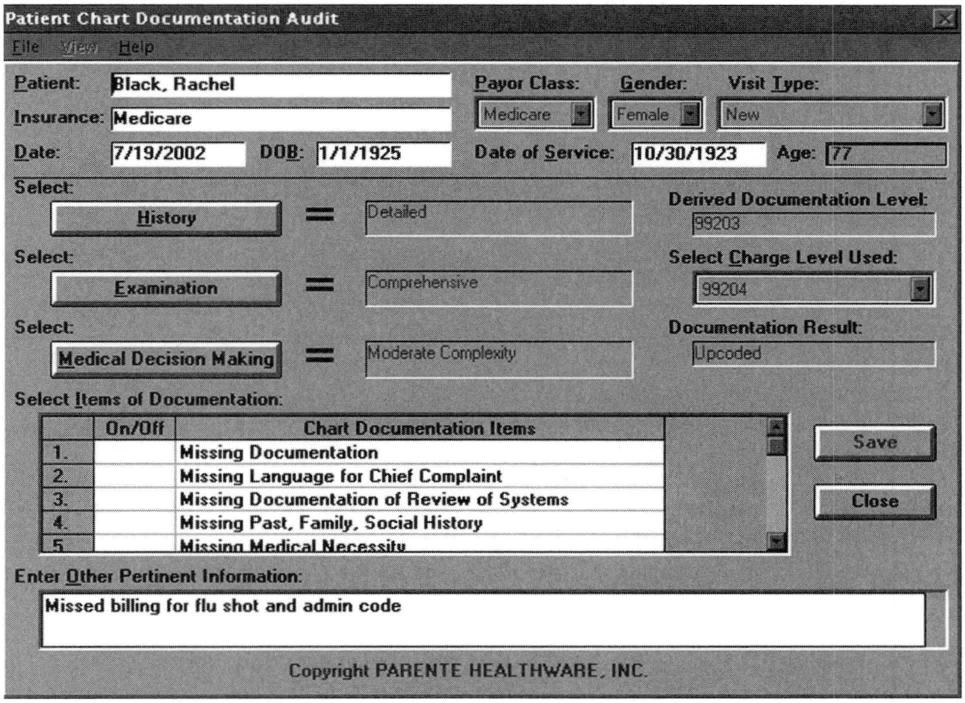

FIGURE 8-11. An example of upcoding. (Courtesy of Parente Healthware, Inc.)

The example shown in Figure 8-12 illustrates that the documentation found in the medical record supports the level of service chosen for billing. However, the use of an incorrect diagnosis code is identified, as well as the use of a rule-out (R/O) diagnosis code on the billing form.

The office manager should be very positive about this correctly coded service when discussing it with the physician. It is important, however, to point out the diagnosis problem. Many physicians do not understand that a rule-out diagnosis code cannot be coded.

The sample downcoding screen (Figure 8-13) shows that the patient was evaluated for an office consultation. The physician chose level 99242 for the level of service. The documentation in the medical record supports the billing of a

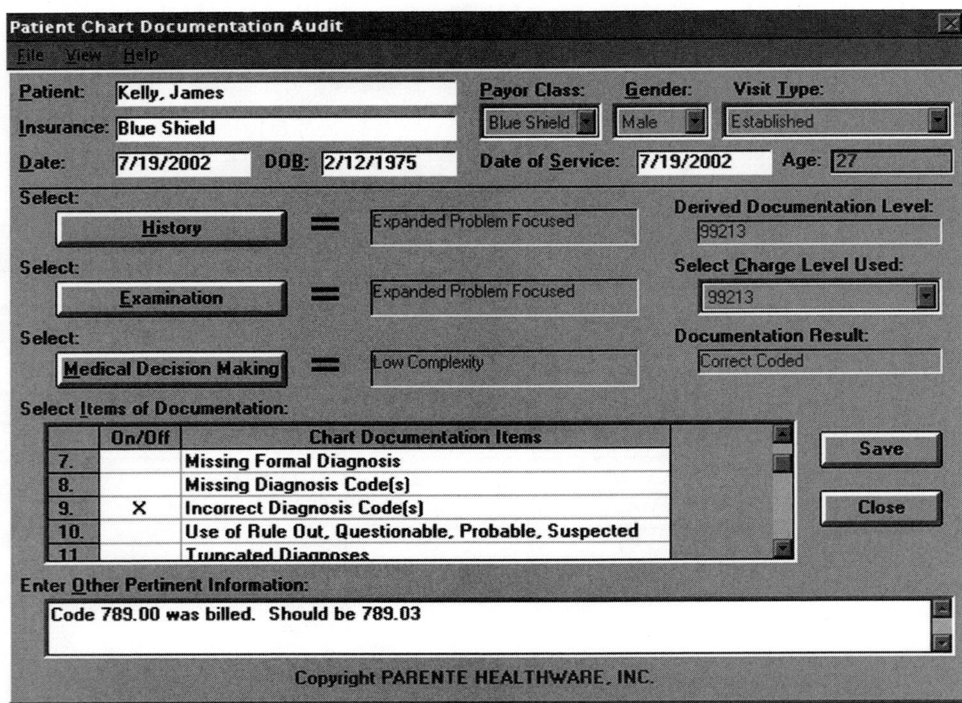

FIGURE 8-12. A correctly coded screen. (Courtesy of Parente Healthware, Inc.)

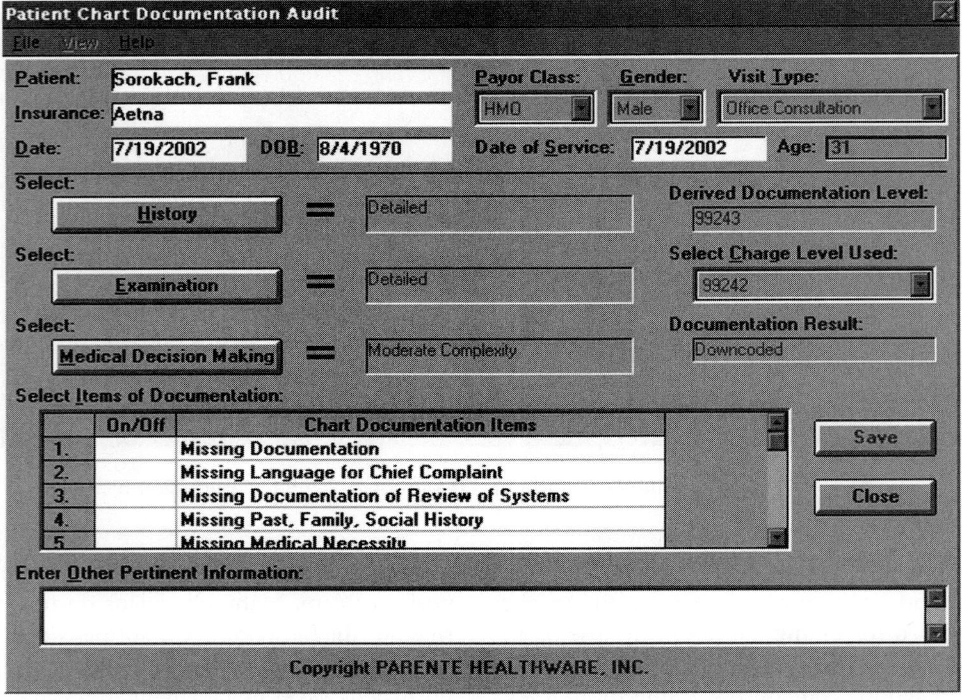

FIGURE 8-13. An example of downcoding. (Courtesy of Parente Healthware, Inc.)

higher level of consultation, level 99243. This downcoding instance demonstrates to the office manager that there was a loss of revenue to the practice. An education and training session with the physician should correct the situation.

Figure 8-14 is an illustration of an incorrect E&M category. The physician chose level 99253 for a hospital consultation. Once the patient's hospital record is audited, it is determined that the visit was actually level 99221, initial hospital service. Physicians often confuse hospital consultations with initial hospital services. It is important for the office manager to understand the difference and to relay the information to the physician via educational sessions or one-on-one interaction. Failure to use the correct code for billing could place the practice at risk should it be audited by a third party.

Figure 8-15 provides a summary of patients and types of visits. Once the audit is completed, the Complete Audit button is selected.

The report is now ready to be printed. This software will compile the information as illustrated in Figure 8-16. By choosing the Yes button in the "Print Audit" screen (Figure 8-17), a report will print. This print screen will provide printing options. The report can then be printed in text format or an Excel spreadsheet illustrating the detailed findings of each audited medical record. An example of the text report and Excel spreadsheet can be found in Appendix I.

In many practices, the office manager is the person responsible for performing the audit function. Using a software program to assist in the auditing process is a tremendous time-saver, because the compilation of information and printing of reports can be completed at the press of a button. When using an audit sheet, the office manager must perform the audit by hand, compile the information, and write the report. Most office managers are already wearing too many hats and therefore prefer it if a software program can save them time. The use of a good software package can be invaluable.

Common Documentation Errors

- Documentation of hospital services does not support any level of billing
- Cookie-cutter documentation via templates that permit overdocumentation and upcoding
- Reason for the visit is not clearly stated or is documented using vague language
- Missing review of systems
- Examinations not properly documented
- Missing provider signature
- Missing documentation of time for time-based codes
- Injections not properly documented

COMMON DOCUMENTATION ERRORS THAT WILL TRIGGER AN AUDIT (OR, HOW TO MEET THE INSPECTOR GENERAL)

The following practices have been known to trigger audits for physician offices:

- Billing all visits with the same one or two codes
- Billing for more testing than other offices of the same specialty in the same geographic location

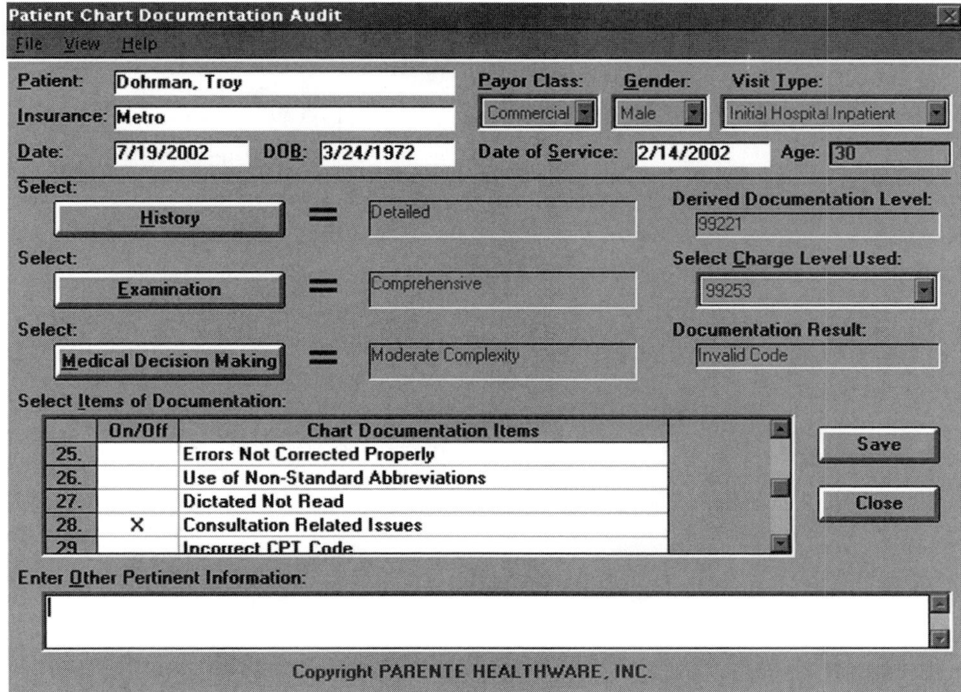

FIGURE 8-14. Screen showing an invalid code. (Courtesy of Parente Healthware, Inc.)

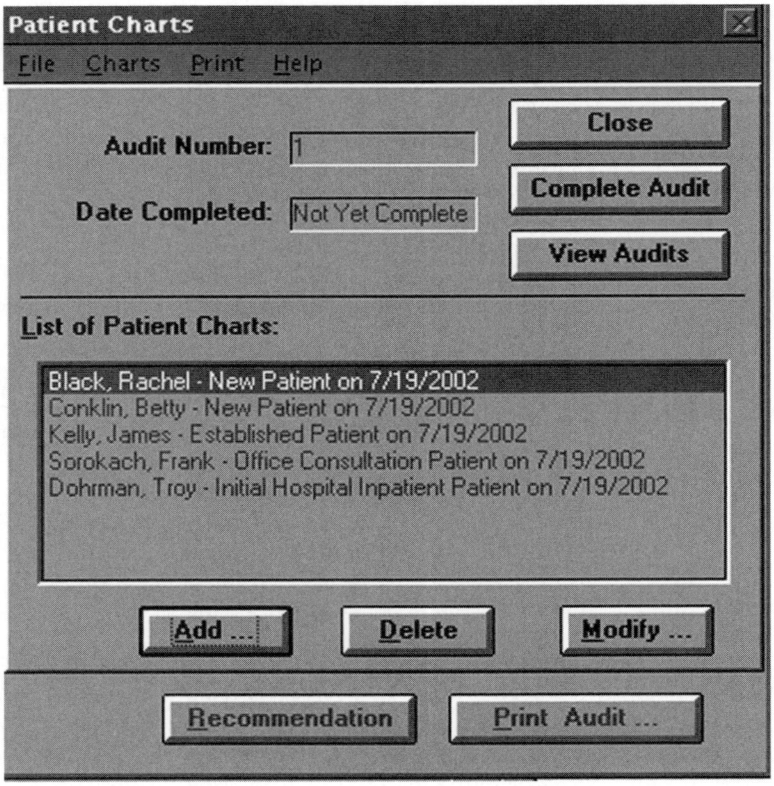

FIGURE 8-15. Patient's chart screen. (Courtesy of Parente Healthware, Inc.)

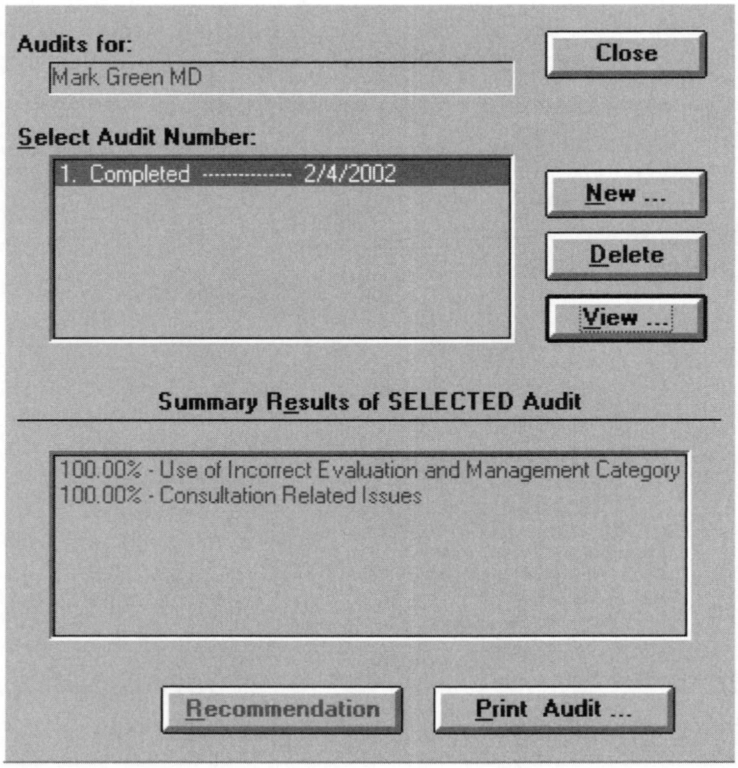

FIGURE 8-16. Audit summary screen. (Courtesy of Parente Healthware, Inc.)

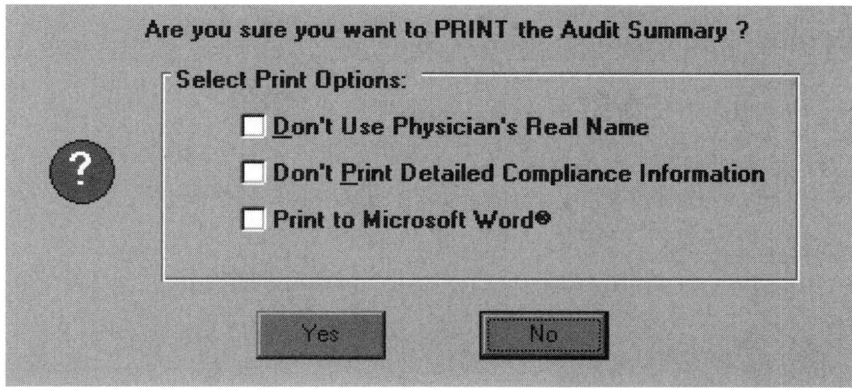

FIGURE 8-17. Print audit screen. (Courtesy of Parente Healthware, Inc.)

- Billing for more injections than other offices of the same specialty in the same geographic location
- Failure to handle waivers, write-offs, credit balances, and so on promptly and accurately

Medicare's Favorites

Medicare has its favorites when it comes to focusing on certain codes for abusive billing practices. The list in Box 8-6 offers a preview of possible areas of concern.

STATISTICS

According to the Office of Inspector General (OIG), in the year 2000 Medicare overpaid providers by $11.9 billion. The overpayments were divided as follows:

Medically unnecessary services: $5.9 billion. A physician was paid $3,305 for hypnotherapy sessions on an Alzheimer's patient. The patient was neither attentive nor cooperative during the initial mental status examination. The services were deemed not medically necessary, reasonable, or appropriate for a 95-year-old patient with Alzheimer's disease who was unable to participate.

Unsupported services: $4.3 billion. A physician's office was paid $800 for office services. The carrier requested copies of the medical records for these services. The medical records did not support the services performed, so the claim was denied.

Upcoding: $1.7 billion. A physician's office was paid $12,344 for initial visits performed in the hospital setting. Review of these claims disclosed that all had been upcoded by one level, and many by two levels.

Noncovered services: $800 million. Medicare cannot be billed for noncovered services such as hearing tests, prescription drugs, and examinations for glasses. One physician billed Medicare for pulse oximetry performed on every patient at every visit. Because these services are considered bundled into the office visit, and many of the patients had no medical necessity for the visit, problems arose.

Education and Training

The audit has been performed and the results obtained; now what? An audit is useless if nothing is done with the information it has provided. If the audit is performed retrospectively, any overpayments should be refunded and an educational session should be scheduled for the physicians and the office staff. If the audit is performed prospectively, changes to the chosen levels should be made immediately and the claims should then be submitted. Again, an educational session should be scheduled for the physicians and staff. Some physicians do not want office staff present at their education session, so it may be necessary to schedule a separate session for the staff. These educational sessions must be mandatory; as the dean of a medical school stated, absence is excusable only by death!

Training sessions should be structured to flow in a logical manner. Many physicians already think that guidelines are in some type of foreign language! The following list provides a structure for physician education that really works:

- Review documentation guidelines
- Identify the three key components
- Discuss history components
- Discuss examination components
- Discuss medical decision-making components
- Illustrate how key components fit into the various levels of E&M services
- Stress the importance of medical necessity
- Provide a "thumbnail" sketch of diagnosis coding

It is helpful if actual physician documentation is discussed. It becomes easier for physicians to understand when they are shown their own personal notes.

BOX 8-6 Medicare's "Top 40" Hit List

Absorptiometry: excessive number of services performed
Ambulatory surgery centers: billing for services that are not covered
Anesthesia: standby anesthesia services (most often done in ophthalmology)
Cataract surgery: excessive preoperative visual acuity services
Coding: excessive use of higher-level codes, such as billing for all comprehensive visits, and excessive use of a single level of care (pattern billing)
Colonoscopy: medical necessity for the test
Consultations: billing for consultations on established patients, referrals made within the same specialty, pattern billing with higher-level consultations
Cryosurgery: excessive coding of the lesion as 3 cm (the size of the freeze area) when the lesion is much smaller
Culture and sensitivity of urine: billing for repeat applications of the test after the organism is identified and sensitivity established
Cystoscopy: billing separately from other endoscopic procedures
Dilation and curettage (D&C): billing on same date as hysterectomy or certain other pelvic surgeries
Durable medical equipment (DME): ignoring billing rules for patients in hospital, skilled nursing facility, or an institution that is part of the hospital
Echo M scans: routine screening is not a covered service
Electrocardiogram (ECG) interpretation: providing medically unnecessary tests to patients before surgery
Endoscopy: performing this procedure instead of less costly studies, such as x-ray studies
Facelifts: billing as removal of fatty tumors
Injections: use of injections during the course of treatment instead of oral medications
IPPB, occasional: the interval between treatments inconsistent with diagnosis or inconsistent with normal treatment frequencies, especially with office patients
Keratosis: excessive billing for removal of sebaceous keratosis
KUB: medical necessity issue when billed separately on the same day as gastrointestinal (GI) and/or C-scan
Laboratory tests: billing for excessive repetition of tests when results are normal
Lesions: billing for excision of physically impossible lesions, that is, those that are too large to be removed in a physician's office
Office visits: upcoding; overutilization, particularly when services rendered were deemed not medically necessary
Patient sharing: surgeons and medical physicians of similar but different subspecialties sharing surgery patients, such as a cardiovascular surgeon and a cardiologist
Place of service: all services provided in the same place of service, having the same diagnosis for all
Portable x-rays: performing one x-ray, billing for two
Power-operated vehicles: questionable medical necessity
Preoperative and postoperative care: billing inside the global fee period
Pulmonary therapy: multiple treatments on inpatients, overutilization of services
Rehabilitation and psychiatric therapy: not following the rule about nonphysician services by employed doctor
Renal dialysis billing for laboratory: test standing orders of questionable necessity
Respiratory therapy: providing too frequently, or when medical necessity is questionable; getting involved in kickback situations
Seat-lift chairs: submitting questionable repair bills; having prescription authorized by a doctor with inadequate knowledge of the patient, certificate of medical necessity forms
Sigmoidoscopy and flexible sigmoidoscopy: medical necessity issue
Standing orders: continuing orders for periodic tests or treatments not medically necessary
Stress testing: overutilization, lack of medical necessity
Transurethral resection of prostate: billing vasectomy as if a separate procedure, on the same day or a different day
Vascular testing: noninvasive medical necessity, overutilization, or lack of documentation
X-rays: fragmentation issues with certain procedures such as angioplasty with multiple vessel studies; brain scan and brain scan with flow study billed on the same day; repeat x-rays that were originally normal; routine x-rays

(From *Part B Answer Book.* Rockville, MD: Part B News, 2002.)
IPPB, Intermittent positive pressure breathing; *KUB*, Kidney, ureter, and bladder.

EXERCISES

MULTIPLE CHOICE

Choose the best *answer for each of the following questions.*

1. What does the S stand for in SOAP?
   a. Symptom
   b. Subjective
   c. Sign
   d. None of the above
2. What modifier is used for teaching physician services between a resident and a teaching physician?
   a. GC
   b. DE
   c. TC
   d. GE
3. One of the codes for an initial hospital service is
   a. 99232
   b. 99222
   c. 99234
   d. 99238
4. Which of the following is *not* an element of the history of present illness?
   a. Condition
   b. Location
   c. Timing
   d. Quality
5. Which of the following is a body area?
   a. Abdomen
   b. Gastrointestinal
   c. Eyes
   d. All of the above
6. A level-four consultation requires the following:
   a. Past, social history
   b. Family, social history
   c. Past, family history
   d. None of the above
7. Which categories of E&M service require three out of three?
   a. Subsequent hospital care
   b. Established office patient
   c. Follow-up consultations
   d. None of the above
8. Which of the following is *not* an element of a social history?
   a. Smoking
   b. Level of education
   c. Family member death
   d. Type of living condition
9. Which of the following is *not* a key component of an E&M code?
   a. Medical decision making
   b. Time
   c. History
   d. Examination
10. Which of the following is *not* a level of examination?
    a. Problem focused
    b. Condition focused
    c. Expanded problem focused
    d. All of the above
11. An extended examination of the affected body area or organ systems and any other symptomatic or related organ system is what level of examination?
    a. Detailed
    b. Problem focused
    c. Comprehensive
    d. None of the above
12. A new patient is one who
    a. Has a new diagnosis
    b. Has not been seen in the practice for the past 3 years
    c. Has not been seen in the practice for the past 2 years
    d. Has not been seen in the practice for the past year
13. What office new patient code is documented as detailed history and examination, low medical decision making?
    a. 99201
    b. 99202
    c. 99203
    d. 99204
14. A consultation in the emergency department of the hospital is
    a. An inpatient consultation
    b. An outpatient consultation
    c. A confirmatory consultation
    d. None of the above
15. Which code is the most commonly used of all E&M services?
    a. 99203
    b. 99253
    c. 99213
    d. 99243
16. Which code is used to report a discharge service of more than 30 minutes?
    a. 99234
    b. 99236
    c. 99238
    d. 99239
17. All services provided by a consultant following an inpatient consultation are reported using which of the following category of codes?
    a. Subsequent hospital visits
    b. Follow-up consultations
    c. Outpatient consultations
    d. None of the above
18. An annual nursing facility assessment is which of the following codes?
    a. 99304
    b. 99310
    c. 99255
    d. 99318
19. Which of the following codes is used to report a discharge from the nursing home lasting 25 minutes?
    a. 99217
    b. 99316
    c. 99315
    d. 99209

20. Which of the following is not one of the "four C's" of an operative report?
    a. Communicative
    b. Comprehensive
    c. Consistent
    d. Complete

TRUE OR FALSE

1. ______ Use of canned reports is a good way for physicians to document operative reports.
2. ______ Teaching physicians can supervise no more than four surgeries at one time to be billable to Medicare.
3. ______ In the SOAP format, the "P" stands for "prognosis."
4. ______ A minor surgery is defined as 10 minutes or less.
5. ______ The range of codes for emergency services is 99281 to 99285.
6. ______ Code 99254 is an inpatient consultation code.
7. ______ Code 99223 is an initial inpatient code.
8. ______ Physicians can use either 1995 or 1997 guidelines for the examination portion of the visit.
9. ______ One must document five or six bulleted items for a detailed examination under 1997 guidelines.
10. ______ Documentation of social history can consist of marital status.
11. ______ There are four types of history.
12. ______ There is a second opinion code that is a consultation.
13. ______ Only body areas can be used toward the documentation of a 1995 comprehensive examination.
14. ______ Consultations require the documentation of all three key components.
15. ______ Documentation of a patient's surgical history is called the past history.
16. ______ Time can only be used to document a procedure.
17. ______ Code 99307 is a code for a nursing facility service.
18. ______ Medical students can document examination, but not history.
19. ______ GE is the modifier used for resident services performed under the primary care exception.
20. ______ SLIDE is a documentation format.

THINKERS

1. Compare and contrast the two documentation formats. Describe which format would be best for the medical practice scenario provided by your instructor.
2. In the following scenario, determine whether the visit is a consultation or a new patient, and explain how you arrive at your decision.

   Kelly Mills was sent to Dr. Sara Class for evaluation of her peptic ulcer disease. Her family physician, Dr. Babinetz, had seen Kelly in the office and needed the expert opinion of Dr. Class regarding her gastrointestinal complaints. Dr. Babinetz reviewed the upper gastrointestinal (GI) study that Kelly brought with her to his office. He will need to order some additional studies and will see Kelly in follow-up in 3 weeks to discuss the results and her prognosis.
3. Describe what a medically unnecessary service is and provide an example of one.
4. List and define the two teaching physician modifiers.

REFERENCES

American Medical Association. *Physicians' Current Procedural Terminology 2008*. Chicago: American Medical Association, 2008.

American Medical Association, *Prepare that Claim*, Chicago, American Medical Association, 2008.

Centers for Medicare and Medicaid Services, Physician Center, *Policies and Regulations*, Washington, DC, 2008.

Documentation Guidelines for E/M Services. Available at www.cms.hhs.gov/mlnedwebguide/25_emdoc.asp.

Guidelines for Teaching Physician, Interns, and Residents, Medicare Learning Network, Centers for Medicare and Medicaid Services, July 2006. Centers for Medicare and Medicaid Services, Medicare Claims Processing Manual, pub. no. 100-04, Chapter 12. Available at www.cms.hhs.gov/Manuals/IOM/list.asp.

McKinnon, P. *Journal of Medical Practice Management*, September/October 2000, Vol. 16, No. 2, pp. 75–76.

Updates to Home and Domiciliary Care Visits related to CPT codes 99321-99350, Medicare Learning Network, Centers for Medicare and Medicaid Services, September 2, 2005.

9

ETHICAL AND LEGAL ISSUES

CHAPTER OUTLINE

Licensing of Health Care Professionals
Properly Trained Staff: A Legal Necessity
Department of Health and Human Services
Abortion: Always a Controversy
AIDS: A Modern Plague
Autopsies
Antitrust Laws: 100 Years Later
Patient Advocacy
Vital Records
Good Medical Records . . . A Legal Asset
Legal Life of Financial Records
Physician-Patient Relationship
Hippocratic Oath
American Medical Association Code of Medical Ethics
Ethics: The Gray Ghost
Legal Aspects of Health Care
Practice Attorney
Patients Who Have Been Abused

CHAPTER OBJECTIVES

After completing this chapter, you will be able to do the following:

- Identify the major legal issues in health care
- Identify risk areas within a medical practice
- Understand the concept of "against medical advice"
- Recognize the importance of good medical records
- Understand the Good Samaritan Law
- Know how to terminate a physician-patient relationship
- Understand medical ethics and end-of-life decisions
- Discuss the importance of confidentiality
- Know the rules and regulations for human immunodeficiency virus (HIV) notification and detection
- Know and understand laws regarding employment
- Understand the purpose for subpoenas and depositions and know how to handle them
- Define *sexual harassment*
- Know what the office manager's responsibility is regarding sexual harassment
- Define *negligence*

LICENSING OF HEALTH CARE PROFESSIONALS

A license is awarded to those who perform competencies in certain specific areas that would not be legal if the individual did not have a license to do so. Individuals obtain a license by passing an examination, through rigorous training, or both. Health care licensing boards and agencies of organizations and states grant individuals permission to practice their trade. Licensing laws limit and control admission to the different health care professions and protect the public from unqualified health care personnel. Each state is responsible for the licensing of health care professionals, such as physicians, dentists, nurses, nurse practitioners, physician assistants, veterinarians, psychologists, and so on. In certain states, even nonmedical professions, such as accountants, barbers, beauticians, funeral directors, architects, engineers, and so on, are required to be licensed. Some advice for all licensed health care professionals:

- Say you don't know if you don't know! Seek the knowledge of a consultant.
- Practice in the field that you have been trained and licensed in, no other.
- Be confident and professional in the presence of patients.
- Confirm all telephone prescriptions in writing.
- Attend continuing medical education workshops.
- Be understanding and listen to all patients.
- Regularly check any medical equipment that is used.
- Maintain complete and accurate medical records.
- Provide quality care and service to all patients.
- Obtain patient consent whenever necessary.

Often the words *licensure* and *certification* are used interchangeably; however, generally certification is not mandatory to be able to practice in your profession. Once a health care professional has obtained a license to practice, he or she must renew that license periodically as deemed by the state that authorized the licensing. Physicians, for example, must demonstrate that they have maintained acceptable standards of professional conduct and medical practice, and must show that they have completed the required number of continuing medical education hours to have their license renewed. *Scope of practice* is a term used by the licensing boards to define the procedures, actions, and processes that are permitted for that specific individual to perform. The scope of practice is limited to procedures in which the individual has proven competence.

There are some instances in which a provider's license is either revoked or not renewed. Should a violation occur, one or more of the following may occur:

- *Probation:* The license is monitored for a specific period of time.
- *Suspension:* The provider may not practice for a specific period of time.
- *Summary suspension:* The license is suspended immediately with evidence that the medical practice presents a threat to public health and safety.
- *Restitution:* The provider must reimburse the patient or other entity for the sum that was improperly obtained.
- *Restriction:* The license is restricted in some way (the provider cannot perform a specific procedure or prescribe certain drugs).
- *Reprimand:* A public reprimand is given.
- *Administrative fine or penalty:* The provider must pay a civil penalty fee.
- *Voluntary surrender of license:* The license is surrendered to avoid further disciplinary action.
- *Denial:* The provider is not granted a renewal.
- *Revocation:* The license is terminated and therefore the provider can no longer practice.

PROPERLY TRAINED STAFF: A LEGAL NECESSITY

Before a patient meets the physician for the first time, he or she progresses through several events that directly affect the patient's experience with the physician. The patient does the following:

1. Makes telephone contact with the medical office to make an appointment.
2. Travels to the office.
3. Finds a place to park.
4. Locates the office if it is in an office building.
5. Arrives at the waiting room.
6. Approaches the desk and is greeted by the receptionist.
7. Has a preliminary visit with clinical personnel.

While progressing through these seven events before meeting with the physician, the patient is arriving at conclusions about the practice. Many things can go wrong before the patient ever meets the physician. Some, such as a long driving distance from the home to the office, or not finding nearby parking on the day of the appointment, cannot be changed. However, some events can be controlled by the office manager and staff.

The importance of a properly trained office staff is greater than most physicians realize. Patients view the staff's attitude as reflective of the office's attitude as a whole. If the patient is greeted by an unfriendly receptionist or a cold and uncaring nurse, the entire visit is off to a bad start. Remember that most patients are unhappy about being at the doctor's office to begin with. Unhappy patient experiences can translate into lawsuits.

Under the legal principle of vicarious liability, the physician is ultimately responsible for the actions of his or her staff. This principle means that not only are employees legally responsible for their actions, but that the physician is also responsible for their actions. Thus the office manager should carefully choose and train all employees. The selection and training process is discussed from a human resources point of view in Chapter 2 from a strictly legal standpoint, there are a few basic areas in which staff training is extremely important:

- Patient satisfaction
- Medical records
- Telephone tactics
- Confidentiality
- Billing and collections

Patient Satisfaction

There are a number of areas, hot spots, where patients become dissatisfied with the practice. The office manager should work to ensure that these problem areas are identified and corrected. Box 9-1 lists 10 of these medical office hot spots, and each one is discussed below.

The Answering Service

The after-hours answering service is a direct reflection on the physician and the office. What the answering service staff says, their attitude toward the patient, and how they process the patient's information can cause unhappiness that may lead to lawsuits. The office manager should sit down with the supervisor of the answering service to establish a policy of how they are to handle calls. This meeting should be documented. Once this has been established, the answering service staff is accountable for any deviation from this policy. It is a good practice to call the office after hours to see how the telephone is being answered. It is a good way to check on the answering service and can identify problems such as the following:

- The phone rang too many times before it was answered.
- The person answering the phone was not courteous.
- The person answering the phone did not take the time to collect the appropriate information from the patient.

BOX 9-1 Ten Medical Office Hot Spots

1. Problems with the answering service
2. Long lag-time to appointment date
3. Failure to return telephone calls
4. Dealing with patients in search of telephone medicine
5. Unfriendly or uncomfortable reception areas
6. Overly long wait in the reception area
7. Lapses in protecting patient confidentiality
8. Operational issues within the billing department
9. Improper handling of medical records and documentation
10. Need for "after-hours" prescription renewals

The office manager should find an answering service that is a good fit, because this is an important function of the office. Patients can be lost when the answering service is unresponsive or dismissive.

Appointment Time Frame

The amount of time a patient waits for an appointment can also be a problem area. If patients have a problem that they feel cannot wait but are unable to secure an appointment in a reasonable amount of time, things can get ugly! If the patient is an established patient, the abandonment issue (discussed later) could very well come into play. Always attempt to give patients appointments in a reasonable amount of time. If there are no available appointments, have the receptionist ask the physician how to handle the situation.

Return Phone Calls

Another issue that may lead to an abandonment lawsuit is not returning patients' calls. Patients who call with problems and do not receive calls back from the physician will leave the practice and seek the care of another physician. This is not only a legal issue, but also borders on an ethical issue and affects the growth of the practice. Most physicians do not want unhappy patients, so all calls should be returned on the same day, if possible.

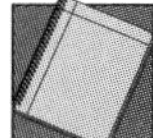

FROM THE EXPERT'S NOTEBOOK

If the patient requires only dosage information or instructions, the office manager, nurse, or receptionist can return the patient's call. Some patients are just lonely and want someone to listen to them. A staff member can easily take over this duty. The physician can direct the calls to the appropriate staff members who have received clear and concise instructions for a reply.

Telephone Medicine

Many patients want to be treated over the phone. They try to eliminate going to the physician's office because they don't want to be bothered or don't want to pay for an office visit. Avoiding telephone medicine is one of the most important policies an office can make, and it should be adhered to no matter how insistent the patient is. Keep in mind the basic principle that the patient must be seen before treatment is rendered. Practicing telephone medicine gives the practice a severe handicap and leaves it open to liability. Simply don't do it!

Reception Area

Having an unfriendly reception area is one sure way of making patients unhappy. Up-to-date magazines, soft music, or even a television can help ease the anxious patient. Having educational reading material available can also be helpful (the "reception area blues" are discussed in Chapter 3). The reception area should be warm and inviting, not cold and sterile. Make it as comfortable a place as it can be.

Prolonged Waiting in the Reception Area

Even if the reception area is cozy, patients do not want to spend a lot of time there. Most patients in a reception area are sick; they just want to be seen and go home. It is important for patients to know that the office is concerned about their time and the office schedule. If situations arise that disrupt the schedule, staff should be trained to advise patients that there has been a problem. Some offices offer coffee or tea at such times. Others ask if the patient wishes to go out for coffee and return a little later. Some patients may wish to be rescheduled. These appointments should be rescheduled in a timely manner.

Confidentiality

Remember . . . voices carry! Office staff should be reminded that gossip is not appropriate in a medical office. Any talk regarding a patient should be private, quiet, and strictly on a professional level. Sitting in the waiting room and hearing staff talking about another patient's hairdo is a sure turnoff. This sounds like a commonsense issue; however, some suits have stemmed from just such instances.

Information that is shared between a physician and a patient for the purpose of medical treatment is considered confidential communication. Any unauthorized disclosure of this information breaches this contractual obligation between the physician and the patient. The vast majority of states have strict regulations regarding the confidentiality of the information physicians receive from their patients. Most state physician-patient statutes are similar to the following:

"No physician should be allowed, in any civil matter, to disclose any information which he acquired while attending the patient in a professional capacity, which enabled him to act in that capacity, which shall tend to blacken the character of the patient, without consent of the patient except in civil matters brought by such patient for damages on account of personal injuries."

If any of these elements are met in the physician-patient relationship, the physician is barred from disclosure of any information without the patient's permission.

The purpose of adopting a physician-patient privilege was to create an atmosphere in which patients could feel secure enough to disclose any information that might pertain to their medical problems. The Principles of Medical Ethics that have been laid out by the American Medical Association (AMA) establish a broader statute of confidentiality than is found in the judicial codes. The AMA code of ethics advocates the confidentiality of all contacts between the medical office and the patient.

There are a few exceptions to the state Duty of Confidentiality statute that are pertinent to daily operations in a medical office. A patient's medical information may be released under the following circumstances:

- The patient files a lawsuit for personal injuries.
- Consent has been obtained.
- The court orders it.
- A third party has requested it.

The patient who files a lawsuit for personal injuries waives the physician-patient relationship by filing suit. This suit allows consent of disclosure of medically related injuries/illnesses. It is not uncommon for patient records to be requested by third parties for the purpose of insurance, employment physicals, and so on. A court may order a patient's medical information in cases of communicable diseases, child abuse, and so on.

Each state has a law regarding the confidentiality of acquired immunodeficiency syndrome (AIDS) testing. The smart medical assistant obtains copies of state guidelines regarding AIDS testing and distributes them to the staff during an office meeting when discussing procedures and guidelines.

In today's high-tech world, we use fax machines for a multitude of purposes. Many offices fax test results, medical records, and so on to hospitals. Insurance companies will even request that medical records be faxed. Confidentiality is a serious issue when using a fax machine to transmit information. It is very important to add a confidentiality notice to the fax transmission cover sheet. This will protect the faxed information from being disseminated or photocopied.

Billing Department

The dreaded billing department . . . where all the "nasty people" work! It is good to concentrate on the bottom line, but billing and collection problems are often the source of legal action against the physician. There must be a balance between hard-nosed and easygoing behavior. Many patients have problems with billing and insurance. Train the staff to start off on the right foot by asking, "How can we help you?"

Medical Records

There are ways in which the medical record can become a liability. Be careful not to release records without proper authorization. Do not allow staff to use abbreviations that they have made up. If abbreviations are necessary, staff should use standard abbreviations. Do not allow staff to use cute or smart-alecky phrases or abbreviations to describe a patient's disposition. This can create problems for the physician should a lawsuit arise, not to mention that it is totally unprofessional. Also, when staff have made a mistake in documentation, do not let them try to "help" by altering a patient's medical record. This could spell disaster! This error should be documented correctly. See Chapter 4 for details on correcting errors.

Prescription Renewals

Institute a policy that all prescription renewals must be documented in the patient's chart. As discussed previously, a stamp can be made for this purpose and is an orderly way to record this information. Train staff to let the physician know if they perceive a problem with a patient's prescription. A pharmacist may call to question a particular prescription or advise the physician that a patient had the prescription refilled last week by another physician. This is very important information and must be immediately passed on to the physician. This information should also be documented in the patient's chart. There should be a policy for staff to follow regarding situations such as these. Beware of patients who just want prescriptions and not an appointment to see the physician.

DEPARTMENT OF HEALTH AND HUMAN SERVICES

The Department of Health and Human Services (HHS) is a part of the executive branch of the federal government. The secretary of HHS reports directly to the President regarding issues of health, welfare, income security plans, policies, and programs. There are five divisions of HHS:

1. Social Security Administration (SSA)
2. Centers for Medicare and Medicaid Services (CMS)
3. Human Development Services (HDS)
4. Public Health Service (PHS)
5. Family Support Administration (FSA)

Social Security Administration

The SSA is directly responsible for the nation's Social Security program. The Social Security fund is supported by employees and employers across the nation. When the earning capacity of an individual decreases because of disability, the fund pays benefits to assist the employee, and when an individual's earning capacity ceases because of death, the fund pays benefits to the individual's family.

Centers for Medicare and Medicaid Services

CMS administers the Medicare and Medicaid programs and the medical care and quality assurance that go with them. This division develops policies and procedures related to program recipients such as hospitals, nursing homes, physicians, and insurance contractors. CMS also works with state governments regarding the needs of medically indigent people. In June 2001, this organization, formerly named the Health Care Financing Administration (HCFA), adopted a new name and developed three separate centers of service:

- The Center for Beneficiary Choices: This branch focuses on the Medicare + Choice program and provides information to beneficiaries.
- The Center for Medicare Management: This branch deals with the traditional fee-for-service program.
- The Center for Medicaid and State Operations: This branch focuses on programs that are administered by the states, including Medicaid, the State Children's Health Insurance Program, and insurance regulations.

Human Development Services

HDS directs programs for children, the elderly, Native Americans, persons with disabilities, and individuals living in rural areas. It develops programs, controls equal employment opportunity and civil rights policies, and supervises research. HDS also directs public affairs.

Public Health Service

The PHS was developed to help protect the nation's physical and mental health. It coordinates with each state the national health policy, associated programs, research, alcohol and drug abuse programs, and enforcement of laws regarding medical devices, safe foods, and safe cosmetics. The Food and Drug Administration (FDA) is part of the PHS. The FDA supervises and controls the introduction of new drugs, foods, cosmetics, and medical devices. Every food and drug product found on store shelves today is regulated by the FDA.

Family Support Administration

The FSA advises the secretary of HHS on the needs of children and families. It directs family support programs in federal, state, and local governments. It directs and coordinates programs for the Secretary of Labor regarding employment and training.

ABORTION: ALWAYS A CONTROVERSY

Abortion is the termination of a pregnancy at a time when the fetus is incapable of sustaining life on its own. Medical professionals today are faced with a twofold problem regarding abortion. They may incur civil liability for refusing to perform abortions, and they may incur criminal liability by performing abortions where they are prohibited by state laws. Many states have placed indirect restrictions on abortions by denying state funding for clinics in which abortions are performed. In dealing with this very controversial issue, you will find that the U.S. Supreme Court often passes the burden of judgment to the states. Any physician who is considering performing abortions should monitor state judicial proceedings closely and should consult with an attorney before making any decisions. Some states require that gestational age and medical necessity be determined, that informed consent be obtained, and that a spouse or parent be notified. Each state has its own laws regarding abortion, and even on a federal level these laws change rapidly.

Personnel problems may arise should your physician decide to perform abortions. Many states issue the "Right of Conscience," a document that informs medical personnel of their right to refuse to participate in abortions, to employees of physicians who have decided to perform abortions. As an office manager, you must be aware that no civil, criminal, administrative, or disciplinary action can be taken against an individual who refuses to aid in an abortion.

Should your physician opt to perform abortions in his or her facility, you must contact the Department of Health in your state to check on the regulations regarding such a facility. Some states require that an Abortion Facility Registration Form be signed and various reports be filed, such as the following:

- Quarterly facilities report
- Report on induced termination of pregnancy
- Report on pathologic examination
- Report on maternal death
- Report on complications during or following abortion

AIDS: A MODERN PLAGUE

Acquired immunodeficiency syndrome (AIDS) poses some of the most serious social, ethical, and economic problems throughout the world. People with AIDS can be afflicted with a wide variety of specific, life-threatening infections and other conditions that are the result of an underlying deficiency in the immune system of infected individuals. AIDS is not a cause of death; it is simply the catalyst of death, in that it destroys the body's capacity to ward off viruses and bacteria that it would ordinarily be able to fight off. The virus that causes AIDS (the human immunodeficiency virus, or HIV) is highly contagious and is found in high numbers in the following groups:

- Homosexual males
- People who use intravenous drugs
- Prostitutes (both female and male)
- People with hemophilia

This disease has caught the attention of the World Health Organization (WHO), and there are now educational programs in every nation in the world. At the time of this writing, it is estimated that between 38 million and 110 million adults and more than 10 million children are infected worldwide. An estimated 50,000 health care workers have contracted HIV through the workplace, according to the Centers for Disease Control and Prevention (CDC). AIDS has already killed more young Americans than the Korean and Vietnam wars combined, and it has now become the leading cause of death for women in the United States between 25 and 40 years of age. No cure has been found for this quickly spreading plague.

Medical offices are liable for transmitting this disease through transfusions of HIV-infected blood, accidents involving needlesticks, and failure to take the appropriate precautions when dealing with HIV patients. States have set up laws governing the health care setting and HIV. The federal government, through its Occupational Safety and Health Administration (OSHA) regulations, is attempting to protect physicians and health care workers from HIV infection.

Because of the social stigma associated with AIDS, it is thought that incidence of the disease is underreported. It is the responsibility of all physicians and hospitals to report their patients with HIV to their county office of the state Department of Health. It is the office manager's responsibility to see that the reporting requirements are fulfilled.

Each state has its own legislation regarding HIV testing. Some states require pretest counseling, some require posttest counseling, and some require both. Office managers should be aware of their state's regulations regarding HIV testing and should educate their staff concerning these regulations.

Generally, physicians and their employees are required to maintain the confidentiality of all HIV-related information. This rule applies whether the information was obtained voluntarily or involuntarily. This information can be disclosed only to the following:

- The patient
- The physician who ordered the test
- Any person designated by the patient to receive such information
- The Department of Health and the CDC
- An individual with a court order
- A funeral director
- A health care worker directly involved in the care of the individual
- Peer review organizations

No health care worker can refuse to treat a patient with HIV. It is necessary, however, for health care workers to protect themselves and other office patients from the transmission of the virus. OSHA regulations regarding barrier methods and employee HIV testing are discussed in detail in Chapter 11.

In addition, there is the risk of harm to patients being treated by HIV-infected health care workers. This is especially important for health care workers who are involved in surgeries, because surgical accidents, such as scalpel cuts or needlesticks, may put patients at risk.

Notification

Now comes the ethical question, Should a physician with HIV notify patients of his or her health status? According to CDC guidelines, health care workers who perform "exposure" procedures should voluntarily test for HIV, and if positive, inform their patients. Many will argue that it is in direct violation of their Fourth Amendment right to privacy. Both patients and health care workers have rights and responsibilities requiring a delicate balance. This is an important issue and not one that can be swept under the carpet for another day.

AUTOPSIES

A licensed physician, usually a pathologist, may perform an autopsy or postmortem examination on a deceased patient within 36 hours after death. Autopsies are done for the following four reasons:

- To establish the cause of death
- To educate
- To serve legal purposes (in which case, they are usually done or ordered by the coroner/medical examiner)
- To maintain quality assurance regarding hospital care (i.e., to make sure the death was not due to error at the hospital)

It is mandatory that the physician or office manager obtain the appropriate authorization before an autopsy is performed. Authorization may be given by the following persons, listed in order of preference:

- The deceased patient (before death) with spousal consent
- Written authority by the deceased
- The spouse of the deceased
- Any adult children of the deceased
- Any adult grandchildren of the deceased
- The parents of the deceased
- The brothers or sisters of the deceased
- The nephews or nieces of the deceased
- The grandparents of the deceased
- The uncles or aunts of the deceased
- The adult cousins of the deceased
- The adult stepchildren of the deceased
- A relative who is next of kin of a previously deceased spouse
- Any other relative or friend with written authorization from the deceased

A coroner does not need to obtain necessary authorization to perform an autopsy. He or she must, however, investigate the circumstances surrounding the death to establish whether the death was the result of a criminal act.

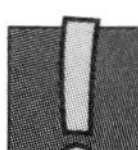

MANAGER'S ALERT

There is never a time when an attending physician can order an autopsy without the necessary authorization!

ANTITRUST LAWS: 100 YEARS LATER

Antitrust laws, first developed when America's businesses were forming alliances to reduce competition, were practically nonexistent in the health care field until 1975. With health care expenditures on the rise, the demand for economical approaches to the delivery of health care is increasing. The growing number of health care professionals and the various alternatives to health care delivery have become major issues today. The Sherman Antitrust Act is the federal law that has come into play in the health care field. The Sherman Antitrust Act consists of two parts:

- Every contract, combination in the form of trust or otherwise, or conspiracy in restraint of trade or commerce among the several states . . . is declared to be illegal.
- Every person who shall monopolize, or attempt to monopolize, or combine or conspire with any other person or persons to monopolize any part of the trade or commerce among the several states . . . shall be deemed . . . guilty of a felony.

In plain English, the first part deals with the type of conduct that may be encountered in the health care industry. The second part deals with monopolies.

Areas of concern for health care include price fixing, limiting new entrants into the area, preferred provider arrangements, exclusive contracts, and so on. Physicians are more likely to be confronted with private, nongovernmental antitrust actions than with governmental actions. The recent antitrust actions by the federal government have focused on physician conduct. In an extended meeting in 1988 between the American Medical Association and the U.S. Department of Justice, it was decided that the government would stop intervening in medical practice to force competition among physicians.

Exclusive Contracts

Physicians practicing in certain specialties often become involved in exclusive contracts for their services with hospitals and insurance companies. These physicians are generally pathologists, anesthesiologists, cardiologists, and radiologists, whose services cannot be provided by other physicians.

These contracts are legal; however, caution should be used when entering into them. Setting up these contracts is generally a complicated process and should not be done without the assistance of the practice attorney.

Price Fixing

As a general rule, physicians practicing in one geographic area should not agree on what prices to charge for services unless they are partners. The physician and the office manager should be cautious when discussing the pricing of medical services with competitors.

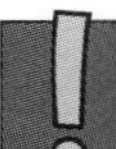

MANAGER'S ALERT

Be very careful when discussing prices with other office managers. It is easy to get caught up in a friendly conversation and to forget that you are giving away trade secrets. It is best to avoid the subject of money altogether.

Moratoriums

Hospitals often institute staff moratoriums, which means they do not allow any further additions to staff. These moratoriums are generally for a specific time period and are lifted at a later date, at which time applications are accepted. Moratoriums must be applied in a nondiscriminatory manner. If your physician is just moving into an area where the hospital has a closed staff, it is imperative that he or she obtain counsel for representation of this issue.

PATIENT ADVOCACY

We read about many consumer movements on a daily basis; however, many people do not realize that this consumer movement has moved into health care. Although this is not a new concept, as consumer movements began in 1899, it is a newer concept when it comes to health care, because health care has always been something personal to a patient, not something complained about, or even taken any legal action about. Life back then was easier, with fewer choices. However, life today requires many choices in a complex world. Patients have become consumers and do not place their physicians on a pedestal. In earlier years, physicians were "gods" who could do no wrong. They were highly respected members of the community. Today, physicians are not above scrutiny and are very aware that they are being closely watched and questioned.

Health care is changing. The small town physician practice has been replaced with large groups who practice very differently. Today's physician can be part of a large group of physicians that can range in number from three to (seemingly) infinity! Technology has changed also with a multitude of tests that can be performed to diagnose even the most obscure conditions. This technology isn't cheap, and therefore the cost of health care is growing at a rate higher than ever before. With all of these changes, it is necessary to develop an understanding of patient advocacy and how physicians and their staff can address the issues of education, sharing of information, and helping patients to understand their rights and responsibilities. To be sure that you are delivering a service that is beneficial to the patient, follow these simple guidelines:

- Always explain in detail and layman's terms when speaking with patients.
- Consider new and better ways to keep patients informed.
- Review and follow the suggestions for better patient understanding through effective communication in Chapter 3.
- Continually update educational materials.

The Patient's Bill of Rights

The American Hospital Association (AHA) published the "Patient's Bill of Rights" in 1973. The AHA wrote the Patient's Bill of Rights to provide more effective care and greater satisfaction for the patient, physician, and hospital. The medical assistant might want to copy this document and place it in the waiting room for patients to either read in the office or pick up and take home.

At the hospital, the Patient's Bill of Rights is generally given to the patient at admission. The physician-patient relationship takes on new dimensions when the patient is in the hospital setting. Not only is the physician responsible for the patient, but the hospital as an institution also accepts responsibility for the patient. The patient's rights should be supported by both the hospital and the physician; they are an integral part of the patient's recovery. Because this document has been prepared by professionals rather than consumers, it would probably be admissible as evidence in a case where the rights of the patient are concerned. The medical assistant might want to develop a particular Patient's Bill of Rights for the medical office. This can be included in the *Patient Information Handbook* or can be made into a pamphlet and placed in the waiting room for patients to pick up. The Patient's Bill of Rights developed by the American Hospital Association is provided in Box 9-2, and the Patient's Bill of Rights developed by the U.S. Advisory Commission on Consumer Protection and Quality in the Health Care Industry is provided in Box 9-3.

VITAL RECORDS

Vital records are considered to be a legal source of primary information about a patient. These records may consist of

BOX 9-2 The American Hospital Association's Patient's Bill of Rights

1. The patient has the right to considerate and respectful care.
2. The patient has the right to obtain from his physician complete current information concerning his diagnosis, treatment, and prognosis in terms the patient can be reasonably expected to understand. When it is not medically advisable to give such information to the patient, the information should be made available to an appropriate person in his behalf. He has the right to know, by name, the physician responsible for coordinating his care.
3. The patient has the right to receive from his physician information necessary to give informed consent prior to the start of any procedure and/or treatment. Except in emergencies, such information for informed consent should include but not necessarily be limited to the specific procedure and/or treatment, the medically significant risks involved, and the probable duration of incapacitation. Where medically significant alternatives for care or treatment exist, or when the patient requests information concerning medical alternatives, the patient has the right to such information. The patient also has the right to know the name of the person responsible for the procedures and/or treatment.
4. The patient has the right to refuse treatment to the extent permitted by law, and to be informed of the medical consequences of his action.
5. The patient has the right to every consideration of his privacy concerning his own medical care program. Case discussion, consultation, examination, and treatment are confidential and should be conducted discreetly. Those not directly involved in his care must have the permission of the patient to be present.
6. The patient has the right to expect that all communications and records pertaining to his care should be treated as confidential.
7. The patient has the right to expect that within its capacity a hospital must make reasonable response to the request of a patient for services. The hospital must provide evaluation, service, and/or referral as indicated by the urgency of the case. When medically permissible, a patient may be transferred to another facility only after he has received complete information and explanation concerning the needs for, and alternatives to, such a transfer. The institution to which the patient is to be transferred must first have accepted the patient for transfer.
8. The patient has the right to obtain information as to any relationship of his or her hospital to other health care and educational institutions insofar as his care is concerned. The patient has the right to obtain information as to the existence of any professional relationships among individuals, by name, which is treating him.
9. The patient has the right to be advised if the hospital proposes to engage in or perform human experimentation affecting his care or treatment. The patient has the right to refuse to participate in such research projects.
10. The patient has the right to expect reasonable continuity of care. He has the right to know in advance what appointment times and physicians are available and where. The patient has the right to expect that the hospital will provide a mechanism whereby he is informed by his physician or a delegate of the physician of the patient's continuing health care requirements following discharge.
11. The patient has the right to examine and receive an explanation of his bill regardless of source of payment.
12. The patient has the right to know what hospital rules and regulations apply to his conduct as patient.

(Developed by the American Hospital Association.)

BOX 9-3 The Patient's Bill of Rights

The following Patient's Bill of Rights was developed in 1998 by the U.S. Advisory Commission on Consumer Protection and Quality in the Health Care Industry.

1. **Information Disclosure.** You have the right to accurate and easily understood information about your health plan, health care professionals, and health care facilitates. If you speak another language, have a physical or mental disability, or just don't understand something, assistance will be provided so you can make informed health care decisions.
2. **Choice of Providers and Plans.** You have the right to a choice of health care providers that is sufficient to provide you with access to appropriate high-quality health care.
3. **Access to Emergency Services.** If you have severe pain, an injury, or sudden illness that convinces you that your health is in serious jeopardy, you have the right to receive screening and stabilization emergency services whenever and wherever needed, without prior authorization or financial penalty.
4. **Participation in Treatment Decisions.** You have the right to know your treatment options and to participate in decisions about your care. Parents, guardians, family members, or other individuals that you designate can represent you if you cannot make your own decisions.
5. **Respect and Nondiscrimination.** You have a right to considerate, respectful, and nondiscriminatory care from your doctors, health plan representatives, and other health care providers.
6. **Confidentiality of Health Information.** You have the right to talk in confidence with health care providers and to have your health care information protected. You also have the right to review and copy your own medical record and request that your physician change your record if it is not accurate, relevant, or complete.
7. **Complaints and Appeals.** You have the right to a fair, fast, and objective review of any complaint you have against your health plan, doctors, hospitals, or other health care personnel. This includes complaints about waiting times, operating hours, the conduct of health care personnel, and the adequacy of health care facilities.

(Compiled by The U.S. Advisory Committee on Consumer Protection and Quality in the Health Care Industry.)

information such as births and deaths. Birth certificates may be necessary in some states to obtain marriage licenses, driver's licenses, passports, and so on. Death certificates are necessary for cashing life insurance policies, Social Security, cemeteries, and so on.

The Birth Certificate

A birth certificate is a document of identity that contains the following information:

- Name of the person at time of birth
- Date and time of birth
- Sex of baby
- Place of birth
- Birth registration number
- Legal names of mother and father

This certificate is generally requested by the hospital nursery shortly after the birth of the baby. Most hospital nurseries have computer links that automatically link to the state government record office, where the birth certificate is stored and copies are released from. This is one of a person's most valuable documents because it is the official identity document that will be used for obtaining other documents throughout the years. This document is used as proof of nationality and age, and is used for obtaining a driver's license, passport, and marriage license. A copy of one's birth certificate can be obtained online for a fee of between $15 and $50 depending on the state of issuance.

Death Certificate

A medical office should maintain a file with blank death certificates. Often, a patient will die in a hospital during a physician's office hours. The funeral director must obtain a death certificate before picking up the body, and often will handle this aspect for the family. If your office does not have blank copies of death certificates, the funeral director generally carries them and will provide you with one. The funeral director will fill out the necessary information on the certificate; however, the physician must write the cause of death on the certificate and sign it. The attending physician at the hospital usually supplies the funeral director with the death certificate. How the death certificate is handled depends on state regulations. It is always a good idea to check with your state for accurate information.

GOOD MEDICAL RECORDS . . . A LEGAL ASSET

The importance of good medical records becomes evident in cases of malpractice. Studies have shown that 30% of malpractice cases result from problems with the patient's medical record. Documentation is a very important part of the defense against a malpractice charge and should not be taken lightly. The medical record is one of the most important pieces of evidence in any malpractice case. Most people find it difficult to remember last week, let alone 5 years ago. This is where a good, complete medical record is invaluable. If it contains proper documentation, a medical record can jog the memory of a physician and help him or her recall the events of patient care.

BOX 9-4 The RALTIC Method for Keeping Medical Records

Relevant
Accurate
Legible
Timely
Informative
Complete

Any strange behavior or personality traits should be documented in the patient's chart. The complexity of the problem coupled with a therapeutic plan of action should be carefully explained in the medical record.

All medical records should be kept by using the RALTIC method (Box 9-4). It is important that information in a medical record be *relevant* (containing nothing superfluous), *accurate* (clear and free of error), *legible* (neat and preferably typed), *timely* (dated and in proper sequence), *informative* (e.g., documenting treatment, prognosis, diagnosis), and *complete* (no omissions).

LEGAL LIFE OF FINANCIAL RECORDS

Retention of financial records is an important issue and should be followed closely by the office manager. The following guidelines will assist the office manager in deciding how long to maintain certain financial records in the medical office. They should be reviewed with the practice accountant for verification.

1. Records to be kept indefinitely
   a. General ledgers
   b. Financial statements
   c. Capital assessment records
2. Records to be kept for 10 years
   a. Payroll register
3. Records to be kept for 7 years
   a. Accounts receivable ledger cards
   b. Remittance advice slips (explanations of benefits)
   c. Canceled payroll checks
   d. Day sheets
4. Records to be kept for 5 years
   a. Bank statements/canceled checks/deposit slips
   b. Records on uncollectable accounts
   c. Time cards or time sheets

5. Records to be kept for 4 years
    a. Payments and reports to the government (e.g., Internal Revenue Service [IRS], state government)
    b. Vendor contracts
    c. All dealings with Medicare
6. Records to be kept for 2 years
    a. Purchase orders
7. Records to be kept for 1 year
    a. Accounts receivable trial balances

PHYSICIAN-PATIENT RELATIONSHIP

Medical care is not an inalienable right that is guaranteed to every individual. The physician has control over the patients he or she chooses to treat. However, once the physician-patient relationship has begun, the patient has the right to expect it to continue unless the physician gives him or her suitable notice that it is going to end. Making an appointment does not constitute a physician-patient relationship, but once the patient arrives in the office, the relationship begins. Because there are no specific laws regarding the beginning of this relationship, most cases are decided by state courts. For example, depending on the court, it is possible (although not probable) that a woman to whom a physician gave medical advice during open house at her children's school could view that encounter as a physician-patient relationship. It is important for the office manager to train staff regarding giving advice to patients. When a staff member offers advice to a patient, the law views this as advice from the physician's agent, creating a duty on the physician's part to treat the patient.

In the following circumstances, a physician can see a patient without entering into a physician-patient relationship:

- Examining a patient for life insurance purposes
- Giving expert opinion for a workers' compensation or disability carrier
- Performing a preemployment physical
- Performing a court-ordered examination

Remember that any emergency treatment that a physician offers must be carried through by the physician. In other words, once a physician accepts an undertaking in an emergency situation, he or she is obligated to the patient. The physician may not neglect or withdraw his or her services unless there is another physician available to continue the patient's treatment.

Abandonment

Abandonment is a physician's severance of the professional relationship with a patient without reasonable notification, and during a period when the physician's services were needed by the patient. Once a physician assumes the care and treatment of an individual, a physician-patient relationship is established. During this established relationship, the physician may not withdraw from the patient without giving the patient enough notice to obtain a new physician.

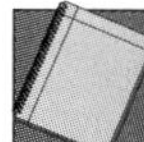

FROM THE EXPERT'S NOTEBOOK

A physician-patient relationship is created when a physician provides care to a patient, either face-to-face or by telephone.

It is the office manager's responsibility to ensure that when the physician is absent from the practice, another physician provides care to the practice's patients. If there is not adequate coverage for the patients during the physician's absence, the physician could be charged with abandonment.

Against Medical Advice

Whenever a patient is unhappy and does not wish to continue treatment with a physician, the patient must sign a form acknowledging that he or she wants to discontinue medical services. All practices should use "against medical advice" forms to protect the physician and legally release the practice from liability from that point forward. A sample template is illustrated in Figure 9-1. A patient cannot be forced to sign this form. Should a patient refuse to sign, the form should be signed and dated by any of the personnel that are present to witness the refusal. The words "signature refused" should then be placed on the form before it is filed in the chart.

Good Samaritan Law

The Good Samaritan Law was developed to protect health professionals when treating persons in emergency situations within the scope of their training. This law varies widely state by state; in most states, immunity is granted only during an emergency. The American Medical Association Web site provides information on this law for all states within the United States and the District of Columbia at www.ama-assn.org/ama/pub/category/15833.

The definition of *emergency* for this purpose is "a combination of unforeseen circumstances that require spontaneous actions to prevent impending danger." However, even with the law on your side, the courts have the final decision as to whether the situation requires spontaneous actions to prevent impending danger. For example, a family physician in Pennsylvania attended to a 21-year-old woman involved in an automobile accident in front of his office. Fearing the car would explode, he believed it necessary to amputate her leg

This is to certify that I am discontinuing medical services at my own insistence and against the advice of my physician, Dr. ____________________. I have been informed of the consequences and dangers of my actions of discontinuing medical services at this time. I assume all responsibility for any results caused by discontinuing medical services, and I hereby release the physician, the practice, and its employees and officers from all liability.

Patient name: ____

Patient signature: ____

I agree to hold harmless the practice, its employees and officers, and my physician from all liability with reference to the discharge of the patient named above.

Patient representative: ____

Date: ____________________

Witness signature/title: ____

FIGURE 9-1. Discontinuing medical services against medical advice.

at the scene in order to pull her from the wreckage. He amputated her left leg, pulled her to safety, and essentially saved her life. She and her family later sued him and won. In this case, the courts found that the patient was not in impending danger and ruled against the physician.

Termination of the Problem Patient

One of the major considerations of dismissing a problem patient is a law protecting discrimination against people with disabilities. This law, the 1990 Americans with Disabilities Act, was designed to prevent discrimination based on disability. A disability is any physical or psychologic problem that makes the individual unable to perform daily life activities. The term *psychologic* is defined legally as any emotional or mental illness. Some physicians have patients with severe psychologic problems whose behavior disrupts the medical office. If a physician decides to terminate the physician-patient relationship with such a patient, he or she could be liable under the 1990 Americans with Disabilities Act. This law specifically addresses professional health care offices. Any noncompliant or disruptive patient with psychologic problems that could be regarded as a disability is protected by this law. However, if it can be proved that a patient is interfering with the care of others, it is possible to terminate the physician-patient relationship under the new law without complications. The office manager should be aware of the law; however, if paper trails are created, and documentation of disruptive acts and verbal abuse to the staff and physician is carefully entered into the patient's medical record, there should be no problems with dismissal.

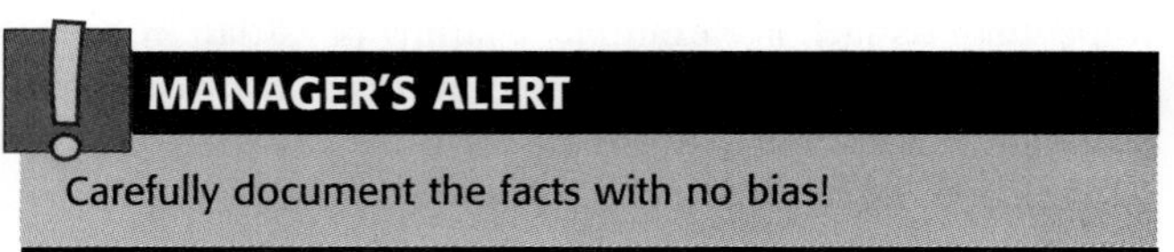

MANAGER'S ALERT
Carefully document the facts with no bias!

Cases have been brought to court for wrongful termination of the physician-patient relationship because of psychologic disability, but to date these cases have been decided in favor of the physician. A 2-week to 1-month notice is recommended for patients to secure a new physician. An attorney will generally recommend that if the physician is terminating a patient for psychologic reasons (e.g., noncompliance, disruptive behavior), the office should not give the patient the exact reason for the termination. Some sample termination letters are shown in Figure 9-2. Any of these letters can be changed to fit the needs of the practice. The office manager should discuss these letters with the physician to be sure that a correct format is used.

Patients who are noncompliant and disruptive, miss appointments, and have drug problems are the most likely to sue a physician. This type of patient should be terminated as soon as a problem develops, because continued care only increases potential liability. The office manager should ask staff members who are involved in the care of patients to point out problem patients. If the physician is not aware of these problems, it is the office manager's job to present the past problems to the physician and feedback from the staff.

The office manager will find that many of these patients do not pay their bills and can sometimes be gently nudged out of the office by continued pressing for payment. These patients do not want to pay, so they dismiss the physician when asked for payment. This eliminates the need for the office to initiate termination action.

Good office staff will often recognize a problem patient in the first call for an appointment, and feedback from the staff should not be ignored. Listen to them! The office is not required to take every patient who calls.

CERTIFIED MAIL DELIVERY: A MUST!

Termination letters should be sent by certified mail with a return receipt requested. One copy of the letter should also be sent by regular mail, and another copy should remain as

Dear Ms. Conklin:
We are no longer able to provide care to you and request that you find another physician within [time period designated by office policy] of the date of this letter. If you have an emergency, we will continue to provide you with medical care for the time period stated above, or you may seek medical care in the nearest emergency room. Once you have obtained a new physician, we will be happy to forward a copy of your medical records to him or her. It will be necessary for you to either sign a Records Release Form or send us a note with your signature and the address of the new physician.

Sincerely,

Alexander Babinetz, M.D.

Dear Mr. Hessler:
I find it necessary to inform you that I will no longer be able to serve as your physician or prescribe medications for you.

The reason for this decision is: ____________________

Because you may need medical attention in the future, I recommend that you promptly find another doctor to care for you. You may want to contact the medical society or local hospital for the names of physicians near you who are accepting new patients.

I will be available to provide you with emergency care until ____________________. This will give you time to obtain a new physician. I will be happy to forward a copy of your medical records to your new physician upon receipt of a signed Records Release Form from the physician.

Sincerely,

Alexander Babinetz, M.D.

Dear Mr. Miller:
Because you have refused to follow our medical advice by signing out of the hospital, we find it necessary to terminate our physician–patient relationship. We feel that we can no longer have a beneficial, therapeutic relationship with you and would be pleased to send your records to the physician of your choice.

If you require medical attention before securing a new physician, we urge you to seek care in the nearest hospital emergency room. We do urge you to seek a new physician as soon as possible.

Sincerely,

Alexander Babinetz, M.D.
for Cardiovascular Specialists

Dear Mrs. Matthews:
I find it necessary to inform you that I am withdrawing from further professional attendance of your medical needs because you have persisted in refusing to follow my medical advice and treatment. Because your condition requires medical attention, I suggest that you place yourself under the care of another physician without delay. If you so desire, I shall be available to attend to you for a reasonable time after you have received this letter, but in no event for more than 5 days from the date of this letter.

This should give you ample time to select a physician of your choice from the many competent physicians in this area. With your approval, I will make available to this physician your case history and information regarding the diagnosis and treatment that you have received from me.

Sincerely,

Alexander Babinetz, M.D.

FIGURE 9-2. Sample patient termination letters.

a permanent part of the patient's medical record. There is a fee for certified mail delivery, but it provides the sender with a receipt bearing the signature of the person who received the letter. This receipt should be kept attached to the copy of the letter in the patient's chart.

To send the letter, the envelope must be attached to a white receipt for certified mail. The receipt must be filled out with the recipient's name and address. A green delivery receipt with the recipient's name and address on one side and your name and address on the other must also be completed. The green delivery receipt will be returned to you as a postcard with the recipient's signature on it. This type of mail service is discussed in Chapter 4.

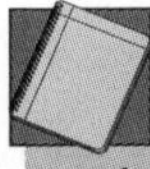

FROM THE EXPERT'S NOTEBOOK

Ask the postal clerk to stamp the front of the envelope with "addressee only/restricted delivery." This ensures that no one else but the patient or designee is allowed to sign for the letter.

Often, certified mail will be returned to the office stating that it was not picked up. Many individuals have debts that result in regular calls and letters from creditors. They generally will not pick up certified mail for this reason. This is why a copy of the letter should be sent by regular mail also. The returned envelope should also be placed in the patient's medical record.

Alternatives to Termination

There are other ways in which the medical office can care for patients who should be terminated but who need further care. Difficult patients who require extensive amounts of testing can be referred to a state teaching hospital or enrolled in a courtesy patient plan at the local community hospital. Any hospital that receives funds from the federal government must provide a certain amount of free and charitable care to individuals with hardships. Many patients are difficult simply because they do not have the funds to obtain further testing. More and more individuals refuse testing because they are unemployed or uninsured. The letter in Figure 9-3 can be sent to patients who find themselves in need of care that they cannot afford.

Informing patients that they are possibly going to be terminated from the physician's practice is another alternative to actually taking the action. Telling patients that they are being considered for termination from the practice because they refuse to take their medications is sometimes enough to motivate them into compliance.

Boomerang Patients

If the practice is old enough, there might be occasion to deal with the "boomerang" patient. Many physicians find themselves in the predicament of being on call in the emergency department and having a dismissed patient appear and require treatment. The physician, who is unable to refuse treatment in this circumstance, should explain to the patient at the time of service that this emergency treatment is on a one-time basis only. The physician should carefully explain that this does not reaffirm their physician-patient relationship. It is good for the office manager to check the bylaws of the hospital before this situation arises to be sure that the physician's actions are in line with them.

HIPPOCRATIC OATH

There are two versions of the Hippocratic Oath, classical and modern. This oath defines principals and ethics for physician and is one of the oldest documents in the world. The classical version of the oath was credited to Hippocrates in the fourth century BCE. Although Hippocrates is believed to be the father of medicine, it is widely believed that the oath was actually written by followers of Pythagoras. No matter who wrote this oath, it is considered to be the rule for practitioners of medicine to follow. The classical version of this oath is provided in Box 9-5.

The modern version of this oath was written in 1964 by Louis Lasagna, Academic Dean of the School of Medicine at Tufts University, and is provided in Box 9-6.

AMERICAN MEDICAL ASSOCIATION CODE OF MEDICAL ETHICS

The American Medical Association (AMA) was founded by Nathan Davis in 1847. Dr. Davis received his doctorate degree in 1837 and began working as a physician in the

Dear Mrs. Casey:

As we discussed during your recent office visit, your condition is still undiagnosed and lies in an area outside my circle of expertise. It could be nothing, or it could be very serious. I will continue to serve as your physician, but you must understand that it is impossible for me to provide you with the kind of care you require if funds are not available for the tests you need. I would like to take this opportunity to refer you to a hospital where you might obtain the testing that is necessary for your care.

Should you wish to follow through with this suggestion, please call my office and my staff will help you make arrangements for your testing.

Sincerely,

Alexander Babinetz, M.D.

FIGURE 9-3. Letter recommending courtesy treatment.

BOX 9-5 Hippocratic Oath

I swear by Apollo Physician and Asclepius and Hygieia and Panaceia and all the gods and goddesses, making them my witnesses, that I will fulfill according to my ability and judgment this oath and this covenant:

- To hold him who has taught me this art as equal to my parents and to live my life in partnership with him, and if he is in need of money to give him a share of mine, and to regard his offspring as equal to my brothers in male lineage and to teach them this art—if they desire to learn it—without fee and covenant; to give a share of precepts and oral instruction and all the other learning to my sons and to the sons of him who has instructed me and to pupils who have signed the covenant and have taken an oath according to the medical law, but no one else.
- I will apply dietetic measures for the benefit of the sick according to my ability and judgment; I will keep them from harm and injustice.
- I will neither give a deadly drug to anybody who asked for it, nor will I make a suggestion to this effect. Similarly I will not give to a woman an abortive remedy. In purity and holiness I will guard my life and my art.
- I will not use the knife, not even on sufferers from stone, but will withdraw in favor of such men as are engaged in this work.
- Whatever houses I may visit, I will come for the benefit of the sick, remaining free of all intentional injustice, of all mischief and in particular of sexual relations with both female and male persons, be they free or slaves.
- What I may see or hear in the course of the treatment or even outside of the treatment in regard to the life of men, which on no account one must spread abroad, I will keep to myself, holding such things shameful to be spoken about.
- If I fulfill this oath and do not violate it, may it be granted to me to enjoy life and art, being honored with fame among all men for all time to come; if I transgress it and swear falsely, may the opposite of all this be my lot.

BOX 9-6 Modern Hippocratic Oath

I swear to fulfill, to the best of my ability and judgment, this covenant:

- I will respect the hard-won scientific gains of those physician in whose steps I walk, and gladly share such knowledge as is mine with those who are to follow.
- I will apply, for the benefit of the sick, all measures that are required, avoiding those twin traps of overtreatment and therapeutic nihilism.
- I will remember that there is art to medicine as well as science, and that warmth, sympathy, and understanding may outweigh the surgeon's knife or the chemist's drug.
- I will not be ashamed to say "I know not," nor will I fail to call in my colleagues when the skills of another are needed for a patient's recovery.
- I will respect the privacy of my patients, for their problems are not disclosed to me that the world may know. Most especially must I tread with care in matters of life and death. If it is given me to save a life, all thanks. But I may also be within my power to take a life; this awesome responsibility must be faced with great humbleness and awareness of my own frailty. Above all, I must not play at God.
- I will remember that I do not treat a fever chart, a cancerous growth, but a sick human being, whose illness may affect the person's family and economic stability. My responsibility includes these related problems, if I am to care adequately for the sick.
- I will prevent disease whenever I can, for prevention is preferable to cure.
- I will remember that I remain a member of society, with special obligations to all my fellow human beings, those sound of mind and body as well as the infirm.

If I do not violate this oath, may I enjoy life and art, respected while I live and remembered with affection thereafter. May I always act so as to preserve the finest traditions of my calling and may I long experience the joy of healing those who seek my help.

state of New York. He was elected to the New York Medical Society and began working on a set of standards for medical education. These standards evolved into the establishment of the AMA in 1847.

The AMA Code of Medical Ethics is maintained by the Council on Ethical and Judicial Affairs. This council consists of seven physicians, one resident, and one medical student and is responsible for the updating of all ethics policies for the AMA. This code was developed in 1803 by Thomas Percival, a physician, philosopher, and writer. When the AMA had its first meeting in 1847, it adopted Percival's code of ethics as the code that would be used by the AMA. This code consists of nine principles and must be followed by all who are members of the AMA:

1. A physician shall be dedicated to providing competent medical care, compassion, and respect for human dignity and rights.
2. A physician shall uphold the standards of professionalism, be honest in all professional interactions, and strive to report physicians deficient in character or competence, or engaging in fraud or deception, to appropriate entities.
3. A physician shall respect the law and also recognize a responsibility of changes in those requirements, which are contrary to the best interests of the patient.
4. A physician shall respect the rights of patients, colleagues, and other health professionals, and shall safeguard patient confidences and privacy within the constraints of the law.

5. A physician shall continue to study, apply, and advance scientific knowledge, maintain a commitment to medical education, make relevant information available to patients, colleagues, and the public, obtain consultation, and use the talents of other health professionals when indicated.
6. A physician shall, in the provision of appropriate patient care, except in emergencies, be free to choose whom to serve, with whom the physician associates, and the environment in which to provide medical care.
7. A physician shall recognize a responsibility to participate in activities contributing to the improvement of the community and the betterment of public health.
8. A physician shall, while caring for a patient, regard responsibility to the patient as paramount.
9. A physician shall support access to medical care for all people.

This code of ethics, as it stands now, was last revised in 2001.

ETHICS: THE GRAY GHOST

Many philosophers, teachers, and theologians agree that there is no objective method of arriving at an ethical decision. When it comes to ethics, there is no right answer, there is just a range of acceptable actions that can be taken. Most hospitals now have ethics committees that guide physicians and other staff members through various situations. These committees can minimize many conflicts between physicians, staff members, and families and help defuse volatile situations when they arise.

Physicians face many difficult ethical choices in today's world of high-tech medicine. The following list identifies some of the many ethical dilemmas faced by physicians:

- End-of-life decisions
- Organ donations
- Confidentiality
- HIV detection and notification
- Mapping of genomes
- Beginning-of-life technologies
- Disclosure of medical errors
- Ethics and the pharmaceutical industry

Care for the Dying

Unfortunately, every office has patients who are battling life-threatening diseases, who have been in pain for so long that they lose the will to live. Medical practices now have a new place to turn for help for these patients: palliative care programs.

These innovative programs are answering the need for end-of-life care that emphasizes humanity, not just technology. They provide warmth and comfort to the dying patient. Palliative care means treating the symptoms of terminally ill patients such as pain, nausea, and depression. Some programs are expanding their coverage to cover all seriously ill people, including those with chronic ailments. The benefit to a patient is that the physicians and nurses are trained in advanced pain relief and include the family as part of the treatment. They will also help the patient decide whether to undergo therapy. When the patient's primary physician is busy seeing other patients, these physicians have the time to sit and talk.

END-OF-LIFE DECISIONS

In the United States, the Patient Self-Determination Act guarantees individuals the right to decide for themselves the limits they wish to set on the use of life-sustaining therapy when they are terminally ill or in a vegetative state. This law came into effect in December 1991. It requires that hospitals, nursing homes, personal care facilities, hospices, home health care agencies, and health maintenance organizations ask patients whether they have prepared an advance directive (also called a *living will* or a *durable power of attorney*) for health care.

The medical office can help patients by understanding the Patient Self-Determination Act and having blank living wills and durable power of attorney forms in their offices. In fact, the law requires that institutions educate staff members and the community about the law. The office manager should instruct the staff on the law and its ramifications in a workshop or seminar. It can be very helpful if all staff are familiar with the law and can aid the physician in educating patients. With all the attention this topic has received in television programs, radio talk shows, newspapers, and magazines, it is unusual for patients to know nothing of these directives. Still, a good medical office will not wait until the last minute to speak to patients about the Patient Self-Determination Act (Figure 9-4). It is a good practice to discuss it before it is actually needed, so that emotions do not cloud the decision-making process. The office manager may want to designate one staff member to finish with the patient after the physician has begun the education process. It is easier if the patient brings up the subject, and this can be gently encouraged by keeping

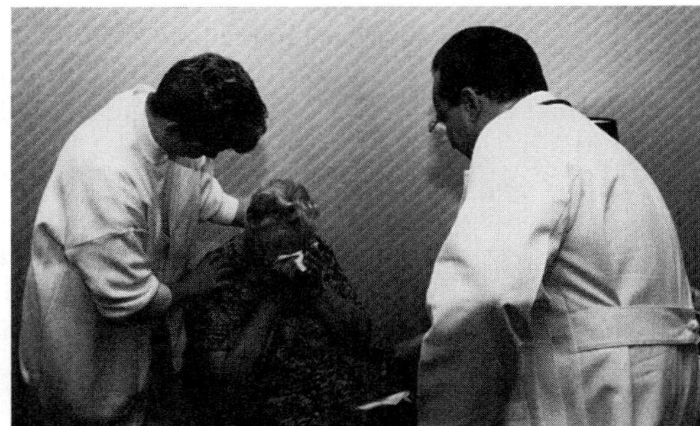

FIGURE 9-4. Discussing end-of-life decisions can be emotional.

As authorized by the Commonwealth of Pennsylvania "Advance Directive For Health Care Act," April 1992.

I, ________________________________, being of sound mind, willfully and voluntarily make this declaration to be followed if I become incompetent. This declaration reflects my firm and settled commitment to refuse life-sustaining treatment under the circumstances indicated below.

I direct my attending physician to withhold or withdraw life-sustaining treatment that serves only to prolong the process of my dying, if I should be in a terminal condition or in a state of permanent unconsciousness.

I direct that treatment be limited to measures to keep me comfortable and to relieve pain, including any pain that might occur by with holding or withdrawing life-sustaining treatment.

In addition, if I am in the condition described above, I feel especially strong about the following forms of treatment:

I do or do not want cardiac resuscitation.

I do or do not want mechanical respiration.

I do or do not want tube feeding or any other artificial or invasive form of nutrition (food) or hydration (water).

I do or do not want blood or blood products.

I do or do not want any form of surgery or invasive diagnostic tests.

I do or do not want kidney dialysis.

I do or do not want antibiotics.

I realize that if I do not specifically indicate my preference regarding any of the forms of treatment listed above, I may receive that form of treatment.

Other instructions:

I do or do not want to designate another person as my surrogate to make medical treatment decisions for me if I should be incompetent and in a terminal condition or in a state of permanent unconsciousness. Name and address of surrogate, if applicable:

Name and address of substitute surrogate (if surrogate designated above is unable to serve):

I made this declaration on the _____day of ______________ (month, year).

Declarant's signature: ______________________________

Declarant's address: ______________________________

The declarant or the person on behalf of and at the direction of the declarant knowingly and voluntarily signed this writing by signature or mark in my presence.

Witness's signature: ______________________________

Witness's address: ______________________________

Witness's signature: ______________________________

Witness's address: ______________________________

(Courtesy of the Delaware Valley Geriatrics Society.)

FIGURE 9-5. Living Will Declaration (for the state of Pennsylvania). (Courtesy of the Delaware Valley Geriatrics Society.)

booklets about the Patient Self-Determination Act in the waiting room. Many patients will become interested in speaking with someone about the act. Each state has developed booklets and forms that can be obtained for use by patients. Figure 9-5 shows Pennsylvania's living will.

DOCTORS ADVISE . . . PATIENTS DECIDE

When a patient has prepared an advance directive, the medical office and the physician can make treatment decisions regarding the aggressiveness of a patient's care. It is very helpful for the physician to take the time to explain advance directives to patients so they clearly understand the ramifications of their decisions (Figure 9-6). Many community centers and church groups are also becoming involved in educating people about the Patient Self-Determination Act.

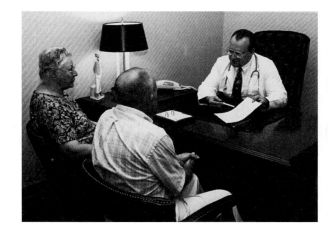

FIGURE 9-6. A physician explains a living will to patients.

Some states do not honor the living will. The office manager must contact the practice's attorney to check on state regulations. The office might be located in a state that honors a durable power of attorney but not a living will. Be it a living will or a durable power of attorney, some form of advance directive is now necessary. Health care providers who comply with valid advance directives are immune from civil and criminal liability. Withholding or withdrawing life-sustaining treatment in compliance with a valid advance directive does not constitute a suicide or a homicide.

This immunity notwithstanding, health care providers are not forced to comply with the advance directive. The advance directive can be revoked at any time and in any manner by the patient, regardless of the patient's physical or mental condition at the time it is revoked. This revocation becomes a part of the patient's medical record.

A different format of living will from that shown in Figure 9-5 is shown in Figure 9-7. It may be changed to follow specific guidelines issued by individual states. Living will and durable power of attorney forms may be obtained from the local medical society.

ORGAN DONATIONS

Most potential organ donors fall under medical-legal jurisdiction. In most cases, the medical examiner is the person responsible for the authorization of the organs or tissues for use by another. According to the United Organ Sharing Network (UNOS), the waiting list is so large that approximately 17 people die each day from that list. As of August 2006, there were 92,715 people on this network awaiting organ and tissue donations. This is an extremely grave situation for children who are in need of an organ or a tissue. They have considerable restraints because of the size of the organs being donated. Unfortunately, the needs of the medical examiner come first with respect to organ donations, and organs often cannot be authorized because of the medical-legal need to keep the body intact. This is especially important in the death of a child, and, of course, those organs are the most valued. More and more people are becoming organ donors; however, this only amounts to about 15% at this time. If a patient has requested that he or she be an organ donor, the medical practice staff should advise the proper authorities in this matter.

The following is a list of important things to know about organ donation:

- Donors can range in age from birth to 75 years old.
- Tissues, such as eyes, skin, bone, and heart valves, can be donated up to 24 hours after death.
- Donation can be considered only after every effort has been made to save a patient's life.
- Organ and tissue donation does not interfere with funeral services.
- Every 30 minutes a new name is added to the transplant waiting list, while an average of six people die every day awaiting organ transplants.
- Patients who are organ donors will have a stamp on their driver's license or a card in their wallet.
- Transplants work. About 80% of all transplants result in patients living full and active lives.
- One donor can save or enhance 50 lives!

This declaration is made this day, ________________ . I, Janet Casey, being of sound mind, willfully and voluntarily make known my desires that my moment of death shall not be artificially postponed.

If at any time I should have an incurable and irreversible injury, disease, or illness judged to be a terminal condition by my attending physician, who has personally examined me and has determined that my death is imminent except for death-delaying procedures, I direct that procedures that would only prolong the dying process be withheld or withdrawn and that I be permitted to die naturally with only the administration of medication, sustenance, or the performance of any medical procedure deemed necessary by my attending physician to provide me with comfortable care.

In the absence of my ability to give directions regarding the use of such death-delaying procedures, it is my intention that this declaration shall be honored by my family and physician as the final expression of my legal right to refuse medical or surgical treatment and accept the consequences from such refusal.

Signed: ***Janet Casey***

The city, county, and state of residence of the declarant is personally known to me, and I believe him or her to be of sound mind. I saw the declarant sign the declaration in my presence (or the declarant acknowledged in my presence that he or she had signed the declaration) and I signed the declaration as a witness in the presence of the declarant. I did not sign the declarant's signature above for or at the direction of the declarant. At the date of this instrument, I am not entitled to any portion of the estate of the declarant according to the laws of intestate succession or, to the best of my knowledge and belief, under any will of declarant or other instrument taking effect at declarant's death, nor am I directly financially responsible for declarant's medical care.

Witness: ***Lynn Giononi***
Witness: ***Lisa Braun***

FIGURE 9-7. A sample living will.

Confidentiality

Information that is shared between a physician and a patient for the purpose of medical treatment is considered confidential communication. Any unauthorized disclosure of this information breaches the physician's contractual obligation to the patient. The vast majority of states have strict regulations regarding confidentiality of the information physicians receive from their patients. Most state physician-patient statutes are similar to the following:

No physician should be allowed, in any civil matter, to disclose any information acquired while attending the patient in a professional capacity, which enabled him to act in that capacity, which shall tend to blacken the character of the patient, without consent of the patient, except in civil matters brought by such patient for damages on account of personal injuries. If any of the above elements are met in the physician-patient relationship, the physician is barred from disclosing any information without the patient's permission.

The purpose of adopting a physician-patient privilege was to create an atmosphere in which patients could feel secure enough to disclose any information that might pertain to their medical problems. The Principles of Medical Ethics issued by the AMA establish a broader statute of confidentiality than is found in the judicial codes. The AMA code of ethics advocates the confidentiality of all contacts between the medical office and the patient.

There are a few exceptions to the states' Duty of Confidentiality statutes that are pertinent to daily operations in a medical office. A patient's medical information may be released in the following circumstances:

- The patient files a lawsuit for personal injuries
- Patient consent has been obtained
- The court orders release of information
- A third party has requested it and the patient has given consent

A patient who files a lawsuit for personal injuries waives the physician-patient relationship by filing suit. This suit implies consent for disclosure of medically related injuries or illnesses. It is not uncommon for patient records to be requested by third parties such as insurance companies and employers. Records can be released to third parties with the patient's consent. A court may order a patient's medical information in cases involving communicable disease and child abuse.

Each state has a law regarding the confidentiality of HIV testing. The smart office manager obtains copies of state guidelines regarding HIV testing and distributes them to the staff during an office meeting when discussing policy and procedure.

In today's high-tech world, we use fax machines for a multitude of purposes. Many offices fax test results, medical records, and so on to hospitals. Insurance companies will even request that medical records be faxed. Confidentiality is a serious issue when using a fax machine to transmit information. It is very important to add a confidentiality notice to the fax transmission cover sheet. This will protect the faxed information from being disseminated or photocopied. A sample confidentiality notice is shown in Box 9-7.

BOX 9-7 Confidentiality Notice for Faxed Information

This facsimile message and the document(s) accompanying this fax transmission may contain confidential information, which is legally privileged and intended only for the use of the addressee named above. If the reader is not the intended recipient or the employee of the intended recipient, you are hereby notified that any dissemination, copying, or distribution of this communication is strictly prohibited. If you received this communication in error, please notify us immediately by fax or telephone and return the original documents to us via the U.S. Postal Service at the above address. Thank you for your help.

HIV Detection and Notification

A wide range of ethical and moral issues surround the HIV epidemic. The following are issues that need to be addressed by the AMA and health care regulatory agencies:

- Mandatory testing of health care workers
- Mandatory screening of patients for HIV
- Confidentiality
- Discrimination

Genome and Beginning-of-Life Technologies

A *genome* is a complete gene set of an individual. In one of the most exciting scientific endeavors in history, scientists have been making radical attempts to alter the basic building blocks of the body and personality by altering genomes. With a patient's genomic information, physicians can intervene and alter the genetic structure before a disease manifests. The concern, however, is that some physicians may use genomic information simply to change people's behavior, not prevent disease.

More pressing for society at this point are issues that this increasing reproductive technology has presented us. The following is a list of issues of which the medical office should be aware:

- The gift procedure
- Fetus harvesting
- Sperm donors
- Egg donors
- Surrogate motherhood
- Abortion of the problem fetus

Beginning-of-life topics and subjects related to the mapping of genomes are not issues that most medical office staff will have to face. They are mentioned here merely to make the office manager aware and to provide a very basic understanding of them.

Disclosure of Medical Errors

Medical errors are the fifth leading cause of death in the United States. These errors result in costs of $29 billion on an annual basis. In a survey by the Institute of Medicine, 95% of physicians reported being a witness to a medical error and 61% of health care professionals believe that errors are often preventable. According to the report, many of the errors are due to mistakes such as poor communication between multiple health care providers and inadequate labeling of drug interactions. This type of error is often preventable with the use of an electronic medical record system that can improve the coordination of care, identify any potential errors, investigate them, and prevent them from happening. The ethical decisions come when a medical error is witnessed; should someone be notified, or should it be overlooked? This is of particular interest to medical students who may witness such errors. It also applies to the staff of a medical practice. After all, the physician is signing their paycheck, so do they want to get involved? If this occurs, it is best to approach the physician and discuss the turn of events.

Ethics and the Pharmaceutical Industry

Much controversy arises about medical practice and the pharmaceutical industry. Physicians and the pharmaceutical industry share a number of common interests. Both parties share the same concerns regarding the medical necessity of drugs, monitoring their use, and drug research. The differences, however, are great. The physician is interested in the care of the patient and any scientific advances that may benefit the patient. Although that is of concern to the pharmaceutical industry, its main focus is the commercial outcome. The three main concerns by both the physician and the community are as follows:

- The possibility that the association of the physician and the pharmaceutical company may lean more toward the goals of the company as opposed to the ethical obligation of the physician to the patient
- The risk that pharmaceutical representative visits and sales pitches will have an effect on the physician's decisions on what drugs to use
- The danger that industry involved in research will lead to skewed data that may prevent independent assessment of data

There seems to be a need for clear-cut procedures that will address such issues as gifts to physicians, sponsorship of conferences, and continuing education activities.

LEGAL ASPECTS OF HEALTH CARE

Consent

Consent is the voluntary agreement by a person who has sufficient mentality to make an intelligent choice to allow something proposed by another. It can be either express or implied. *Express consent* is a verbal or written agreement to undergo a medical procedure. *Implied consent* is consent implied by some type of action or inaction by silence that leads to the presumption that consent has been given. Consent must be obtained from the patient, or from a person authorized to be a delegate of the patient, before any medical or surgical procedure can be done. Touching a patient who has not given consent to be touched could be considered battery. It is necessary to give patients sufficient information, in a form that they can understand, before asking them to make health care choices. Informed consent requires that patients have full understanding of that to which they have consented.

IMPLIED CONSENT

Implied consent exists in emergencies, when immediate action is required to save a patient's life. An emergency situation "trumps" the need for a signed consent and provides the health care professional permission to provide treatment. If and when it may be necessary to protect the life or the health of a patient, it is important to document the need to treat before obtaining an informed consent from the patient.

INFORMED CONSENT

Informed consent is when the physician is obligated to disclose information to the patient regarding a service or procedure so that the patient can make an informed decision as to whether or not to proceed. The patient must have a thorough understanding of the consent. Informed consent must be documented by way of explanation of the service or procedure and the risks involved. It cannot be waived because of a patient's anxiety. Informed consent is valid for 30 days from the date that it is signed. In cases where treatments are planned in advance, such as chemotherapy, consent may be obtained for the treatments to be provided up to 6 months in advance. An informed consent must contain the following five elements:

- The diagnosis of the patient
- The purpose of the proposed treatment/procedure
- The possible risks and benefits of the proposed treatment/procedure
- Possible alternatives to the proposed treatment/procedure
- The possible risks of not receiving the treatment/procedure

CONSENT OF A MENTALLY ILL PATIENT

It is not possible for a patient who is mentally ill to consent to treatment. In this case, it is necessary to obtain consent from the patient's legal guardian. If there is no legal guardian, the court is petitioned to give permission to treat.

CONSENT OF A MINOR

When medical treatment is rendered to a minor, the physician must obtain consent of the minor's parent or guardian (someone standing in loco parentis) before performing a service or procedure.

The only exception to this rule is if the child has an immediate need for care and is in an emergency situation. Parental consent is not necessary if the minor is married or emancipated (free from traditional social restraints). Most states permit a minor in this circumstance to provide consent that is considered by the letter of the law. Many states have passed legislation permitting treatment for pregnancy, sexually transmitted diseases, and drug dependency without consent of the parents. The reason for this leniency is that the government is concerned that minors with these conditions will not seek care should it require the consent of the parents and that it is more important to provide care to minors in need. Health care personnel in each state must follow the state guidelines when dealing with minors.

LACK OF CONSENT

In a case where the patient is competent, yet there is not consent, treatment would be considered battery. Patients have the right to be informed of the risks and benefits of services and procedures that may be recommended by their physicians. The medical practice should have a policy regarding the patient's rights and informed consent.

Authorization for Release of Information

In order for a physician practice to release medical information regarding a patient, there must be a written consent by the patient to do so. Patients can revoke their consent at any time by submitting their wishes in writing to the physician practice. According to the Health Insurance Portability and Accountability Act (HIPAA) (45CFR Sec. 164.502), patient authorization is not required for release of health information under the following scenarios:

- Treatment of illness or injury
- Legal request such as a subpoena or warrant
- Approved research program
- Request of family members
- Civil and criminal proceedings
- Medical record audits
- Payment
- Public health
- Circumstances of domestic violence
- Organ donation procurement

Patient authorization must be obtained to use protected health information (PHI) for marketing or employment issues. The privacy rule of HIPAA does not preempt any state laws, so it becomes very important to research the appropriate state law. All patients must sign a consent in order to be treated.

GUIDELINES FOR AUTHORIZATION FORMS

Each form should contain, at a minimum, the following information:

- The name of the individuals to whom the disclosure can be made
- The date or date range that the authorization expires
- The name of the physician practice that will be disclosing the information
- A signature line for the individual's signature and date the form was signed
- A detailed summary of the information that may be disclosed
- A line stating that this authorization may be revoked by the individual by way of written direction

Reportable Diseases/Incidences

A reportable disease is one that is considered to be a threat to public health. Should a physician encounter a diagnosis of one of the reportable diseases, it is necessary for the physician to report the diagnosis to the local health department or the Department of Health in the state in which it was diagnosed. The following is a list of the most common diagnoses that must be reported:

- AIDS/HIV infection
- Chickenpox
- Chlamydial infections
- Encephalitis
- Food poisoning
- Giardiasis
- Gonorrhea
- *Haemophilus influenzae*
- Hepatitis A, B, and C
- Legionellosis
- Malaria
- Meningitis
- Mumps
- Pertussis
- Poliomyelitis
- Rabies
- Rubella
- Salmonellas
- Shigellosis
- Syphilis
- Tetanus

Although not a threat to public health, all cancers need to be reported to a cancer registry for tracking purposes. Each state compiles its own list of reportable diseases.

There are also certain conditions or incidences that require physician reporting. These are deemed reportable based on state guidelines. Some of these conditions are as follows:

- Impaired drivers (impaired vision, epilepsy)
- Impaired physicians
- Injuries as a result of a deadly weapon (defined as any weapon used to produce bodily harm and cause death or serious bodily injury).
- Abuse (elderly, child, spousal)
- High blood alcohol levels
- Stillborn births
- Deaths
  - Occurring 24 hours after discharge from hospital
  - As a result of violence
  - From an unknown cause

Each state compiles its own list of reportable conditions or incidences.

Negligence

It is a serious mistake for a practice to assume that it will never be sued. A high degree of skill and strict adherence to the code of professional ethics are not enough to guarantee that a practice won't be subject to a malpractice suit. Suits based on negligence generally require a patient to prove the case with expert medical testimony. A bad medical outcome is not necessarily proof of negligence. The patient's attorney must show that the damages sustained by the patient were due to an error that would not have been committed by a physician exercising reasonable care and skill in accepted standards of care. A physician is responsible not only for his or her personal care of a patient, but also for the care provided by his or her employees. It is extremely important for a physician to have adequate malpractice insurance to cover such episodes, should they occur.

LOWERING THE CHANCES OF A SUIT

Negligence is the commission or omission of an act that a reasonably prudent person would not or would do under any given circumstance. This conduct, which is caused by heedlessness or carelessness, deviates from accepted standards of care. There is no sure way to guard against a lawsuit; even the best physicians are threatened at some time in their careers. Why do patients sue? Dissatisfaction—that is key! Maintaining good relations with patients is a way to minimize malpractice suits. Many suits arise from unhappy patients who feel that the physician didn't care or the staff was rude.

Patients want a physician who is available, cares, and listens to them. They want an office staff that is warm, caring, efficient, and professional in every way. All patients believe their problem is an emergency, regardless of whether the staff agrees. Well-trained office staff always listen, and never give patients the impression they are not important or their problem is not urgent. Often the decision to initiate a suit is encouraged by a neighbor across the street, a family member dealing with guilt, or a person with a financial crisis in the family. Chapter 15 discusses many ways the office can promote patient satisfaction. Many suits can be prevented by simply making it a point to maintain good relationships with patients. Table 9-1 lists state statutes of limitation for malpractice and wrongful death charges.

Following are seven ways to prevent malpractice suits:

1. Maintain accurate medical records.
2. Have a risk management plan.
3. Provide patient services based on standards of care.
4. Maintain good rapport with patients.
5. Have prescription renewal policies in place.
6. Show respect for patients and their families.
7. Strive for good treatment outcomes.

The legal importance of keeping good medical records has already been discussed in this chapter. In addition to keeping accurate records, it is necessary for the office to develop a good risk management plan and stick to it! Solid foundations for medical care and good rapport with patients are a must; they can alleviate many unpleasant situations. The need for a good prescription policy has already been discussed; however, it's not enough simply to have a written policy. You must abide by it . . . no exceptions! Having respect for patients and their families is one of the most important things the office can do to prevent malpractice suits. Treat patients and their families as you would want to be treated, and you will never go wrong. Good outcomes, of course, are what everyone wants, but they are not always possible. Everyone must recognize this while continuing to do the very best they can.

FORMS OF NEGLIGENCE

Negligence can take the following forms:

- Malfeasance
- Misfeasance
- Nonfeasance
- Malpractice
- Criminal negligence

Malfeasance is the execution of an unlawful or improper act. *Misfeasance* is the improper performance of an act, resulting in injury to another. *Nonfeasance* is the failure to act, when there is a duty to act, as a reasonably prudent person would act. *Malpractice* is the negligence or carelessness of a professional person. *Criminal negligence* is a reckless disregard for the safety of another. It is the willful indifference to an injury that could follow an act.

TABLE 9-1 State Statutes of Limitation for Alleging Malpractice or Wrongful Death

STATE	MALPRACTICE	WRONGFUL DEATH
Alabama	2 yr	2 yr
Alaska	2 yr	2 yr
Arizona	2 yr	2 yr
Arkansas	2 yr	3 yr
California	1 yr	1 yr
Colorado	2 yr	2 yr
Connecticut	2 yr	2 yr
Delaware	2 yr	2yr
District of Columbia	3 yr	1 yr
Florida	2 yr	2 yr
Georgia	2 yr	2 yr
Hawaii	2 yr	2 yr
Idaho	2 yr	2 yr
Illinois	2 yr	2 yr
Indiana	2 yr	2 yr
Iowa	2 yr	2 yr
Kansas	2 yr	2 yr
Kentucky	1 yr	1 yr
Louisiana	1 yr	1 yr
Maine	2 yr	2 yr
Maryland	3 yr	2 yr
Massachusetts	3 yr	3 yr
Michigan	2 yr	2 yr
Minnesota	2 yr	3 yr
Mississippi	2 yr	2 yr
Missouri	2 yr	3 yr
Montana	5 yr	2 yr
Nebraska	5 yr	2 yr
Nevada	2 yr	2 yr
New Hampshire	6 yr	2 yr
New Jersey	2 yr	2 yr
New Mexico	3 yr	3 yr
New York	2 yr	2 yr
North Carolina	3 yr	2 yr
North Dakota	2 yr	2 yr
Ohio	1 yr	2 yr
Oklahoma	2 yr	2 yr
Oregon	2 yr	2 yr
Pennsylvania	2 yr	2 yr
Rhode Island	3 yr	3 yr
South Carolina	6 yr	6 yr
South Dakota	2 yr	3 yr
Tennessee	1 yr	1 yr
Texas	2 yr	2 yr
Utah	4 yr	2 yr
Vermont	3 yr	2 yr
Virginia	2 yr	2 yr
Washington	3 yr	3 yr
West Virginia	2 yr	2 yr
Wisconsin	3 yr	3 yr

DEGREES OF NEGLIGENCE

Ordinary negligence

Ordinary negligence is the failure to do what a reasonably prudent person would do under the circumstances, or the doing of that which a reasonably prudent person would not do under the circumstances.

Gross negligence

Gross negligence is the intentional or wanton omission of care that would be proper to provide, or the doing of that which would be improper to do.

Subpoenas

Physicians are often asked to provide testimony in cases. An attorney cannot force a physician to do so unless the physician is served with a subpoena, which makes it mandatory for the physician to appear or surrender medical records (whatever the subpoena specifies). Failure to comply with or answer a subpoena may result in the physician being held in contempt of court, which can end in jail time.

A *subpoena* is a legal order that requires that a person or documents appear before the court. Subpoenas can be requested by the following people:

- Attorneys
- Judges
- Law enforcement officials

The main parts of a subpoena are as follows:

- A reference number
- The names of the plaintiff and defendant
- The date, time, and place to appear
- The name, address, and telephone number of the opposing attorney
- The documents requested, if the subpoena is for records

A plaintiff is the party who brings a suit seeking damages. A defendant is the party against whom a suit is brought. In a criminal case, the defendant is the person accused of committing a crime.

Subpoenas can be served by the following:

- Attorney
- Sheriff
- Process server
- Court clerk

A *subpoena ad testificandum* orders a person to appear at a trial to give testimony. Failure to appear can result in contempt of court. A bench warrant can be issued if the witness fails to appear. A *subpoena duces tecum* is a written notification for records, documents, or other evidence described in a subpoena. Failure to bring the appropriate documents can also be considered contempt of court and carries with it a penalty of fines and/or imprisonment.

If a subpoena is served to a physician or an employee of a practice, it is imperative to immediately contact the practice attorney. The attorney will provide guidance from there.

GUIDELINES FOR HANDLING SUBPOENAS

- IMMEDIATELY tell management (supervisor and/or physician) that you have received a subpoena. Don't ignore it; it is a legal document that can land you in jail or result in fines.
- IMMEDIATELY, AT THE DIRECTION OF THE PHYSICIAN, CALL THE ATTORNEY FOR THE PRACTICE TO REPORT RECEIVING THE SUBPEONA.
- DO NOT DESTROY any information, whether it be medical or financial in nature.
- The receptionist who received the subpoena should note the date and time that it was served and how it was served.
- The practice attorney will provide directions on how to handle this subpoena.

Some common legal terms are defined in Box 9-8.

Respondeat Superior

Respondeat superior is legally defined as "Let the master answer," which means that the employer is responsible for the actions of his or her employees; thus the physician is held legally accountable for the actions of any and all employees working in the medical office. This is also referred to as *vicarious liability,* that is, the employer is

BOX 9-8 Legalese

Affidavit: A sworn voluntary statement given before an official authorized to administer an oath.
Allegation: A statement that a person expects to be able to prove.
Attestation: The act of witnessing a document in writing.
Bona fide: In good faith, honestly, without knowledge or intent of fraud.
Captain-of-the-ship doctrine: The physician is responsible for the negligent acts of other professionals because the physician had the right to control and oversee the totality of the care provided to the patient.
Caregiver: One who provides care to a patient.
Civil law: Body of law that describes the rights and responsibilities of individuals. It does not deal with crimes.
Complaint: The first statement by the plaintiff against the defendant; the complaint states a reason for the suit.
Consent: One person agrees to allow someone else to do something.
Counterclaim: Defendant's claim in opposition to a claim of the plaintiff.
Decedent: Deceased person.
Deposition: A method of discovery before the trial that consists of statements of fact from a witness under oath with a question-and-answer period. Such statements are admitted into evidence.
Do-not-resuscitate order: Directive to a physician to withhold cardiopulmonary resuscitation in the event a patient goes into cardiac arrest.
Durable power of attorney: Legal instrument enabling an individual to act on another person's behalf. In health care, it gives authority to make a medical decision for another.
Euthanasia: Causing the merciful death of a person suffering from an incurable condition.
Guardian: Person appointed by the court to protect the interests of and make decisions for a person who is incapable of making his or her own decisions.
Incompetent: Incapable of making rational decisions on one's own; this determination is made by a court.
Informed consent: Consent given by the patient after being fully advised of the potential risks and benefits of a service or procedure.
Living will: Document whereby an individual expresses in advance his or her wishes regarding the use of life-sustaining treatment in the event the patient is incapable of making decisions.
Next of kin: People who by law would be the close blood relatives of the decedent.
Nuncupative will: Oral statements made in anticipation of death. Intended as a last will.
Ombudsman: Person who is designated to speak and act on behalf of a patient, especially in regard to the patient's daily needs.
Palliative care: Care that keeps a person comfortable but is not intended to prolong life.
Perjury: False testimony under oath.
Respondeat superior: "Let the master answer"; the employer is responsible for the acts of an employee who is acting within the scope of employment.
Standard of care: Conduct that is expected of an individual in a given situation.
Statute of limitations: Legal limit on the time allowed for filing a suit in civil matters.
Suit: Court proceeding in which one person seeks damages or other legal remedies from another.
Tertiary care: Highly specialized care provided in a major medical center.
Writ: A written order that is issued to a person requiring the performance of some specified act or giving authority to have it done.

liable for the wrongful acts of his or her employees. The wrongful act must occur during the course of employment to be a respondeat superior liability issue. The medical assistant in a medical practice is not liable for the acts of other employees as long as he or she was not involved in the actual act itself.

Deposition Demands

The time may come when an office manager is called on to provide a deposition in a lawsuit between a physician and a patient. Other members of the staff might be summoned also, so it is important to understand the few basic steps in giving a deposition.

Before giving a deposition, prepare an updated copy of your resume in case it is required by legal counsel. Review any documents in which you had a hand, including telephone logs, medical records, and financial statements. Meet with the practice attorney or malpractice insurer's attorney who will be representing you. Review the plaintiff's complaint and the defendant's answer, so you are clear on the issues.

At the deposition, wait until a question has been asked in full before attempting to answer it. Answer only the question that was asked; don't provide any extra information. If you do not understand the question, ask the attorney to repeat or rephrase it. Tell the attorney if you are not sure you understand the question. If you become tired or feel confused, ask for a break to confer with your attorney. Never answer a question with a guess. If you do not know the answer, say so. Be honest! The practice attorney will be able to guide you in the areas that are critical to the case. The key to giving a good deposition is to be clear, accurate, and truthful at all times.

Delegation of Duties

An office is more efficient when various duties are delegated to paraprofessionals; however, by doing this, the office could open itself to liability. The delegation of routine duties can sometimes become a headache for both the office manager and the physician. One way to prevent this problem is to stay well within the limits of the law. Any time an office manager or physician asks an employee to perform a task that is in a gray area (such as running an errand to pick up the physician's special surgery eyeglasses from the optician), the office exposes itself to potential problems.

Civil Law

Civil law protects the rights and responsibilities of individuals. This type of law does not involve crimes, only actions between two parties. One area of civil law that affects health care is contract law.

CONTRACT LAW

A contract is an agreement between two parties and can be either written or oral. The purpose of the contract is to define the agreement so that it can be legally enforced. There are eight types of contracts:

- Express (written or oral)
- Implied
- Voidable
- Executory
- Executed
- Enforceable
- Unenforceable
- Contracts for realty, goods, or services

Elements of a Contract

There are three elements of a valid contract:

- The offer—An offer has to be communicated to be accepted.
- The consideration—This is the legal benefit of the contract.
- The acceptance—On acceptance of the offer, a contract is formed.

Tort Law

A tort is a breach of contract committed against a person or property for which the court provides a ruling in the form of an action for any damages that have occurred. The purpose of the tort law is to preserve the peace between the individuals, to find fault for the wrongdoing, to discourage the wrongdoer, and to compensate the injured person.

Statute of Limitations

The statute of limitations is the legal limit on the time that is allowed to file a suit in a civil court. This time frame is measured from the time of the wrongdoing or the time when a reasonable person would have discovered it. If a case is filed later than the allowed time frame, the case cannot proceed. Many technical rules apply with the statute of limitations and are determined by the state.

Mediation and Arbitration

Mediation takes place when a third party, the mediator, attempts to work out a settlement between both parties. The mediator cannot force a settlement. Arbitration is when both parties maintain their positions, but agree to submit their differences to a panel for resolution.

Criminal Law

Criminal law is imposed on behavior that is beyond the acceptable human and institutional behaviors. A crime is an act that is punishable by law. Crimes are classified as misdemeanors and felonies. Misdemeanors are punishable by less than 1 year in prison and/or a fine. An example of a misdemeanor is driving under the influence of alcohol. Felonies are a more serious crime, such as a murder or rape. These crimes are punishable by imprisonment in a state or federal penitentiary for more than 1 year. An infraction is a minor violation that is only punishable by the payment of a fine. A parking ticket is considered an infraction of the law.

Sexual Harassment

The legal concept of sexual harassment originated in 1964 with the Civil Rights Act, which prohibited discrimination on the basis of sex. In 1975, a case was filed by women who claimed verbal and physical harassment by a manager. Unfortunately, the courts ruled that the Civil Rights Act did not cover such cases and it was dismissed. In 1977, a case was brought wherein a woman claimed that she lost her job because she would not accept the sexual advances of her boss. In this case, the court ruled that this discrimination did indeed fall under the Civil Rights Act of 1964. In 1980, the Equal Employment Opportunity Commission (EEOC) provided guidelines that prohibit unwelcome advances, either verbal or physical. These guidelines also define a condition referred to as "hostile workplace." The courts upheld cases of hostile workplace due to harassment in 1986. In 1991, a Florida court ruled that provocative pin-ups hung in the workplace are a form of harassment and ordered them removed. California also got deeply involved in 1991, stating that all cases of hostile workplace should be evaluated using a "reasonable woman standard" and not a "reasonable person standard." In 1993, the Supreme Court upheld that a workplace may be determined hostile even in the absence of objectively measured hostility: the perception of abuse is sufficient. Although most cases involve harassment of females, males can also be the victims of sexual harassment.

It is not uncommon to pick up a newspaper and read about a sexual harassment case in the workplace. This seems to be a problem running rampant in medicine; many physicians have been charged with sexual harassment in the medical office setting. There must be an office policy in place to prevent sexual harassment and sexual harassment charges. This policy should include a requirement that a medical assistant, nurse, laboratory technician, or other clinical employee accompanies the physician into the examination room when examining a patient (Figure 9-8).

Sexual harassment comes in various forms; the office should prepare a written policy regarding patients, staff, and sexual harassment. Always remember: do not exhibit any type of behavior that could be misconstrued. It is the office manager's job to protect the physicians and staff by ensuring that they know how to treat patients appropriately. It is also the office manager's job to protect employees from sexual harassment.

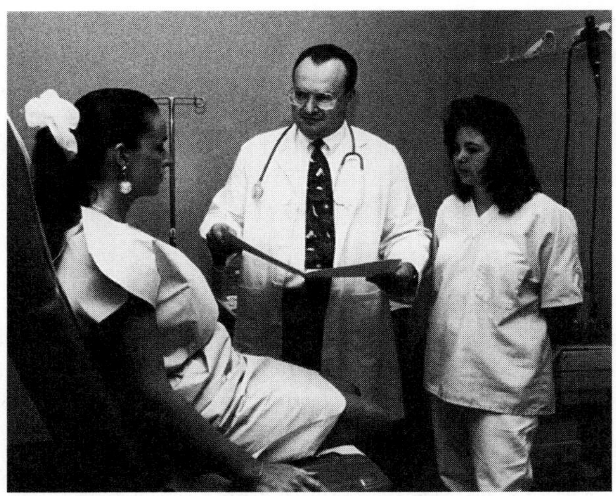

FIGURE 9-8. The physician should have an assistant present in the examination room.

Employment Law

In today's legal environment, even small practices must be concerned about abiding employment laws. All office managers should therefore understand the implications of the following federal and state employment laws:

- **National Labor Relations Act of 1935.** This act, also known as the Wagner Act, was designed to protect employees' rights to organize and bargain. This act ensures that an employer must bargain in good faith with all unions involved in a dispute.
- **Fair Labor Standards Act of 1938.** This act provides for overtime for an hourly employee who works more than 40 hours in a work week. It requires that the employee be paid no less than 1.5 times her or his regular hourly rate for each hour over 40. This overtime requirement does not apply to executives, professionals, and administrative employees. This act has also established equal pay for equal work (Equal Pay Act of 1963).
- **Labor Management Relations Act of 1947.** This act, also known as the Taft-Hartley Act, was designed to prohibit unfair labor practices by unions by protecting workers' positions from union officers. It maintains a balance between company management and the union.
- **Labor Management Reporting and Disclosure Act of 1959.** This act is also known as the Landrum-Griffen Act. It was designed to regulate internal union practices and to develop a bill of rights for union members.
- **Equal Pay Act of 1963.** This act, also known as the Wage Discrimination Act, was designed to prevent wage discrimination between the sexes for employees working under the same conditions, possessing the same skill sets, and exerting the same amount of effort and responsibility.

- **The Civil Rights Act of 1964.** This act, also known as Title VII, is credited with providing the most far-reaching legislation regarding fair and equitable employment. This act prohibits discrimination based on race, color, religion, sex, or national origin. Out of this act, the Equal Employment Opportunity Act of 1972 was conceived.
- **Executive Order 11246.** This order, which is also known as the 50/50 Rule, requires that all businesses having federal contracts of more than $50,000 and employing more than 50 people develop affirmative action programs.
- **Age Discrimination in Employment Act of 1967.** This act prevents discrimination against workers ages 40 to 70. It protects these workers from discrimination in hiring, retirement, wages, and other areas of employment.
- **Uniform Guidelines on Employee Selection Procedures.** These guidelines were issued in 1970 by the EEOC, Office of Personnel Management, Department of Justice, and Department of Labor. They assist employers and employment agencies in prohibiting discrimination against employees based on race, color, religion, sex, and national origin.
- **The Occupational Safety and Health Act of 1970.** This act was designed to provide for employee health and safety on the job. This act was amended in 1976 to include that employers must maintain a log of all injuries and illnesses that occur on the job. This log must be kept for 5 years, and all records regarding injuries and illnesses must be maintained for the duration of the worker's employment.
- **Equal Employment Opportunity Act of 1972.** This act was designed to enforce equal employment opportunity. It can be used to prosecute employment discrimination cases in federal courts.
- **Vocational Rehabilitation Act of 1973.** This act was designed to protect the handicapped against discrimination. The definition of handicapped refers to employees with physical disabilities, emotional disturbances, alcoholism, and drug addictions.
- **Employee Retirement Income Security Act of 1974 (ERISA).** This act was developed to maintain minimum federal standards for pension plan benefits. It is used to develop guidelines for companies that have pension plans.
- **Pregnancy Discrimination Act of 1978.** This act was designed to protect employees from discrimination on the basis of pregnancy, childbirth, or related conditions. It requires that all pregnant women be treated the same as other employees, and forbids firing or denying a promotion to an employee because of pregnancy.
- **Immigration Reform and Control Act of 1986.** This act was developed to provide a series of checks and balances by verifying an employee's citizenship or immigration status. It prohibits discrimination based on national origin.
- **Americans with Disabilities Act.** The Americans with Disabilities Act (ADA), which was signed into law in 1990 and amended in 1992 and 1994, protects individuals with disabilities in employment situations, transportation situations, and public accommodations. It replaced the Rehabilitation Act of 1973. This law protects the rights of all people in the United States who have physical and mental disabilities. These protections include requiring that changes be made in restrooms for easy access, that tables accommodate patients in wheelchairs, and that accommodations be made available for the hearing and sight impaired, to name a few. There may be some instances in which a physician practice must provide a hearing interpreter; however, there are no regulations that mandate such services. The ADA does not mandate the use of interpreters in every instance. The physician practice can choose alternatives to interpreters as long as there is effective communication between the hearing-impaired patient and the physician. Acceptable alternatives are written materials, lip reading, and note taking. The physician practice makes the final decision regarding the use of an interpreter or other alternative; however, this should be done with the wishes of the patient in mind. If an interpreter is used, the physician practice is responsible for the payment for the interpreter. The cost cannot be passed on to the patient and becomes part of the overhead expense of the practice. There may be a tax break of up to 50% of the cost of the interpreter; however, the practice accountant should be consulted on this issue. Figure 9-9 shows an office where a special ramp was installed to accommodate patients with disabilities.
- **Older Workers Benefit Protection Act of 1990.** This act specifically prohibits employers from denying benefits to older employees. It developed and currently maintains standards for claims filed under the Age Discrimination Act.
- **The Patient Self-Determination Act of 1990.** This act was developed to protect the rights of patients to make

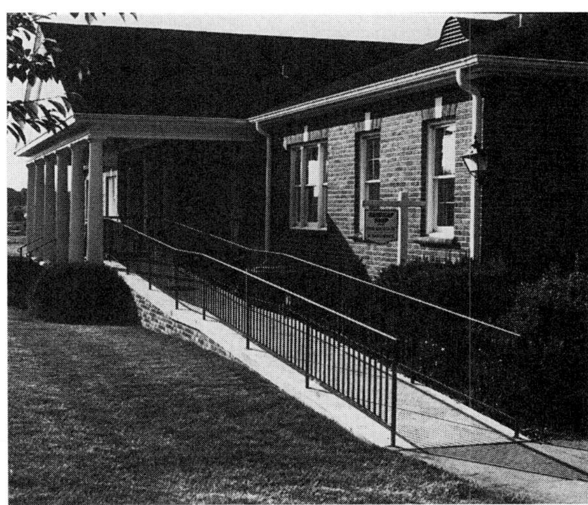

FIGURE 9-9. A ramp used by patients with disabilities.

decisions regarding their own health care, including the right to accept or refuse medical or surgical treatment.

- **Family and Medical Leave Act of 1993.** This act was designed to provide employees with additional benefits in time of personal crisis. It provides unpaid leave to care for a newborn baby, to care for a sick family member, or for employees' own health problems. Employers are required to hold the employee's position or provide the employee with a position that is of like status, pay, and responsibility. Figure 9-10 provides a request form for this leave of absence.
- **Workers' compensation laws.** Workers' compensation laws protect employees who are injured on the job. Any employee who is injured while performing job-related duties may sue the employer for injuries sustained, and many employers are required to maintain insurance coverage for such injuries. This law is based not on negligence, but rather on the employee-employer relationship. This law varies from state to state.

Limited English Proficiency Patients

The Department of Health and Human Services released regulations in 2003 requiring physicians to provide and pay for interpreters in their practices. It developed four factors that providers must weigh in determining the appropriate response to limited English proficiency (LEP) patients:

1. Number or proportion of LEP persons eligible to be served or likely to be encountered
2. Frequency with which the LEP individuals come in contact with the provider
3. Nature and importance of the program, activity, or service provided by the provider to people's lives
4. Resources available to the provider and the costs associated with these resources

This guidance in 2003 replaced a more strict guidance that was issued the year before. Any physician who accepts Part B payments must follow this guidance.

Employee name: ____________________

Employment status: ______Full-time ______Part-time

Start date of requested leave: ______________

End date of requested leave: ______________

Purpose:

_____ Medical condition

_____ Care of spouse, child, or parent

_____ Newborn care (birth to 12 months)

_____ Adoptive care (birth to 12 months)

_____ Foster care (birth to 12 months)

_____ Other:

____

____

____

____

____

____

I understand that family/medical leave will be granted in accordance with the law. I understand that my employer may request certification of any of the above conditions. If I do not return to work on the expected date of return, I will no longer be considered an employee. I understand that I will be required to use all sick, personal, and vacation time. I understand that upon my return I will assume my position or one that is equivalent to it. I understand that my employment will be terminated if I am unable to return to work once I have exhausted all leave granted me by the Family and Medical Leave Act.

______________________ ______________________

Employee signature Date

FIGURE 9-10. Family and Medical Leave Act Request Form.

Employment at Will

The *employment at will doctrine* states that employment is at the will of either the employer or the employee, and that employment can be terminated by either party at any time without reason. This law is usually not applicable in today's society. Some medical practices have evolved into sophisticated businesses, and many courts have reassessed this doctrine. At-will terminations can cause time-consuming and expensive legal battles, and juries side with the terminated employee almost 75% of the time. It is best to create a paper trail to document problems with an employee, and reasonable attempts to reconcile these problems. Only when such attempts have failed should you relieve an employee of his or her position.

Other Regulations

The office manager should also know about the following regulations, details of which are found in Chapter 7:

- Fraud and Abuse Amendments of 1972
- Anti-kickback Statute of 1974
- Antifraud and Abuse Amendments of 1977
- Civil Monetary Penalties of 1981
- Medicare and Medicaid Patient and Program Protection Act of 1987
- Safe Harbor Regulations of 1991–2001
- Self-Referral Prohibitions (Stark Law) of 1989–1996
- Omnibus Budget Reconciliation Act of 1989
- Health Insurance Portability and Accountability Act of 1996
- Balanced Budget Act of 1997
- Publication of Office of Inspector General's (OIG's) Provider Self-Disclosure Protocol, 1998
- Publication of OIG's Rulemaking, 1999
- Safe Harbor Regulations, 1999
- Final Rule: HIPAA Privacy Regulations, 2000
- Stark II Regulations, 2001

PRACTICE ATTORNEY

Because our society is litigious, it is important to have a qualified, knowledgeable attorney available. The practice attorney should be well informed in the field of health care in addition to business. Your lawyer should be called on for advice regarding employment, tax, and business issues; government regulation in regard to health care; and insurance law. If your lawyer is not familiar with an issue he or she is asked to handle, he or she might consult with a partner or associate.

The task of the medical office manager is to help the office obtain an attorney by carefully evaluating various legal firms, their fees, and their knowledge of health care issues. The following is a short list of areas in the medical practice where an attorney's help may be needed:

- Physician contracts
- Retirement and profit-sharing plans
- State and federal legislation
- Health insurance plans
- Partnership and corporation formation
- Office and equipment leases
- Managed care contracts
- Representation of the physician in collection cases
- Representation of the physician in hospital matters
- Employment issues

Ask about attorney fees and areas of expertise. Attorney fees can be an unpleasant surprise if the office is not quick to establish a foundation for charges. Some attorneys negotiate their fees; they are not carved in stone. Agree on the parameters of payment from the outset and carefully monitor services and charges. Lawyers can be flexible. Understand that if you are told that a fee agreement is "iron-clad," you may find that the attorney meant "what we agreed on, plus expenses."

Ask what the firm charges for making photocopies, filing documents, and doing research. Interview several attorneys before hiring one for the job. After all, your attorney will be making decisions and giving advice that will affect your business.

PATIENTS WHO HAVE BEEN ABUSED

Each state has laws protecting physically and verbally abused individuals. Health care professionals are required in most states to report such suspected abuse. This abuse can involve children, adults, or the elderly.

It is imperative for the office manager to research state laws and to be aware of reporting obligations in the event that a situation should arise in your practice. All states have laws against child abuse. Most states have laws that protect the informant, and some states have laws for failing to report suspected child abuse. The practice attorney can be very helpful in providing this information.

The following employees of a medical practice have a responsibility to report incidents of abuse:

- Physicians
- Chiropractors
- Podiatrists
- Optometrists
- Nurses
- Social workers
- Mental health professionals

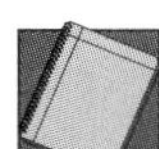

FROM THE EXPERT'S NOTEBOOK

Any person reporting abuse must do so in good faith that the facts reported are true to the best of his or her knowledge.

Child Abuse

It is often a challenge to determine abuse in children; what constitutes abuse is difficult to determine because children are naturally prone to injury. They play hard and fast, which may result in bruises, red marks on the skin, scratches, and even broken bones. These injuries are often due to accidents. There are cases, however, where serious physical injury is intentionally inflicted by a parent or other individual. For example, "shaken baby syndrome" is a common abuse found with infants. Children cry and cannot be comforted; parents cannot quiet them, become frustrated, and, without thinking, shake the baby or child violently. This can result in serious injury or even death. The medical office should be aware of child abuse and report any suspicious injuries or illnesses. Individuals who may be involved in abusing children include the following:

- Parents
- Siblings
- Babysitters
- Boyfriends/girlfriends
- Other relatives
- Neighbors
- Friends

Elder Abuse

Forty-three states have protective laws for the elderly. This type of abuse is not reported as often as child abuse, even though it may occur just as often! According to the Senate Subcommittee on Elder Abuse, only one case of elder abuse in eight is reported, versus one in three cases of child abuse. Medical practice personnel must be aware of elder abuse when treating older patients.

Elder abuse can manifest itself as physical, verbal, or emotional abuse, including acts of neglect. The most prevalent of these three abuses are the verbal and emotional forms. Elder abuse is most commonly found in nursing facilities.

EXERCISES

MULTIPLE CHOICE

Choose the best *answer for each of the following questions.*

1. The commission or omission of an act that a reasonably prudent person would not or would do is
   a. Negligence
   b. Retribution
   c. Vengeance
   d. Self-help
2. The policy that temporarily denies new appointments to a hospital medical staff is called
   a. Moratorium
   b. Exclusive contract
   c. Restraint of trade
   d. Reduced market approach
3. The physician is liable for the negligent acts of her or his clinical staff under the doctrine of
   a. Res ipsa loquitur
   b. Umbrella policy
   c. Respondeat superior
   d. Deposition
4. The order that calls for a document to be produced by the medical office is called
   a. Summons
   b. Subpoena duces tecum
   c. Writ
   d. Bench order
5. Malpractice is negligence by a
   a. Physician
   b. Registered nurse
   c. Pharmacist
   d. All of the above
6. When a provider's license is revoked or not renewed, what may occur?
   a. Suspension
   b. Restitution
   c. Restriction
   d. All of the above
7. Which of the following affects patient satisfaction?
   a. Physician does not return patient phone calls
   b. Prolonged time in the reception area
   c. Difficulties with the billing staff
   d. All of the above
8. Which of the following is not a division of the Department of Health and Human Services?
   a. Family Support Administration
   b. Centers for Medicare and Medicaid
   c. Health Care Administration
   d. Social Security Administration
9. Which division directs programs for children?
   a. Public Health Service
   b. Human Development Service
   c. Social Security Administration
   d. None of the above
10. Physician office staff should be aware of the "Right of Conscience" when the physician performs which of the following procedures?
    a. Electrocardiogram
    b. Abortion
    c. Adoption
    d. Genome testing
11. An autopsy is usually performed by a
    a. Pathologist
    b. Radiologist
    c. Gerontologist
    d. None of the above
12. Who of the following can give authorization for an autopsy?
    a. Spouse
    b. Parents
    c. Adult cousin
    d. All of the above

13. Which of the following is not found on a birth certificate?
    a. Sex of baby
    b. Names of grandparents
    c. Place of birth
    d. Legal name of mother
14. Which of the following documents must be signed by the attending physician before a deceased patient's body can be picked up by the funeral director?
    a. Writ of death
    b. Funeral summons
    c. Death certificate
    d. None of the above
15. The physician's severance of the professional relationship with a patient without reasonable notification is
    a. Abandonment
    b. Termination
    c. Against medical advice
    d. None of the above
16. How many versions of the Hippocratic Oath are there?
    a. One
    b. Two
    c. Three
    d. Five
17. The American Medical Association was founded by
    a. Andrew Still
    b. Apollo
    c. Nathan Davis
    d. Edward Koop
18. Which of the following is an ethical dilemma for a medical practice?
    a. Disclosure of medical errors
    b. End-of-life decisions
    c. Beginning-of-life technologies
    d. All of the above
19. Under HIPAA, no patient authorization is required for
    a. An insurance request
    b. A research program
    c. Medical record audits
    d. A subpoena
20. Which of the following is a reportable disease?
    a. Chickenpox
    b. Gonorrhea
    c. Rabies
    d. All of the above

MATCHING

Match the following acts and administrative orders with their better-known names.

1. _____	Labor Management Reporting and Disclosure Act	A. Title VII
2. _____	Labor Management Relations Act of 1947	B. Landrum-Griffen Act
3. _____	Equal Pay Act of 1963	C. Wage Discrimination Act
4. _____	Civil Rights Act of 1964	D. 50/50 Rule
5. _____	Executive Order 11246	E. Taft-Hartley Act

TRUE OR FALSE

1. _____ Appointment time frames are never a problem area in physicians' offices.
2. _____ Physicians would rather treat patients on the phone than see them in the office.
3. _____ The Human Development Service directs programs for Native Americans.
4. _____ There are 43 states with protective laws for the elderly.
5. _____ The address of the opposing attorney is part of a subpoena.
6. _____ A subpoena duces tecum orders a person to appear at a trial for testimony.
7. _____ Malpractice cases are never the result of a problem with a medical record.
8. _____ *Malpractice* is the failure to act, when there is duty to act, as a reasonably prudent person would act.
9. _____ *Misfeasance* is a form of negligence.
10. _____ The Patient Self-Determination Act helps employees with benefits at a time of crisis.
11. _____ The Family and Medical Leave Act helps employees with additional time off for a personal crisis.
12. _____ The office manager would enlist the help of the practice attorney with physician contracts.
13. _____ Almost all elder abuse is reported.
14. _____ Abuse can be emotional in nature.
15. _____ *Nonfeasance* is the improper performance of an act resulting in injury to another.
16. _____ There are three degrees of negligence.
17. _____ Food poisoning is a reportable disease.
18. _____ It is not necessary to date an authorization form.
19. _____ When the patient is mentally ill, the legal guardian must give consent for treatment.
20. _____ The AMA Code of Ethics was developed by Thomas Percival in 1803.

THINKERS

1. Mrs. Reynolds passed away during the night in the nursing home. What is the physician's responsibility, if any, at this point?
2. A patient has become noncompliant, failing to take prescribed medications and to go for requested testing. The physician believes that it is in the best interest of the patient to obtain a new physician to whom the patient will listen. How would the office manager handle this situation?
3. Someone from the sheriff's office has just served a subpoena duces tecum to the office. What is the office's responsibility at this point?
4. In a medical practice scenario provided by your instructor, list some ways in which you would use the practice attorney.
5. Your office has interviewed an individual for a position at the front desk. This applicant is in a wheelchair. The assistant office manager tells you that you do not have to make special provisions for this applicant if you decide to hire him. What are your responsibilities to this applicant, if any? Explain your reasoning.

REFERENCES

Bauman, S.M. "What's Law Got to Do with It?" *Archives of Family Medicine*, Vol. 8, No. 4, July/August 1999, pp. 22–24.

Bloche, G.M. "Fidelity and Deceit at the Bedside." *JAMA*, Vol. 283, No. 14, April 2000, pp. 31–34.

Clark, L. "When and When Not to Protect Patient Privacy." *Medical Economics*, May 1991, pp. 99–109.

Crane, M. "The Medication Errors That Get Doctors Sued." *Medical Economics*, November 1993, pp. 36–41.

Delmar, D. "Be Wary of Legal Pitfalls When Dismissing Problem Patients." *Physicians Financial News*, June 1991, pp. 1, 31.

Gibbons, R.V., Landry, F.J., Bouch, D.L., et al. "A Comparison of Physicians' and Patients' Attitudes towards Pharmaceutical Industry Gifts." *Journal of General Internal Medicine*, 1998, Vol. 13, pp. 151–154.

Institute of Medicine, *Identifying and Preventing Medical Errors*, The National Academies, Washington, D.C.

Kanoti, G. "The Toughest Ethical Choices Encountered by Physicians." *Physician's Management*, May 1992, pp. 71–79.

Kirschner, M. "How Advance Directives Can Ease Your Burden." *Medical Economics*, April 1992, pp. 75–87.

Luxenberg, S. "How to Tell When Your Lawyer Is Overcharging." *Medical Economics*, September 1993, pp. 92–97.

Mabon, R. "How to Do a Discovery Deposition." *Group Practice Journal*, November/December 1993, p. 49.

Medical Group Practice: Legal and Administrative Guide. Aspen Health Law and Compliance Center. Gaithersburg, MD: Aspen Publishers Inc., 1999.

Murray, D. "Dismiss a Patient, Invite a Lawsuit?" *Medical Economics*, August 1993, pp. 57–70.

Pozgar, G.D. *Legal Aspects of Health Care Administration*. 8th edition. Rockville, MD: Aspen Publishers, 2001.

Schorr, B. "The National Practitioner Data Bank: A Case of Overkill?" *Physician's Management*, January 1993, pp. 109–121.

Sopko, S. "Complying with the Disabilities Act." *The Office*, July 1993, pp. 31–32.

Tannenbaum, R., & Berman, M. "Why Even Patients Who Like You Will Sue You for Malpractice." *Physician's Management*, April 1993, pp. 85–97.

Wold, C. "The Art of Malpractice Risk Management." *Physician's Management*, February 1993, pp. 57–68.

10

HEALTH CARE TECHNOLOGY

CHAPTER OUTLINE

CHAPTER OBJECTIVES

After completing this chapter, you will be able to do the following:

- Identify the parts of a computer
- Negotiate a computer contract
- Choose the proper computer for a medical practice
- Understand the reason for parallel processing
- Develop a patient encounter form
- Analyze the different types of medical practice software
- Recognize the importance of different computer-generated reports
- Comprehend the benefits of computerized medical records
- Recognize the importance of the Internet

COMPUTERS IN THE WORKPLACE

"Our computer system is very updated. It gives no information to those who need it, and plenty to those who don't!"

—ANONYMOUS

Computers affect all of us in our daily lives. They are changing our work habits today just as the telephone has changed people's work habits over the past century. Computers help us gather, organize, process, and store information. As in any industry, it is vital for a medical office manager to be computer literate because we live in a fast-paced information age of high technology. Buying a computer has become much like purchasing any appliance for your home. If it has the features you need, you will make better use of it. In today's health care environment, computer technology is indispensable.

The past two decades have seen greater emphasis placed on the management aspects of the medical office. Today, medical offices are finding that they cannot operate without the use of a computer as they become more prevalent in everyday tasks. Furthermore, with the ever-increasing costs of health care, the proper use of technology is one way to effectively and efficiently manage the costs associated with running a medical office.

There are many uses for a computer system in the medical office (Figure 10-1). You will find that once a computer system is in place, uses often arise that go beyond the original purposes. One example is the way people have been able to use existing computer systems and networks to make e-mail the number one means of business communication today. Other examples of effective computer usage include the following:

- Billing
- Age analysis of accounts
- Claims processing

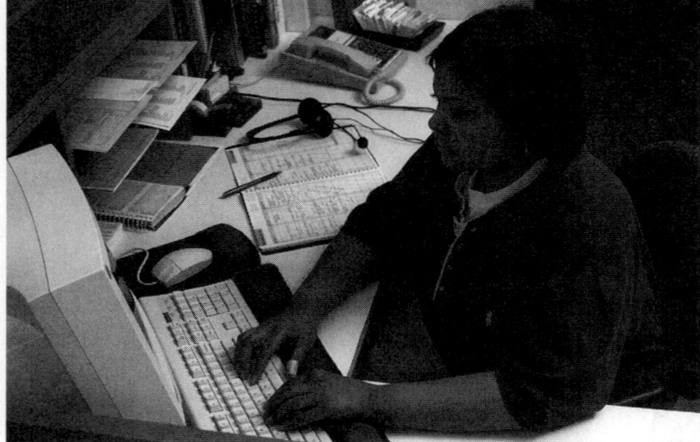

FIGURE 10-1. The computer has become an invaluable asset to the employees of a medical office.

- Collection letters
- Reminders
- Appointment scheduling
- Recall lists
- Accounting functions
- Employee vacations and sick days
- Inventory
- Ability to generate reports
- Word processing
- Access to national databases
- Access to hospital computers
- Drug interactions
- Research
- Patient education
- Medical records
- Policies and procedures
- Referring physician lists
- Continuing medical education (CME) programs
- Label and envelope printing
- Check writing
- Prescription writing
- Electronic claims
- Preparation of the deposit slip
- W-2 forms
- Hospital records
- Profiles by patient demographics
- Profiles by diagnosis and procedure
- Literature retrieval
- Retirement plans
- Interoffice memos
- Correspondence
- Internet access
- PowerPoint presentations

COMPUTER ANATOMY

It is almost inevitable today that the medical office manager will at some point be faced with buying a new computer or be charged with the responsibility for upgrading existing systems. As a result, it is important to be familiar with the terminology surrounding computer usage. If comparing a computer to a human, the hardware would be equated to the parts of the body, which do the physical work. The software would be equated to the workings of the mind; it does the thinking.

Hardware: Includes all of the physical parts of the computer system:

- The processor
- The monitor
- The hard drive
- Random access memory (RAM)
- Keyboard/mouse
- Modem
- Network interface card

- Printers
- Floppy disk/Zip/CD/DVD drives

Software: Software is the set of instructions without which the computer can do nothing. When you type an instruction on the keyboard, the software interprets that instruction and follows it, giving you the information that you requested. Many different software programs are available that meet the needs of the medical office.

Software can be categorized in four ways for the purposes of a medical office:

- The operating system, such as Microsoft Windows
- General office software, such as Microsoft Office
- Microsoft Internet Explorer
- Medical industry–specific software

The following terms describe the components of a computer:

Processor: The processor is the circuit chip that gives the computer the ability to process information. Several generations of processors can be found in computers being used today. Processors are described in two ways. First is the name given by the manufacturer:

- Pentium
- Celeron
- Athlon

This identifies processors by the manufacturer and technology that went into the process of creating it. Second is the number of Hertz (abbreviated Hz) of the processor. This indicates the actual speed of the processor. Current processors run at millions (mega) and billions (giga) of Hertz. Of course, the faster the chip, the more efficiently the computer runs.

Monitor: The monitor is the screen. Monitors are categorized by the viewing size of the screen and can be purchased from 15-inch viewable space to 21-inch viewable space. The larger the viewing size of the monitor, the more pixels can be viewed. *Pixels* are the smallest addressable unit on the screen. The higher the number of pixels, the clearer the graphics of a computer will appear.

Hard drive: This is the component of a computer that stores the information. It is a small metal box inside the computer that contains disks capable of long-term information storage. In humans, it can be likened to long-term memory. Hard drives can range in size from 1 gigabyte up to 40 gigabytes. One gigabyte is equivalent to 1 billion bytes of information, but by today's standards is a small amount of information.

Byte: A byte is a group of eight bits that is used to represent a single letter, number, or symbol in a computer. The *bit,* short for binary digit, is the fundamental unit of storage in all computers.

Megabyte: A megabyte is 1 million bytes of computer storage.

RAM: Short for *random access memory* and also referred to as simply *memory.* RAM the primary set of memory chips used to store data or instructions that can be altered by the user. It can be likened to short-term memory in humans. RAM is identified in bytes, and can range from 4 megabytes (MB) to 2 gigabytes (GB) in size today, depending on the machine. Newer machines are capable of holding much more RAM than older machines. A simple guide is that the more memory, the better the machine will perform. More memory will most notably improve the performance of Microsoft Windows and software that performs computations.

Keyboard and mouse: The keyboard and mouse are referred to as *input* devices because they are the primary means for putting information and commands into the computer. Keyboards are mostly universal in the layout of the keys; the greatest choices today concerning these devices are whether a more traditional design is preferable to the more ergonomic designs that are now available.

Modem: The modem is the device that allows a computer to send information over a telephone line. Modems can be used to communicate with specific systems that insurance companies and hospitals may use, or for the more widespread use of connecting to the Internet. Modems are offered in baud rates, which today include models that can be purchased in 33.6 kilobits per second (kbps) and 56 kbps. A problem frequently encountered is that the age of the existing phone lines may prevent modems from obtaining optimal data transfer speeds.

Baud: A baud is the number of signal changes in a communications channel per second, which controls the speed at which communications are transferred.

Printer: Printers are available in varied shapes, sizes, and speeds. The printer's function is to produce a hard copy (a paper document) of the information in the computer. The laser printer is the top-of-the-line printer, is the most popular printer today, and produces a finely finished product. Other types of printers include dot matrix and ink-jet printers. Dot matrix printers traditionally have been used to generate large reports (Figure 10-2). Ink-jet printers are less expensive than laser printers and have color printing capability, but lack the speed and fine quality of laser printers. However, as technology ages, it becomes less expensive. It is now possible to purchase a small laser printer for approximately $150 and a color laser printer for approximately $600. Furthermore, the long-term costs associated with printing, which include the ink or toner, are far less with a laser printer than with an ink-jet printer.

One other aspect to consider when reviewing the printer needs for the office is the *digital copier.* Copiers can be networked to allow you to print to them directly. This is especially useful if you need multiple copies of a document. The benefits include faster document prints and much lower associated costs in terms of toner usage. Ultimately, it can be much less expensive to print to a digital copier

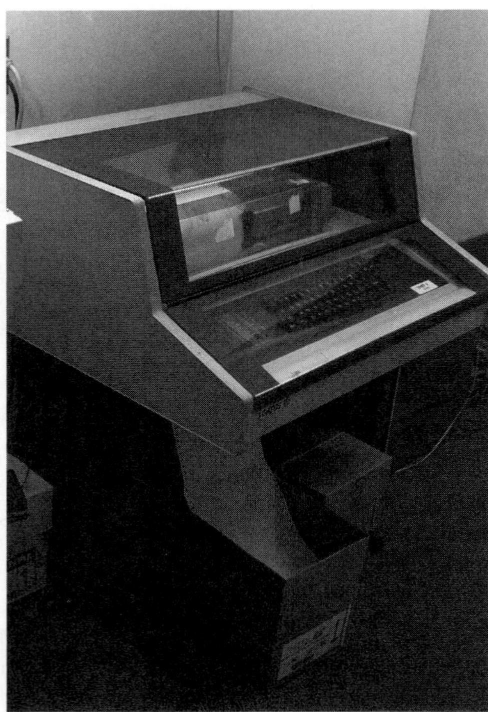

FIGURE 10-2. A large printer used for printing insurance forms and patient encounter forms.

than to an ink-jet or even a laser printer. Also, the technology has evolved to the point where the copiers manage document flow quite well so that printed and copied documents do not get mixed together.

Floppy disk/Zip/CD/DVD/Flash drives: These devices use media referred to as discs to transfer data from one computer or system to another or simply as a means of backing up data. Floppy and Zip disks are smaller media, holding up to approximately 1.5 MB for floppy disks and between 250 MB and 2,000 MB for Zip disks. CD and DVD discs are optical drives. A CD can store up to 700 MB of data and a DVD can store 4.7 to 10 GB of data. A flash drive is a memory stick that is connected to a computer via the universal serial bus (USB) port. A flash drive can store anywhere from 32 MB to 64 GB. Samsung has plans to release a 100 GB drive in the near future.

Backup tape: Backup tapes are cartridges that have a large capacity of several gigabytes of data. These are crucial because this media type allows you to create a repository for your data that fits into the palm of your hand. Easy storage and transportation means that a highly effective method of storing data can be developed. In addition to tape backups, there are now several online services for doing what tape backup drives accomplished without the necessity to manage the individual media. This means it is more efficient because there is a lesser chance that human error will cause a data loss in the short term. Clearly, backing up data is the most important single function because companies have become more dependent on their computer systems.

Network: A *network* is a group, or groups, of computers that are linked together. This can include all of the computers within an office, all of the computers within a health care system, and even all of the computers on the Internet. Any time computers have the ability to share data or hardware devices such as printers, they are considered networked together. Computers that are linked have *network interface cards* that allow them to speak to each other. When computers are properly networked together, they can share files such as appointment scheduling, billing functions, and even peripheral devices such as scanners and printers. There are two types of networks:

- Ethernet
- Wireless

The Ethernet (hard-wired) network is faster than a wireless network, and it is more secure than a wireless network. For a hard-wired network, the computer company will have to run a series of wires throughout the office where computers will be placed. The can be expensive, but is part of the cost of doing business.

Battery Backup

It is important to have equipment in place in case of a power outage or power surge. The computer system should be plugged into a power supply that provides a certain amount of uninterruptible time in the case of a power outage or power surge. This power supply, or battery backup, is as simple as purchasing a battery backup at your local office supply store. Battery backups can range in price based on the amount of time that you need to properly "power down." The battery backup is the Cadillac of power strips. The battery backup should also have surge protection in the event of an electrical surge from the power company.

COMPUTER SECURITY

Security is a very important aspect of the computer network that rarely receives the amount of attention needed. All companies should employ good security in their networks, but the medical field has an added level of need because of the degree of concern surrounding patient confidentiality. Confidentiality is a Health Insurance and Portability Accounting Act (HIPAA) issue that was discussed in previous chapters.

Computer misuse is a common occurrence in today's society. For instance, an employee who wishes to know the salaries of all staff, including the physician, or a disgruntled employee who wishes to retaliate over the lack of a raise may access sensitive information and use it to cause trouble. The best defense against computer fraud is to use a password-protected system. Most networks use a security format that allows management to control where employees can access necessary programs or data. Those without proper privilege who attempt to gain access are denied. These systems can be configured so that passwords can be permanent, or they can be changed on a periodic basis, whereby they expire after a certain date and time. New passwords are issued at that time.

NEGOTIATING THE CONTRACT

Each computer vendor will use a standard sales agreement when selling its computer system. Computer companies are competitive and hungry for your business. Keep this in mind, as well as the following ground rules, and negotiate a good purchase price for your office.

- Always involve your practice attorney. Listen and follow his or her advice!
- Make sure all promises made by the vendor are written out and signed by the vendor.
- Push for a delay in payment. Don't agree to make the final payment on the system until the system has been in place for at least 1 month. This will give you time to get the bugs out!
- Hold the vendor to a specific date by which the computer should be up and running to your satisfaction. If this date arrives and the computer hasn't been completely set up, you want to be able to walk away from this deal, and be able to seek out new vendors.
- Specify damages for which your vendor will be responsible should the computer not perform to your satisfaction. It is best if you can negotiate a clause that states that the vendor is responsible for legal fees if it comes to the point of legal action.
- Ask the vendor to specify in writing that the system proposed has not been sold to anyone else for less money.

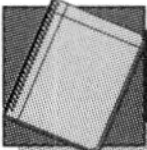

FROM THE EXPERT'S NOTEBOOK

The vendor will be more cooperative if the final payment is being withheld until you are satisfied!

PURCHASING THE COMPUTER

Purchasing Software

Determining the software package, or group of software programs, needed to perform the many tasks within your office is the first step. To make this determination, find out for what functions the physician intends to use the computer. Make a list of the individual tasks and then begin searching for the appropriate software packages available. It is not as important to determine the exact software needed before purchasing a computer as it once was. However, it is vital to know exactly what you want the software to do, so be thorough in studying your office's needs and the prospective packages you are looking at. If possible, arrange a demonstration from the software vendor to see how it works and also to ask questions about how it fits the needs of the practice. Involve the office computer expert in the software decision-making process to determine if the software meets the technical standards of the office.

SOFTWARE OPTIONS

Medical software programs perform a multitude of functions. Some of these functions are as follows:

- Appointment scheduling
- *International Classification of Diseases* (ICD) coding
- *Current Procedural Terminology* (CPT) coding
- Correct Coding Initiative (CCI) editing software
- Patient information
- Billing
- Insurance form generation
- Envelope and postcard addressing
- Label addressing
- Electronic submission of claims to insurance companies
- Missing insurance information
- Generation of deposit slips and audit trails
- Practice analysis
- Hospital/physician interface
- Recall and letter notices
- Clinical and drug histories
- Word processing
- Credit and collections packages
- Patient ledger accounts
- Chart tracking
- Payroll
- E-mail (electronic mail)
- Inventory control
- Medical records transcription
- Office management packages
- Patient encounter form printing
- Year-end statements
- Tracking packages
- Practice marketing
- Medical records

The most important of these functions are the patient billing and insurance functions. The software you purchase should be able to track accounts, age accounts, edit accounts, and resubmit them. It should also be able to submit insurance claims electronically. There was a time when electronic submission was simply an option. It is not an option any longer. Paperless claims are required by Medicare and all significant insurance companies today.

Like many specialty packages, the aforementioned options have been offered for years and can be tailored to fit the needs of each individual medical office. Companies can customize packages to be convenient and easy to use. When thinking about having a program customized for your office, always check on the cost of the service, because it can be quite expensive. With some research, you may be able to find a system that closely meets your needs without the added expense of customization.

SOFTWARE SUPPORT

When purchasing software, it is vitally important to have good technical support. The software company you select should always be available and should be extremely knowledgeable about the software program you have selected (Figure 10-3). Not everyone is computer literate, and this must be kept in mind when purchasing a software package. It is an easier task to computerize the office if the software is user friendly.

> **MANAGER'S ALERT**
>
> Always ask for references so that the practice can verify information about the computer, the software, and the support behind it.

Your software support people will become your best friends. Before purchasing a software package, ask for references for the support people and check with these references on the quality of the support provided. It is important that they are accessible. Generally, you will find that phone support is delivered in one of two ways:

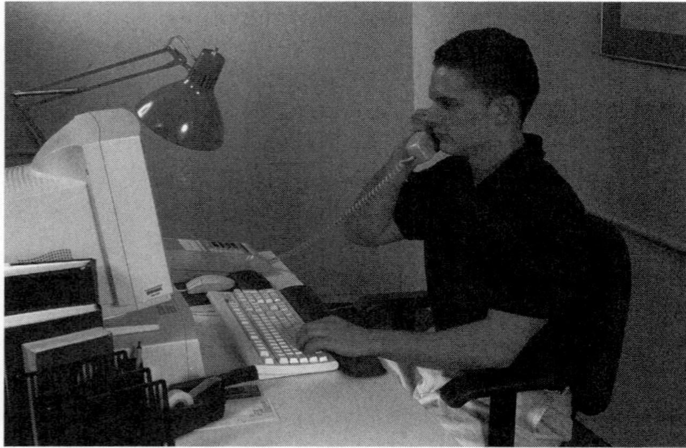

FIGURE 10-3. A software company's hotline operator is always friendly and eager to help customers.

- Leave a message and a technician will return your call.
- When you call you immediately get through to a support person.

Some companies employ both methods, using the second as advanced technical support and the first as lower-level support. Some companies only employ one method or the other. You will find that smaller software manufacturers will generally force you to leave a message, whereas larger software companies such as Microsoft employ a more immediate response system. A reasonable response time if your vendors employ a message system is 4 hours.

Whichever method your software manufacturer uses, research how much technical support will cost you. Some manufacturers include it in the price of the software, but more commonly you must purchase technical support, either on a per incident basis or in blocks of time.

Purchasing Hardware

HARDWARE OPTIONS

When shopping for hardware, buy a system that is more system than you need at that time. If your office is new to computerization, the office will see more and more ways to become more efficient with the use of the computer. Buying a larger system allows for practice growth, faster speed, and less hassle.

HARDWARE SUPPORT

Hardware support is just as important as software support. It is important to know how much "downtime" the computer system has. Call the references and ask, "Have you had much downtime with your XYZ computer system?" This is important, especially if the printer jams and you are in the middle of running your monthly statements. Some vendors may give you a false sense of security, so it is important to ask other medical offices who are using the same equipment. Some hardware problems can be corrected easily by following instructions given over the telephone by a hardware technician. Get to know your hardware technician; someday you might need help in a hurry, and being friends will help get her or him to your office sooner! Most individuals working as hardware and software technicians are knowledgeable and quick to respond.

TRAINING AND ORIENTATION

It is critically important to have the staff properly trained in the use of not just computers, but all office technology. Often, the systems within an office don't yield their full return on investment because not all users are aware of their capabilities. Furthermore, inadequate training can be a major source of severe stress for employees in the context of technology. To prevent these problems, have the office employees become involved in the quest for new computers and technology systems from the beginning. Allow them to be part of the decision-making process so that they are mentally prepared to make changes in the system. When considering training, determine if on-site training is available, and couple it with off-site classroom training if necessary. If possible, allow the staff to make the determination of what training and how much will be needed. Again, if staff members are not comfortable with the technology, it will not be fully utilized.

PARALLEL PROCESSING . . . A CRUTCH?

Parallel processing consists of running the old computer system or the manual system simultaneously with the new computer system. Running a parallel system can provide the office with benefits and problems. It can be helpful in identifying problems when they arise as a result of the addition or changing of systems. However, because the operations are bound to be different, it is almost impossible to compare any results from tasks that have been performed, and the chance of making errors is much greater. In addition, it places extra stress on the staff because of the extra work involved in performing the same tasks twice. Parallel running of systems should not exceed more than 4 months. After 4 months have gone by, any bugs or glitches that might have been in the new system will have been worked out and employees will need to fly solo.

The Old System to the New

If the office already has a computer in place and is in need of an upgrade, there are several options to consider. There are two main ways to accomplish this awesome task: run parallel systems or balance-forward all information into the new system.

As mentioned in the preceding section, running parallel systems means that you run both the new and old systems simultaneously. You simply pick a date at which time you will enter any new charges into the new system only. The only data entry done on the old system would be the application of charges to existing bills.

If you choose to use the balance-forward method, any unpaid balance in the old system would be converted to the new system by a one-line entry stating, "Balance forward." There would be no details of the services rendered on the new system except for the new services entered. All of the details from the old system can be printed to hard copy, backed up onto a disk or tape backup, and then purged.

Hard copies and data backups should be maintained until it is determined that they are no longer needed. Also, most software today includes utilities for importing data from other systems. The primary problem with this is that often the data do not fit perfectly into the new system and may ultimately be unreliable. It is wise to test the data import function thoroughly before making the live switch to the new system.

If the practice is changing from a manual system to a computerized system, the staff can spend extra time entering the patient demographics before the system goes live, which is the day you start using the new system.

GOING ELECTRONIC

Filing Insurance Claims Electronically

Electronic insurance claims are submitted via telephone lines and take only a short time to transmit. Software on the computer translates, edits, and formats the specific data according to the requirements of each specific insurance carrier.

Before purchasing electronic claims submission software for the office, there are a several things to consider.

- Ask other practices of your choice if they have any experience filing claims electronically. Ask if you can come to see their system in operation.
- Contact the insurance carriers with whom you would be filing claims electronically and ask them for recommendations of qualified vendors.
- Consider attending the next professional meeting to speak with vendors and look at their presentations.
- Ask the office's health care consultant, if the office has one, for recommendations on qualified vendors.
- Ask the vendor how long it has been involved with electronic claims submissions.
- Ask the vendor for the names of offices for which it has installed electronic claims systems.
- Call these offices and ask them about the vendor's service and support.
- Ask about charges associated with these electronic claims packages.
- Ask about the cost of service contracts.
- Ask about updates on the software.
- Ask whether training is available for the staff and physician.

Handling the Tickler System

The tickler system is a method that the practice uses to recall patients to the office for various reasons—an annual physical, an annual Papanicolaou (Pap) smear, a follow-up examination after the removal of a polyp, and so on.

Manual tickler systems usually take the form of 3 × 5–inch index cards filed by the months of the year. However,

TABLE 10-1 Tickler File Uses

Follow-up on test results	65.2%
Notify patients of test results	60.4%
Wellness (examinations, vaccinations, etc.)	43.3%
Chronic disease management	38.0%

they can be much more efficiently done on a computer. For example, the computer can be programmed to pull the names of all patients who had a physical in June of last year and print a reminder that can be mailed in May of this year. It can send collection notices to all patients with an overdue balance of 60 days or longer.

According to a survey by the Medical Group Management Association (MGMA), 67.6% of medical practice tickler files are computerized. Index cards are used by 26.6%, and 19.3% use a flagged medical record system. This same study showed how practices use their tickler files (Table 10-1).

Generating Letters

Just as it does with the tickler system, a computer will automatically print correspondence that is preprogrammed into the system at the request of the user. For instance, if a patient passes away, the user can print out a preprogrammed letter of condolence to the family with the push of a few buttons. However, it is always best to send a personal, handwritten note.

By accessing a patient referral letter, the user can generate and print out a thank-you letter to the physician or patient who provided the referral. Figure 10-4 shows a computer-generated recall letter. The more you use the computer's letter-generating capability, the more uses you will think of for it.

Printing Data Mailers

As discussed in Chapter 6, there is a difference between data mailers and patient statements. The data mailer is either a four-part or six-part one-piece bill that is generated from the computer. The mailer prints the patient's bill and the address on the envelope at the same time. A front sheet is attached so that the medical biller can see what was printed on the bill on the inside of the mailer. The front sheet can be easily removed and thrown away after review of the bill. All that is needed to mail the bill to the patient is a stamp. If you are thinking of using data mailers, make sure the printer you have is a workhorse and is able to handle the thickness of the data mailer. The amount of space on a data mailer is limited, so if you wish to print a lot of information regarding services and payments, it might be better to consider a patient statement.

March 24, 2002

Ann Smith
100 Main Street
Springtown, State 22222

Dear Ann:
Our records show that you are overdue for your yearly physical. Please call our office at 222-1234 at your earliest convenience to set up an appointment.

It is very important that you understand the necessity for a yearly examination. Your vital statistics will be monitored and yearly tests will allow us to keep your current health status in a controlled state. We know that you have a busy schedule, but won't you take time out to do something for yourself? Call and schedule your appointment soon.

Sincerely,

Alexander Babinetz, M.D.

FIGURE 10-4. Sample computer-generated recall letter.

Performing the End-of-Day Backup

Every computer trainer will emphasize the importance of the end-of-day backup. If files are not backed up onto a disc or tape at the end of every day, there is a possibility of losing all the work that was done on the network or computer for that day. If you have a backup and something happens to the computer the next day, it is easy to restore the lost data by simply placing the disc or tape into its drive and restoring the file(s) from the last backup. No matter how little the volume of work performed, it is still important to perform the backup. Fortunately, most backup tape drives include software that can automate the backup process by allowing you to program the desired parameters of the backup job. You simply have to change the tape and ensure that one is sent off site on a regular basis. The software does the rest of the work. Also, there are now Internet-based systems that charge a very competitive monthly fee to back up your data right over the Internet to their systems without the need of any media. This method will most likely be prevalent in the future.

DESIGNING THE PATIENT ENCOUNTER FORM

As was stated in Chapter 3, the patient encounter form is another name for the superbill. Once you have chosen the type of hardware and software you are going to use, you need to consider the type of forms for your new system. Many vendors supply the forms necessary for your use. If not, they will supply you with names of suppliers where you may purchase forms.

One of the most important forms you might want to design is the fee slip, or patient encounter form. It needs to include such areas as the following:

- Patient demographics
- Account balance
- Evaluation and management (E&M) codes
- Procedure codes
- Laboratory and x-ray codes, if applicable
- Diagnosis code
- Date for return appointment
- Name, address, and phone number of provider of service

Some offices include an area for procedures that need to be scheduled. Other offices include an area for the physician's signature. The best part about all of this is that you can customize and change your form as often as needed.

PATIENT DEMOGRAPHICS

This area of the fee slip/patient encounter form should include the following information:

- Patient's name
- Patient's address
- Patient's phone number
  - At work
  - At home
- Patient's date of birth
- Patient's insurance company
  - Primary
  - Secondary
- Patient's insurance numbers

ACCOUNT BALANCE

This area of the fee slip/patient encounter form should include the balance due on the patient's account. It is advisable to show the balance in the following areas:

- Due by patient
- Due by insurance
- Previous balance
- Today's charges

This area can be extremely helpful when outstanding balances are due. The area shows the amount the patient owes, so that it can be collected at the time of the patient's appointment.

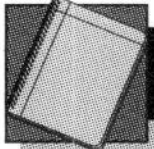

FROM THE EXPERT'S NOTEBOOK

The balance due area can be highlighted before the patient visit to remind the staff that there is a bill to collect!

EVALUATION AND MANAGEMENT CODES

This area should include all levels of service E&M codes. The physician's choices will be much easier when he or she is able to see the various levels from which to choose. The levels should include the following:

- New-patient codes
- Established-patient codes
- Consultations (referred by another physician)
- Confirmatory consultations
- Preventive medicine codes

PROCEDURE CODES

This area should include the procedures most commonly provided in the office. The electrocardiogram and fiber-optic sigmoidoscopy are examples.

LABORATORY AND X-RAY CODES

This area should include any laboratory or x-ray studies that would be performed in the medical office, such as complete blood count, urinalysis, or x-ray.

DIAGNOSIS CODES

This area should include the diagnoses most commonly used in the office. There should also be ample room left for additional diagnoses to be written in. This should include V codes and E codes when applicable.

DATE OF NEXT APPOINTMENT

This is the area of the form where the physician communicates to the front-desk personnel when the patient is to return for a follow-up appointment. The physician might want to see the patient for follow-up in 6 weeks or maybe not for 3 months. This can be written by the physician in this area.

NAME OF PROVIDER

This area illustrates who provided the service to the patient. It can be printed or handwritten, but is an essential part of the form because all carriers require the identity of the provider of the service. This field would contain the physicians in the group, plus any other provider of service such as a nurse practitioner or physician's assistant.

DESIGNING THE HOSPITAL TRACKING FORM

A form similar to the fee slip/patient encounter form can be designed for use with hospital patients. The following areas should be included on the hospital tracking form:

- Patient's name
- Patient's date of birth
- Admission date
- Discharge date

- Authorization/precertification number
- Insurance company
  - Primary
  - Secondary
- Insurance numbers
- Diagnosis code area
- Procedure code area
- Total charge area
- Physician's signature area

PATIENT'S NAME/DATE OF BIRTH

This area should include the patient's name with middle initial and the patient's date of birth. The date of birth is especially important, because there might be two patients with the same name in the hospital at the same time.

AUTHORIZATION/PRECERTIFICATION NUMBER

This number is required by some insurance companies for payment of the hospital stay. It is important to include this number on the billing sheet so that the billing department can access it.

DIAGNOSIS CODES

Space for diagnosis codes can be provided on the hospital tracking form in two ways. One way is to designate an area where diagnoses can be written in by the physician or biller. They *must* be in order of priority. It is sometimes helpful to set up the diagnosis code area as follows:

Diagnosis:

1. ______________________
2. ______________________
3. ______________________
4. ______________________

It is important to remind the physician that diagnosis coding is her or his responsibility. It is unfair, and illegal, to expect billing personnel, or even clinical personnel, to be able to choose the diagnosis of the patient.

Another way to provide space on the hospital tracking form for diagnosis codes is to provide a list of common diagnoses with blanks in front to prioritize them. Additional open space must be left for diagnoses that are not listed. This is not always the best way to set up the diagnosis section of the hospital tracking form. Hospital diagnoses can be too numerous to mention, and depending on the specialty, it may be too difficult to set it up in this manner. An example would be as follows:

_____530.11 Reflux esophagitis
_____689.2 Cellulitis, nonspecific
_____786.59 Chest discomfort
_____724.5 Backache, unspecified
_____244.9 Hypothyroidism
_____451.2 Deep vein phlebitis

Generating Reports

Many financial reports and other types of reports can be generated by the computer system. These reports can be used to assess the practice's financial status, or to track the number of new patients seen. The computer also can produce many statistics that can be helpful for forecasting the future of the practice. The following is a partial list of reports that can be produced:

- Accounts receivable aging analysis
- Patient master file
- Analysis of patient demographics
- Listings of charges, payments, and adjustments by month-to-date (MTD) and year-to-date (YTD)
- Location master file
- Analysis of referring physicians
- Audit trails
- Billing reports
- Master insurance file
- Analysis of procedures
- Analysis of diagnoses
- Productivity report

The computer screens and corresponding reports shown in Figures 10-5 through 10-10 illustrate how a report is chosen from the computer and what the final product looks like.

There are specialty software packages designed to provide payroll and tax services. They keep track of all business transactions and their effects on the assets and liabilities of the practice. They maintain daily records of deposits and withdrawals, print balance statements, and print the checks for both payroll and payables. These functions should have limited accessibility to users so that only authorized individuals may access them.

Managing Prescriptions

If you have the right software, you can use the computer to manage the office prescriptions. You can print prescriptions and track the medications, saving the physician valuable time and improving the quality of care. Patients' allergies can be clearly displayed on the computer screen to avoid the improper prescribing of medication. Medication conflicts and medication-mandated laboratory work can also be flagged in the computer system. Prescription renewal alerts can be established for every patient, and a complete list of the patient's medication, with directions and precautions, can be given at each visit.

With this type of software, physicians can easily choose a medication from a list of medications in the database and tailor it to the parameters necessary for that individual patient. The capabilities of checking and double-checking are phenomenal, and therefore the percentage of errors is decreased. Medication interactions are promptly pointed

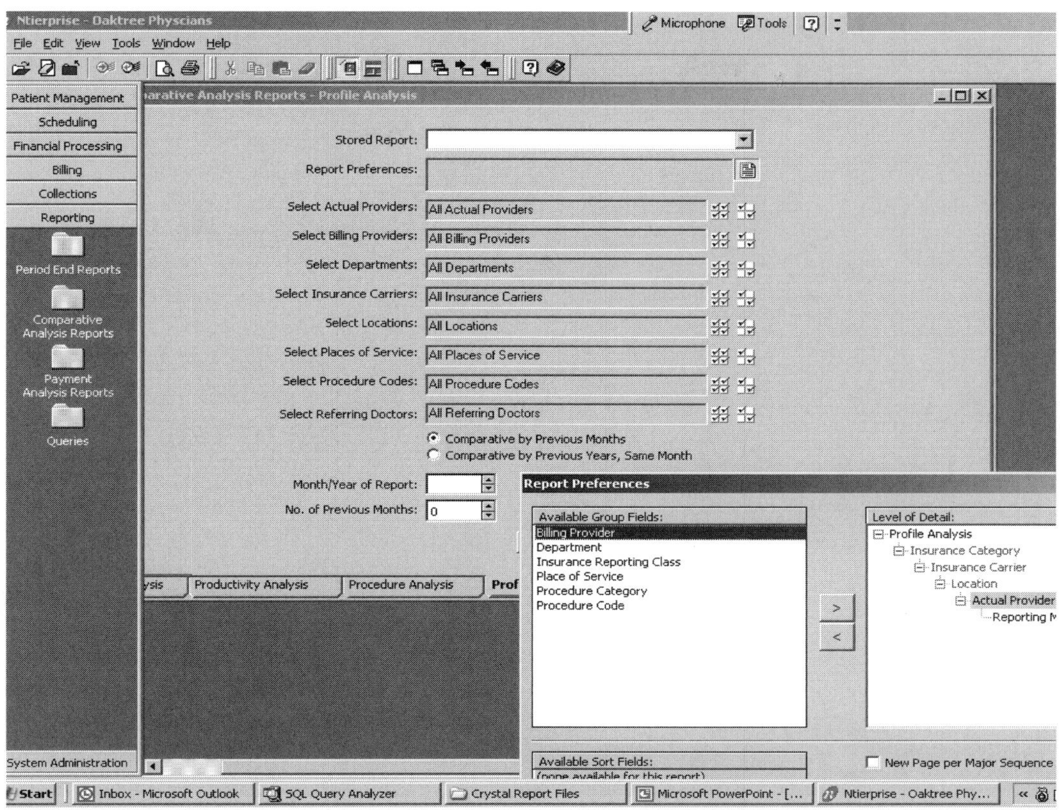

FIGURE 10-5. Various ways to generate a physician productivity report. (Courtesy of Compusense, Inc.)

out if the physician prescribes a medication that interacts with another. This software not only prints out the appropriate prescription, but also places an entry of the medication prescribed into the patient's record. Access to these programs can be limited to protect patient confidentiality.

OFFICE SOFTWARE

The practice should have some type of "office" software such as a word processing software, a spreadsheet software, and even perhaps some type of database or slide show software. Word processing products may be WordPerfect or Microsoft Word. Spreadsheet products may be Microsoft Excel or Lotus. Microsoft Access works great as a database product, and for preparing presentations, Microsoft PowerPoint can't be beat. Whatever your choice, it is important to be able to have those software packages available. It may be necessary to open a document from someone that requires Excel or Word. Many practice management software packages also offer Microsoft Office or Office Suite along with their product. A spreadsheet program can be very helpful to the office manager in a variety of situations. A word processing program would be used to prepare meeting agendas, memos about changes in billing procedures, preparation of job descriptions, development of policies and procedures, and so on.

FROM THE EXPERT'S NOTEBOOK

Be sure to *always* save any document you are working on, whether it be a Word document or a spreadsheet. Closing the document without saving it first will cause the information to be lost.

Coding Software

In Chapter 6, the use of coding software to prevent incorrect coding was discussed briefly. The advantages of using coding software were discussed, but not actually how the software works. Using Flash Code as an example, a brief description of the benefits and of coding software and how easy it is to use is described.

Flash Code is coding software used for rapidly finding, documenting, and validating the codes required for

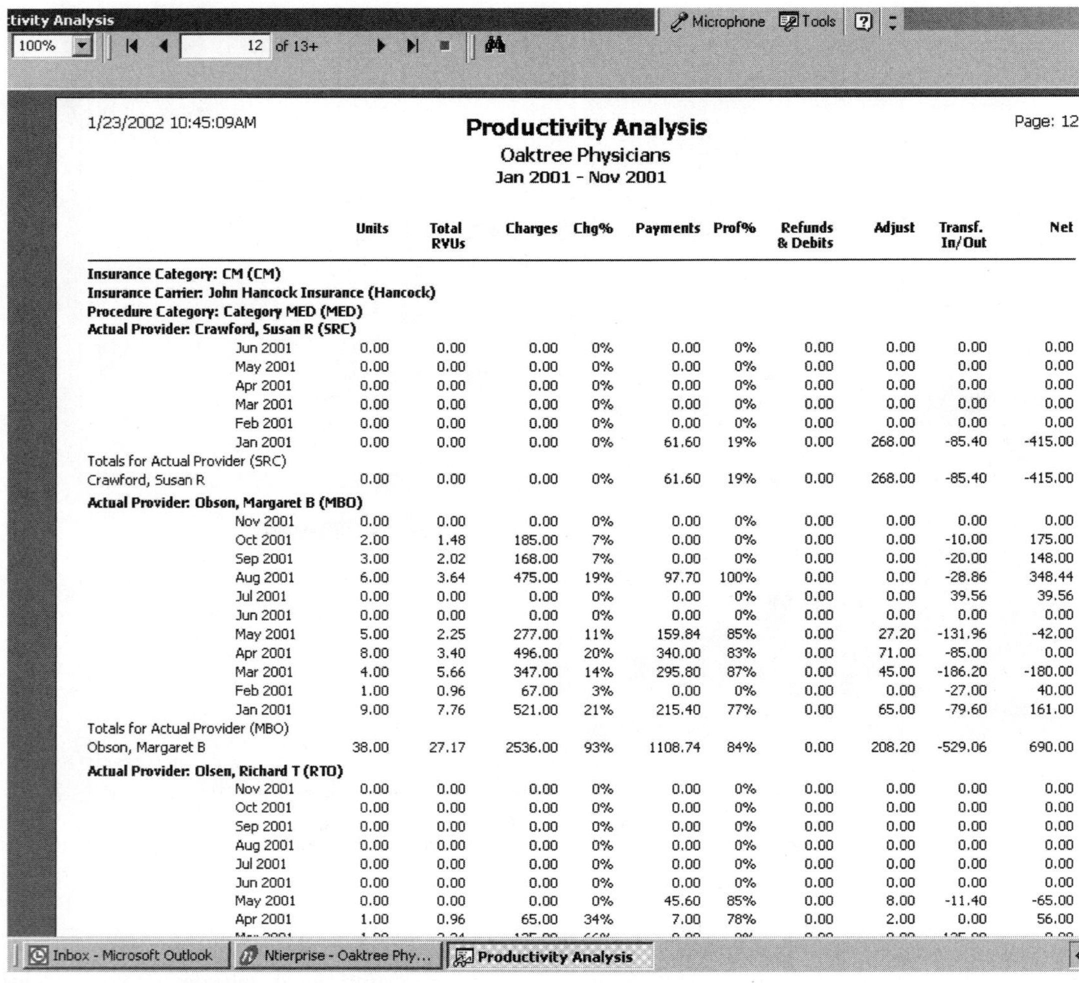

1/23/2002 10:45:09AM | Page: 12

Productivity Analysis
Oaktree Physicians
Jan 2001 - Nov 2001

	Units	Total RVUs	Charges	Chg%	Payments	Prof%	Refunds & Debits	Adjust	Transf. In/Out	Net
Insurance Category: CM (CM)										
Insurance Carrier: John Hancock Insurance (Hancock)										
Procedure Category: Category MED (MED)										
Actual Provider: Crawford, Susan R (SRC)										
Jun 2001	0.00	0.00	0.00	0%	0.00	0%	0.00	0.00	0.00	0.00
May 2001	0.00	0.00	0.00	0%	0.00	0%	0.00	0.00	0.00	0.00
Apr 2001	0.00	0.00	0.00	0%	0.00	0%	0.00	0.00	0.00	0.00
Mar 2001	0.00	0.00	0.00	0%	0.00	0%	0.00	0.00	0.00	0.00
Feb 2001	0.00	0.00	0.00	0%	0.00	0%	0.00	0.00	0.00	0.00
Jan 2001	0.00	0.00	0.00	0%	61.60	19%	0.00	268.00	-85.40	-415.00
Totals for Actual Provider (SRC)										
Crawford, Susan R	0.00	0.00	0.00	0%	61.60	19%	0.00	268.00	-85.40	-415.00
Actual Provider: Obson, Margaret B (MBO)										
Nov 2001	0.00	0.00	0.00	0%	0.00	0%	0.00	0.00	0.00	0.00
Oct 2001	2.00	1.48	185.00	7%	0.00	0%	0.00	0.00	-10.00	175.00
Sep 2001	3.00	2.02	168.00	7%	0.00	0%	0.00	0.00	-20.00	148.00
Aug 2001	6.00	3.64	475.00	19%	97.70	100%	0.00	0.00	-28.86	348.44
Jul 2001	0.00	0.00	0.00	0%	0.00	0%	0.00	0.00	39.56	39.56
Jun 2001	0.00	0.00	0.00	0%	0.00	0%	0.00	0.00	0.00	0.00
May 2001	5.00	2.25	277.00	11%	159.84	85%	0.00	27.20	-131.96	-42.00
Apr 2001	8.00	3.40	496.00	20%	340.00	83%	0.00	71.00	-85.00	0.00
Mar 2001	4.00	5.66	347.00	14%	295.80	87%	0.00	45.00	-186.20	-180.00
Feb 2001	1.00	0.96	67.00	3%	0.00	0%	0.00	0.00	-27.00	40.00
Jan 2001	9.00	7.76	521.00	21%	215.40	77%	0.00	65.00	-79.60	161.00
Totals for Actual Provider (MBO)										
Obson, Margaret B	38.00	27.17	2536.00	93%	1108.74	84%	0.00	208.20	-529.06	690.00
Actual Provider: Olsen, Richard T (RTO)										
Nov 2001	0.00	0.00	0.00	0%	0.00	0%	0.00	0.00	0.00	0.00
Oct 2001	0.00	0.00	0.00	0%	0.00	0%	0.00	0.00	0.00	0.00
Sep 2001	0.00	0.00	0.00	0%	0.00	0%	0.00	0.00	0.00	0.00
Aug 2001	0.00	0.00	0.00	0%	0.00	0%	0.00	0.00	0.00	0.00
Jul 2001	0.00	0.00	0.00	0%	0.00	0%	0.00	0.00	0.00	0.00
Jun 2001	0.00	0.00	0.00	0%	0.00	0%	0.00	0.00	0.00	0.00
May 2001	0.00	0.00	0.00	0%	45.60	85%	0.00	8.00	-11.40	-65.00
Apr 2001	1.00	0.96	65.00	34%	7.00	78%	0.00	2.00	0.00	56.00

FIGURE 10-6. Office managers can use this productivity report to advise the physician on the volume and types of services and procedures performed during a period. (Courtesy of Compusense, Inc.)

medical billing. This particular software contains three basic reference books:

1. *International Classification of Diseases*, Ninth Revision, Clinical Modification (ICD-9-CM) diagnosis codes. This book is composed of four sections:
   - ICD codes (arranged numerically; approximately 15,000 of them)
   - ICD index (arranged alphabetically, approximately 73,000 entries)
   - Table of drugs and chemicals (approximately 4,600 drugs with six columns of data each); these drugs reflect causes of illness rather than drugs used for patient care
   - Table of neoplasms (1,725 neoplasms with six columns of data each)
2. *Physicians' Current Procedural Terminology* (CPT) procedure codes. This book contains three sections:
   - CPT codes (arranged numerically; just under 8,000 of them)
   - CPT index (arranged alphabetically, approximately 27,000 entries)
   - CPT guide (contains modifier information and guidelines for CPT code use)
3. *The Healthcare Common Procedure Coding System* (HCPCS) procedure/supply codes. This book has two sections:
   - HCPCS codes (arranged numerically; approximately 3,000)
   - Table of drugs (1,300 entries for drugs used in patient care)

There is no alpha index as the index entries are nearly identical to the codes.

ICD-9 codes are categorized into three-digit families (Figure 10-11). Codes that are billable have a red light, indicating that the user has reached the end of the road. Green lights indicate that the user has reached a fork in the road. At this point, more descriptive codes are displayed by clicking the green light or the "4" in order to

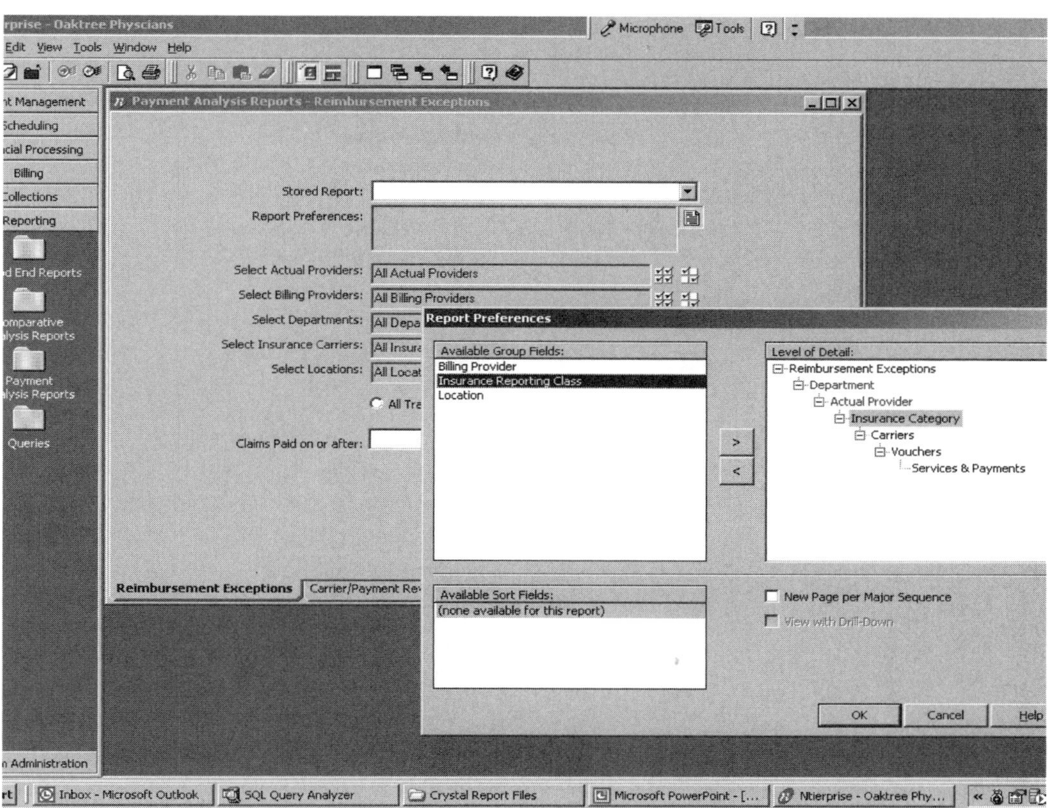

FIGURE 10-7. Various ways to generate a reimbursement report. (Courtesy of Compusense, Inc.)

display four-digit codes. This will prevent the billing of truncated diagnosis codes. A truncated diagnosis code is one that requires a fourth or fifth digit for billing.

The search screens allow for partial word AND searches, as well as numeric searches. Ranges of codes can be found by placing "..." between the beginning and ending number. The type of code displayed in the found set can be restricted to three-, four-, or five-digit codes, as well as only codes specific enough for billing (red codes) (Figure 10-12).

When using the CPT function of the program (Figure 10-13), there are additional navigational buttons to choose from. These buttons identify the various categories, which are illustrated with six CPT headings: Evaluation and Management, Anesthesia, Surgery, Radiology, Path/Lab, and Medicine codes. In addition, the Alpha divisions of the HCPCS codes can also displayed. An alpha division refers to the division among the codes based on the first letter of each code. Various letters represent various categories of codes. For example, J codes identify drug codes, D codes identify dental procedures, etc. Both fee schedules and edit check information can be accessed from this screen.

Clicking on the dollar amount displays a screen that allows the user to view Medicare fees calculated to the penny based on the location of service (hospital versus nonhospital), geographic location, and other factors used by the government to calculate the allowable fee for most CPT codes (Figure 10-14). In addition, the codes for Durable Medical Equipment and Laboratory Services have been added, by state, in order for the user to be aware of the costs involved in ordering these tests. A physician practice might not use this feature as much as the others. The rules for using modifiers are also displayed.

Clicking over the starred field (*) will allow the user to see a variety of codes that fall into many categories. These codes have special instructions unique for their selected group. These instructions or the affected codes can be displayed, and then exported or printed (Figure 10-15).

The correct coding initiative edits are used by the government to detect potentially fraudulent billing. This layout displays the codes that fall into this category (Figure 10-16). Intelligent feedback will be shown in later screens.

ICD-9 codes that are required for billing with specific CPT codes are found in Local Medicare Review Policy bulletins. When the ABN button is black, a policy with specific ICD-9 codes applies. By clicking the ABN button, the ICD-9 codes can be displayed (Figure 10-17). In addition, the user can enter any ICD-9 code to see if it matches codes in the list.

In many cases the user simply wants to use Flash Code to find codes quickly and easily. However, some users want to enter a series of codes and then have Flash Code validate the codes against government rules. To perform this task, a series

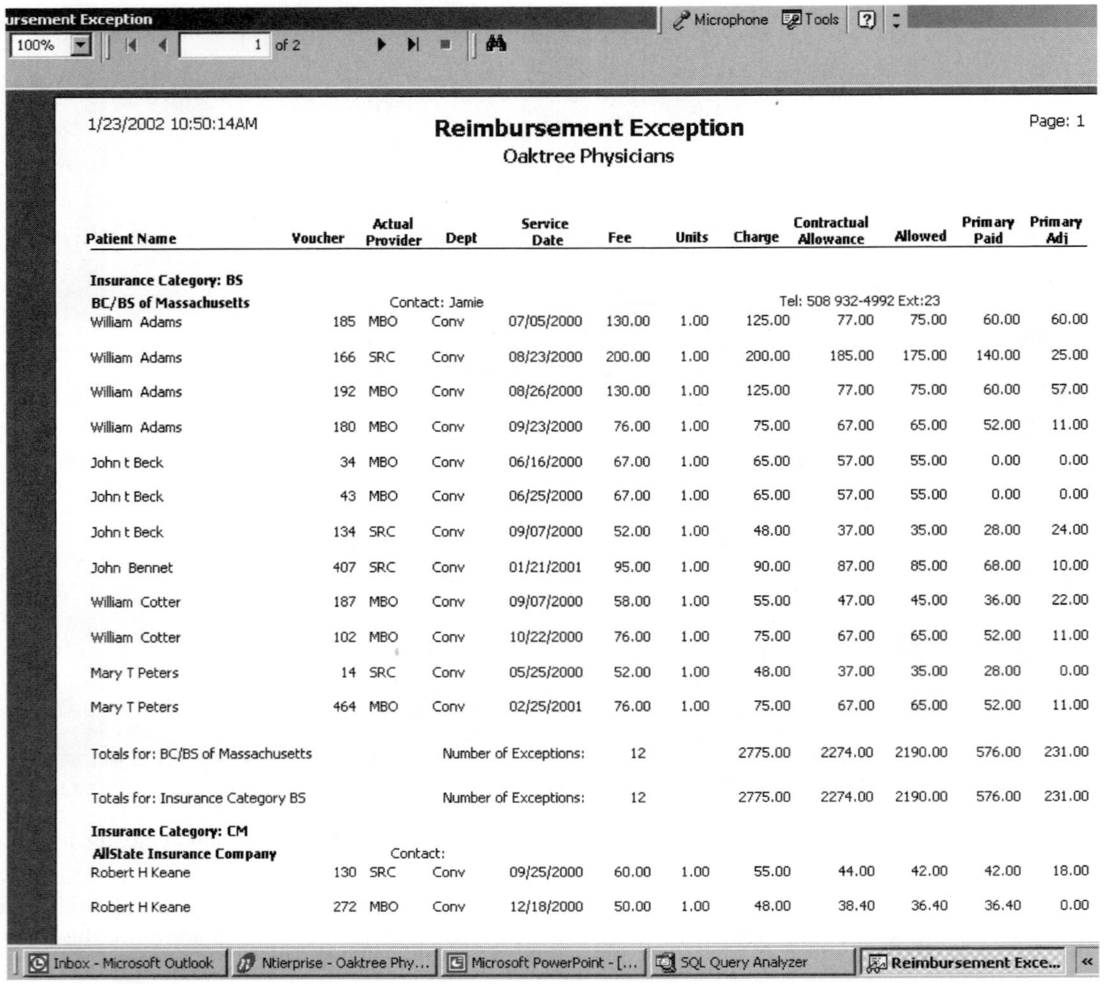

1/23/2002 10:50:14AM — **Reimbursement Exception** — Page: 1

Oaktree Physicians

Patient Name	Voucher	Actual Provider	Dept	Service Date	Fee	Units	Charge	Contractual Allowance	Allowed	Primary Paid	Primary Adj
Insurance Category: BS											
BC/BS of Massachusetts		Contact: Jamie					Tel: 508 932-4992 Ext:23				
William Adams	185	MBO	Conv	07/05/2000	130.00	1.00	125.00	77.00	75.00	60.00	60.00
William Adams	166	SRC	Conv	08/23/2000	200.00	1.00	200.00	185.00	175.00	140.00	25.00
William Adams	192	MBO	Conv	08/26/2000	130.00	1.00	125.00	77.00	75.00	60.00	57.00
William Adams	180	MBO	Conv	09/23/2000	76.00	1.00	75.00	67.00	65.00	52.00	11.00
John t Beck	34	MBO	Conv	06/16/2000	67.00	1.00	65.00	57.00	55.00	0.00	0.00
John t Beck	43	MBO	Conv	06/25/2000	67.00	1.00	65.00	57.00	55.00	0.00	0.00
John t Beck	134	SRC	Conv	09/07/2000	52.00	1.00	48.00	37.00	35.00	28.00	24.00
John Bennet	407	SRC	Conv	01/21/2001	95.00	1.00	90.00	87.00	85.00	68.00	10.00
William Cotter	187	MBO	Conv	09/07/2000	58.00	1.00	55.00	47.00	45.00	36.00	22.00
William Cotter	102	MBO	Conv	10/22/2000	76.00	1.00	75.00	67.00	65.00	52.00	11.00
Mary T Peters	14	SRC	Conv	05/25/2000	52.00	1.00	48.00	37.00	35.00	28.00	0.00
Mary T Peters	464	MBO	Conv	02/25/2001	76.00	1.00	75.00	67.00	65.00	52.00	11.00
Totals for: BC/BS of Massachusetts			Number of Exceptions:		12		2775.00	2274.00	2190.00	576.00	231.00
Totals for: Insurance Category BS			Number of Exceptions:		12		2775.00	2274.00	2190.00	576.00	231.00
Insurance Category: CM											
AllState Insurance Company		Contact:									
Robert H Keane	130	SRC	Conv	09/25/2000	60.00	1.00	55.00	44.00	42.00	42.00	18.00
Robert H Keane	272	MBO	Conv	12/18/2000	50.00	1.00	48.00	38.40	36.40	36.40	0.00

FIGURE 10-8. Office managers can use this reimbursement report to track reimbursements by various insurance carriers. (Courtesy of Compusense, Inc.)

of codes are copied into the clipboard, then run through the validation checker (Figure 10-18). In this case a Thyroid Stimulating Hormone, TSH (CPT Code 84443), is ordered.

On validation, it is shown that there are ICD-9 codes required for billing (Figure 10-19). The list of codes is presented to the user so that an appropriate code is selected for billing.

In this case two incompatible CPT codes, 12001 and 12002, are selected for billing (Figure 10-20). Flash Code evaluates the payment schedule and instructs the user to drop the "component part" code 12001, since these two codes cannot be billed together. In certain instances, CPT codes can be billed together if an appropriate modifier is used. When this occurs, Flash Code displays the modifier list so that the user can make a selection.

Flash Code also evaluates ICD-9 codes for specificity. In this case 873 is a green light code and must be taken to a higher level of specificity (Figure 10-21).

Clicking the view button will allow the user to see more specific codes associated with 873 (Figure 10-22). The user can select the code that matches. If a code is green, the next level of more specific codes will be displayed.

This software has many additional features not listed in this text. These features illustrate that a well-written coding application can help you in many ways and catch mistakes before the claim gets submitted.

MANAGER'S ALERT

The use of coding software is *no* substitute for physician participation in choosing the correct CPT, HCPCS, and ICD-9 codes.

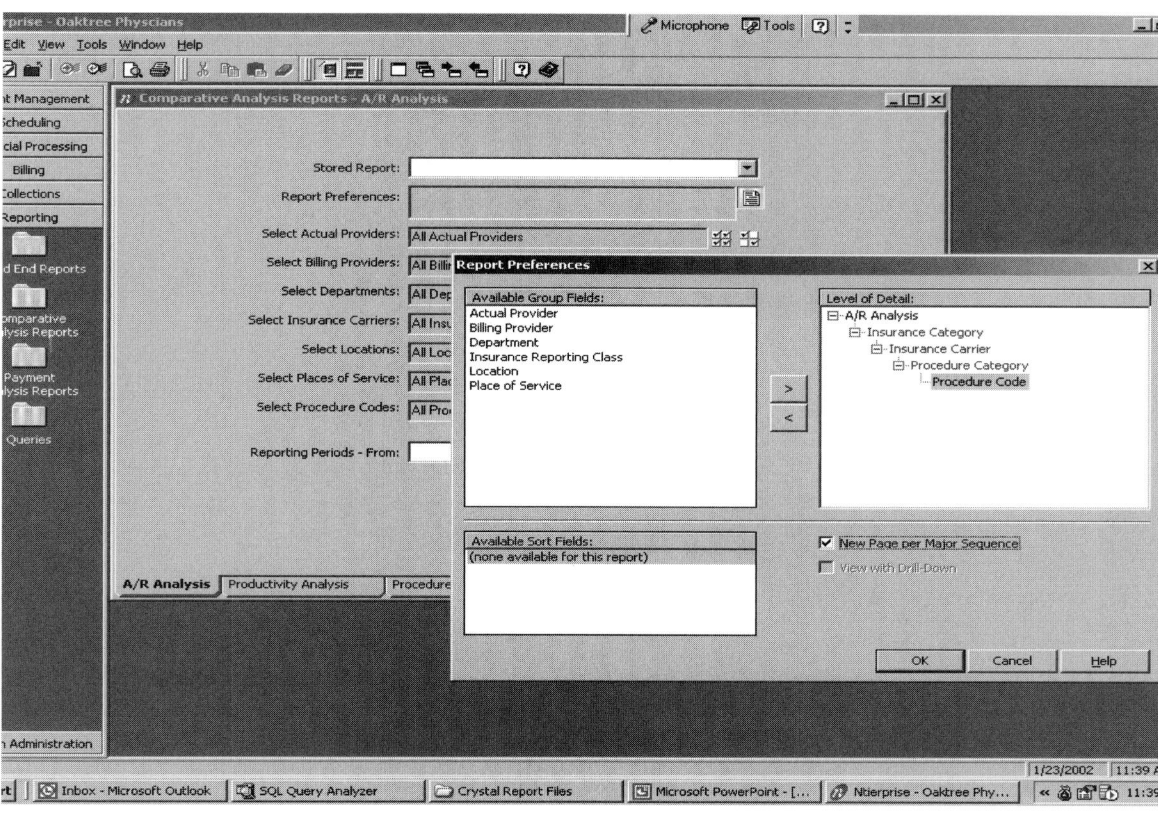

FIGURE 10-9. Office managers can use this accounts receivable (A/R) report to collect outstanding fees. (Courtesy of Compusense, Inc.)

THE ELECTRONIC MEDICAL RECORD

An electronic medical record (EMR) is one that is in a digital (electronic) format. The first EMR was developed in the early 1990s by Richard Dick, Elaine Steen, and Don Detmer, authors of the book *The Computer-Based Patient Record: An Essential Technology for Healthcare.* Its adoption has been rather slow; recent studies show that the number of physician practices that have implemented an EMR has doubled over the past few years, although a study by Massachusetts General Hospital and George Washington University Hospital found that only one in four physicians in the United States uses an EMR. Health care technologies should reduce cost, improve quality, and enhance patient safety.

An EMR should be highly flexible; after all, that is what technology is all about. It should adapt to the needs of each individual practice by providing different information captures for pediatrics versus neurology, for example. Obviously, the information requirements for these two practice specialties are different. A good EMR will reconfigure itself to meet the specific needs of both specialties. It should serve not only the large medical practices, but the smaller practices as well. An EMR should serve the needs of a 100-physician multispecialty practice the same as a 2-physician dermatology practice. The right EMR will do the following:

- Increase the availability of the patient's medical history and preserve accuracy
- Facilitate clinical research by providing comprehensive views of health care delivery
- Provide diagnostic and therapeutic problem-solving support
- Increase efficiency of the staff by reducing time spent retrieving information
- Eliminate overhead and administrative costs associated with paper transfer and storage
- Maintain a comprehensive legal record of patient care
- Ensure confidentiality of patient data through the use of passwords

Possible Factors for Failure

Four factors may affect the success of the implementation of an EMR:

- Lack of understanding of EMRs
- Lack of commitment to the project

1/23/2002 10:56:51AM — **A/R Analysis** — Page: 2

Oaktree Physicians

Jan 2001 - Nov 2001

	Prev A/R	Charges Charge%	Payments Profile%	Refunds & Debits	Adjust	Trans-In	Trans-Out	New A/R # Days
Insurance Category: HM (HM)								
Totals for Insurance Carrier (HMO Blue)								
HMO Blue	82.00	440.00 2%	287.70 87%	0.00	42.70	72.60	109.20	155.00 51
Totals for Insurance Carrier (Tufts)								
Tufts Health Plan	283.00	2625.00 15%	1787.00 88%	0.00	247.56	0.00	873.44	0.00 0
Totals for Insurance Category (HM)								
HM	365.00	3065.00 17%	2074.70 85%	0.00	359.56	141.90	982.64	155.00 228
Insurance Category: MD (MD)								
Totals for Insurance Carrier (MD OH)								
Medicaid of Ohio	0.00	282.00 2%	128.00 80%	0.00	32.00	0.00	0.00	122.00 0
Totals for Insurance Category (MD)								
MD	0.00	282.00 2%	128.00 80%	0.00	32.00	0.00	0.00	122.00 0
Insurance Category: MR (MR)								
Totals for Insurance Carrier (MC B)								
Medicare Part B	441.60	2694.00 15%	1165.10 57%	0.50	881.80	20.80	644.60	465.40 201
Totals for Insurance Carrier (Medicare)								
Medicare	0.00	429.00 2%	294.56 83%	0.00	60.80	0.00	73.64	0.00 0
Totals for Insurance Category (MR)								
MR	441.60	3123.00 17%	1459.66 61%	0.50	942.60	20.80	718.24	465.40 96
Insurance Category: Self-Pay (Self-Pay)								
Totals for Insurance Carrier (Self-Pay)								
Self-Pay	480.10	760.00 4%	2486.37 93%	0.00	178.32	3587.68	156.70	2006.39 243
Totals for Insurance Category (Self-Pay)								
Self-Pay	480.10	760.00 4%	2486.37 93%	0.00	178.32	3587.68	156.70	2006.39 243

Inbox - Microsoft ... | Ntierprise - Oaktre... | Microsoft PowerPo... | SQL Query Analyzer | Crystal Report Files | A/R Analysis

FIGURE 10-10. Various ways to generate an accounts receivable (A/R) report. (Courtesy of Compusense, Inc.)

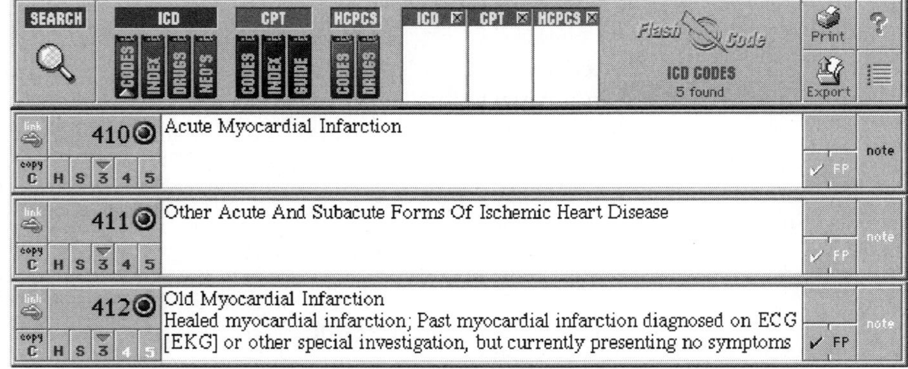

FIGURE 10-11. ICD-9-CM code screen showing specific and nonspecific codes. (Courtesy of Flashcode, Inc.)

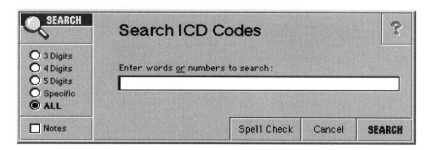

FIGURE 10-12. ICD-9-CM search screen used to select appropriate diagnosis codes. (Courtesy of Flashcode, Inc.)

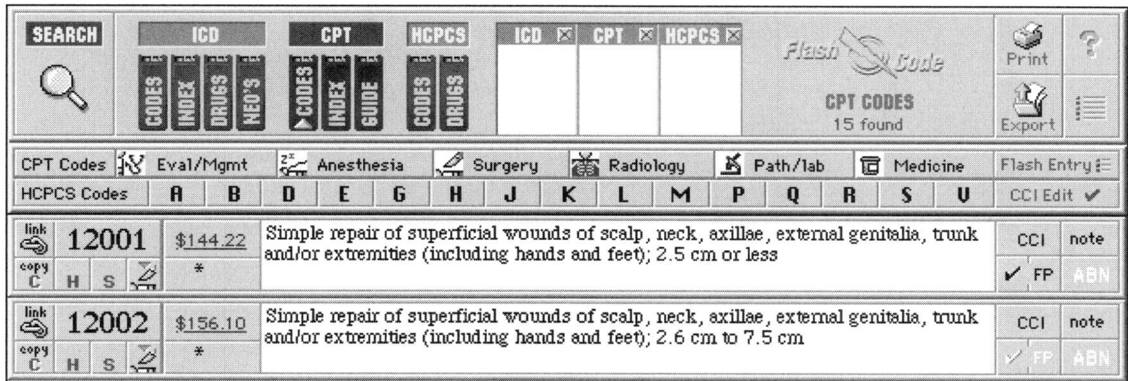

FIGURE 10-13. CPT code screen with detail screens just a click away. (Courtesy of Flashcode, Inc.)

- Lack of communication among the physician, the staff, and the EMR vendor
- Lack of office preparation for the project

LACK OF UNDERSTANDING OF EMRs

When talking about "going electronic," the office manager should begin to research the various EMR products that are available. Much of the initial research can be performed online. Once the office manager has been educated on the basics of an EMR, it is time to call some of the vendors and set up appointments to meet with them to discuss their product.

LACK OF COMMITMENT TO THE PROJECT

If the practice is serious about implementing an EMR, everyone must be committed to the endeavor. There will be a breakdown in the success of the project if everyone is not committed.

LACK OF COMMUNICATION AMONG THE PHYSICIAN, THE STAFF, AND THE EMR VENDOR

It is important to be sure to have clear communication between the EMR vendor and the practice that is purchasing the EMR product. There is no room for misunderstandings, because they can be costly and the practice may end up with a product that does not work for it. Put the needs, concerns, and wants in writing. Review them, make changes, and then discuss with the EMR vendor.

LACK OF OFFICE PREPARATION FOR THE PROJECT

It is most important to the project of implementing an EMR to be prepared, because it can be a trying but rewarding experience. The office manager should prepare a blueprint for this very important project with details and time frames outlined. The staff should be "in the loop" during the entire process, and this change should always be seen as positive. Change can be difficult for anyone, but when a positive spin is placed on the EMR, it can have surprising results. If the staff is not kept informed, there could be fear of the unknown, which will put a negative spin on the project.

How to Buy an Electronic Medical Record

Not all EMRs are alike, so it is important to understand the components and operations of a few different EMRs before making a choice for your practice. The following checklist provided by Misys Healthcare Systems can be used as a guide in evaluating EMR systems:

- Does the EMR complement the current workflow of the practice?

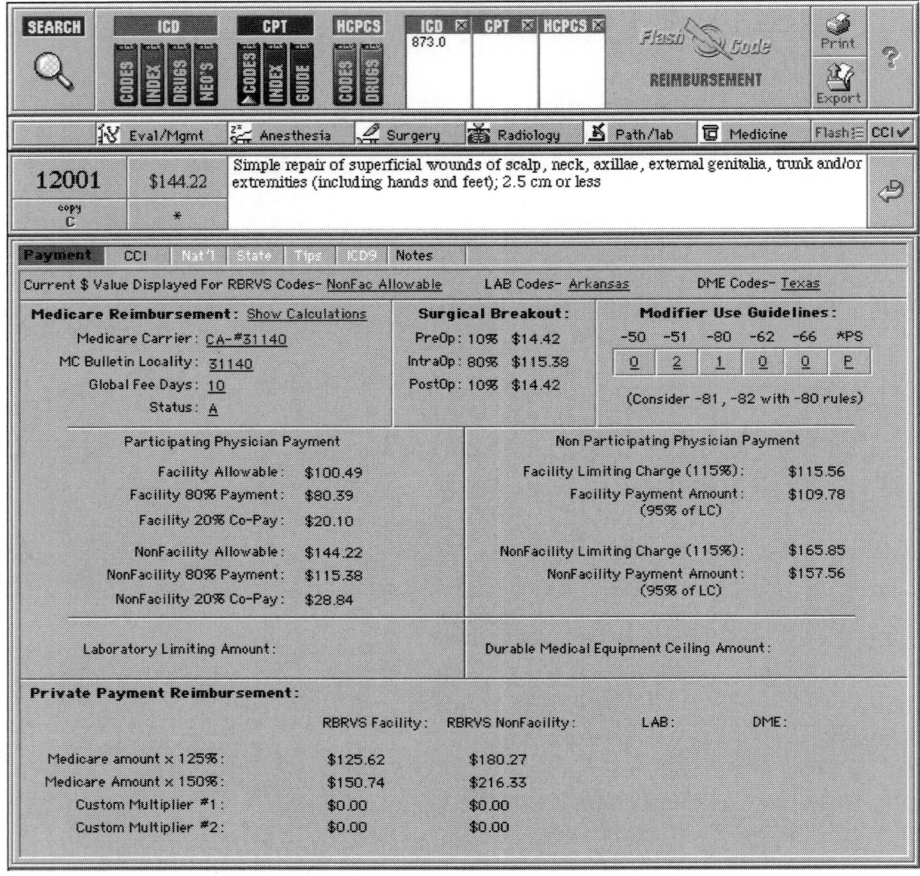

FIGURE 10-14. Reimbursement screen containing drop-down lists for selecting region-specific information. (Courtesy of Flashcode, Inc.)

- Does the EMR work well for my specialty? Will it require any customization to fit my practice?
- Does the EMR require each physician to document in the same manner, or can some physicians continue to dictate their notes?
- Are there certain components that must be purchased as a package, or do I have the flexibility to pick and choose?
- Where did the design information come from? Were physician, nurses, or other health care professionals involved in the development?
- Will this EMR generate revenue for the practice? Can it help the practice to reduce inefficiencies and make it more productive? Can it help provide quality patient care?
- Is the EMR compatible with the currently used practice management system, or do I have to replace it?
- Who installs the system? What about training—does the EMR require on-site or off-site training?
- What kind of support is available to the practice? What are the time frames?
- Is the company stable?
- Are there any specialties similar to mine using this EMR? Can you provide references? Any in the area?
- Tell me about your research and development. Will the product continue to change? How frequently do you anticipate releasing updates and new versions? Is the cost included in the purchase price?

An EMR that fits the practice will provide templates that will allow the physician to quickly and accurately document a patient's service or procedure. It will allow for easy patient registration and 24/7 access to patient charts. Documentation is easily transformed into correspondence to others, eliminating the need for costly transcription. Some systems are not specialty focused and contain a "one size fits all" template that is required to meet the needs of all specialties. If the practice is spending the money for an EMR, make sure to get one that works the best for your practice; don't settle for a general system that may not work for your specialty. Many systems provide templates that allow for the physician to simply document by using a series of "clicks" through the medical record. For example, the history portion in most systems is a series of drop-down lists except for the chief complaint and history

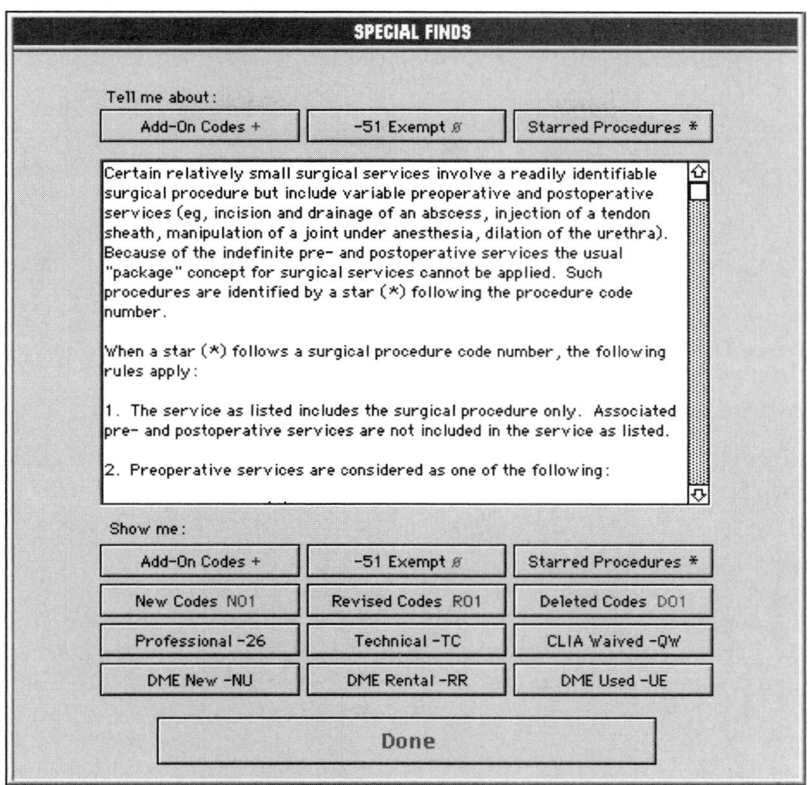

FIGURE 10-15. A "special finds" screen provides the user with all new, revised, deleted, or special groups of codes. (Courtesy of Flashcode, Inc.)

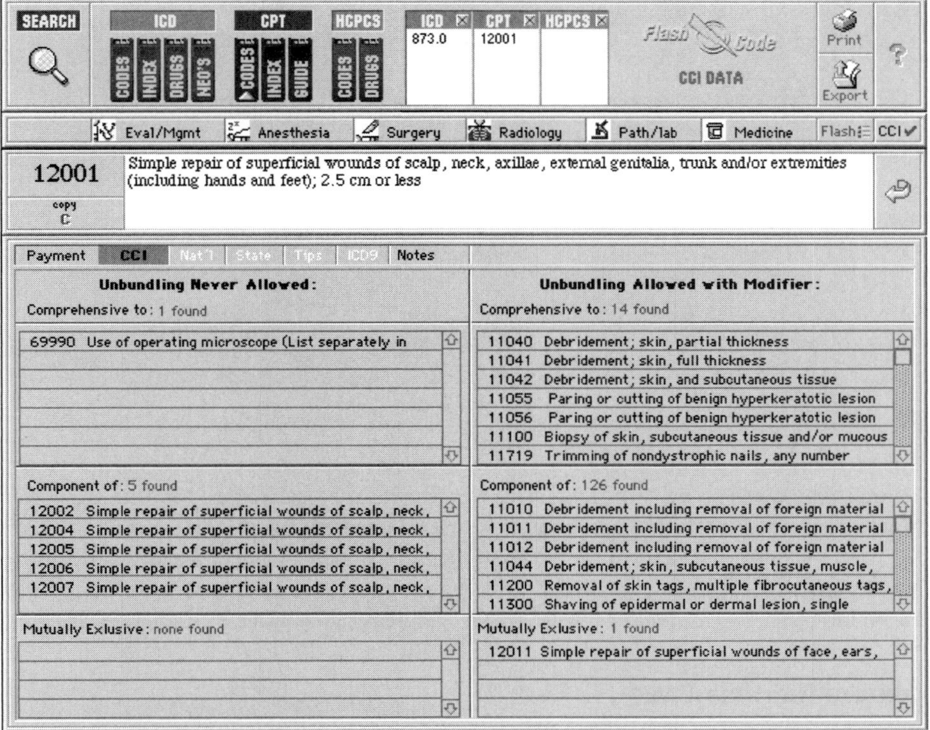

FIGURE 10-16. This screen provides the user with bundling information for the code chosen. (Courtesy of Flashcode, Inc.)

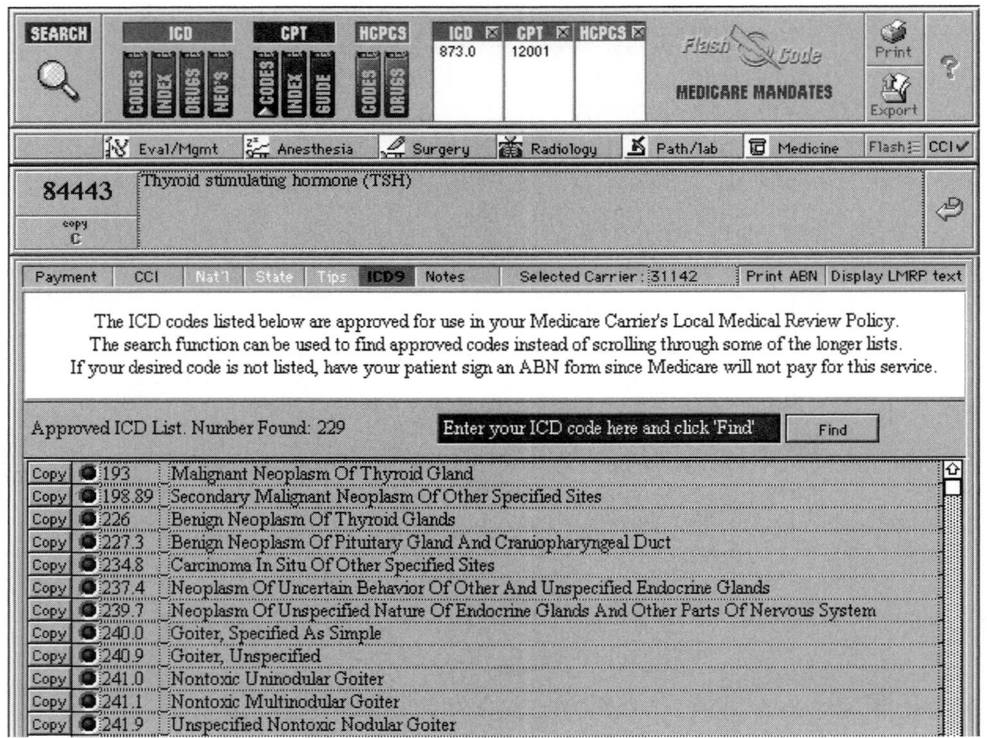

FIGURE 10-17. Screen providing related information from a Local Medical Review Policy bulletin, which will help a practice to ascertain whether an Advanced Beneficiary Notice should be signed. (Courtesy of Flashcode, Inc.)

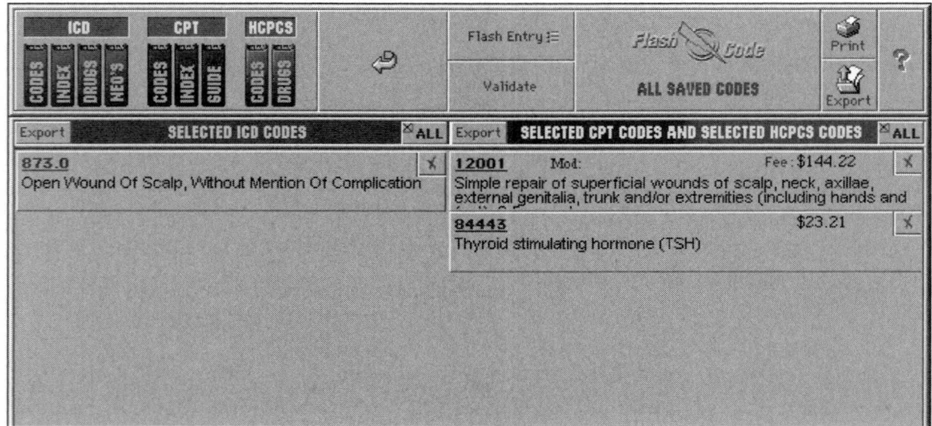

FIGURE 10-18. This screen lets the user save ICD-9-CM and CPT codes. (Courtesy of Flashcode, Inc.)

of present illness sections. These are called "free text" areas where the physician can type the reason for the visit and the history behind that complaint. The examination section can easily be documented by a series of "clicks," and the medical decision making can be "clicked" as well.

Fraudulent Documentation via EMR

Do we make documentation so easy that levels of E&M services are rising? Are they supported by the documentation in the medical record? Is that documentation accurate? It has been found that some providers of service find it too easy to "click" off items in the drop-down boxes whether or not they were reviewed or examined. There are an increasing number of higher levels of history and examination with the implementation and use of the EMR. Is it medically necessary to perform a complete review of systems and complete past, family, and social history for a patient with a sprained ankle as a result of playing basketball? Is it medically necessary to perform a comprehensive

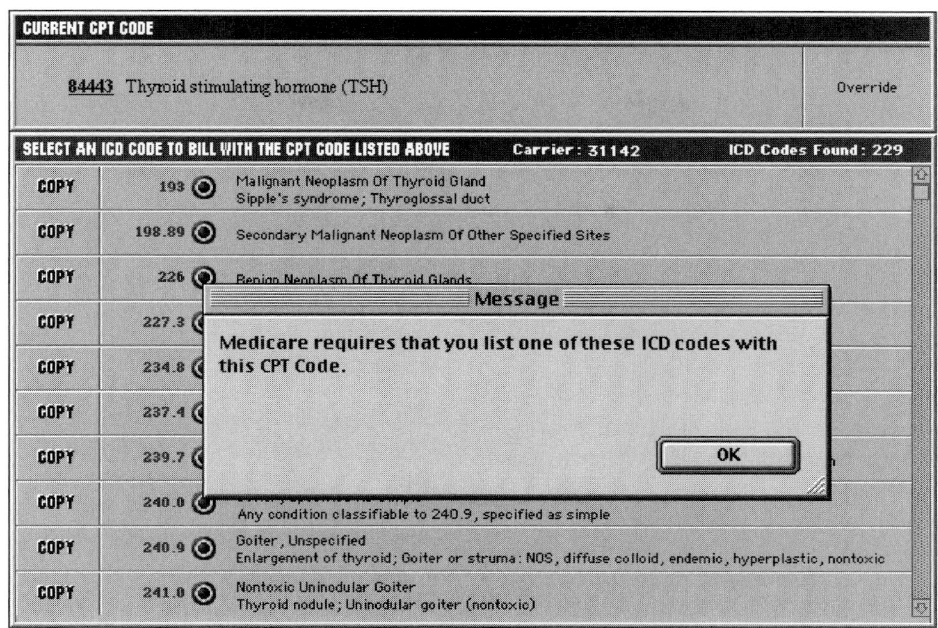

FIGURE 10-19. This screen lists the ICD-9-CM codes that are approved for use with the CPT code chosen, per LMRP. (Courtesy of Flashcode, Inc.)

examination on a patient who has an earache? In physician practices where last year's medical record audit results identified detailed histories and examinations, these same medical record audits are not showing billings of comprehensive levels of history and examination. Remember, only "click" on what you do. Maybe the phrase "Don't 'click it' if you didn't do it!" will take the place of the old, but true, "If you didn't document it, you didn't do it!"

Printing EMRs

Portions of the medical record can be printed from their computerized forms. Some physicians want to update medical records when they are in hard copy, not computer based. Some employees and physicians are resistant to change, and therefore find comfort in hard-copy records. Some practices do not have enough computers or laptops to go around, and it becomes necessary to print some medical records for entry into the computer at a later date. When copies of an EMR are made, there is a risk of having multiple pages and it becomes easy to lose track of the document that has the most recent entries. Having the possibility of different versions of the same medical record is dangerous for the practice and the patient.

Hard copies can also cause confusion when the format of the printout changes. Copies of EMRs printed with different versions of the same software may look different. This can be especially troublesome for court documents. They may be the same but appear different, which is a problem for lawyers to explain. Making a pdf of the document is a good solution when records are printed and should not be changed in any way. One important rule to remember is, *Don't document on printed copies of an EMR.*

E-Discovery

Attorneys are finding loopholes in EMRs that would not exist in a paper record. With the growth of EMRs, health care lawyers and health information technologists predict the number of "e-discoveries" to increase significantly in the next decade. E-discovery can reveal a lot about a record's reliability as evidence due to hidden time stamps that are embedded in the programming. E-discovery grants lawyers access deep into the malpractice case electronic records, which may provide information pertinent to a lawsuit. This data, referred to as digital Easter eggs, or metadata, is lying there waiting to be discovered. Metadata captures something that paper documents can't: the time that the entries themselves were made. Metadata can do more than capture the time entry, it can show when a document was accessed, who looked at it, and if it was altered from its original format. It tells a lot about the integrity of the medical record and its reliability as evidence in the case. Because of this, e-discovery requests for metadata will increase as it becomes known. The medical practice staff will need to familiarize themselves with this metadata and how to access it as the importance and availability of this data is discovered. The staff will need to know how to store, manage, and access the information. The following

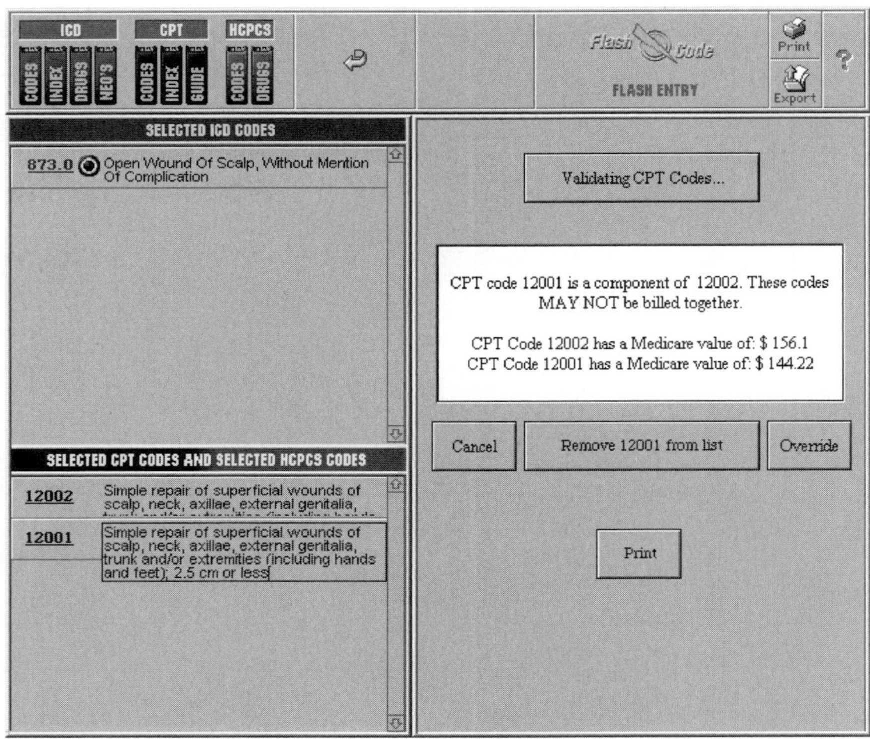

FIGURE 10-20. Screen identifying codes that cannot be billed together. (Courtesy of Flashcode, Inc.)

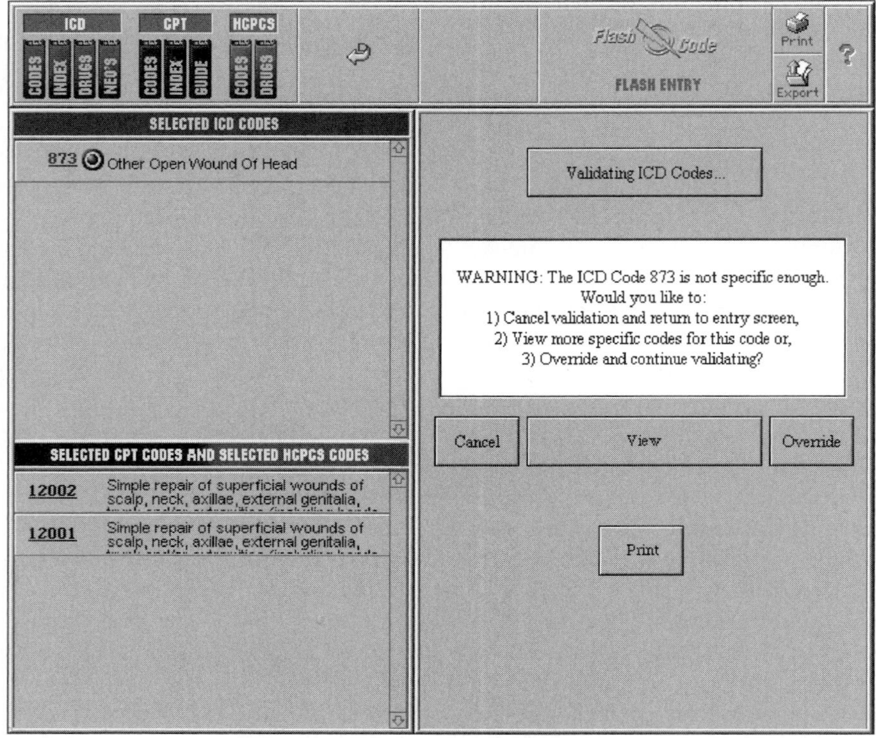

FIGURE 10-21. Screen identifying ICD-9-CM codes that require a fourth or fifth digit. (Courtesy of Flashcode, Inc.)

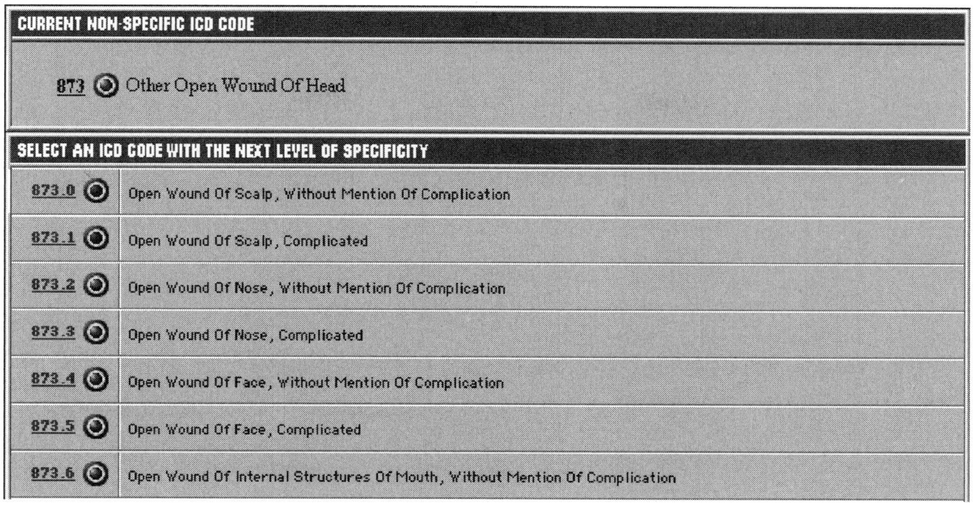

CURRENT NON-SPECIFIC ICD CODE	
873	Other Open Wound Of Head

SELECT AN ICD CODE WITH THE NEXT LEVEL OF SPECIFICITY	
873.0	Open Wound Of Scalp, Without Mention Of Complication
873.1	Open Wound Of Scalp, Complicated
873.2	Open Wound Of Nose, Without Mention Of Complication
873.3	Open Wound Of Nose, Complicated
873.4	Open Wound Of Face, Without Mention Of Complication
873.5	Open Wound Of Face, Complicated
873.6	Open Wound Of Internal Structures Of Mouth, Without Mention Of Complication

FIGURE 10-22. Screen prompting the user to obtain the most specific ICD-9-CM code. (Courtesy of Flashcode, Inc.)

checklist will help the physician practice to prepare for e-discovery:

- Search the Internet for articles on e-discovery and learn all that you can about the topic.
- Review the practice's information management plan if there is one. If there isn't one, think about preparing one.
- Review the policy and procedure manual regarding all policies about EMRs.
- Review the policy and procedure manual regarding the life of the electronic record, the storage, and the destruction.
- Arrange a meeting with the physician(s), management team (office manager, assistant office manager, billing department manager/supervisor, etc.) to discuss the implementation of an e-discovery policy.
- Designate one person within the practice whose responsibility it will be to handle all requests for metadata.

Remember: If you store it, it's probably open to e-discovery!

THE TIE THAT BINDS THE MEDICAL OFFICE AND THE HOSPITAL

Information systems are providing the infrastructure for the health care entity of the future. They address the daily functions of both the hospital and the office and play a major role in patient care. Each entity must have the support of the other in an effort to increase quality care and decrease costs. Medical offices are more efficient when a computer system linked to the hospital's computer system can transfer all of the necessary data to resolve both administrative concerns and health care information. This system is used to review laboratory and x-ray reports that once never seemed to make it to the office, saving office staff time in calling to obtain the report while the patient is waiting in the office. Billing and insurance information can also be easily shared by both the hospital and the office. This can eliminate claims denials or delays due to incorrect insurance information provided by either the hospital or the office. The office hospital billing staff no longer has to go to the hospital medical records department or the billing department for billing and insurance information.

HANDHELD DEVICES

Everybody loves gadgets! However, this handheld gadget is also a timesaver, reduces errors because of bad handwriting, increases revenues due to a more efficient charge capture process, and makes physicians more efficient and more productive. Handhelds come with many names: Palm, Palm Pilot, Pocket PC, Blackberry, PDA, and so on. A Harris Interactive Health Care group poll revealed that in 2005, 83% of the people surveyed were favorable to the idea of using monitoring devices for home use, 78% were favorable to the idea of adopting electronic medical records, and 75% responded favorably to personal digital devices to be used for the purpose of recording information. It is believed that these devices will reduce the cost of health care while increasing the quality of care of the patient. Many improvements have been made that have increased the portability and ease of use of portable medical devices. The term PDA stands for personal digital assistant or personal data assistant. There are many uses for PDAs, including charge capture for services rendered, transcription, obtaining results of tests and procedures, e-mail, prescription writing, and maintaining the physician's schedule.

Some features for prescription writing involve ease of use, drug interactions and contraindications, daily updates from the Internet, and individual information about the patient in question. Once the physician has decided on the prescription that is to be issued, the information can be beamed to the office printer to be filed in the patient chart and to the pharmacy of the patient. There are companies on the Internet, such as Skyscape, that sell entire books that can be downloaded into PDAs. Some downloads for handhelds include the following:

- InfoRetriever is a collection of several evidence-based databases. It will simultaneously search Griffith's Five-Minute Clinical Consult, InfoPoems synopses, Clinical Rules and Calculators, Numbers Needed to Treat, Abstracts of Cochrane Systematic Reviews, and Evidence-Based Practice Guideline Summaries.
- Diagnosaurus is a free differential diagnosis tool containing over 1,000 diagnoses from McGraw Hill. One may browse by symptom, disease, organ system, or all entries.
- Harrison's On-line can be accessed and selected chapters and updates can be saved for convenient access.
- NLM mobile can search Medline via the handheld unit. Provides PICO template, downloadable versions of books from the NCBI bookshelf, and MD on Tap.
- SUNY Upstate Family Medicine provides a spreadsheet full of useful Web links.
- Epocrates Rx is a free drug reference tool that includes over 3,300 brand name and generic drugs, dosing, interactions, adverse reactions, and pricing and has a multichecker for multiple drug interactions.
- Medical Mnemonics is a free database of medical mnemonics to help remember important details.
- Group on Immunization Education is free software that includes Shots 2007 and a quick reference guide to the 2007 Childhood Immunization Schedule.
- Adobe Reader for Pocket PC is a free download that enable pdf files to be read on a handheld.
- Family Practice PDA is free software that includes an OB Wheel, Archimedes free medical calculator, and a pneumo calculator.
- Medical Eponyms is a free database that contains over 1,500 common and obscure medical eponyms with descriptions.
- Unbound Surgery offers comprehensive information that is specifically engineered to provide detailed, focused answers to diagnostic and therapeutic surgical questions.
- mobileMICROMEDEX searches four clinical databases for drug information, alternative medicine information, disease information, and toxicology information.

Many physicians today find that handhelds are as necessary as their stethoscope! There is no way that physicians can keep all of that information in their heads. With the advantages of allowing physicians to spend more time with their patients and decreasing the chances of medical errors, it can be expected that there will be an increase in handheld acceptance. According to an article in the *Seattle Post-Intelligencer* in August 2007, about 55% of the physicians in the United States currently use a mobile device such as a PDA, smart phone, and so on, and about one third of all medical schools now require new students to have this technology. According to physicians, this up-and-coming technology is used more at large hospitals and medical schools than in smaller physician practices.

PHYSICIANS AND THE INTERNET

Many physicians and office managers use the Internet on a daily basis. Most professional or management journals can now be found online. Medical office personnel can simply print out the articles they want to read. But even with the Internet, it is time consuming to search for specific articles and information. The Internet provides not only research information, but also information regarding new medications and techniques. Physicians and office managers can search for appropriate educational workshops that they may want to attend. They can print the conference information, such as hotels, agenda, dates and times, and so on. Once a decision has been made to attend, they can register online. They can then find a hotel and book a room, find a flight, if necessary, find a rental car, and find good restaurants, without leaving their chair.

Of the 257 primary care physicians that were surveyed by Ziment Associates Inc., 75% replied that they use the Internet routinely to look up medical information such as drug or new product information. Further, 68% replied that they regularly gather information about a treatment or disease and 48% routinely read journals and other publications online.

Navigating the Internet can be difficult and time consuming. Many people get lost and have a difficult time searching for information. This is why many physicians will ask the office manager to "pull up" information for them from the Internet. Some tips for navigating the Internet for medical research are as follows:

- When searching the Internet, be aware of who the author of the information is and who paid for its publication (just as you would with an article you would read in a print journal).
- Use databases such as the National Library of Medicine's Medline and CancerLit to collect abstracts of articles that may be needed.
- Get online access to full-text articles through as many journal Web sites as possible. That may mean registering at the Web sites of journals to which the physician subscribes or calling the medical library at the

hospital to gain user identifications and passwords for journals to which your office or physician subscribes.
- Consider subscribing to an online service for physicians that offers full-text journal articles.
- Ask for help from medical librarians.

To Search or Not to Search, That Is the Question

Have you ever tried to search the Internet, knowing there is a ton of information on that subject, but you just can't find it? Here are some helpful hints to keep in mind when searching:

- Enclose phrases in quotation marks.
- Use the "+" sign to make sure that a specific term is included. Example: diabetes mellitus + National Health Institute retrieve only pages about diabetes and the National Health Institute.
- Use the "-" (minus sign) to exclude unwanted terms. Example: diabetes mellitus - National Health Institute retrieves only pages about diabetes that do not include the National Health Institute.
- Pay attention to case, using lowercase most times. Capital letters are taken literally, whereas lowercase letters are case insensitive. Example: "aids" retrieves items such as hearing aids, audiovisual aids, and acquired immunodeficiency syndrome (AIDS). But AIDS in all capital letters only retrieves items with AIDS in capital letters.
- Some search engines allow truncation of terms using an asterisk (*). Typing "pediatr*" will retrieve pediatric, pediatrics, pediatrician, and pediatricians.
- Follow a search engine's home page for hints and instructions. Every search engine is different.

EXERCISES

MULTIPLE CHOICE

Choose the best *answer for each of the following questions.*

1. Which of the following is *not* a common use for a computer in a medical office?
   a. Word processing
   b. Billing
   c. Games
   d. Electronic medical record
2. Which of the following is considered computer hardware?
   a. Keyboard
   b. Mouse
   c. Hard drive
   d. All of the above
3. What is the smallest addressable unit on a computer screen?
   a. Pixel
   b. Bit
   c. Byte
   d. RAM
4. A megabyte is how many bytes of computer storage?
   a. One thousand
   b. One hundred thousand
   c. One million
   d. One billion
5. RAM stands for
   a. Random access memory
   b. Resource available access
   c. Resource access monitoring
   d. None of the above
6. Which of the following is considered to be an input device?
   a. Monitor
   b. Mouse
   c. RAM
   d. None of the above
7. The most popular printer used in medical practices today is a/an
   a. Dot matrix printer
   b. Ink-jet printer
   c. Laser printer
   d. None of the above
8. Which of the following is the most important software function?
   a. Recall notices
   b. Scheduling
   c. Reports
   d. Billing
9. A tickler system is used to
   a. Remind patients that it's time for an appointment
   b. Notify the physician about her or his schedule
   c. Schedule patient appointments
   d. All of the above
10. Which of the following would not be found on a patient encounter form?
    a. Account balance
    b. CPT codes
    c. Patient name
    d. Emergency contact
11. Which of the following would not be considered patient demographics for the patient encounter form?
    a. Patient's date of birth
    b. Patient's weight
    c. Patient's insurance company
    d. Patient's name
12. Which area of the patient encounter form should show a balance when applicable?
    a. Due by patient
    b. Previous balance
    c. Today's charge
    d. All of the above
13. Which of the following would not be found on a hospital tracking form?
    a. Patient's name
    b. Spouse's name
    c. CPT code
    d. Diagnosis code

14. An EMR will
    a. Improve quality of care
    b. Reduce cost
    c. Increase efficiency
    d. All of the above
15. Which of the following is not a factor for failure of an EMR?
    a. Lack of understanding
    b. Lack of commitment
    c. Lack of resources
    d. Lack of communication
16. Metadata is often referred to as a/an
    a. Palm pilot
    b. Christmas tree
    c. Easter egg
    d. None of the above
17. Helping lawyers to find loopholes in EMRs is done with
    a. E-discovery
    b. E-law
    c. E-lawyer's helper
    d. None of the above
18. One of the biggest issues identified in metadata is
    a. The time stamp
    b. The documentation
    c. Billing code
    d. The examination of the patient
19. What symbol is used when searching the Internet?
    a. Asterisk
    b. Star
    c. Exclamation point
    d. Dollar sign
20. According to an article in August 2007, what percentage of physicians use a mobile device?
    a. 50%
    b. 55%
    c. 75%
    d. 35%

TRUE OR FALSE

1. _____ Some software packages can provide tax services.
2. _____ The modem contains the "memory" of the computer.
3. _____ A network exists when you place a lot of computers in one room.
4. _____ To store large amounts of information, the office should use a CD.
5. _____ When negotiating a contract, involve the physician, not the attorney.
6. _____ The billing function is one of the most important functions of the medical office computer.
7. _____ Software support is not important; only hardware support is important.
8. _____ A computer tickler system is better than a manual system.
9. _____ A tickler system is used to remind the physician of personal appointments, such as dental appointments and haircuts.
10. _____ A computer system linked to the hospital is an asset to the physician office.
11. _____ Current processors run at billions of Hertz.
12. _____ There is more space on a CD than on a floppy disc.
13. _____ Parallel processing is when you are doing billing and scheduling at the same time.
14. _____ Offices should print several copies of the EMR.
15. _____ The expression "Don't click it if you didn't do it!" refers to finding information on a PDA.
16. _____ A palm pilot is a type of handheld device.
17. _____ Free software is available for handheld devices.
18. _____ Use of handhelds by physicians allows for more efficient charge capture.
19. _____ An Easter egg is another name for an EMR.
20. _____ E&M codes should be printed on a patient encounter form.

THINKERS

1. Describe ways in which a physician or medical office can use the Internet.
2. Using the previously distributed medical practice scenarios, list the computer features that are important for your practice.
3. Using the previously distributed medical practice scenarios, design a patient encounter form for your practice.
4. Explain the issues with e-discovery.

REFERENCES

Mason, J., Information Based Medicine, *Seattle Post –Intelligencer*, August 13, 2007.

Cross, M. "Online Odyssey: Medical Research and the Internet." *Internet Health Care Magazine*, October 2000, pp. 54–58.

Dick, R., Steen, E., & Detmer, D. *The Computer-Based Patient Record: An Essential Technology for Healthcare*. Committee on Improving the Patient Record, Washington, DC: Institute of Medicine of the National Academies, 1997.

Dimick, C. "E-Discovery." *Journal of AHIMA*, May 2007.

EMRs Buyer's Guide: Considerations for Practices Evaluating EMRs. Raleigh, NC: Misys Healthcare Systems, 2004.

Farber, L. *Encyclopedia of Practice and Financial Management*. Oradell, NJ: Medical Economics Books, 1988.

Landholt, T. *Automating the Medical Record*. Norcross, GA: The Coker Group, 1999.

PDA Downloads and Wireless Resources for Handheld Devices in Healthcare. Retrieved from www.upstate.edu/library/internet_new/pda.php

PDA's in Health Care. Charleston, SC: Medical University of South Carolina Library, 2007.

Simkin, M.G. *Discovering Computers*. Dubuque, IA: William C. Brown Publishers, 1990.

Taylor, H., & Leitman, R. "Health Care News." *Harris Interactive*, Volume 1, Issue 25, August 15, 2001.

Tappert, E. "Improve Practice Productivity." *Group Practice Journal*, May/June 1992, pp. 25–26.

Whinnery, S. "Electronic Claims Submission Helps Group Practice Cut Costs." *Group Practice Journal*, July/August 1989, pp. 26–58.

11

SAFETY AND HEALTH

CHAPTER OUTLINE

CHAPTER OBJECTIVES

After completing this chapter, you will be able to do the following:

- Understand the purpose of the Occupational Safety and Health Administration (OSHA)
- Follow OSHA guidelines as they pertain to a medical practice
- Develop a checklist for a medical practice's OSHA readiness
- Understand the priorities of an OSHA inspection
- Identify and define OSHA violations
- Understand and discuss the Clinical Laboratory Improvement Amendments of 1988

EMPLOYEE SAFETY

Employees should be given training so that there will be minimal accidents in the medical office. As new equipment is purchased or there are changes in supplies or older equipment, each employee should be advised of the changes and should be retrained. Each employee should be given a safe, clean place in which to work. Once this space has been provided, it is the responsibility of each employee to maintain his or her space, to keep it neat and clean, and to keep it safe. There should be no cords hanging or lying on the floor where someone could trip over them. Any problems with buckling carpets should be fixed immediately. The office building should also be maintained. If the sidewalk to the front door is cracked, fix it. If the door continues to blow shut, fix it or replace it *before* someone gets hurt. If an employee is injured while at work, he or she is entitled to workers' compensation. Workers' compensation laws are mandated by each state. The office manager should research the law in her or his state because state laws vary widely from state to state.

Employees who are injured at work are entitled to reasonable medical care with weekly compensation for the time that they are not able to work. The amount of compensation is based on the date and the type of injury that they sustained. Patients receiving workers' compensation benefits are urged to return to work as soon as possible. If Judy works in the medical office full time, but also works at the nursing home every other weekend, she must notify the physician practice that she has additional monies from the second job. The office manager should develop an incident report that should be completed for every accident that takes place. These forms should not be part of the employee's file; instead, they should all be kept in one place in a separate file. This form should contain the following information:

- The name of the employee
- The name of the person making this report (usually the office manager)
- The age and date of birth of the employee
- The location of the accident
- A short description of the accident
- The signature of the person writing the report
- The disposition of the employee's treatment (treated by the practice physician, sent to the hospital, etc.)
- The signature of the employee

This form should also be adapted for patients or caregivers who may have sustained injuries while visiting the practice.

The practice should have a policy on employee safety that includes the following information:

- How and when to report the accident
- How to complete an incident report

NATIONAL PATIENT SAFETY GOALS

On June 1, 2007, the Joint Commission's Board of Commissioners approved the 2008 National Patient Safety Goals. In 2008, the new goals (3E, 16, and 16A) have a 1-year phase-in period that includes all expectations for planning, development, and testing at months 3, 6, and 9.

- **Goal 1:** Improve the accuracy of patient identification.
- **Goal 1A:** Use at least two patient identifiers when providing care, treatment, or services.
- **Goal 1B:** Before the start of any invasive procedure, conduct a final verification process to confirm the correct patient, procedure, and site, using active, not passive, communication techniques.
- **Goal 2:** Improve effectiveness of communication among caregivers.
- **Goal 2A:** For verbal or telephone orders or for telephone reporting of critical test results, verify the complete order for the test results by having the person receiving the information record and read back the complete test results.
- **Goal 2B:** Standardize a list of abbreviations, acronyms, symbols, and dose designations that are not to be used throughout the organization.
- **Goal 2C:** Measure and assess, and, if appropriate, take action to improve the timeliness of reporting, and the timeliness of receipt by the responsible licensed caregiver, of critical test results and values.
- **Goal 2E:** Implement a standardized approach to hands-off communications, including an opportunity to ask and respond to questions.
- **Goal 3:** Improve the safety of using medications.
- **Goal 3C:** Identify and, at a minimum, annually review a list of look-a-like and sound-a-like drugs used by the organization, and take action to prevent errors involving the interchange of these drugs.
- **Goal 3D:** Label all medications, medication containers (e.g., syringes, medicine cups), and other solutions on and off the sterile field.
- **Goal 3E:** Reduce the likelihood of patient harm associated with the use of anticoagulation therapy.
- **Goal 7:** Reduce the risk of health care–associated infections.
- **Goal 7A:** Comply with current World Health Organization (WHO) hand hygiene guidelines or Centers for Disease Control and Prevention (CDC) hand hygiene guidelines.
- **Goal 7B:** Manage as sentinel events all identified cases of unanticipated death or major permanent loss of function associated with a health care–associated infection.
- **Goal 8:** Accurately and completely reconcile medications across the continuum of care.

- **Goal 8A:** There is a process of comparing the patient's current medications with those ordered for the patient while under the care of the organization.
- **Goal 8B:** A complete list of the patient's medications is communicated to the next service provider when a patient is referred or transferred to another setting, service, practitioner, or level of care within or outside the organization. The complete list of medications is also provided to the patient on discharge from the facility.
- **Goal 9:** Reduce the risk of patient harm resulting from falls.
- **Goal 9B:** Implement a fall reduction program, including an evaluation of the effectiveness of the program.
- **Goal 10:** Reduce the risk of influenza and pneumococcal disease in institutionalized adults.
- **Goal 10A:** Develop and implement a protocol for administration and documentation of the flu vaccine.
- **Goal 10B:** Develop and implement a protocol for administration and documentation of the pneumococcus vaccine.
- **Goal 10C:** Develop and implement a protocol to identify new cases of influenza and to manage an outbreak.
- **Goal 11:** Reduce the risk of surgical fires.
- **Goal 11A:** Educate the staff, including operating licensed independent practitioners and anesthesia providers, on how to control heat sources and manage fuels with enough time for patient preparation, and establish guidelines to minimize oxygen concentration under drapes.
- **Goal 12:** Implement applicable National Patient Safety Goals and associated requirements by components and practitioner sites.
- **Goal 12A:** Inform and encourage components and practitioner sites to implement the applicable National Patient Safety Goals and associated requirements.
- **Goal 13:** Encourage patients' active involvement in their own care as a patient safety strategy.
- **Goal 13A:** Define and communicate the means for patients and their families to report concerns about safety, and encourage them to do so.
- **Goal 14:** Prevent health care–associated pressure ulcers.
- **Goal 14A:** Assess and periodically reassess each resident's risk for developing a pressure ulcer, and take action to address any identified risks.
- **Goal 15:** The organization identifies safety risks inherent in its patient population.
- **Goal 15A:** The organization identifies patients at risk for suicide.
- **Goal 15B:** The organization identifies risks associated with long-term oxygen therapy, such as home fires.
- **Goal 16:** Improve recognition and response to changes in a patient's condition.
- **Goal 16A:** The organization selects a suitable method that enables health care staff members to directly request additional assistance form one or more specially trained individuals when the patient's condition appears to be worsening.

WHAT IS OSHA?

The Occupational Safety and Health Act of 1970 was enacted by Congress to establish national protocols and standards for occupational health and safety. The Occupational Safety and Health Administration (OSHA), a division of the Department of Labor (DOL), issues standards that must be followed by all employers and employees and conducts site visits to ensure compliance with those standards. These regulations are critically important to all medical offices, clinics, ambulances, and hospitals. Presented with the following statistics, Congress was led to create this legislation:

- Job-related accidents accounted for more than 14,000 worker deaths each year
- Nearly 1.5 million workers became disabled each year due to workplace injuries
- New cases of occupational diseases each year were estimated at 300,000

With this information in mind, a bipartisan Congress passed the 1970 law "to assure so far as possible every working man and woman in the nation safe and healthful working conditions." Since that time, this act has had a profound effect on workplace safety, and accidents and injuries have declined.

It is necessary for medical office managers to know OSHA's regulations and to follow them strictly. Under federal law, OSHA has the right to inspect all private health care facilities and hospitals in all 50 states, the District of Columbia, Puerto Rico, and U.S. territories. Federal agencies, including military bases and veterans' hospitals, may also be inspected.

OSHA'S ROLE IN SAFETY AND HEALTH

As part of the U.S. Department of Labor, OSHA was created to accomplish the following:

- Develop and enforce mandatory job safety and health standards
- Maintain a reporting and record-keeping system to monitor job-related injuries and illnesses
- Encourage employers and employees to reduce workplace hazards and implement or improve safety and health programs
- Provide for research in occupational safety and health

- Establish training programs to increase the number and competence of Occupational Safety and Health personnel
- Establish separate but interdependent responsibilities and rights for employers and employees to achieve better safety and health conditions
- Provide for state-level Occupational Safety and Health programs in those states that want to control their own programs

The Occupational Safety and Health Act does not apply to self-employed individuals, farms where only family members are employed, or certain industries that are regulated by other federal agencies. Federal, state, and local governments are not covered, because they have an internal process for handling such issues.

HISTORY OF OSHA'S DEVELOPMENT OF BLOODBORNE PATHOGEN STANDARDS

OSHA's involvement with medical practices began in 1983, when it issued a set of voluntary regulations intended to decrease the risk of occupational exposure to the hepatitis B virus (HBV). Since then, the regulation of medical workplaces has increased slowly but steadily. In 1986, the American Federation of State, County, and Municipal Employees petitioned OSHA for emergency temporary standards to reduce workers' risk of contracting certain infectious diseases. That petition eventually led to the development of the bloodborne pathogen regulations that were put into effect officially in 1992.

In 1987, the U.S. Department of Labor and the U.S. Department of Health and Human Services issued a joint advisory notice urging employers to institute universal precautions set forth by OSHA wherever workers might have contact with blood or other potentially infected fluids. They also published an advance notice of their intention to initiate a rule-making process aimed at reducing occupational exposure to HBV. In 1988, OSHA started sending selected advisors on fact-finding inspections of medical offices, and in May 1989 OSHA published a bloodborne disease proposal. Receiving increasing pressure from the public to "do something" about acquired immunodeficiency syndrome (AIDS), in 1989 Congress began holding hearings on the proposed new OSHA rules. In March 1991, Congress increased the financial penalties for workplace noncompliance with these rules, and in October of that year it directed OSHA to issue the bloodborne disease regulations by December 1, 1991. Finally, on December 6, OSHA published its bloodborne pathogen standards in the *Federal Register.*

OSHA'S BLOODBORNE PATHOGEN STANDARDS

The final OSHA standards regarding exposure to bloodborne pathogens are important to all medical facilities that pose a risk of exposure to infectious materials and bloodborne pathogens. Settings that are found to be noncompliant are subject to penalties in the thousands of dollars per incident. Since the implementation of OSHA's final ruling on the bloodborne pathogen standards in January 1992, federal OSHA agents have visited hundreds of medical-surgical hospitals in the United States and have found thousands of violations of these standards.

These regulations require medical facilities to develop the following documents and programs:

- Hazard communication plan
- Exposure plan
- Medical waste management plan
- Housekeeping policies
- Personal protective measures
- General safety precautions
- Fire safety plan
- Staff development/in-service training program

GUIDELINES OF THE OCCUPATIONAL SAFETY AND HEALTH ADMINISTRATION

Hazard Communication Plan

The purpose of a hazard communication plan is to help employees understand the policies and procedures the practice has adopted in response to OSHA's Hazard Communication Standard of 1987. This standard is also known as the "Right-to-Know Law." Employees must be informed of hazardous chemicals in their place of employment, and they must be made aware of the health risks associated with these chemicals. Employers must develop a labeling and tracking system to identify all hazardous chemicals, their purpose, and their location. One staff member should be appointed to be in charge of OSHA compliance. This employee should make and post a list of all hazardous materials in the office setting. The following items are often overlooked when developing this list:

- Printer or copy machine cartridges
- Typing correction fluid
- Glass and surface cleaner
- Antibacterial soaps
- Chemicals used for instrument cleaning
- Furniture polish

As you can see, even ordinary household items are considered hazardous and should be treated as such.

There must be a material safety data sheet (MSDS) for each hazardous chemical in the office. MSDSs can be obtained from chemical manufacturers; most companies have them on file and can easily put one in the mail to you. They also can be downloaded from the Internet. These sheets should be kept together in a binder labeled "MSDS—Material Safety

Data Sheets." The potential risks of all hazardous chemicals in the office should be discussed in a meeting with all personnel.

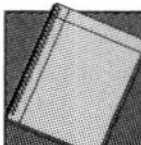

FROM THE EXPERT'S NOTEBOOK

Many MSDSs are available on the Internet, so check there first before reinventing the wheel.

An OSHA hazard communication plan also requires medical offices to do the following:

- Report accidents and incidents (use an exposure incident report)
- Post notices of new and revised MSDSs for 10 days on an employee bulletin board
- Inform contractors of hazardous chemicals

Exposure Control Plan

An exposure control plan is one of the most important plans mandated by OSHA; the requirement was adopted in 1991. The purpose of this plan is to prevent or control employee exposure to blood, body fluids, and other potentially infectious materials. The office's exposure control plan must be written and available to all employees. It must be reviewed and updated annually and should include provisions for staff training. The purchase of any new equipment or the addition of a new procedure requires an update of the plan. The exposure control plan consists of the following components, any of which can be inspected by OSHA at any time:

- Exposure determination
- Compliance regulations
- HBV vaccination
- Postexposure evaluation
- Hazards communication to employees
- Record-keeping requirements

Determining which jobs entail a risk of exposure to infectious materials is a part of exposure determination. The office manager must list any position that involves risk of exposure to infectious materials, and must describe the risk based on the employee's function and duties. Any protective equipment used by employees should also be described.

To comply with OSHA regulations regarding exposure control plans, the office manager must ensure that the procedures and policy manual contains sections on the following:

- Biohazard labeling
- Classification of exposure categories
- Engineering controls
- Exposure determination
- Needlesticks and cuts
- Injury on the job
- Incidence of exposure to blood/body fluids
- HBV immunizations
- Protective equipment

BIOHAZARD LABELING

Biohazards must be labeled with a biohazard symbol or by using red bags or red containers (Figure 11-1) to warn employees of potential hazards. Any contaminated waste, containers of regulated waste, refrigerators, freezers, or other containers used to store, transport, or ship blood or other potentially infectious materials must be labeled. Standard warning labels can be purchased that include the universal biohazard symbol followed by the word "Biohazard." The label must be fluorescent orange or orange-red, with lettering or symbols in a contrasting color, and must be affixed to the container. Red bags or containers may be substituted for specific labeling.

Labeling is not required for the following:

- Containers of blood, blood components, and blood products that have been labeled as to their contents and released for transfusion or other clinical use that have been screened for HBV and the human immunodeficiency virus (HIV) before their release
- Individual containers of blood or other potentially infectious materials that are placed in secondary labeled containers during storage, transport, shipment, or disposal
- Specimen containers in a facility that uses standard precautions when handling all specimens

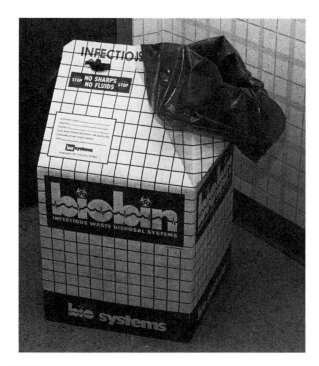

FIGURE 11-1. Waste management container for infectious material. (Courtesy of BioSystems.)

- Laundry bags or containers in a facility that uses standard precautions for handling all laundry
- Regulated waste that has been decontaminated

CLASSIFICATION OF EXPOSURE CATEGORIES

The classification of exposure categories is a written list of job categories that expose employees to bloodborne pathogens. To create this list, the office manager first defines all duties, tasks, and procedures of each and every position in the office that puts an employee at risk of exposure. From this list, the manager then develops a classification of related jobs. If all employees within a specific job classification perform the same pathogen-exposing duties, a list of specific tasks and procedures for each position is not required. For instance, if the office employs three nurses, it is necessary to develop only one job classification that encompasses all three positions.

ENGINEERING CONTROLS

Engineering controls are used to eliminate or minimize employee exposure. These controls include isolating employees from hazards such as sharps, by using sharps containers or self-sheathing needles. Because needlestick injuries occur from a variety of devices, no single device or policy can prevent all needlestick injuries.

One effective engineering control is to forbid the practice of recapping or removing contaminated needles by hand unless there is no feasible alternative or recapping is required during a specific medical procedure. Procedures that require recapping or removing contaminated needles by hand include drawing blood gases (which is never done in an office setting) and administering incremental doses of medications to a patient (which does sometimes occur in a medical office). Mechanical devices and plastic shields are available for such purposes. Bending, shearing, or breaking contaminated needles is prohibited.

All needles must be placed in a sharps container for proper disposal. Although some sharps containers are reusable, it is better to use disposable ones in an office setting. These containers must be easily accessible to employees. For example, they must be located next to the phlebotomy chair, not across the room. In examination rooms, they should be located near the examination table area where they would be most commonly used. Examination room sharps containers should be tamper-proof, denying access to used needles (Figure 11-2).

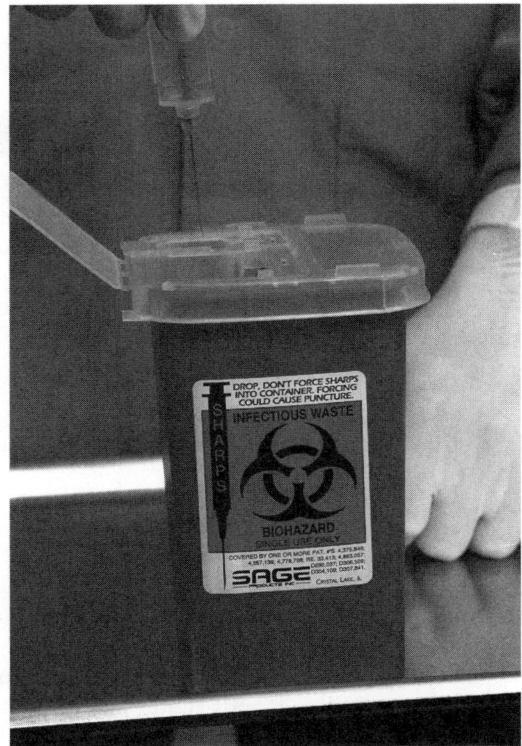

FIGURE 11-2. A tamper-proof disposable sharps container.

EXPOSURE DETERMINATION

Exposure determination involves many components. Administration of HBV vaccine is one component of this category and is discussed in detail later in this chapter. Should an exposure occur, a confidential medical examination and documentation are immediately required. The employee must identify the patient source, and that patient's blood must be tested as soon as possible after consent is obtained to determine HIV or HBV infectivity. Any information on the patient's HIV or HBV test must be provided to the evaluating physician. A copy of the OSHA guidelines must be on-site, readily available, and followed exactly.

PROTECTIVE EQUIPMENT

The use of protective equipment is an important factor if a laboratory is located in the medical office. A technician must wear gloves during the phlebotomy process. (The only exception to this rule is phlebotomy performed in volunteer blood donation centers.) If an employee is allergic to the gloves, the employer must provide an alternative such as hypoallergenic gloves, glove liners, powderless gloves, or simply a different brand of glove. Whatever it takes, the office is required to solve the problem!

Face and eye protection is required when there is a potential for splashing, spraying, or spattering of blood or other potentially infectious materials. Prescription glasses may be used as protective eyewear as long as they are equipped with solid side shields. If protective eyewear is chosen instead of a face shield, the eyewear must be worn in combination with a mask to protect the nose and mouth.

Personal Protective Measures

The purpose of a personal protective measures plan is to minimize occupational exposure to bloodborne pathogens through the use of personal protective equipment (PPE) and effective safety procedures. PPE is clothing and equipment designed to protect health care workers from direct exposure to blood, body fluids, and other potentially infectious materials. Physicians and office managers should be aware that OSHA mandates the use of PPE by all employees directly involved with patient care. The staff must be provided, at no cost to themselves, the equipment required by OSHA, including the following:

- Gloves
- Eye shields
- Resuscitation bags
- Masks or face shields
- Mouthpieces
- Splash guards
- Gowns and laboratory coats
- Protective jumpsuits
- Eye-wash stations
- Surgical caps or hoods
- Shoe coverings, when appropriate
- A sign stating that "Standard Precautions are in Effect"

There are many types of PPE from which to choose, but you must ensure that the equipment effectively prevents blood and other liquids from coming into contact with your staff and their clothing. All employees are required to use PPE unless they refuse because, in their personal or professional judgment, they believe that using the equipment would prevent the delivery of quality health care, endanger public safety, or pose an increased hazard to their safety or the safety of a co-worker. Should these situations arise, they must be carefully documented. Most offices make the use of this equipment mandatory.

The physician or office manager must ensure that all necessary protective gear is available in the proper sizes, that it is clean and laundered, and that disposable gear is properly disposed of after it has been used. The physician or office manager is also responsible for the repair and replacement of any equipment that is no longer effective. The office manager must ensure that all employees use PPE appropriately to eliminate the risk of exposure.

OSHA requires procedures for the following issues:

- Handling and disposing of used needles
- Classification of exposure categories
- Employee health programs
- Hand washing
- The use of gloves and gowns
- The use of masks
- Capillary blood sampling

Medical Waste Management Plan

The purpose of a medical waste management plan is to protect the public and environment by preventing improper storage, handling, and disposal of infectious medical wastes. The plan should cover the following topics:

- Categories of waste
- Disposal of sharps
- In-service training
- Medical waste containers
- Preparation of medical waste for pickup
- Weighing, storing, and tracking medical waste

Housekeeping Policy

The OSHA housekeeping policy requires employers to maintain sanitary conditions in the workplace. Schedules should be implemented for appropriate cleaning of rooms where body fluids are present. Housekeeping employees must wear appropriate PPE while cleaning off blood, body fluids, or other potentially infectious materials and during decontamination procedures. Disinfecting must be performed with a chemical germicide. The office manager should have a workable housekeeping procedure in place at all times. This means that the office should always be clean and sanitary. There should be a written schedule for any method of decontamination. The materials necessary to dispose of contaminated material must be readily accessible. OSHA has issued specific regulations for the treatment of contaminated laundry, and they must be followed to the letter.

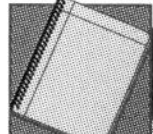

FROM THE EXPERT'S NOTEBOOK

Regular household bleach in a 1:10 dilution can be used for disinfecting. This method has been approved by OSHA and is less expensive than commercially purchased solutions. Bleach solutions must be made fresh daily.

General Safety Precautions

OSHA requires a general safety precautions plan to ensure a safe working environment for all employees. Each office should have safety policies and procedures regarding employee health, exposure categories, first-aid kits, hazardous and toxic substances, protective equipment, and smoking.

Fire Safety Plan

Each office must develop a fire safety plan that contains written policies and procedures regarding the following:

- Exits and exit signs (Figure 11-3)
- Fire alarm pull stations
- The sound of the fire alarm
- Fire drills and classes on how to use a fire extinguisher

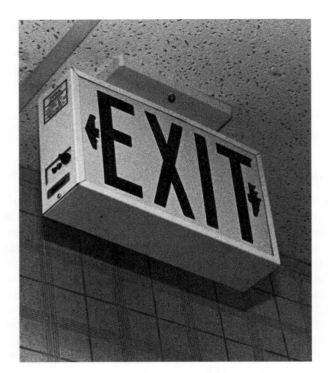

FIGURE 11-3. Illuminated emergency exit sign. (Courtesy of Gastrointestinal Specialists, Inc.)

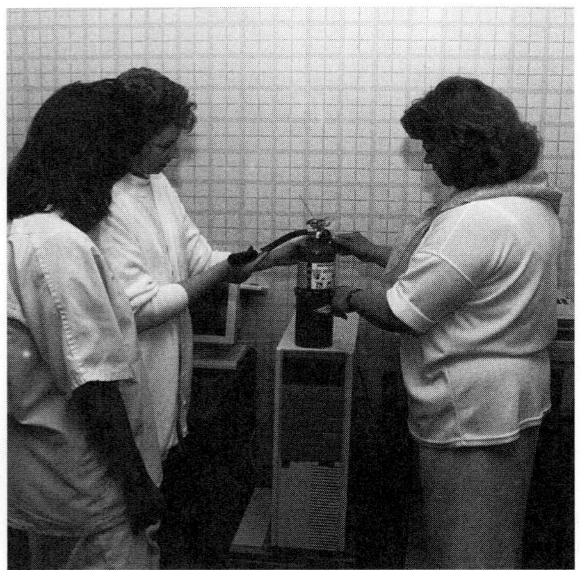

FIGURE 11-4. The office manager demonstrates the proper use of the fire extinguisher.

- Fire extinguishers (Figure 11-4)
- Fire prevention
- Floor plans
- Hazardous areas
- Inspection of heat and air conditioning systems

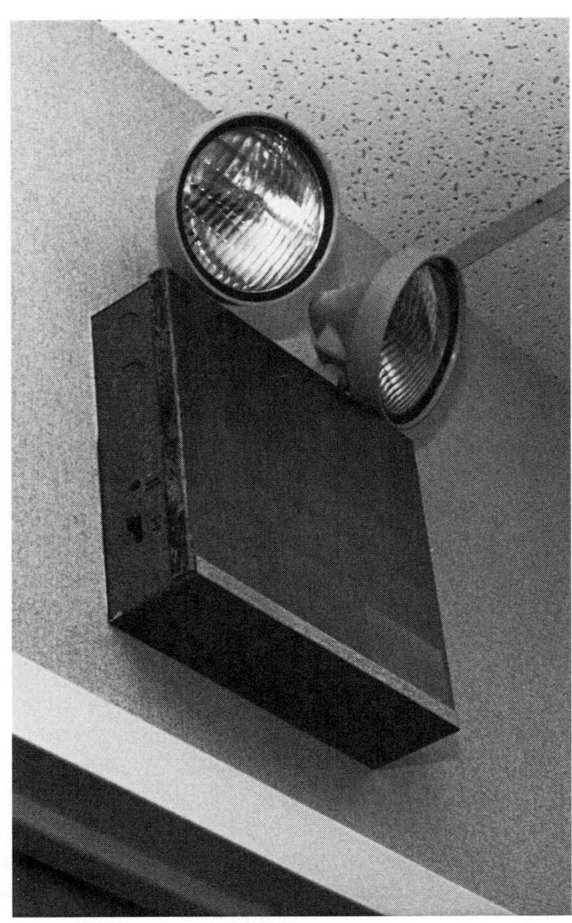

FIGURE 11-5. Emergency lighting. (Courtesy of Gastrointestinal Specialists, Inc.)

- Testing of fire alarms
- Testing of sprinkler systems
- Treatment of the injured
- Methods of evacuation
- Missing persons
- Discovering a fire
- Emergency telephone numbers
- Emergency lighting (Figure 11-5)
- Compliance
- Employee training

Staff Development/In-Service Training Programs

One of OSHA's most important functions is developing standards for the education and training of employees. Providing employee training is a vitally important part of complying with OSHA regulations. Training must be provided to employees at the beginning of their employment and annually thereafter. Every employee at risk of exposure to blood or other infectious materials must participate in these training sessions. No one may be excused! These training sessions must be provided during working hours and before a new employee starts a position. Training must consist of the following elements:

- Epidemiology and symptoms of HBV and HIV infection
- Modes of transmission of HBV and HIV
- Exposure control plan
- PPE
- Standard precautions
- HBV vaccine
- Procedures to follow should exposure occur
- Signs, labels, tags, and color coding denoting biohazards
- Compliance

All medical offices must follow OSHA's standard precautions and document all training. Therefore employees should assume that all materials are infectious and are to be dealt with according to the procedures required by standard precautions.

OSHA Office Manual

OSHA regulations outline the engineering that should be used to reduce the chances of occupational transmission of infectious diseases (e.g., a venipuncture recapping device). Equipment must be checked regularly to ensure proper functioning. The regulations mandate that controls be in place to reduce the risk of exposure.

One of the most obvious work practice controls is proper hand washing. Each medical office should have facilities that are easily accessed by the staff. The physician is responsible for ensuring that all employees wash their hands at the appropriate times.

Another mandated work practice control is the proper disposal of sharps. These regulations now state that syringes should not be recapped, bent, or removed. It is strictly prohibited to shear off or break a contaminated needle. The only exception to this rule is to provide information that there was no alternative to recapping available to the employee. All sharps must be placed in appropriately marked containers until they are picked up for processing. Some states have a similar regulation for sharps disposal, according to the Department of Environmental Resources. Sharps containers must be labeled with orange and black stickers that read "Biohazard."

Many other commonsense procedures are included in OSHA rules and regulations, including the following:

- Eating or drinking in areas where occupational exposure could occur is prohibited.
- Storage of food and drink in refrigerators, freezers, shelves, cabinets, or other places where infectious materials might be stored is prohibited.
- Pipetting or suctioning of blood or potentially hazardous material by mouth is prohibited.
- Packaging infectious materials in any container that is not leak-proof or labeled is prohibited.
- The use of "Biohazard" labels is mandatory.
- HBV immunizations/evaluations must be administered when employees have been exposed.
- Application of cosmetics or lip balm and handling of contact lenses in an occupational exposure area is prohibited.

Physician offices are required to make the HBV vaccine available at no cost to all employees who have a risk of occupational exposure. The only exceptions are employees who have already received the vaccination, employees who have demonstrated that they are immune through an antibody test, and employees who for medical reasons cannot accept the vaccine. If an employee refuses the vaccine, the physician or office manager must obtain his or her signature on the appropriate employee consent form. A sample of this form is shown in Figure 11-6.

The HBV vaccine should be administered after the employee has received training in the prevention of occupational exposure and within 10 working days of the start of employment. Office managers should be aware of these time constraints and be available to train the new employee within the first week of his or her employment. The regulations do not require that an employee specify a reason for refusing vaccination; however, documentation is always helpful when OSHA inspectors are at the door. Employees who refuse the vaccine are allowed to change their mind at any time during the course of their employment; if they do, the physician is obligated to provide this vaccine at no cost.

MANAGEMENT RESPONSIBILITIES

As an office manager, you must have a full understanding of OSHA, because it is your responsibility to ensure that the practice meets OSHA expectations. The following is a checklist for office managers:

- Provide a safe and healthful workplace free from recognized hazards that are likely to cause death or serious physical harm to employees.
- Be familiar with OSHA standards and make copies available to employees on request.
- Educate all employees about OSHA, and post the OSHA safety and health poster.
- Inspect the office to be sure it conforms to the standards.
- Minimize or reduce hazards.
- Be sure employees have well-maintained PPE.
- Identify potential hazards with color codes, posters, or labels.
- Establish and update operating procedures.
- Provide training.
- Report any accident that results in hospitalization of five or more employees. This report must be made within 48 hours of the accident.

I understand that due to the nature of my position, there is a risk of occupational exposure to blood or infectious materials. I understand that I may be at risk of acquiring hepatitis B virus (HBV) infection. I have been given the opportunity to be vaccinated with the HBV vaccine at no cost to myself and have received information regarding HBV. The following information has been explained to me:

1. I may request HBV antibody testing before deciding whether to receive the HBV vaccine.
2. If I am found to be immune to HBV by antibody testing, my employer is not required to offer to me the HBV vaccine.
3. If I refuse the HBV vaccine and at a later date decide to accept the vaccine, I may do so at that time in accordance with the policies governing HBV immunizations and at no cost to myself.

I have been informed that the side effects of this vaccine might include the following:

1. Soreness at injection site	2. Local reaction	3. Rash
4. Fatigue	5. Joint pain	6. Headache
7. Dizziness	8. Fever	

I hereby [ ] accept [ ] refuse the HBV vaccine.

Employee signature: ______________________ Date: __________

Prescreening date: ______________

Results: ______________________________________

Dates of vaccination

1st: ____________ 2nd: ____________ 3rd: ____________

I certify that the above-named individual received a copy of the HBV information sheet and has been fully explained the contents. I certify that I reviewed with the above-named individual our established HBV immunization policy and procedures.

__________ ______________________ ________________

Date Signature Title

FIGURE 11-6. Hepatitis B immunization consent form.

- Keep good records of work-related injuries and illnesses.
- Allow employees access to OSHA information at a reasonable time.
- Do not discriminate against employees who have exercised their rights under OSHA.
- Post any OSHA citations near the involved area and allow them to remain there until the violation has been cleared, or for 3 days, whichever is longer.

MANAGER'S ALERT

Ignorance of OSHA-mandated responsibilities is no excuse. Both management and employees must accept responsibility!

EMPLOYEE RESPONSIBILITIES

Employees have responsibilities also. These responsibilities must be communicated to employees during training sessions. Follow this checklist for the responsibilities you will need to emphasize during training:

- Employees must comply with OSHA standards.
- Employees must wear the prescribed protective clothing and equipment.
- Employees must report any hazardous conditions to the office manager.
- Employees must report any job-related injury or illness to either the office manager or a practice physician.
- Employees must cooperate with OSHA compliance officers conducting an inspection.
- Employees must exercise their rights under OSHA.

IS YOUR OFFICE "OSHA READY"?

Understanding what will take place during an inspection can eliminate any initial panic you are likely to experience when an OSHA inspector unexpectedly arrives. Once you've undergone your first inspection, you will find the next one much more bearable! An OSHA inspection can occur at any time during office hours. Being prepared for this inspection will help eliminate chaos and will allow the inspection to proceed smoothly and efficiently. Any information needed regarding OSHA regulations can be obtained through OSHA's Web site and various publications. Also, OSHA will provide consultants to help practices become compliant. This service is offered free of charge. Office managers should acquaint themselves with these regulations. According to a Supreme Court ruling, OSHA may not conduct an inspection without the employer's permission. Keep in mind, however, that OSHA can obtain a search warrant for an inspection. It is best to allow OSHA personnel to inspect without the need for such a warrant. They will not be confrontational, but will be professional and courteous.

The OSHA inspector will do the following:

- Check for the posting of the OSHA safety and health poster.
- Ask to see the OSHA manual.
- Review the OSHA log of injuries for the current year and 2 prior years.
- Inspect for compliance with specific OSHA standards affecting your medical practice.
- Comment on obvious hazards noted during an office tour.
- Inquire about the existence of a basic safety and health program at your office.

Inspection

OSHA inspections consist of three parts:

Initial meeting: The inspector interviews the physician.
Walk-through: Office compliance is assessed. Employees are sometimes interviewed privately.
Final meeting: The physician is informed of any apparent violations.

INITIAL MEETING

During the initial meeting, the inspector asks to see the exposure control plan. This plan must be complete, accessible, and presentable. It must be reviewed and updated annually or whenever changes in job classifications or risk of exposure occur. Keep this in mind: 90% of all violations found in medical offices are the result of inadequate exposure control plans.

WALK-THROUGH

The walk-through is where the inspector checks office procedure for compliance with OSHA regulations. Some inspectors go so far as to observe a patient procedure to evaluate the use of PPE and work practice policies. The inspector also asks to see procedures for waste disposal and housekeeping policies. If the office contains a laboratory, the inspector will observe the collection, handling, and disposal of blood and its components for compliance with OSHA regulations.

FINAL MEETING

During the final meeting the inspector presents a list of violations and discusses how they will be resolved.

Violations and Penalties

The inspector reports any violations to OSHA, which compiles a compliance report and prepares any appropriate citation. If the medical office receives a citation, it is given 15 days in which to file an appeal. A hearing is then scheduled before an administrative law judge, at which time a determination will be made. A list of OSHA regional offices is provided in Box 11-1.

Penalties for OSHA violations range from $70 to $70,000 for each violation cited. The amount is based on the severity of the violation and its impact on infection control. There are four categories of violations:

1. Willful
2. Serious
3. Repeat
4. Other

Each violation is judged individually, and good intentions will not keep an office from receiving a citation and fine. The office manager is responsible for monitoring and controlling the compliance of the office and should therefore take a good, hard look at all office policies and procedures to ensure that they comply with OSHA regulations.

Five Priorities of an OSHA Inspection

OSHA has developed a system of priorities to help them in their inspections, with the first being the most serious.

First Priority: Imminent Danger. This category is reserved for conditions where there is reasonable certainty that an employee is exposed to a hazard that can cause death or serious physical harm immediately or before the danger can be eliminated.

Second Priority: Catastrophes and Fatal Accidents. Catastrophes and fatal accidents include incidents resulting in hospitalization of five or more employees or the death of a single employee. These incidents must be reported to OSHA within 48 hours for investigation, even when no violation of a regulation has occurred. Such accidents are investigated to ensure that they will never happen again.

Third Priority: Employee Complaints. An employee may report (anonymously, if desired) alleged violations or unsafe working conditions. Employee complaints are the most common cause of OSHA inspections.

Fourth Priority: Programmed Inspections. Programmed inspections are aimed at high-hazard industries, occupations, or substances. Special emphasis programs may also be developed for commonly reported accidents.

Fifth Priority: Follow-up Inspections. A follow-up inspection determines whether the violation has been corrected. "Failure to Abate" violations can carry stiff penalties.

BOX 11-1 OSHA Regional Offices

Region 1 (CT, MA, ME, NH, RI, VT)
U.S. DOL/OSHA
JFK Federal Bldg., Room E340
Boston, MA 02203
617-565-9856
Fax: 617-565-9827

Region 2 (NJ, NY, PR, VI)
U.S. DOL/OSHA
201 Varick Street, Room 670
New York, NY 10014
212-337-2339
Fax: 212-337-2371

Region 3 (DC, DE, MD, PA, VA, WV)
U.S. DOL/OSHA
Gateway Building, Suite 2100
3535 Market Street
Philadelphia, PA 19104
215-861-4900
Fax: 215-861-4904

Region 4 (AL, FL, GA, KY, MS, NC, SC, TN)
U.S. DOL/OSHA
Sam Nunn Atlanta Federal Center
61 Forsyth Street, SW, Room 6T50
Atlanta, GA 30303
404-562-2281
Fax: 404-562-2295

Region 5 (IL, IN, MI, MN, OH, WI)
U.S. DOL/OSHA
230 South Dearborn, Room 3244
Chicago, IL 60604
312-886-7034
Fax: 312-353-8478

Region 6 (AR, LA, NM, OK, TX)
U.S. DOL/OSHA
525 Griffin Street, Room 602
Dallas, TX 75202
214-767-4736 ext. 238
Fax: 214-767-4760

Region 7 (IA, KS, MO, NE)
U.S. DOL/OSHA
1100 Main Street, Suite 800
Center City Square
Kansas City, MO 64105
816-426-5861
Fax: 816-426-2750

Region 8 (CO, MT, ND, SD, UT, WY)
U.S. DOL/OSHA
1999 Broadway, Suite 1690
Denver, CO 80202-5716
303-844-1600 ext. 309
Fax: 303-844-1616

Region 9 (American Samoa, AZ, CA, Guam, HI, NV, Trust Territories of the Pacific)
Technical Assistance
U.S. DOL/OSHA
71 Stevenson Street, Room 420
San Francisco, CA 94105
800-475-4019
Fax: 415-975-4319

Region 10 (AK, ID, OR, WA)
U.S. DOL/OSHA
1111 Third Avenue, Suite 715
Seattle, WA 98101-3212
206-553-5930
Fax: 206-553-6499

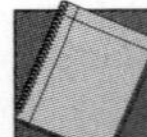

FROM THE EXPERT'S NOTEBOOK

Generally, medical practices do not experience many OSHA inspections, and practices with fewer than 10 employees will not be inspected because of their low Standard Industrial Classification code rating.

Common Violations of the Bloodborne Pathogen Standards

The following is a list of the most common violations of the bloodborne pathogen standards found during OSHA inspections over a 1-year period:

- Improper storage containers were used for nonsharps waste.
- The exposure control plan did not include the method and schedule for implementing a standard.
- Work surfaces were inappropriately decontaminated.
- Signed refusal of the HBV vaccine was not available.
- Employees did not comply with standards for use of PPE.
- HBV vaccine was not available.
- Containers of regulated waste were improperly labeled.
- A written exposure control plan was not available.
- A list of job classifications for all employees exposed was not available.
- A list of tasks being performed when employees were exposed was not available.
- Hand washing was not performed properly.
- Face protection was used improperly.
- A written schedule for cleaning and decontamination of an area was not available.

- Documentation that employees were trained within 90 days was not available.
- Name of person who trained staff on OSHA regulations was not documented.

CLINICAL LABORATORY IMPROVEMENT AMENDMENTS OF 1988

The amendments to the Clinical Laboratory Improvement Act (CLIA) set forth performance requirements for laboratories. These rules and regulations were amended in 1993 with the final version of performance requirements. In-office laboratories are now subject not only to state but also to federal regulations. Each physician-owned, hospital, or independent laboratory is responsible for payment of a compliance fee. This fee varies from state to state and is based on an hourly rate determined by each state government, as opposed to the average amount.

The CLIA inspection process is focused on the quality of laboratory services provided. CLIA inspections are intended to provide on-site education regarding accepted laboratory procedures. They are also intended to determine whether a laboratory is compliant with CLIA standards and will aid in the decision to issue certificates. During this inspection, laboratory personnel may be asked to perform procedures, show the inspector all areas of the laboratory, and provide requested documentation. These inspections are conducted by regional surveyors from the Centers for Medicare and Medicaid Services (CMS) and by state agency personnel. CMS will provide written guidelines to assist regional surveyors and state agency personnel with federal inspections. These guidelines are available from the National Technical Information Service at 703-487-4650 (regular orders) or 1-800-553-6847 (rush orders); request "Appendix C," document #PB-92-146-174. This information also can be accessed via the Internet.

DISASTER PLANNING

The terrorist attacks of September 11, 2001, are still fresh in our minds. It is the office manager's responsibility to prepare the office for such a disaster and for natural disasters such as floods, earthquakes, tornadoes, and hurricanes. Such events force us to think about developing a strategy for patients who may need care in a disaster situation.

Steps to Take in a Disaster Situation

The best way to deal with a disaster is to be ready for it. Natural disasters and catastrophic accidents can happen anywhere; other disasters, such as terrorist attacks, typically occur in well-populated, urban areas. No matter where you live, it is important to be disaster-ready. The following steps will guide the office manager through the process of disaster preparation:

- Identify potential risk.
- Store computer backup tapes off-site.
- Store emergency supplies off-site.
- Develop an evacuation plan.
- Develop a plan for patient care off-site.
- Ensure that your insurance policy does not exclude certain disasters.
- Develop a plan for contacting patients, vendors, and employees' families.

The first step is to identify how much risk there is. Obviously, if the practice is located in New York City, risk is much greater than a practice located in Iowa. Check your insurance policies to ensure that coverage is not limited to office contents, but also covers loss of income should a disaster occur.

When the computer is backed up each evening, a copy of the backup tape should be stored off-site at a safe and accessible location. Identification of this site may be the most difficult part of the plan. A complete hard-copy list of patient names, addresses, and phone numbers should also be kept off-site. This may be necessary in the event that patients need to be contacted.

Once this off-site location has been determined, the following supplies should also be stored there:

- Insurance forms
- Paper, pencils, pens
- Petty cash
- Small kit of clinical equipment, including thermometer, blood-pressure cuff, stethoscope, adhesive bandages, antibiotic creams, gauze and Ace bandages, tape, casting supplies (if you have them), *Physicians' Desk Reference* (PDR), cell phone and charger, batteries of all sizes, patient list, flashlights, urine dip sticks, hurricane lamp with oil, hard candy, and samples of medications.

Assign an individual to handle the phone call to the police or fire department should an emergency occur. Set up a clear plan that designates which employees are in charge of patient and staff evacuation. Allow employees with children to leave so that they can relocate them to a secure situation.

Design a plan to ensure that patients can still receive care if needed. This can be done via an alternative location (perhaps an office satellite that is not affected by the disaster), or by a covering physician who is not affected by the events.

It is important for the office manager to maintain open and honest communication with all employees during a disaster. It may be necessary to provide employees with counseling after this stressful situation.

EXERCISES

MULTIPLE CHOICE

Choose the best *answer for each of the following questions.*

1. Under federal law, OSHA can inspect in only how many states?
   a. 12
   b. 50
   c. 44
   d. None of the above
2. OSHA falls under which federal department?
   a. Department of Health and Human Services
   b. Department of Labor
   c. Department of Justice
   d. Department of Safety
3. Which of the following is *not* part of OSHA regulations?
   a. Exposure plan
   b. Housekeeping policy
   c. Trauma policy
   d. Fire safety plan
4. Which of the following would *not* be considered a hazardous medical office material?
   a. Copy machine cartridges
   b. Typing correction fluid
   c. Furniture polish
   d. Saline solution
5. Which of the following is *not* a component of the exposure control plan?
   a. HBV vaccination
   b. Record-keeping requirements
   c. Compliance regulations
   d. Fire safety
6. Items classified as protective equipment include
   a. Mouthpieces
   b. Socks
   c. Scarves
   d. All of the above
7. A household item that can be used to disinfect the office is
   a. White vinegar
   b. Bleach
   c. Cider vinegar solution
   d. Laundry detergent
8. The proper way to handle sharps is to
   a. Bend the needle down and throw it into the sharps container.
   b. Recap the needle and throw it into the sharps container.
   c. Shear off the needle with cutting utensils and throw it into the sharps container.
   d. Throw the whole assembly into the sharps container.
9. If an employee refuses an HBV vaccine, what must take place?
   a. The employee must sign a release stating refusal of vaccine.
   b. Nothing special needs to be done.
   c. The employee must be counseled regarding refusal.
   d. The employee must take the vaccine anyway.
10. Which of the following does *not* take place during an OSHA inspection?
    a. Initial meeting
    b. Discussion of terms
    c. Final meeting
    d. Walk-through
11. Which of the following is *not* a category that can be cited with an OSHA violation?
    a. Repeat
    b. Serious
    c. Other
    d. Initial
12. The amount of workers' compensation received by the patient is based on
    a. The patient's age
    b. Date and type of injury
    c. Gender and type of injury
    d. None of the above
13. An incident report form should contain
    a. Name of person making the report
    b. Location of accident
    c. Name of employee
    d. All of the above
14. Each year the Joint Commission's Board of Commissioners releases the
    a. Joint Commission Report
    b. National Commission Report
    c. National Patient Safety Goals
    d. National Joint Commission Report of Safety
15. Which of the following is a goal of the report released by the Joint Commission's Board of Commissioners?
    a. Improve accuracy of patient identification
    b. Improve effectiveness of communication among caregivers
    c. Standardize a list of abbreviations, acronyms, symbols, and dose designations
    d. All of the above

TRUE OR FALSE

1. _____ OSHA was developed in 1970 as part of the Department of Health and Human Services.
2. _____ Correction fluid is considered a hazardous material.
3. _____ A biohazard is an antibiotic that some patients may be allergic to.
4. _____ Engineering controls should be a section of the exposure control plan.
5. _____ Common white vinegar used to clean the office coffeepot can also be used for disinfecting the office.
6. _____ The purpose of personal protective measures is to ensure that you do not infect the patient.
7. _____ Physician offices are not required by OSHA to provide HBV vaccine for employees.
8. _____ Medical practices are high priorities for OSHA inspections.
9. _____ Employees are required to sign HBV consent forms whether they are accepting the vaccine or refusing it.
10. _____ OSHA requires a procedure for answering the phone.

THINKERS

1. List five policies that should be covered in the medical waste management plan.
2. There has been an explosion in a building on your block. The police have arrived at your office and state that the block must be evacuated. Identify the steps that you as the office manager should take after learning of this situation.
3. In preparation for an earthquake, what items should be in your disaster supply kit? Explain the reasons each item is necessary.
4. An employee has accidentally stuck himself with a needle after drawing blood on a patient. The employee comes to you totally distraught. What does OSHA mandate that you do?

REFERENCES

Cavalli, K. "Is Your Office Ready for an OSHA Compliance Inspection?" *Physician's Management*, July 1993, pp. 94-95.

Chaff, L. *Health and Safety Management for Medical Practices.* Chicago: American Medical Association, 2001.

Federal Register, December 1999, pp. 64175-64181.

Medical Group Practice Legal and Administrative Guide. Gaithersburg, MD: Aspen Publications, 1999, pp. 6.1-6.71.

Nielsen, R.P. *OSHA Regulations and Guidelines: A Guide for Health Care Providers.* Albany, NY: Delmar, 2000.

Tompkins, N. *A Manager's Guide to OSHA.* Menlo Park, CA: Crisp Publications, 1993.

12

RESPONSIBILITIES OF THE MANAGER

CHAPTER OUTLINE

CHAPTER OBJECTIVES

After completing this chapter, you will be able to do the following:

- Understand the importance of a good physician-administrator relationship
- Differentiate among the types of office managers
- Discuss the goals and management principles of an office manager
- Understand the importance of good leadership skills
- Identify the different management styles
- Recognize the signs of an impaired physician
- Comprehend the importance of a policy and procedure manual
- Understand how physicians are credentialed

- Use the practitioner data bank
- Identify the components of a successful staff meeting
- Discuss the purchasing process
- Understand the benefits of buying versus leasing
- Explain the daily operational issues of a medical office
- Recognize the signs of employee theft
- Help plan the building of a medical facility
- Discuss the issues involved in a medical office relocation

MISSION STATEMENT FOR THE MEDICAL OFFICE

The philosophy of the medical office is an integral part of its success. This philosophy, or *mission statement,* should be brought to all employees' attention so that they have a clear understanding of the conscience of the practice. The mission statement is generally written by the physician(s) and office manager and simply spells out the philosophies of the practice and the rules and regulations by which the office means to uphold this philosophy. This is very important when an office is attempting to retain employees and avoid a high turnover rate. The anxiety and time involved every time the office manager must replace an employee are not to be taken lightly; having a clear mission statement about the office philosophies may help make the office objectives easier to attain. A sample mission statement that can be personalized to fit any medical practice is shown in Chapter 15, Box 15-5.

THE PHYSICIAN-ADMINISTRATOR RELATIONSHIP

"Whenever you hear that everything is going as planned, somebody is either a fool or a liar." —TED LEVITT, MANAGEMENT GURU

The challenge of blending the efficacy of treatment with appropriate financial decisions has never been more pressing than today. Pressures on physician practices increase from hospitals, payers, government regulations, and, most of all, patients. Physicians must graduate from medical school and be ready to accept not only the clinical challenges but also the business challenges of medical practice. They must be able to integrate clinical and financial data in their practice. This becomes difficult for physicians, who have been trained to focus on the patient, one-to-one, and to provide the best care possible for that patient. This is the way they want to practice medicine. How many times have you heard the physician say, "I just want to take care of my patients!" This is where the abilities of the office manager/administrator come into play.

Office managers are trained to multitask. They can do many things at once, making one decision after another. Their most important role is one of partnership with the physician. They must guide the physician and maintain the business side of the practice. With medicine changing daily, it is important for the office manager to be well informed and to keep abreast of all changes relating to the physician practice. Dr. Arnold Relman of *The New England Journal of Medicine* wrote in 1991, "the health care system, formerly a social service that was the responsibility of dedicated professionals and not-for-profit facilities, has become a vast, profit-oriented industry." Almost two decades later, it has only gotten more profit oriented. In *Hospital Forum Magazine,* an article by Simendinger and Moore regarding a study of physician-administrator cooperation identified characteristics that should be present in both the physician and the administrator:

- Honesty and trust
- Energy and hard work
- Compatibility
- Enthusiasm
- Intelligence

Relationships between physicians and administrators will always be a challenge as we face different personality types and the often conflicting demands of each job.

In a study done by the Medical Group Management Association (MGMA), the major frustrations of the physician-administrator relationship were identified as follows:

- Problem solving and decision making at meetings
- Employees who do not follow office policy
- Interpersonal conflicts and communication problems
- The introduction of change
- Influencing decisions and policies
- Motivating the board

This study identifies that decision making, combined with knowledge and creativity, is a must for any relationship to succeed.

It is most important to have a good working relationship with the physician. It may not be a relationship that is built easily; it requires the hard work of both parties. It is important to understand clearly what the physician expects. Find out from the physician what the goals of the practice are, what the goals of the office manager's position are, what the responsibilities of the position are, and whether there are any obstacles that may prevent you from doing a good job. It is only after you have obtained full and clear answers to these questions that you will be able to be both effective and productive.

Getting a new idea across to the physician requires excellent timing and the right content. If you have a strong, open relationship with the physician, it is easier for the development of new ideas for the practice. If a strong relationship does not exist, you might first want to work on that aspect before attempting to go further. Show the physician that you are a capable, dependable, and responsible manager with the best interests of the practice in mind at all times. Help the physician to make the best and most effective use of her or his time, and keep the lines of communication open at all times. Communication is "circular"—it is not only the importance of the message, but the importance of feedback. Ask the physician on a regular basis if there is anything you can do to help make the day better. Recognize when the physician is having a bad day and ask if there is anything you can do. This will be greatly appreciated, and the physician with insight will be pleased that you can recognize a bad day and are willing to help to make it better. It is important to realize that the result of any interaction with the physician should always be a mutually positive outcome, not who wins or loses. Problems between physicians and administrators should be resolved privately and quietly, not through a shouting match in the hallway! If the physician continues to remain angry, often it is best to walk away and discuss it further at a later date. Timing is everything!

After the solid relationship has been established, carefully choose a time to present your new idea. Timing is a critical factor in whether your new idea is accepted. Don't present the physician with a new idea as she or he is racing down the hall toward the hospital! There is no formula for determining when the window of opportunity is open. After working with a physician for a while, you will able to sense when the time is right to spring a new idea on her or him. In addition, have documentation available to back up your idea, and present it in such a manner that will evoke a positive response from the physician (Figure 12-1). If your presentation requires handwritten material, keep it clear and short. Nobody has the time to read a large amount of material, so your success will depend in part on whether you can present your information completely, yet briefly. Practice the presentation before attempting it on the physician; this will help you identify any flaws or glitches in it.

The Physician...Part of the Team

The position of the physician is changing. The position of physician has moved from the top of the chart to a member of the team (Figure 12-2).

There is a spectrum of physicians that fall into three categories. The first is the physician who has no respect for anyone, including the office manager. This physician feels godlike and expects others to take care of details. Then there is the physician who is very comfortable handing over considerable responsibility to others and who is glad that someone else is taking care of important matters such as billing and personnel. Last but not least are physicians who are just coming out of residencies. These physicians have been formally introduced to the concept of being part of a team and respect the various team members and the part that they play in the care of the patient.

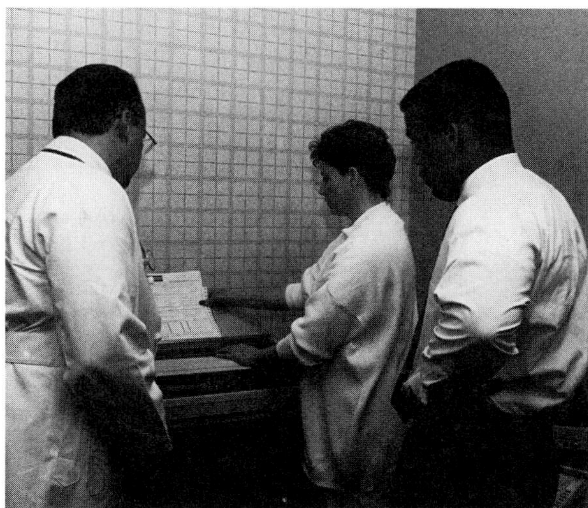

FIGURE 12-1. The office manager brings the computer transmission dilemma to the physician's attention.

This is the dramatic evolution that the physician role has taken. Physicians have been used to being "ego stroked." They always felt superior because they chose a career that has worthwhile purpose and because they deal with life-and-death issues every day. Anyone who for years has had the opportunity to save lives will feel godlike—whether it is a physician, a nurse, or a medical assistant. The problem is that this godlike persona translates into everything a physician does. In a medical office, a physician retains the decision-making power in medical and business matters. She or he is used to being the smart one in the office who delegates to the staff. Now patients are pressuring medical offices to improve patient care. This involves the whole team, and physicians now play the part of a team member.

A HARD ACT TO FOLLOW

It is not easy to step into someone else's shoes. Facts are, the staff probably liked the last office manager and are not easily swayed into accepting a replacement. The manager who held this job previously may be a hard act to follow. It is difficult

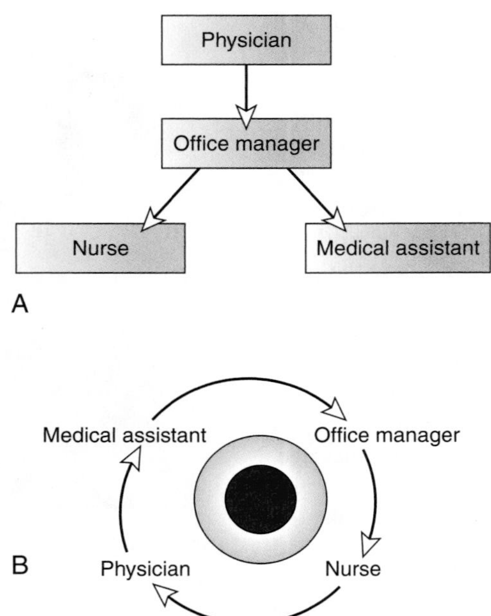

FIGURE 12-2. The physician has moved from the top of the chart (**A**) to a member of the team (**B**).

to overcome self-doubts and prove yourself under adverse conditions. Staff members will be resistant to changes, saying, "But we always did it this way!"

When you are trying to fill these big shoes, the worst battle will be within yourself. There is generally a buildup of anxiety and self-doubt that far exceeds the resistance from staff members. Remind yourself of all the positive things that you are doing, counsel yourself, and downplay the fears. You know you would not be there if you were not qualified to do the job! Avoid justifying your decisions and actions. When you are told that the other way was better, simply tell the staff that you appreciate their suggestions and will consider them. Tell them that your way of doing things may be a little different, and say it firmly. The staff members will eventually come around. Make sure that the wide range of emotions that you feel every day are controlled. Your success is tied directly to your self-discipline. Failing to keep your emotions under control can cause problems. Look secure and confident, and the staff members will soon see you that way!

The Problem Manager

In many articles and books regarding managers, supervisors, and bosses, the unspoken implication is that bad ones are few and far between. Not so, says psychologist Mardy Grothe, co-author of *Problem Bosses: Who They Are and How to Deal with Them.* There are more bad ones than good ones! The vast majority of people polled said they had experienced difficulties with a boss or manager. Let's face it, the medical office manager will usually not win a popularity contest; however, an environment of mutual respect and friendliness will work. Such an environment can be stymied by employee behaviors that can make an office manager cranky. The following is a partial list of types of employees you can expect to put you in a cranky mood:

- Employees who insist on talking to you even though you are actively involved in a telephone conversation
- Employees who insist on talking and asking questions at the same time
- Employees who constantly whine or complain
- Employees who stampede for the front door at the end of the day
- Employees who give matter-of-fact answers when really they are unsure
- Employees who take forever to say something
- Employees who insist on standing at the office door when you return from vacation, wanting all the details of the trip. . . meanwhile there are mounds of paperwork waiting for attention
- Employees who don't produce a requested piece of information until you ask them for it a second time
- Employees who have an excuse for everything
- Employees who are chronically late
- Employees who always have an emergency
- Employees who are always "sick"

The Novice Manager

Of all the problem managers today, the most common seems to be the office managers who have been promoted into their management position without proper training, experience, and education. To avoid being this type of manager, it is important to develop a list of areas, such as creating the budget or interviewing job applicants, where inadequacies seem to be prevalent. Sign up for workshops and seminars (at the office's expense) to gain skills in these areas. Once you have attended these courses, you will have more confidence and feel generally better about the position. It is also important to not stay in your office; get up and walk around all areas of the office. Stop and ask individual employees how they are doing. Ask them about their work. Be seen!

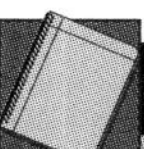

FROM THE EXPERT'S NOTEBOOK

A good office manager is a "working" office manager. An individual who knows what the staff is doing is a successful and effective office manager.

The Wimp

The wimpy office manager has a difficult time dealing with conflict and making a firm decision. This office manager is afraid to ask an employee to perform a certain task and often performs the task herself or himself. This manager cannot handle employee conflicts and would rather have the employees slug it out before getting involved! To avoid being this type of manager, again consider taking a seminar or workshop on personnel management. Weekly or monthly staff meetings will also help you feel more comfortable with facing the staff. To get some of the confidence you need, meet with the physician for feedback on the practice's expectations.

The Task Master

Some office managers think the more hours worked, the more work done. This is not always the case. Frustrated employees will fill time with paper shuffling if they are asked to stay and work long hours. Look for ways for each employee to be more productive and efficient during the time allotted for her or him. Perhaps a reassessment of job descriptions would be helpful. In addition, do not expect all workers to work at the same speed, and understand that employees have responsibilities outside the office that also require their attention.

The Phantom

The phantom manager makes an appearance at the office, does one or two things, and then leaves. This forces employees to address their questions and suggestions for alternatives to an empty chair, usually by sticking Post-It notes on it. To manage, you must be there! It is unfair to expect employees to make unqualified judgments and decisions because of an absent "leader." You know the old saying: "The band cannot play without the bandleader. How would the trumpets know when to come in?"

The Intimidator

Intimidators attempt to make themselves feel better about their own inadequacies by controlling and bullying the employees. They correct an employee in front of others, causing an embarrassing situation for the employee. The old saying "You can catch more flies with honey than you can with vinegar" seems to fit here. It doesn't help any situation to be nasty. Any reprimanding should be done in your office with the door closed; it should never be done in public. Behavior like this will cause low morale and a chronic staff turnaround problem.

TWELVE SIGNS OF A GREAT OFFICE MANAGER

1. Communicate openly, honestly, and regularly with the employees. Be approachable and show caring and concern for each employee.
2. Don't tolerate a slacker. All employees have to hold their own and be accountable for their work.
3. Refuse to pick favorites and ignore others. Employees should be rewarded based on a job well done, not because they are a friend of the office manager.
4. Give and receive feed back on projects and ideas. Listen to how employees who are doing the job think it can be done better.
5. Promote balance for each employee between work and home life. A good employee knows that the practice wants the employees to have a good balance.
6. Handle conflict by going to the source and refuse to avoid it. All conflict should be addressed in a timely fashion.
7. Avoid gossip and negative feelings. Focus on the positive and the staff will follow by example.
8. Provide deadlines and help staff with prioritizing their work.
9. Don't employ bullies! Protect employees from bullying behaviors and strive to maintain a pleasant work environment.
10. Recognize and reward the accomplishments of the staff.
11. Don't use the staff as stepping stones. Put the success of the staff ahead of personal success.
12. Have integrity. Always do what's right.

THE FOUR GOALS OF A MEDICAL OFFICE MANAGER

1. Patient quality of care
2. Happy employees
3. Achievement of goals
4. Proficient and profitable

Quality is important in any product or any service. If the product or service a business provides is not of high quality, the business will lose customers. A medical office is no different. Providing a happy environment for employees to work in is a key to successful office management. Happy employees are more productive employees and take pride in their accomplishments. The achievement of goals results in proficiency and profitability for the practice. In Box 12-1, you will find a blueprint for achievement.

AREAS OF EXPERTISE

The competent office manager possesses expertise in three important areas:

- Clinical
- Financial
- Psychologic

Clinical Knowledge

Knowledge of the clinical aspects of a medical practice can be most helpful to an office manager. It can be helpful in understanding the triage of patients to be seen by the physician and in determining the correct code for the service provided. Having some type of clinical background can be as important as having a business background, depending on the type of medical practice.

BOX 12-1 Blueprint for Achievement

BELIEVE while others are doubting
PLAN while others are playing
STUDY while others are sleeping
DECIDE while others are delaying
PREPARE while others are daydreaming
BEGIN while others are procrastinating
WORK while others are wishing
SAVE while others are wasting
LISTEN while others are talking
SMILE while others are pouting
COMMEND while others are criticizing
PERSIST while others are quitting
—William Arthur Ward

Financial Knowledge

Knowledge of finances is another major aspect of the office manager's competence. Physicians are concerned about revenues and expenses, as well as about patient care. To many physicians, an important responsibility of the medical office is to keep an eye on the bottom line. It is necessary for physicians to know the overhead costs, the turnaround time of billing, and other financial ratios to be able to budget for the coming year, and it is the office manager who gives them these vital pieces of financial information.

Psychologic Knowledge

Personnel management is the most difficult part of the medical office manager's job. Many managers say it would be easy to manage a medical office, were it not for personnel problems. These, unfortunately, are a reality. The medical office manager should be a counselor and an advisor to the staff. She or he should be able to make decisions that achieve what's good for the office and yet address some of the needs of the employees. This is discussed in detail in Chapter 2. Psychologic knowledge can also come in handy when dealing with physicians and other contacts, such as hospital employees, patients, salespersons, and others. As Priscilla Gross of the American Medical Association once said, "A personnel manager should possess a sensitive ear, a caring heart, and the skin of a rhinoceros."

MANAGEMENT PRINCIPLES TO LIVE BY

Many people have had ideas about management. Some of these ideas have endured, and some have not. The following are eight management ideas that have withstood the test of time:

Miles' Law: Where you stand depends on where you sit. Miles' Law forces the manager to focus on the big picture, negotiating and building strengths. According to Miles' Law, the manager builds a sense of teamwork by walking around. Don't just sit at your desk; walk around, talk to employees, get updates.

Parkinson's Law: An activity expands to fill the time allotted to it. In 1957, an English historian found that the more people who were hired, the more work they created, without necessarily increasing the office's output. A corollary to this law is that activity speeds up as a deadline approaches.

GIGO: Garbage in, garbage out. An anonymous, frustrated computer operator coined this phrase to account for the fact that a computer's output is totally dependent on what's put into it. Likewise, the output of any project is totally dependent on the quality of input (the people, materials, budgets, and information).

The Law of Effect: Behaviors immediately rewarded increase in frequency, and behaviors immediately punished decrease in frequency. The educational psychologist E. L. Thorndyke believed that timely feedback is one of the manager's most powerful motivators. The Law of Effect is a particularly suitable tool for a proactive manager. Catch employees in the act of victory and thank them on the spot. Just as quickly point out mistakes when you find them. But always remember to be tactful.

The Peter Principle: People tend to be promoted until they reach a level beyond their competence. A best-seller entitled *The Peter Principle* proposed this simple explanation as to why competent performers become less effective when promoted.

Pareto's Law (the 80/20 Rule): The significant elements in any group usually constitute only a small portion of that group. Pareto, an Italian engineer, developed the law of the "trivial many" and the "significant few." Eighty percent of your productivity comes from 20% of your effort.

The Pygmalion Effect: Our expectations for others condition our behavior toward them, which in turn affects how they behave. According to this law, if you believe your employees are lazy and apathetic, you will respond with minimal delegation and trust. They, in turn, will fail to improve, and you will end up with a group of employees who really are lazy and apathetic.

Murphy's Law: If anything can go wrong, it will. Murphy's Law warns us to always have a contingency plan. This law is most evident when you attempt to implement change in the office. Try to anticipate your employees' objections to an innovation and defuse them before they arise.

All of these laws contain a common thread: the admonition to treat people well. This is also known as the Golden Rule.

LEADERSHIP VERSUS MANAGEMENT

How people function during instability and change is characteristic of leadership. How people function while accomplishing objectives, coordinating staff, and monitoring workflow is characteristic of management. Leadership and management balance each other. Important components of effective leadership are

- Skills
- Knowledge
- Talents
- Competencies

Skills can be defined as an ability or a proficiency that can be transferred from one individual to another. *Knowledge* is what you have learned, your training and background. *Talents* are the abilities that you are born with; they cannot be learned. They influence behavior and thoughts. *Competencies* are skills that are essential to perform certain functions. There are essential leadership skills to be used in health care. These skills contain a set of related skills that are commonly referred to as a *skill set*. The following skill sets are the most commonly used in health care:

- Delegation—a set of skills for assigning tasks
- Counseling—a set of skills to maximize outcomes in employment
- Budgeting—a set of skills to effectively plan and implement a budget
- Negotiating conflict—a set of skills to effectively assess and manage conflict
- Performance—a set of skills for influencing team development and performance
- Commitment—a set of skills for assessing the causes of decreased commitment
- Motivation—a set of skills for assessing the cause of decreased motivation
- Decision making—a set of skills that provide the medical office manager with the ability to think strategically
- Evaluation—a set of skills for assessing personal and organizational resources and their effects on the medical office

LEADERSHIP AND THE MEDICAL OFFICE MANAGER

"Leaders are like eagles. They don't flock. You find them one at a time."
—ANONYMOUS

In a medical practice, leadership skill is crucial not only because patients, physicians, and staff members expect it, but also because quality improvement demands it. Who is a leader? A leader is a person who is assertive, resilient, proactive, charismatic, innovative, focused on the big picture, and quality oriented and who puts these traits into the service of inspiring and guiding employees through day-to-day operations. Employees' success in performing their duties relies on four factors:

- What the manager says
- How the manager says it
- Whether the manager believes it
- How the manager acts

Creative leadership will be accomplished by directing the efforts of others in an effective, innovative way to accomplish the goals of the practice. Results are one way to measure the success of your method. Truly successful leaders also look for changes in attitude and commitment on the part of the employees. With effective leaders, employees will perform at the same level regardless of whether or not you are there to supervise them.

Management Styles

Ohio State University conducted research on different management styles (which are sometimes referred to as leadership styles) and the effectiveness of each. It identified four management styles (Box 12-2) that office managers should recognize and try out before attempting to establish when to use each type of style.

STYLE 1: DIRECTING

Directing managers give their employees a lot of direction and little support. They

- Set goals and expectations
- Set plans for action
- Control the decision process
- Determine evaluation methods
- Provide specific directions

This style is appropriate in a crisis or emergency situation, where there is little or no time for consultation or evaluation of the problem. It is not recommended for day-to-day personnel management.

STYLE 2: COACHING

The office manager, when using this style, obtains more feedback from the employee than is obtained from the directing style. The coaching style also encourages motivation. The amount of direction the manager gives remains high because the employee is still learning the job. Coaching managers

- Set goals and action plans but still consult with the employees
- Encourage two-way communication between themselves and their staff
- Explain the big picture—why things are done a certain way
- Give lots of feedback, both positive and negative
- Make final decisions and evaluate performance
- Continuously teach, train, and provide direction

The coaching style is most effective with employees who are still learning their jobs and need encouragement to maintain their motivation. This management style involves a great deal of hands-on training.

STYLE 3: SUPPORTING

When they adopt this style of management, office managers

- Share responsibility for problem solving with the staff
- Delegate some goal-setting and decision-making tasks
- Involve the employees in performance evaluations
- Listen and provide feedback
- Encourage self-evaluation and independence

This style allows seasoned employees to solve their own problems. The amount of direction given is reduced, because the employees know their jobs. The manager wants to encourage more independence.

STYLE 4: DELEGATING

When managers use this type of style, they "free up" time that can be used for other tasks that only management can perform. Delegating managers

- Team up with the employees to set individual goals
- Encourage the employees to monitor and evaluate their own work
- Demonstrate trust and confidence in the employees by encouraging independent thought and action
- Allow the employees to take responsibility and give them full credit

As stated previously, by training staff and then motivating them, the medical office manager frees up time to do other necessary tasks, such as planning the overall goals of the practice and the budget for the practice. A good leader provides stimulation, encouragement, support, and inspiration to all employees, allowing them to grow and achieve. Some believe that at this point, the manager gives up supervision in favor of consultation. It is good to encourage employees to solve their own problems in their own ways and to come to you only when these ways have failed. In other words, "Come to me with solutions to your problems!" This approach to management can be risky, but it is beneficial in that you reap the benefits of energized and empowered employees.

BOX 12-2 Management Styles

Style 1: Directing
High directive
Low supportive

Style 2: Coaching
High directive
High supportive

Style 3: Supporting
Low directive
High supportive

Style 4: Delegating
Low directive
Low supportive

Characteristics of a Creative Manager

"Leaders should spend no more than four hours a day in their offices. The rest of the time, they should be out with their people. They should be talking with employees and getting feedback on problem areas. They should be patting people on the back!"

—LECTURER PERRY M. SMITH

CARING FOR EMPLOYEES' PSYCHOLOGIC HEALTH

Part of being a creative manager is realizing that all employee efforts and accomplishments must be recognized. Always thank employees for a job well done. It's a good idea to say "Goodbye and thank you" at the end of the day. This is called caring for employees' psychologic health. Don't indulge in careless and picky criticism. It is destructive to your employees and to the general office environment.

REMOVING EMPLOYEES WHO ARE ROADBLOCKS TO EFFICIENCY

By the same token, incompetence is not to be tolerated. You have the responsibility to run an efficient office, and employees who ultimately stand in the way of your meeting this responsibility must be removed. This can be a difficult task, but it can be done with grace. These employees are generally nonproductive, troublemakers, or both.

SEEING THE BIG PICTURE

It's good to see the details, the "small picture," but a progressive office manager is also constantly concerned about the "big picture." An office manager with long-term vision is a valuable asset to the medical office.

BOOSTING EMPLOYEE MORALE

People are hungry for opportunities to grow. They crave advancement, responsibility, and opportunity. The most effective way to boost employee morale is to provide the best working environment possible. There are seven key issues in creating such an environment:

1. Appreciation
2. Involvement
3. Social environment
4. Management concern
5. Management loyalty
6. Working environment
7. Everybody needs attention

Table 12-1 identifies areas with the most negative impact on employee morale. Table 12-2 identifies the best remedies for low morale.

MOTIVATION

"Motivation is a fire from within. If someone else tries to light that fire under you, chances are it will burn very briefly."

—STEPHEN R. COVEY

TABLE 12-1 Areas with the Greatest Negative Impact on Employee Morale

ISSUE	AS NOTED BY MANAGEMENT	AS NOTED BY EMPLOYEES
Lack of open, honest communication	52%	30%
Failure to recognize employee achievements	21%	27%
Micromanaging employees	17%	16%
Excessive workloads for extended periods	7%	23%

TABLE 12-2 Best Remedies for Low Morale

REMEDY	AS NOTED BY MANAGEMENT	AS NOTED BY EMPLOYEES
Unexpected rewards	38%	34%
Holding team-building sessions	17%	13%
Providing monetary rewards for exceptional performance	13%	33%
Communication	11%	0%
Recognition programs	7%	0%
Providing additional days off	4%	16%

Motivation is the circumstance that prompts a character to act in a certain way or that determines the outcome of a situation or work. It is the reason that explains or partially explains why a character thinks feels, acts, or behaves in a certain way. Harvard professor B. F. Skinner was an influential American psychologist, author, inventor, advocate for social reform, and poet. His research on human behavior suggests that individuals are motivated by different needs both in their careers and in their personal life. There are six motivational theories that can help medical office managers to get the most from their employees:

- Reinforcement theory
- Expectancy theory
- Theory X and theory Y
- Hierarchy of needs
- Two-factor theory
- Learned needs theory

The reinforcement theory by B. F. Skinner shows that behavior that is rewarded is likely to be repeated. Realizing that employees are motivated by rewards tells office managers that they should provide the kinds of rewards that are meaningful to their employees. This can be accomplished by a simple "thank you."

The expectancy theory emphasizes the importance of having and achieving a goal. This theory by Victor Vroom identifies that individuals are motivated to act because of the expectation that their behavior will lead to a specific reward. Expectancy is the employee's view of whether or not the employee's efforts will lead to the required level of performance necessary to attain a reward.

Theory X and theory Y are two sets of assumptions that managers hold about human nature. This theory by Douglas MacGregor describes that assumptions determine employees' views of motivation. Theory X employees are found to be pessimistic. Theory X describes employees who dislike work and avoid it whenever possible. This is generally due to little or no ambition. With theory Y, employees work willingly without any type of external control. They look for responsibility and opportunities to be productive. Theory Y employees are found to be optimistic.

The hierarchy of needs states that under the right circumstances, employees will work productively and positively. This theory by Abraham Maslow identifies that employees' needs are the motivational forces of behavior. These needs are the factors that drive people to seek fulfillment. Maslow describes five sets of needs (Figure 12-3):

- Physiologic
- Safety
- Love and belonging
- Self-esteem
- Self-actualization

This hierarchy is especially important when dealing with employees as they require more than a salary to meet the first two levels of the pyramid (physiologic and safety). They also need interaction to meet love and belonging needs and require respect to meet self-esteem needs. Medical office managers must keep this in mind when establishing tasks and employment conditions. Keeping this in mind will generate higher psychologic and economic rewards.

The two-factor theory was developed by Frederick Herzberg and is based on motivators and hygiene factors. He defines *motivators* as

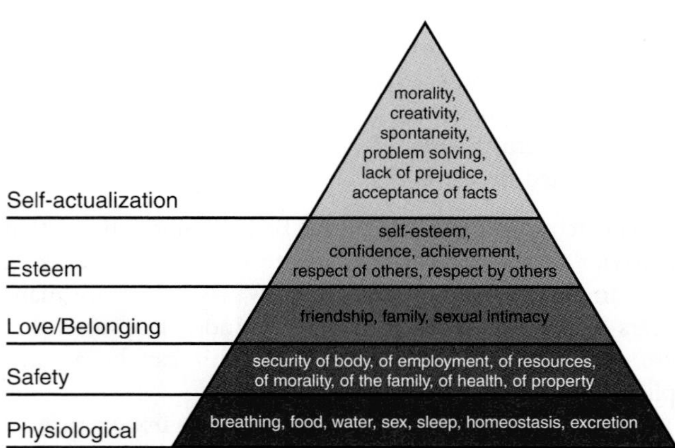

FIGURE 12-3. Maslow's hierarchy of needs.

- Recognition
- Advancement
- Growth

He defines hygiene factors as

- Job security
- Salary
- Working conditions

Failure to meet any of these can result in dissatisfaction. Herzberg found that the most important hygiene factor is money. Medical office managers should keep this in mind when structuring the pay scales for the employees. Employees require a certain pay level to meet basic physiologic and safety needs, so limiting or eliminating pay raises or incentive programs can easily demotivate employees. In today's world, job insecurity is also a demotivator.

Learned needs theory discusses three core needs:

- Power
- Achievement
- Affiliation

This theory of David McClelland theorizes that needs are developed and learned over a period of time. Employees with a need for power like to be in charge of situations and individuals. They can become effective managers or supervisors in a medical office. As an effective medical office manager it is important to recognize this need for power within certain employees and to empower them so they have some control over their jobs.

Achievement drives job performance, which is especially of interest to a medical office manager. These employees love a challenge and will shine in an environment of competition. They will look for ways to be more productive. These employees should be given positions that are challenging. Employees with the need for affiliation need a sense of belonging and want to be liked by everyone.

Commitment

Commitment is defined as the act of binding oneself both intellectually and emotionally to a certain course of action. It is a message that makes a pledge. There are varying levels of commitment that range from extremely low to extremely high. They are as follows:

Deep commitment—Employees who are deeply committed have a deep sense of purpose and find meaning in their work. They make a difference.

Personal ambition—Employees with personal ambition work hard and know how to work the system to achieve their own personal goals and ambitions.

Concerned but limited sense of power (CLSP)—Employees who are concerned are technically competent and care about quality, but feel that they are victims of society.

Formal commitment—Employees with formal commitment do only what is required and will not extend themselves beyond the minimum.
Retired on the job—Employees who are retired on the job are actively hiding from work and responsibility. They make excuses for their poor performance.
Alienated—Employees who are alienated exhibit mistrust of the physician and management, co-workers, or patients.
Actively hostile—Employees who are actively hostile avoid being fired and are antimanagement.

According to a study by M. O'Malley (2000), 43% of employees are highly committed during their first year of employment. This percentage drops to 34% by the fourth year and stays the same for 20 years. Committed medical office employees are motivated to maintain a connection, whereas uncommitted employees produce work that barely meets minimum standards (Box 12-3). Turnover rates in health care are generally between 25% and 40%.

The best way to ensure employee commitment is to implement an office environment of trust, economic independence (pay them what they are worth), and productivity.

DEALING WITH EMPLOYEES' INFLEXIBILITY

When a medical office has just opened, employees' roles are generally loose and flexible. In addition, communication is usually good, because the office is small. When the office starts becoming experienced, roles start to become more defined, and when the office starts growing, rules and procedures are developed to ensure consistency and quality. As the office manager, you may begin to think in terms of positions, rather than in terms of the people in them. Keep in mind that once employees have been doing a task a certain way for a long time, they are likely to fight change. Simply giving them a new telephone will send some employees into a frenzy. It may be difficult for these employees to adapt to changes that you, as a creative leader, wish to make. When implementing changes, involve employees, but beware of inflexibilities and proceed with caution. Changes can be made—maybe not quickly, but they can be made.

BOX 12-3 Characteristics of Committed and Uncommitted Employees

Characteristics of Committed Employees
- Pleasant
- Hard working
- Productive
- Act in the office's best interest
- Stay employed at that office

Characteristics of Uncommitted Employees
- Remote
- Aloof
- Take advantage of all time off
- Defensive and oppositional
- Will leave for a different job without another thought

BALANCING THE NEED FOR EMPLOYEE TRUST

Trust is vital to good leadership. However, fulfilling this trust cannot overrule the need to do whatever is necessary for the good of the office. Some decisions may be very difficult to make. As an example, you might agree to change the position of an employee to a recently opened different position. After interviewing new candidates, you feel the office would run smoother if the new employee would take the open position because of her or his qualifications, and the established employee would stay in the position she or he is in currently. This can be disappointing for the employee, and there is always a risk of that employee resigning. It is always important to do what is in the best interest of the office, but weigh all consequences before making a decision.

TEACHING YOUR STAFF

Good leadership in a medical office depends greatly on teaching. Leaders must be teachers, willing to share insights, skills, and experiences with their staff and helping them to grow as employees.

MANAGING THE DEMANDS ON YOUR TIME

Time management and organization are integral components of effective management. You will find that your travel plans, telephone calls, mail, and schedules can easily get out of hand. Staying busy and working longer hours do not always solve the problem. The discipline to control your schedule is what is needed.

PHYSICAL STAMINA

Without stamina, you cannot be a good leader. It is wise to build some type of exercise program (jogging, swimming, racquetball, etc.) into your schedule, so that you can get some relief from stress. The demands of a medical practice can take their toll on an office manager in a short period of time. Many gyms employ physical trainers, which will help the office manager to develop a personal workout program that best suits her or his needs.

RUNNING A MEETING

Another sign of creative management is knowing how to run a meeting. This is discussed later in this chapter, but the following are a few basics to remember: Good leaders are actively involved in the meeting, express their views and concerns, know how to draw conclusions and wrap up the meeting, and set the date and agenda for the next meeting.

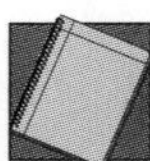

FROM THE EXPERT'S NOTEBOOK

It is essential to keep meetings on a strict time schedule. Everyone at the meeting has a busy schedule, so start on time and finish on time!

ABILITY TO LAUGH

Humor can be a great reliever of tension. You should let your employees know that work is not so important that you can't sit back and laugh a little. Don't confuse humor and laughter with making fun of someone, however. Humor delivered with a sharp tongue and off-color humor are totally unacceptable!

RISK TAKING AND RELIABILITY

Risk taking is sometimes an essential part of decision making. However, it is important to always listen to all sides before making any decisions. Many decisions cannot wait, and there are times when office managers must implement these decisions rather quickly. The office manager should understand what would be the best and the worst possible outcomes of the decision, weigh them carefully, and then, with the consistency of the past, make a quick, solid decision. It is important to realize that there is an element of risk involved every time an office manager needs to make a snap decision. However, the office staff are aware that the office manager makes all decisions with a certain amount of consistency and they begin to rely on that element of the office manager's persona. Office managers should be careful when making commitments to these decisions and should realize that a nondecision, in itself, is also a decision. Reliability is a component of a good office manager and must be present to provide strength and stability to the office.

FLEXIBILITY AND INTEGRITY

Flexibility and integrity are also essential to the medical office manager. The best office managers are those with open minds and a willingness to consider new ideas. Even more important than flexibility is integrity. In fact, of all the qualities a good office manager should have, integrity is probably the most important. Good leaders do not talk about integrity—they simply operate at its highest level. Integrity must be ingrained in all staff members and must be supported by you and the physician.

Box 12-4 lists several leadership qualities that a good manager should have. After reading this list, try to evaluate what qualities you possess that are strong or weak. Try to work on the weak qualities to improve your leadership capabilities and to secure your position as a competent medical office manager.

BOX 12-4 Leadership Qualities of the Medical Office Manager

- Is honest and sincere.
- Uses delegation effectively.
- Has respect for employees and elicits respect from them.
- Is empathetic.
- Is fair.
- Is committed to the goals of the practice.
- Realizes the importance of patient satisfaction.
- Has good communication skills and is an active listener.
- Encourages and rewards good work by staff members.
- Is straightforward and consistent in behavior.
- Is able to admit mistakes and use them as learning experiences.
- Has good counseling skills.

BE HUMBLE...APOLOGIZE

When an office manager admits to a mistake, it becomes a positive experience for both the employee and the office manager. If you never admit to a mistake, you give the impression of being inflexible.

This hard-core approach to mistakes is no longer considered the right way to manage. The office manager of the future must soften up and admit mistakes. For instance, if you blame someone for taking a file and then find it in *your* briefcase, you should simply say, "I'm sorry I blamed you. I found it." Admitting a mistake does not portray weakness; it often improves the relationship between the office manager and the employees. The staff will appreciate your honesty when you admit to a mistake, which in turn will build teamwork and cooperation in the office. No one is perfect; we all make mistakes. A good manager does not worry about constantly saving face.

Professional Societies

MEDICAL GROUP MANAGEMENT ASSOCIATION

The Medical Group Management Association (MGMA) is a valuable source of information and services for medical office managers, administrators, and hospital management personnel. It supplies up-to-date statistics regarding the business side of medicine and advises individuals on national and global developments. The MGMA has developed a strong network that can aid an office manager in the following areas:

- Library resources
- Management consulting services
- Group practice insurance plans
- Government relations resources
- Placement services
- Educational programs

You can contact the MGMA at the following address:

Medical Group Management Association
104 Inverness Terrace East
Englewood, CO 80112-5306
1-877-275-6462
www.mgma.com

PROFESSIONAL ASSOCIATION OF HEALTH CARE OFFICE MANAGERS

The Professional Association of Health Care Office Managers (PAHCOM) is an organized association that caters to small medical groups and solo practices. This organization supplies office managers with the following:

- Salary surveys
- Educational topics
- Newsletters
- Changes in legislation

PAHCOM's published newsletter has valuable articles that will help you with the day-to-day operation of the medical office. For membership information, contact them at the following address:

Professional Association of Health Care Office Managers
461 East Ten Mile Road
Pensacola, FL 32534-9712
1-800-451-9311
www.pahcom.com

THE IMPAIRED PHYSICIAN

An impaired physician is one who suffers from substance abuse, mental illness, or any type of mental deterioration. Some states require that physician incompetencies be reported to state and/or federal agencies, and perhaps require the physician to participate in an impaired physician program. To determine if your state requires this type of reporting, the practice attorney should be consulted. If the practice is a solo physician practice, you are faced with a dilemma. Since there is no other physician within the practice to go to, this impairment must be reported to the practice attorney.

An impaired physician becomes a threat to the family unit also. Some of the aspects of this "family disease" are as follows:

- Denial
- Separation
- Spouse/child abuse
- Children/school problems
- Legal problems
- Extramarital affairs
- Divorce

Alcoholism is the most common disease of the impaired physician. Alcoholism is a primarily chronic disease characterized by impaired control over drinking, preoccupation with alcohol, use of alcohol despite adverse consequences and distortions in thinking, and, most notably, denial. Even though this is a treatable disease of addiction, it is a chronic, progressive, and usually 100% fatal disease if unrecognized and untreated.

Signs of Alcohol Abuse

The office manager should be aware of the following signs of alcohol abuse:

- Smell of alcohol on breath or in perspiration
- Red-faced and/or prominent capillaries over cheeks and nose, especially if still present in winter
- Development of a bluish-red bulbous nose
- Fiery red palms with redness still present when hands are held upward
- Bloodshot eyes
- Profuse sweating when others are comfortable, especially if individual is not overweight
- Known medical problems such as hypertension, ulcers, or gout, yet is treating herself or himself
- Use of strong cologne or always has a breath mint in her or his mouth
- Hands shake or tremble in the morning
- Handwriting worsens
- Erratic behavior—from compassionate to abrupt and caustic in short order
- Generally more irritable, especially if someone comments on her or his drinking pattern
- Quick to blame others (e.g., patient, patient's family, nurses, and other physicians)
- Sloppy charting and dictations
- Makes rounds or does dictations at odd hours of the day or night
- Consults on everything, lets specialists formulate the treatment plan but rarely refers the patient to another physician
- Always late, not showing up when or where expected, cancels appointments or operating room schedule
- Cannot be reached on call or will not come in

The Other Addiction

Another addiction is drug use. An *addiction* is defined as a disease process characterized by continued use of specific psychoactive substances despite physical, psychologic, or social harm. It creates a pathologic relationship to mood-altering experiences, events, or things that have life-damaging consequences such as family and work. All addiction-prone drugs are used at least initially for positive effects and because the user believes that the short-term benefits surpass long-term costs. Once initiated, the drug permits entry to a reinforcement system, accessed by self-administration. This provides the user with an experience that the brain equates with profoundly important events such as eating, drinking, and sex.

It may be difficult to identify chemical dependency because the impaired physician is usually in denial. Sometimes there is a conspiracy of silence from family, friends, employers, and employees. A physician's job is usually affected last. Behavioral warning signs to watch for when hiring a new physician or new employees consist of the following:

- Reluctance to have a physical examination
- Vague work references
- Padded job applications, overqualified for job
- Late for interview

SIGNS OF DRUG ADDICTION

The office manager should be aware of the following signs of drug addiction:

- Red eyes
- Constricted or dilated pupils
  - Constricted pupils result from opiates
  - Dilated pupils result from cocaine, stimulants, and marijuana
- Constant nasal congestion, sinus problems, nosebleeds, or an itchy nose with frequent rubbing
- Sore throat, hoarseness (results from cocaine and marijuana)
- Chronic cough (results from marijuana and smoked cocaine)
- Extreme talkativeness and rapid speech (results from cocaine and stimulants)
- Slowed, deliberate speech or slurring (results from benzodiazepines and barbiturates)
- Frequent flulike symptoms, abdominal cramping, and diarrhea (results from opiates)
- Shift between agitation, anxiety, and paranoia to normal and even pleasant behavior (any drugs, once withdrawal occurs)
- Violent behavior or physically aggressive (results from cocaine and PCP)
- "Laid-back" behavior (results from marijuana, opiates, and benzodiazepines)
- Depression (results from benzodiazepines and barbiturates, and after cocaine use)
- Acute seizures (results from cocaine use or withdrawal from benzodiazepines, Demerol, or alcohol)
- Reduced attention to detail
- Unexplained blood on shirt or scrub suits
- Being seen in less desirable parts of town
- Avoidance of colleagues with few meaningful discussions and little eye contact
- Frequent accidents
- Chronically late and unreliable
- Competitiveness wanes

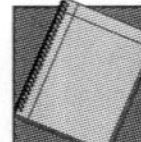

FROM THE EXPERT'S NOTEBOOK

Drug use stimulates further use! All addictive drugs are reinforcing!

Sexual Misconduct/Harassment

Sexual misconduct and sexual harassment are other problems associated with an impaired physician. Some of the signs of this type of behavior are as follows:

- Complaints about unchaperoned examinations "filter" out to nurses and other patients
- Physician accused of inappropriate touching of patients and/or staff
- Unusual breast examinations while undraped or standing up
- Physician discussing examination of a patient's genitalia with nurses or technicians after the examination
- Sexually explicit or suggestive subjects mentioned to nurses or technicians
- Hugging or kissing patients as part of "therapy"
- Seeing patient alone in office after hours or socializing with patients after hours
- Prescribing controlled substances to patients with known or suspected drug abuse problem
- Covering up the sexual misconduct of a partner
- Having a romantic relationship with any current or past patient
- Blatant affairs commonly known to the community

Psychiatric Disorders

Impaired physicians are also driven by psychiatric and behavioral disorders. Signs of these behaviors include the following:

- Depression
- Chronically angry or passive-aggressive behavior
- Many physical complaints with no organic cause
- Extreme paranoia
- Very poor record keeping or is a stickler for documentation
- Quick to assign blame to others, especially ancillary personnel in the office
- Refuses to admit that she or he could be wrong (i.e., severe professional arrogance)
- Works long hours with high rate of productivity, or works at a snail's pace with a lack of balance
- Is aloof and has only a few or no friends

Behavioral Disorders

- Is generally one of the most intelligent physicians in her or his group or on the hospital staff

- Is intolerant of what she or he believes to be "substandard" medical care
- Is vocal to hospital authorities, newspapers, and peers and will make her or his voice known to all who will listen
- Is usually at least partially right in an argument but overreacts on almost every occasion
- Is often backed by other members of the hospital staff because they wish they had the same degree of "courage"
- Has a sense of entitlement and bristles at the very thought of your questioning her or his abilities or behaviors
- Is quick to threaten a lawsuit and may actually file one
- Loves to provoke other professionals, usually with caustic criticism
- Does not learn from mistakes because she or he cannot admit to making one
- Has significantly more complaints written to authorities by patients and ancillary personnel
- A physician with a behavioral disorder must be taken to the highest level of authority before being willing to consider a change of behavior

Each state medical society has a physicians health program. To reach the one in your state, contact the state medical society.

POLICY AND PROCEDURE MANUALS THAT WORK

The office procedure and policy manual is an important tool of the manager of a medical office. Any medical practice consultant will tell you that a manual should be found in every medical office. This manual explains the policies of the office and tells employees what is expected of them. The office will run more smoothly and misunderstandings between employees and management will be kept to a minimum. Every manual should cover the following key areas:

- An introduction
- A mission statement (i.e., the vision of the practice)
- The office's address and phone number
- The name and address of the hospital where the physician is on staff
- Office hours
- Gossip
- Confidentiality
- Orientation and training period
- Employee evaluations
- Employee benefits
- Sick time
- Maternity leave
- Compassion leave
- Vacation policy
- Continuing education
- Discipline, resignation, and termination
- Lunch periods and breaks
- Smoking policy
- Jury duty
- Part-time employment
- Parking
- Employee grievances
- Snow days/inclement weather
- Personal phone calls
- Conduct and appearance
- Workstation appearance
- Public relations
- Job descriptions
- Holidays
- Pay schedule
- General questions

The policy manual should be updated on a regular basis. When the practice moves, increases in size, or changes management, it is necessary to make the appropriate changes in the manual. Always keep the sentences in your manual short and clear. It is important not to send confusing messages to the employees. Make certain to review the manual with each employee.

Try to avoid acronyms and abbreviations. Most people will avoid reading large paragraphs, so keep them as short as possible.

Each manual should include a listing of the employment laws that the practice follows. Below is a listing of pertinent laws. You will find a discussion of these laws in Chapter 9.

EMPLOYMENT LAWS

- National Labor Relations Act of 1935
- Fair Labor Standards Act of 1938
- Labor Management Relations Act of 1947
- Labor Management Reporting and Disclosure Act of 1959
- Civil Rights Act of 1964
- Age Discrimination Act of 1967
- Occupational Safety and Health Act of 1970
- Equal Employment Opportunity Act of 1972
- Vocational Rehabilitation Act of 1973
- Employee Retirement Income Security Act of 1974
- Pregnancy Discrimination Act of 1978
- Executive Order 11246
- Immigration Reform and Control Act of 1986
- Americans with Disabilities Act (ADA) of 1990
- Older Workers Benefit Protection Act of 1990
- Family and Medical Leave Act of 1993
- Uniform Guidelines on Employee Selection Procedures

THE HEALTH CARE CONSULTANT

More and more physicians' offices are calling on the expertise of the health care consultant. This consultant is asked to observe the day-to-day workings of the office, the personnel, and, yes, even the physician, with the purpose of identifying areas that need to be more productive and efficient. To work successfully with a health care consultant, the office staff, the office manager, and the physician must be committed to the overall good of the office. Health care consultants are brought on board for advice on the following:

- Starting a practice
- Closing a practice
- Expanding a practice
- Staff attrition
- Problems caused by decreased patient volumes
- Problems caused by recession and government changes that affect the office bottom line
- Problems with personnel turnover
- Investments and taxes
- Compliance plan development and implementation
- Risk assessment
- Overall operational reviews
- Fee schedule updates

It is important to remember that the health care consultant is not the enemy, but rather a partner who is attempting to solve the practice's problems. A qualified consultant can tell the physician whether the office needs an insurance agent, a billing service, an investment advisor, or a lawyer. There are many medical practice management consulting firms in the United States. Both the office manager and the physician should interview a number of consultants, so that the person who best fits the needs and vision of the practice is selected. When you are interviewing the consultant, note whether the consultant asks the appropriate questions and whether the consultant listens to answers that are given. Does the consultant act anxious to help or distracted? Ask about backup resources and about individual experience. Ask the consultant about her or his approach to the problems presented. Not all consultants take the same approach.

Most consultants will not charge you for the initial interview (which can take more than an hour), but be certain that fees are discussed before signing any contract. Beware of the consultant who comes in with a lower fee. You get what you pay for! Pick a consultant whose fee is in the same general range as the others. Make certain that the terms of the contract are clear so as to avoid problems later. By the end of the interview, a good consultant not only will have helped the physician and manager understand their objectives, but also will have a tentative plan for achieving them.

Consultants bill for their services in one of two ways: either by the hour or by the project. Once the practice's objectives have been identified, the consultant who bills by the hour states a time frame in which the objectives can be accomplished and quotes a fee for that time. Health care consultant fees may range from approximately $100 an hour to $300 an hour. This rate includes time spent in the office, in travel, doing research, and preparing reports for the practice. A 3-month project for a consultant to come into an office and evaluate it could cost as much as $10,000, depending on the types of services the consultant performs. Consultations regarding practice location and office layouts can be even higher in cost.

Consultants will try to disrupt the practice as little as possible, while continuing to become knowledgeable about all aspects of the practice. The office should be open to the suggestions for improvements that the consultant makes. You hired the consultant for her or his expertise, so use it! Smart consultants know their limitations; when they are faced with questions that require an expertise they don't have, they contact the appropriate person and obtain the answer. Generally, good consultants have a broad base of specialists in different areas of health care and business on whom they can call for information. By bringing on a practice consultant, the office is reflecting an innovative, progressive philosophy for strengthening the practice.

Health Care Consultant Scrutiny

According to the *Federal Register,* in July 2001 the Health and Human Services Office of Inspector General issued a special advisory regarding consultants. Beware of consultants who state that they are endorsed by Medicare. The government doesn't endorse anybody! Follow these simple rules to ensure that the consultant you choose is "top notch":

- Ask for references. Ask for a listing of the consultant's last five clients for projects similar to yours. Keep in mind that anyone on their list will probably give a good referral, or they wouldn't be on the list.
- Hire consultants who will "speak up"—even if their advice is not what the physicians want to hear.
- Ask about their knowledge base. Do they understand the regulations? If they are from a different area, are they aware of the local billing policies for your area? Ask where they get their information from.
- Ask how long they have been a consultant. How long have they been with the firm? How long has the firm been in business?

Abiding by these simple steps may help to choose the correct consultant for your practice. Take the time to do it right, because it can be costly if you don't!

A PROJECT LIST THAT CAN KEEP YOU ON TARGET

On a normal day, office managers can find themselves working on as many as 10 different projects. With the constant interruptions from both staff members and the physician, managers may find it difficult to keep track of the various projects on which they are working. A project list can help office managers stay on schedule for completion of each project. This simple list specifies the project name, the starting date, the finishing date, and an area for comments regarding that project.

A sample of a blank project list is shown in Figure 12-4. It can be photocopied and used as is, or it can be customized to fit the individual needs of any office. The purpose of this list is simply to remind the office manager that certain projects are still on the table and must get some type of closure soon. Projects such as developing or revising the policy and procedure manual can take a long period of time. An office manager should not have open projects on this list for more than 3 months. Another reason for keeping an accurate project list is that it is useful at performance review time. You can present this list to the physician as an accurate account of your work for the year.

PHYSICIAN CREDENTIALING

Physician practices must constantly complete credentialing forms for insurance carriers and hospitals so that the physician is recognized as competent and qualified to treat their patients. Credentialing also is used to renew medical privileges, such as patient admissions to the hospital where the physician is on staff. The office manager may want to assume this responsibility, or it may be delegated to another employee.

Once a physician has been hired, it is essential that the practice begin the credentialing process immediately. Uncredentialed physicians cannot bill for reimbursement of services if the credentialing process has not been completed.

One software package, Plan Manager, by National Credentials Corporation, can save a practice approximately 65% of its credentialing time by automating the process. This automated process allows the practice to enter the information into a database one time only. All forms to be completed are then scanned into the software, and the software does the rest. The accompanying screens illustrate this credentialing solution.

This main screen (Figure 12-5) contains a navigator bar with the various tables contained in the database. Information is divided into the following categories:

Project	Time Started	Time Finished	Comments

FIGURE 12-4. Office manager's project list (blank sample).

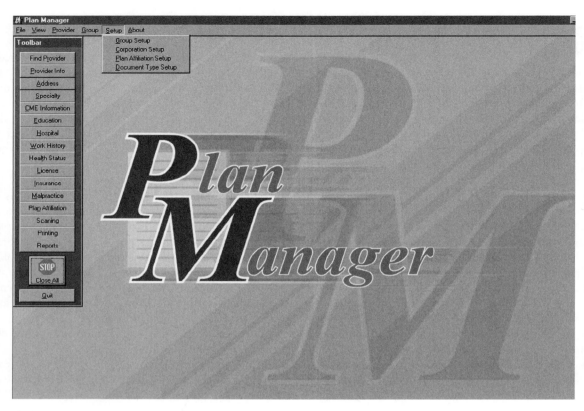

FIGURE 12-5. Main screen with button links to the program functions and tables. (Courtesy of Innovated Medical.)

- General information
- Address
- Specialty
- Continuing medical education (CME) information
- Education
- Hospitals
- Work history
- Health status/adverse actions
- License
- Insurance carriers
- Malpractice history
- Plan affiliation/ownership information

The data entry screen (Figure 12-6) is where information is entered one time and only requires maintenance after that.

This document-scanning screen (Figure 12-7) allows for licenses, Drug Enforcement Administration (DEA) certificates, malpractice face sheets, board certifications, and so on to be scanned and attached to the appropriate provider. With this particular company, a scanner is included in the price of the software so the practice does not have to purchase one.

General applications such as Medicare, Medicaid, and many others are included in this software, along with area hospitals or networks that are required by the physician practice. Once all of the information is entered, the office manager would simply choose the appropriate physician (if two or more are entered) and print the completed form (Figure 12-8).

From the screen in Figure 12-9, the office manager is able to print reports on each physician within the system. Various reports include document expirations, affiliation status by provider, group affiliation status by provider, group affiliations, rosters, CME summaries, malpractice suit summaries, and many more.

Many practices are struggling with finding the time to complete the credentialing process on each of their physicians. Automation is a management solution for the physician practice.

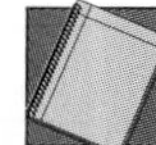

FROM THE EXPERT'S NOTEBOOK

Always make copies of all credentialing forms before they are mailed because often they do not get to their final destination! It is easier to recopy with the information at hand than to have to start all over again.

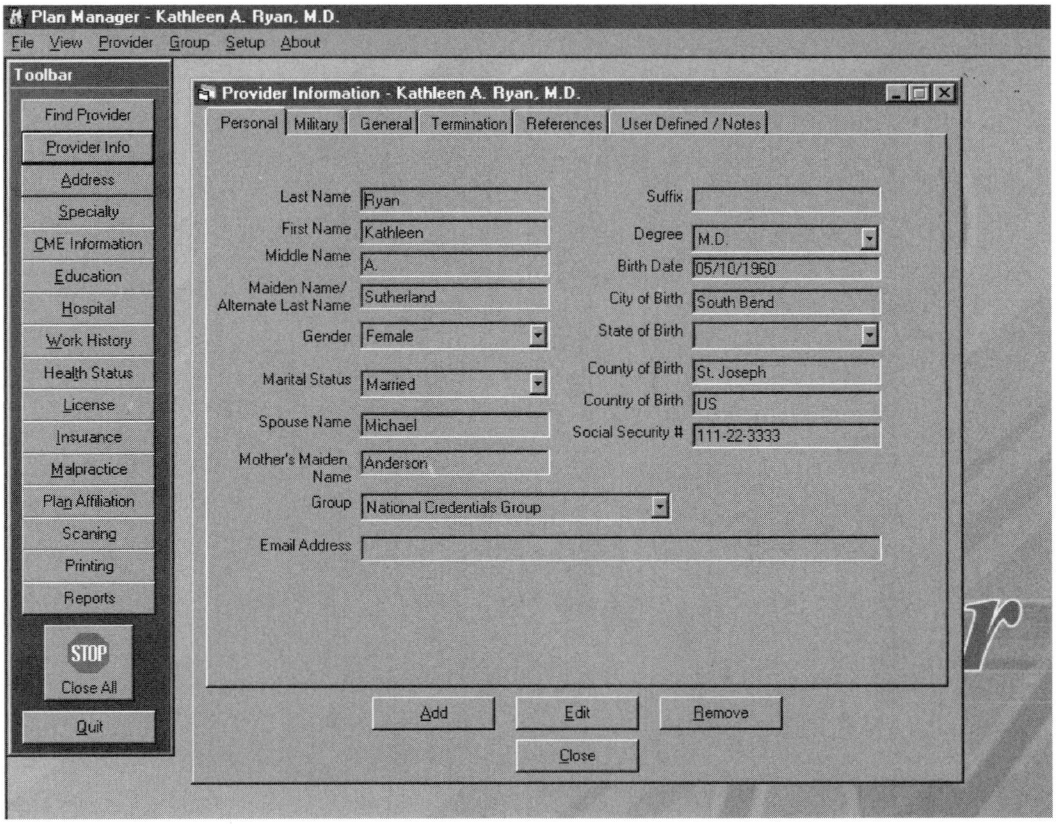

FIGURE 12-6. Provider data entry screen of provider demographics. (Courtesy of Innovated Medical.)

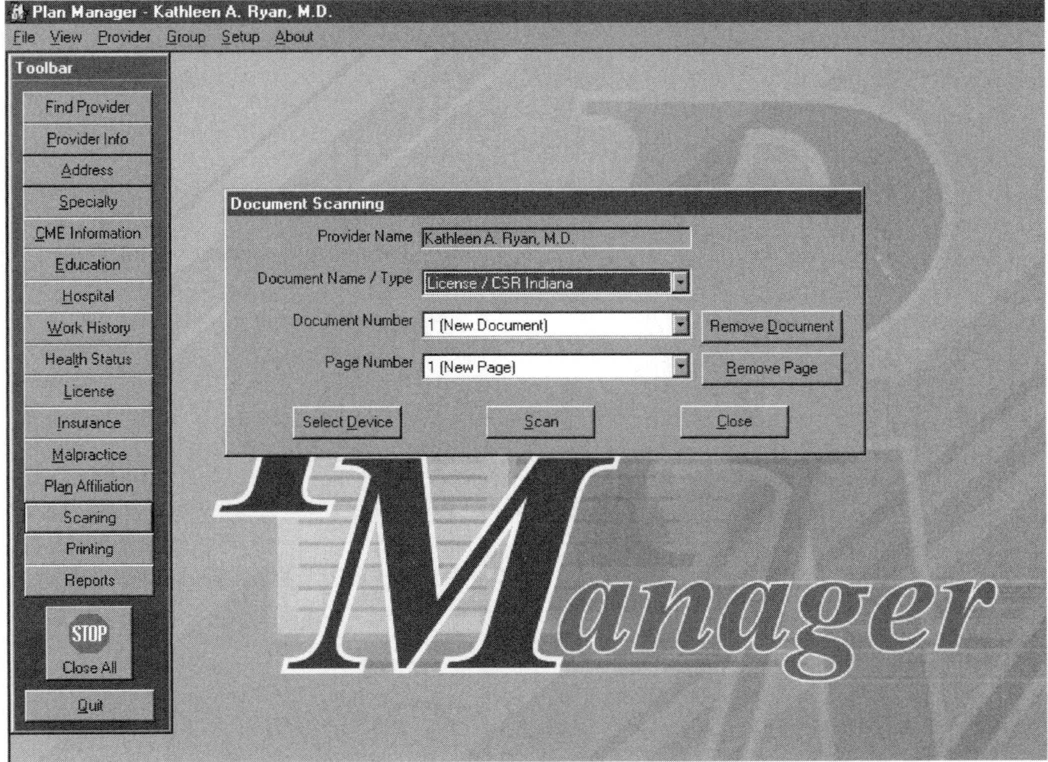

FIGURE 12-7. Document-scanning screen allowing all necessary documents to be scanned for future use. (Courtesy of Innovated Medical.)

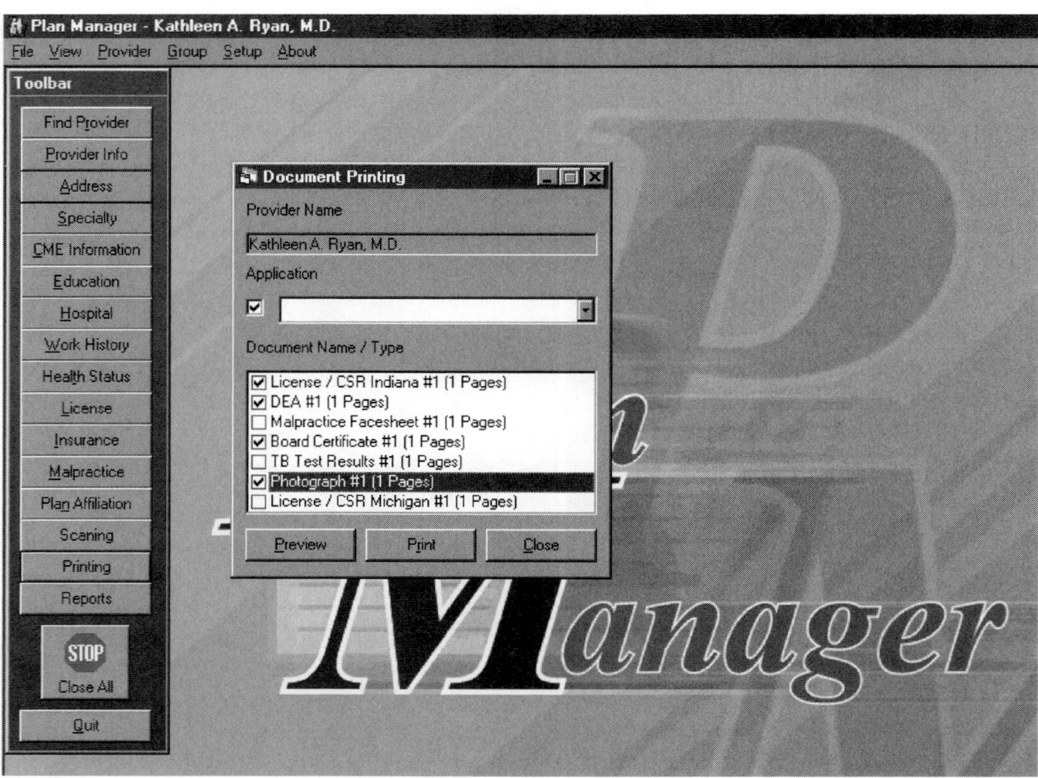

FIGURE 12-8. Printing screen for selecting documents from an easy-to-use pull-down menu. (Courtesy of Innovated Medical.)

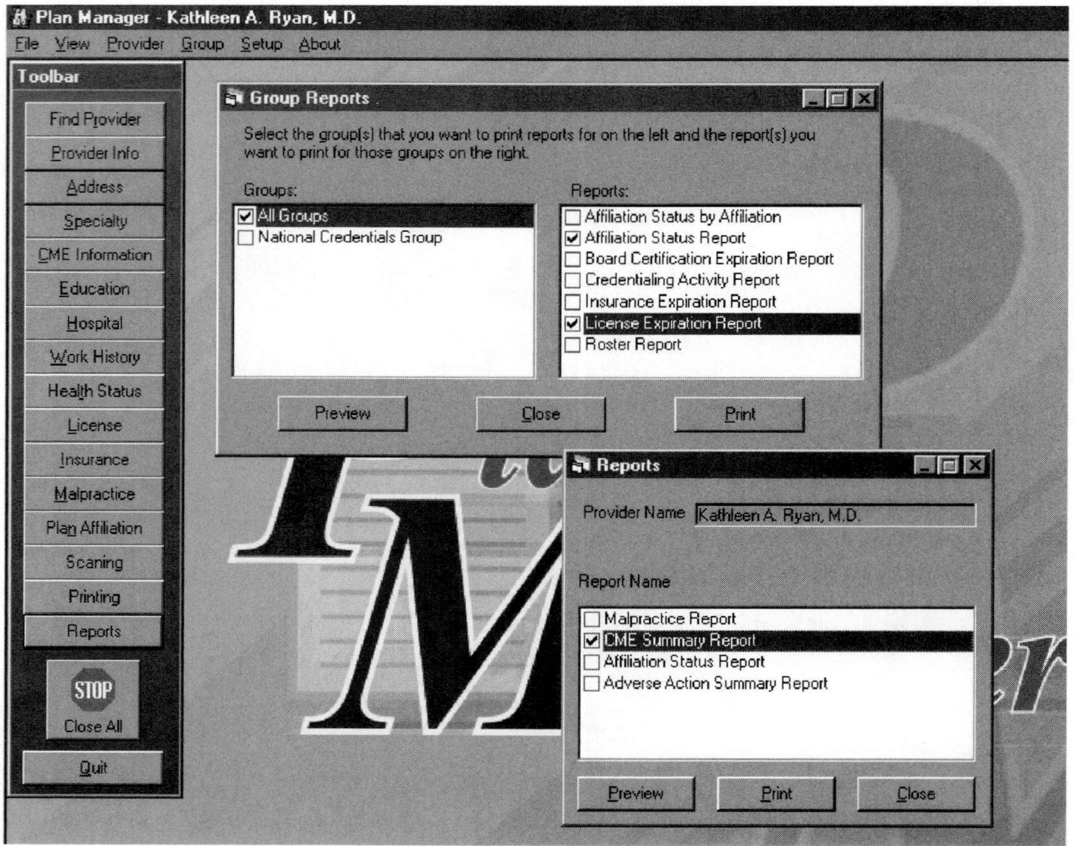

FIGURE 12-9. Screen allowing the user to print reports on each physician entered in the database. (Courtesy of Innovated Medical.)

The Physician Demographics Sheet

The Physician Demographics Sheet comes in handy for many tasks. This sheet can be prepared by you or by any one of your staff who has access to the appropriate information. The Physician Demographics Sheet contains information necessary for recredentialing of the physician for either insurance companies or hospitals. A completed Physician Demographics Sheet contains the following items:

- Physician's name
- Physician's date of birth
- Physician's place of birth
- Physician's Social Security number
- Physician's medical license number
- Physician's DEA registration number
- Physician's CME information
- Name of the physician's malpractice insurance company
- Physician's education
- Positions held by the physician
- Physician's tax ID number
- Office's address
- Office's hospital affiliations

These are the items generally requested on recredentialing forms. If a sheet containing this information is already in the office manager's file, an employee can simply copy the sheet and attach it to the form. Office managers and office staff not in the know have spent many hours completing recredentialing forms. By using this method, a recredentialing form can be completed in just minutes. The staff will still have to copy medical licenses, DEA registration, and malpractice face sheets to attach and mail along with the form, however.

CONDOLENCES

As we hurry through our busy day, going from one task to another, we do not always appreciate those around us. A kind word expressed at the time of a personal loss can mean so much to your patients. Some offices that acknowledge the loss of a patient or family member of a patient find their thoughtfulness is greatly appreciated.

The office should have a policy as to how to handle the death of a patient. Condolences might be handled differently, depending on how long the patient was with the practice and how often the patient was seen. Some offices send flowers or cards. A few offices even attend the viewing and funeral. The most common way to express condolences is to send a condolence letter to the surviving spouse or family. This letter should be short but should offer support, sympathy, and caring at this difficult time. Families of the deceased appreciate that the office took the time to send a note of sympathy. This can be done by the office manager or by another staff member at the direction of the office manager. Before composing the letter, check with the physician to see if there is a special note that she or he would like to include. If not, type the letter and place it on the physician's desk for a signature. Make sure that the letter offers the staff's condolences also.

MEMO WRITING MADE EASY

It takes about an hour for the average person to write a memo successfully. Many office managers do not have that kind of time. If your computer has the basic office programs, you will probably have templates that you can use for the format of your memo. For those managers not familiar with this program, follow these directions to the templates:

1. File (pull down menu in top bar).
2. New.
3. A window will appear with various tabs for templates such as memo, fax pages, resumes, letters, agenda, and so on. If your practice does not have this capability, there are a few short steps that can ease the pain of memo writing forever. If you follow these steps, your memos will be polished and will produce the intended results.

Step 1: Know Your Purpose

The first step in memo writing is to determine what it is you want to accomplish. Decide what it is you want to say, and say it! Start by writing, "I'm writing to tell you that" and then continue with your thought. After you have finished, go back and delete the first six words. This should make an excellent start for your memo.

Step 2: Keep It Short and Get to the Point

The second step in memo writing is to keep it short. Mystery novels may hold someone's attention, but a long memo won't. No one has the time or the desire to read long, rambling memos. State what you want to say as clearly and simply as possible. Don't belabor the point you are trying to make; ask for the action at the beginning of the memo. One way to make sure that you are keeping it short is to imagine that you are sending a telegram and have to pay for every word! After finishing a part, go back and reread it; you might be able to delete even more. As Blaise Pascal said, "I have only made this memo long because I have not had time to make it shorter!"

Step 3: Avoid Catchy Phrases

A memo is not the place to be flip or cute. Often, what comes across as witty wordplay to you while you're writing will just be bothersome to the people reading your message. Write the memo as if you were speaking in person to the person(s) receiving the memo. Your memo is a reflection of you, so be professional.

Step 4: Maintain a Backlog of Successful Memos

Keep copies of other memos so that you can refer to them, if necessary. You can often find the style you need by reading other people's memos. Also, keep any previous memos that you think are excellent pieces of expression. You can turn to them should you ever have a sudden case of writer's block. If you are computerized, these memos can be kept on the hard drive of your computer, which eliminates the need for filing space.

Step 5: Personalize the Memo

Everyone likes attention, and everyone likes to be remembered. If you are sending the same memo to more than one person, take a minute to jot a quick note on each one to personalize it for each recipient. The sincerely flattered person is the person who will be disposed to help you in the future if you need a favor. If you are using your computer for this memo, personalization is easy, as you can quickly change the name of the recipient and reprint the memo.

Step 6: Make It Easy for the Recipients to Give Feedback

Make it easy for everyone who receives your memo to respond to it by inviting the recipients to simply write their answer on your memo and send it back. This will save time and result in quicker responses.

MANAGING DESK CLUTTER

As discussed in Chapter 2, everyone has her or his own work style. Some say that desk clutter is a sign of a highly creative process going on. Others say that desk clutter does nothing but promote missed meetings, misplaced messages, late reports, and so on and that "a neat desk is an organized mind." Organization is very important to a medical office manager. The lack of it can defeat even the best managerial skills. A good office manager makes it a practice to have on her or his desk only what is being worked on at that time. Once that project is finished, the file should be closed and put away. It is then time to move on to the next task. Edwin Bliss, author of *Getting Things Done: The ABC's of Time Management,* states, "No matter how important all your projects may be, you can only concentrate on one at a time. Everything else is a distraction." This does not say that an office manager should not multitask. All office managers must learn to multitask or they will have a difficult time getting projects accomplished. A good habit to get into is to clear your desk before leaving the office at the end of the day. Delegate, dump, or do each project that was sitting there for the entire day. Having a cluttered desk constantly reinforces the fact that there are projects to be done but no time now to do them. The manager ends up playing mental shuffleboard, moving files around from spot to spot, always thinking about them. This is distracting and steals time from the current project.

If not addressed immediately, desk clutter can result in the following problems:

- Lost files and disks
- Errors and incomplete information
- Low morale
- Delays in completing work
- Confusion

The office manager is sometimes to blame for clutter in the office. Perhaps there is a need for additional closet space or shelving. This is not the fault of the employee. The office manager should be continually evaluating the needs of the office and should be addressing any storage needs that may arise. An office manager cannot expect an employee to keep an area neat if there is no room to store supplies, equipment, or personal belongings.

BUSINESS FILES

All business records should be kept in a separate file cabinet in the office manager's private office. This cabinet should be in a secure area and should remain locked at all times. This cabinet or system should be fireproof to protect its valuable contents. Business records that should be stored in this file include the following:

- Lease or deed for the office
- Property insurance policy for the office
- Health insurance policy for employees
- Pension and profit-sharing statements and guidelines
- Financial records
- Checkbook and deposit slips
- Petty cash
- Prescription blanks
- Employee records
- Physician's on-call schedule and vacation schedule
- Equipment booklets and warranties
- Tax records
- Files containing the physician's
  - Medical license
  - DEA registration
  - Current CME certificate

  - Malpractice policy
  - Updated curriculum vitae
  - Personal correspondence
- The office manager's personal correspondence

STAFF MEETINGS

"Diplomacy is the art of letting somebody else have your way."

—DAVID FROST

The main objective of the medical office staff meeting is to instill a team spirit so that staff members will work together to create a more efficiently run office. Monthly meetings should be worked into the schedule and should not be canceled for any reason. These meetings may or may not include the physician. Some medical offices have found that they get more accomplished when the physician is not present. Others say the opposite. It is best to hold meetings both ways to see which works best for your office. Employees will not freely give up their own time for these meetings, so they must be scheduled during their working hours. It is best to block off an hour or so during a workday and have the answering service answer the telephone. Some offices schedule meetings during lunch. Usually these offices will order lunch to be delivered for the staff.

Problems with individual staff members should not be addressed in staff meetings; these should be discussed privately. If a meeting is held to discuss a change in policy, do not ask the staff for their approval; instead, explain the change firmly and ask staff members for input on how to make the new policy successful. Successful meetings mean exchanges of ideas. Be careful not to lose control of the meeting, however, by being too open-minded. Always be positive about some aspect of the staff's work. Too many negative assessments may cause low morale and reticent behavior.

Meeting Planning Checklist

1. Before the meeting, decide the general purpose of the meeting and then the specific objectives of the meeting. Set clear, reasonable due dates for each task that will be assigned at the meeting.
2. Determine the degree of decision sharing and group autonomy. Is this a recommendation group or a decision-making group?
3. Choose the type of meeting format: roundtable discussion, brainstorming, consultative, directive, nondirective, and so on.
4. Choose who will and will not participate.
5. Select those who might perform a task during the meeting, such as taking the minutes, chairing the meeting, and so on.
6. Schedule the time, place, and duration of the meeting as appropriate to the task and purpose.
7. Determine how and when participants will be briefed as to their individual meeting responsibilities—by telephone, written notice, e-mail, and so on.
8. Determine any audiovisual aids, overhead projector, PowerPoint projectors, flip charts, and so on that might be needed and make arrangements for them to be at the meeting place.
9. Develop an agenda and distribute it before the meeting if possible.
10. Order food if scheduled as a lunch meeting.

Keep this list available for all meetings and use it as a reference. A meeting action plan should be completed during every meeting, so that the office manager will know which task is to be completed by whom and when. A sample meeting action plan is shown in Figure 12-10.

Getting Them There. . . On Time

No one likes meetings that go on forever. This can be partially eliminated if everyone arrives on time. It is not fair to others if repeat offenders constantly breeze in 15 minutes after the meeting started. Be sure to post the date, time, and place of the office meeting to give everyone proper notice. Then there can be no excuses. You may find that sometimes scheduling a meeting at an odd time will help people remember it. For example, a meeting that would normally be scheduled for 9:00 AM could be scheduled for 9:45 AM.

Another way to cure latecomers is to discuss important items first. Latecomers can also be motivated to be on time if items of their interest are scheduled for the beginning of the meeting. If you issue an agenda a few days before the meeting, staff members can see what is to be discussed and when. It can also be helpful to involve staff members in the meeting. Perhaps they can report on new coding ideas or new ideas for appointment scheduling. This does wonders for office morale, can be a pleasant learning experience for everyone, and creates the desire to be on time where once there was none.

If none of these ideas seem to work on chronic latecomers, take them aside and discuss the problem privately. Emphasize that it is not only that they are habitually late, but that their input is important to the group and very much needed.

Conducting Effective Staff Meetings

It is important to start the meeting at the designated time, even if all members of the staff are not present. Starting the meeting on time conveys the seriousness and formality of the meeting. Always close the door when starting the meeting. This reinforces the meeting's importance and indicates that any intrusion after this point is disruptive. As mentioned, use a format whereby the most important information is covered first.

Date: ________________

Action to Be Taken	Person Responsible	Deadline

Key Issues

____

____

____

____

____

____

Recorder: ______________________________

FIGURE 12-10. Meeting action plan.

After a while, regularly scheduled office staff meetings can become unproductive, because they are routine to the staff. At this point, meetings should not discuss work in progress. Instead, have each staff member hand in a written update of the project or task on which she or he is currently working, and focus the meeting on issues such as marketing, patient satisfaction, and teamwork.

An effective manager holds staff meetings at odd times, as already mentioned, and just before lunch (Figure 12-11). Holding the meeting just before lunch ensures that staff will stick to the matters at hand. In addition, think about your office's appointment schedule before scheduling a meeting.

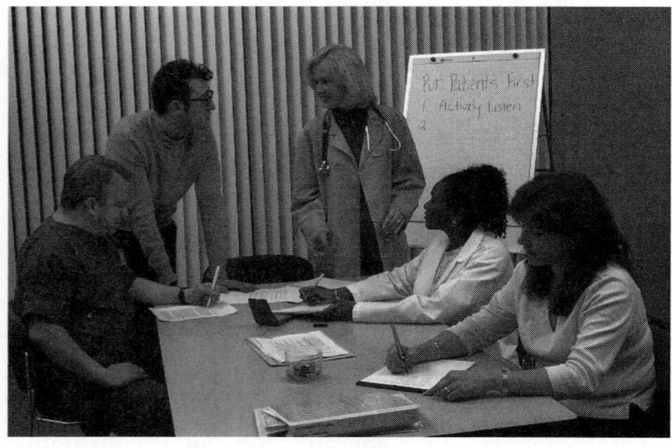

FIGURE 12-11. The office manager conducts an informative staff meeting.

At US Healthcare, the president issued a policy that no staff meetings of three or more could be held between 9:00 AM and 4:00 PM, because this was their busiest time. It made no sense to have staff meetings to discuss better customer relations when the customers needed the staff at that time.

Keep the topics specific, because broad topics can cause the group to lose focus. If the office is large enough to have department heads, meetings with department heads should be scheduled before meetings with the rest of the staff. When writing the agenda, be sure to be specific. For instance:

- The wrong type of agenda listing: **Item III) Marketing Strategies**
- The right type of agenda listing: **Item III) New Marketing Strategy: Patient Information Booklets**

A specific agenda helps the meeting stay on course and keeps the staff members focused. As mentioned, give the staff members the agenda before the meeting, so that they might prepare statements and opinions. In addition, always issue follow-up notes after the meeting that outline what was discussed, what was decided, and how it is to be handled. This way, all staff members are clear as to the role they play in completing this task. When something is written in black and white, it is less easy for employees to say they misunderstood.

An effective meeting leader is like a talk show host. Try to get each member's input without jeopardizing the focus. To do this, simply word questions specifically instead of generally. In other words, ask, "Ann, how does this change in data entry affect your position?" instead of "Ann, what do you think?" A specific question requires a specific answer, and the meeting is kept under control. When people get off track, gently but firmly pull them back on track by stating, "That's very interesting, but how does that relate to our issue?" They will see that they were a bit off the subject and will apologize, allowing the meeting to move on.

It is a good idea to allow time at the end of the meeting for an open forum. This is generally a 15-minute session in which any staff member can bring up a topic for discussion, with the understanding that it must be brief. If the topic is too long, discussion of it can be finished in the office manager's office after the meeting.

Visual aids always help get a point across. The office manager can use a variety of items: flip charts, slides, or handouts. Slides should be used for large groups, and flip charts and handouts for smaller groups. The important thing to remember is that if they see it, they retain it.

PATIENT'S BILL OF RIGHTS

The American Hospital Association (AHA) published the "Patient's Bill of Rights" in 1973. The AHA wrote the Patient's Bill of Rights to provide more effective care and greater satisfaction for the patient, physician, and hospital. The office manager might want to copy this document and place it in the waiting room for patients to either read in the office or pick up and take home. At the hospital, the Patient's Bill of Rights is generally given to the patient at admission. The physician-patient relationship takes on new dimensions when the patient is in the hospital setting. Not only is the physician responsible for the patient, but the hospital as an institution also accepts responsibility for the patient. The patient's rights should be supported by both the hospital and the physician; they are an integral part of the patient's recovery. Because this document has been prepared by professionals rather than consumers, it would probably be admissible as evidence in a case where the rights of the patient are concerned. Box 12-5 presents the AHA's Patient's Bill of Rights. The office manager might want to develop a particular Patient's Bill of Rights for the medical office. This can be included in the *Patient Information Handbook* or can be made into a pamphlet and placed in the waiting room for patients to pick up. A sample Patient Bill of Rights for a medical office is shown in Box 12-6.

PRACTICE MERGERS

Many have predicted that there will be a merging of medical practices across the United States in response to the current climate in the health care field of government regulation and decreased reimbursement. Some believe that the market will force all physicians to join some type of group practice and the days of the solo practitioner will be gone. Regardless of the external forces being applied to the medical practice, there are some definite advantages to practice mergers:

- Centralized billing
- More efficient bill collection
- Group purchase discounts
- Overhead economies of scale
- Better quality total management
- Practice transition

To get to these advantages, however, some storms must be weathered. A major problem occurs when two incompatible practices merge. It is best to determine compatibility before taking this big step. It is like a marriage; the only difference is that it involves more personalities, which makes it even worse! There are three major areas to assess before a merger should take place: finances, employees, and fee schedules.

Finances

The finances of the two practices should be assessed and compared. Each practice's history of collections, accounts receivable, adjustments, and productivity should be included in this assessment. Information should be obtained from the accountant regarding liabilities. The office managers can share information such as overhead and billing turnaround times. Discussion of issues such as Medicare participation and managed care participation is essential. Retirement plans, employee medical insurance plans, and profit sharing also need to be addressed. The office manager should work closely with the physician, the accountant, the lawyer, and the other practice's counterparts. It is in the office manager's best interests to cooperate completely during this transitional period.

Employees

Employees and their salaries must be considered. If the merger takes place, there will be duplication of many positions among the practices. The position and salary structures should be analyzed along with the benefits package that each office offers. Developing new policies and salaries can be difficult, but consensus must be worked out before any merger takes place. Consideration should be given to valuable staff who have been employed for many years. Of course, each practice wants to keep its own employees, so this can be a very difficult aspect of the merger. Often, the employees who are retained are those who are the most cost-effective for the practice. As an office manager, the best position to take is to be pleasant and as helpful as possible and have a positive outlook about the merger process. This will be of great benefit.

BOX 12-5 The American Hospital Association's Patient's Bill of Rights

1. The patient has the right to considerate and respectful care.
2. The patient has the right to obtain from his [or her] physician complete current information concerning his diagnosis, treatment, and prognosis in terms the patient can be reasonably expected to understand. When it is not medically advisable to give such information to the patient, the information should be made available to an appropriate person in his behalf. He has the right to know, by name, the physician responsible for coordinating his care.
3. The patient has the right to receive from his physician information necessary to give informed consent prior to the start of any procedure and/or treatment. Except in emergencies, such information for informed consent should include but not necessarily be limited to the specific procedure and/or treatment, the medically significant risks involved, and the probable duration of incapacitation. Where medically significant alternatives for care or treatment exist, or when the patient requests information concerning medical alternatives, the patient has the right to such information. The patient also has the right to know the name of the person responsible for the procedures and/or treatment.
4. The patient has the right to refuse treatment to the extent permitted by law, and to be informed of the medical consequences of his action.
5. The patient has the right to every consideration of his privacy concerning his own medical care program. Case discussion, consultation, examination, and treatment are confidential and should be conducted discreetly. Those not directly involved in his care must have the permission of the patient to be present.
6. The patient has the right to expect that all communications and records pertaining to his care should be treated as confidential.
7. The patient has the right to expect that within its capacity a hospital must make reasonable response to the request of a patient for services. The hospital must provide evaluation, service, and/or referral as indicated by the urgency of the case. When medically permissible, a patient may be transferred to another facility only after he has received complete information and explanation concerning the needs for, and alternatives to, such a transfer. The institution to which the patient is to be transferred must first have accepted the patient for transfer.
8. The patient has the right to obtain information as to any relationship of his hospital to other health care and educational institutions insofar as his care is concerned. The patient has the right to obtain information as to the existence of any professional relationships among individuals, by name, who are treating him.
9. The patient has the right to be advised if the hospital proposes to engage in or perform human experimentation affecting his care or treatment. The patient has the right to refuse to participate in such research projects.
10. The patient has the right to expect reasonable continuity of care. He has the right to know in advance what appointment times and physicians are available and where. The patient has the right to expect that the hospital will provide a mechanism whereby he is informed by his physician or a delegate of the physician of the patient's continuing healthcare requirements following discharge.
11. The patient has the right to examine and receive an explanation of his bill regardless of source of payment.
12. The patient has the right to know what hospital rules and regulations apply to his conduct as patient.

Courtesy of the American Hospital Association.

BOX 12-6 One Practice's Patient's Bill of Rights

In our years of practice, we have often heard patients complain about doctors. We have tried to live by certain principles. We have decided to write them down for you.

- A patient has the right to know what his or her illness is and what trouble it is likely to cause.
- A patient has the right to have the illness explained in ordinary English, not medical terms.
- A patient has the right to know the treatment options, the advantages and disadvantages of each, and what each will cost.
- A patient has the right to know the doctor's qualifications and experience.
- A patient has the right to consult other doctors without me being insulted or angry that the patient wants another opinion.
- A patient has the right to understand my fees.

I have also tried to live by these standards:

- I will spend a patient's money as wisely as if I were spending my own. I will look for and recommend the least expensive way of solving my patient's problems.
- I will not recommend surgery unless the patient needs help that only surgery can provide.
- If a patient feels I have not provided him or her with my best efforts, I will refund the money he or she paid me—no questions asked. I can't guarantee results of treatment, but I can guarantee you my best efforts to treat you honestly and fairly.

Fee Schedules

The fee schedules and coding, both procedural and diagnostic, of both practices should be considered and compared. The newly formed practice will need a uniform fee schedule. The office manager might want to suggest to the physicians that a management consultant be brought in to review both offices' fee schedules and advise. Existing computer systems and billing systems need to be evaluated by either the office manager or a management consultant. The coding practices of both offices should be studied and a single list of codes created.

Time for the Attorney

Once fee schedules, employees, and finances have been carefully examined and decisions have been made, it is time to contact an attorney to handle other issues: corporate structure, assets, management, compensation, and buyouts. These are not a part of the office manager's duties and should be passed on to the practice attorney. There are no easy mergers, but the most important factor is the compatibility of the physicians. If they are not happy, no one else will be!

Operational Review Plan

Office managers should continually evaluate the practice for efficiency, productivity, and profitability. The following checklist can be followed to ensure completeness in performing this review:

- Annual review of mission statement
- Review of staffing ratios
- Review of job descriptions and performance evaluations
- Review of patient satisfaction forms
- Review of physician satisfaction forms
- Review of expenses
- Review of policy and procedure manual
- Review of currently used forms
- Review of patient flow and daily operations (appointments, telephone, messages, etc.)

These items should be routinely monitored and measured. They should provide insight into practice efficiency and should identify any areas that may need further evaluation.

SNAP DECISIONS: HARMFUL OR HELPFUL?

A good manager is a good decision maker. Decisiveness inspires support, intimidates any opposition, and gives you control. Sometimes a not so great decision made quickly is better than a good decision made slowly. There's something to be said for people who care enough to always do their best; however, nine times out of ten, an adequate decision made in a timely fashion is worth a lot more than an agonized but late perfect choice. Movement in any direction brings a new perspective to any situation, making the right decision more apparent. The following decision-making guidelines can help you be more decisive:

- Know that you might blow it
- Calculate the risks
- Know that you can be flexible
- Defer your decision, if uncertain
- Don't get hung up on fact finding, but do your homework
- Know when to proceed with caution
- Break out of your usual thought patterns
- Search for a solution
- Respect hunches and gut feelings
- Ask an expert

NATIONAL PRACTITIONER DATA BANK

The Health Resources and Services Administration started the National Practitioner Data Bank in 1990. The purpose of this data bank is to collect and disclose adverse actions taken against health care practitioners, providers, and suppliers. It collects the following types of information:

- Exclusions from federal and state health care programs
- Licensure and certification actions
- Health care–related criminal convictions
- Civil judgments
- Other adjudicated actions or decisions

Malpractice insurers, hospitals, and state licensing boards began sending information about physicians and dentists, mostly reports of malpractice insurance payouts, adverse information that was uncovered during credentialing, and licensure decisions. The organizations allowed to query the data bank are hospitals, medical societies, licensing boards, and certain health maintenance organizations.

There is some concern regarding the confidentiality of the information stored in the National Practitioner Data Bank. Most believe that this bank comes with many problems, such as erroneous accusations and mix-ups of records. It is best to advise the physician to check periodically on the status of her or his record. The physician is supposed to be notified if someone deposits data on the individual in question, but the physician is not notified of withdrawals of information. To find out who has been looking at the physician's file, the office must fill out a form available from the bank. Photocopies are not accepted. The address of this bank is as follows:

National Practitioner Data Bank
P.O. Box 6048
Camarillo, CA 93011-6048
www.npdb.com
E-mail: npdb-hipdb@sra.com

Hospitals often "tap" the bank when credentialing new physicians for admittance to the staff of their hospital. This practice is beneficial to the hospital and its staff members. This bank was designed because of the public's concern about physicians who were guilty of poor medical practice and were relocating to another state to continue these same poor medical practices. The following is the information that goes into the bank on each physician:

- Name and address
- Work address
- Social Security number
- Date of birth
- Name of each professional school attended
- Each professional license number and state where issued
- DEA number
- Names and addresses of hospitals of affiliation

In reference to malpractice cases, the following additional information is stored:

- Site where claim has been filed and the case number
- Date and description of the acts or omissions that gave rise to the claim
- Date and description of the case and the amount of the judgment

In reference to sanctions by licensing boards and peer review bodies, this additional information is stored:

- Description of the acts, omissions, and other reasons for the board's actions or limitation of clinical privileges
- Description of the sanction, the date it was imposed, and the date it went into effect

PHYSICIAN'S CV: THAT FIRST IMPRESSION

Many physicians don't realize the importance of the professional look of a curriculum vitae (CV). *Curriculum vitae* is Latin for "a short account of one's career and qualifications" prepared typically by an applicant for a position. Obviously, physicians use their CV when they are on a job search, but a physician's CV is also used for other purposes, such as the following:

- When the physician has been invited to lecture (for example, by a drug company), the sponsoring party will circulate her or his CV as a form of advertisement.
- Hospital medical staff offices make the physician's CV a part of her or his file.
- Law firms using the physician as an expert witness request a copy of the physician's CV.

The physician should be made to realize the importance of this document; after all, it is her or his professional biography. You can help the physician prepare her or his CV. Be sure that the heading is clear and specifies the physician's name, address, and phone number. The CV should be in a logical and chronologic order. The standard form for the CV is as follows:

- Heading
- Education
- Postgraduate education
- Certification
- License
- Experience
- Honors
- Publications

Remind the physician not to leave gaps in the CV. If she or he spent a year traveling around Europe, this trip should be listed. Such gaps can also be listed as "sabbatical" or "personal leave." Any unexplained gaps can look suspicious, so try to be thorough when developing the CV. Remember, this is the first impression of the physician—make it good!

COMMUNICATION ESSENTIALS

Pager

For many physicians, the cell phone has taken the place of the pager, however, there are still physicians who carry both the pager and the cell phone. Pagers can be used in the hospital setting, where some cell phones cannot. To make the physician's life more bearable, consider some of the following factors before purchasing a pager:

- Always get the smallest pager possible. Believe it or not, wearing a pager all day can get heavy and tug on clothing. The physician will appreciate your thoughtfulness.
- Purchase a pager that not only beeps, but vibrates. This is especially helpful to physicians when they are attending or giving a lecture, reading a bedtime story to their youngest, or intently listening to an irregular heartbeat.
- Purchase a pager that stores messages. This is especially helpful when the physician is in surgery or in transit between the office and the hospital. Usually physicians have car phones, but many prefer to answer routine messages when they arrive at their destination.
- Don't give the pager number to anyone unless the physician instructs you to.
- Maintain a good relationship with the answering service. This is very important, because they will happily hold messages and will learn how to triage your calls.
- Advise the physician to obtain a cellular phone. This can save a hassle if indeed the physician is paged for an emergency. The cellular phone eliminates the necessity of finding a pay phone while in transit.
- Education of the patient is most important when attempting to make a pager system work for you. This can be done through the *Patient Information*

Handbook. In the handbook, you should explain the office's policy regarding patients' routine questions about their conditions and their medications. Patients should be asked to keep routine questions for the next business day and not ask the answering service to page the physician during off hours.

Cell Phone

All physicians have cell phones. Even the kids in school have cell phones! This is a great way to keep in touch with the physician. Most office managers will just call the physician on the cell phone instead of using the pager. Pagers must be used when the physician is in the hospital because most hospitals will not allow cell phones to be used. Some cell phones may interfere with hospital equipment, which could be life threatening for a patient. Most hospitals post signs on their doors asking for all cell phones to be turned off before entering. Many physicians use a Blackberry or Treo as their link to the outside world. It provides cell phone, access to their e-mail, access to the Internet, and so on.

Lost in Translation

The United States has long been a melting pot for people of Hispanic, Slavic, Asian, Indian, Anglo-Saxon, and many other cultures. Medicine is currently grappling with a surge of patients who don't speak English. Many barriers inhibit communication between patients and physicians, but none is more serious than the inability to communicate in a common language. Health care workers often find themselves in the waiting room asking for the friends or family of a patient to serve as an interpreter. Many hospitals have hired telephone interpreters or bilingual staff members in an effort to provide the best quality of care for all non–English-speaking patients. Having a translator who is not well versed in the language of medicine comes with its own set of problems. Explanations getting lost in translation are a constant worry. The best solution, of course, is to use trained medical interpreters. They can be borrowed from hospitals and clinics as the need arises or can even be found in the yellow pages.

The telephone company has special telephone services for people with either a hearing or speech impairment. The customer service guide at the beginning of the telephone book explains all the details necessary for offices in need of these services.

Even with the help of a good interpreter, treatment of non–English-speaking patients can be tricky. Always speak directly to the patient, as if there were no interpreter in the room. This will help to establish a bond with the patient. Allow the interpreter to get the patient's whole story and *then* relate it to office personnel and the physician. Sentence-to-sentence translation becomes difficult in a medical setting. After the physician and the office personnel have given instructions to the patient, have the translator ask the patient to repeat them. This will help to avoid any misunderstandings. Any time information is conveyed through another, there is a possibility the information will be distorted, diluted, or completely erroneous. Remember the childhood game "Whisper Down the Lane"? The first child whispered a phrase to another child, who whispered it to another, and so on down the lane. By the time the last child heard the phrase it had become totally distorted. What started out as "I'm going to the movies after school" had become "I'm quitting school to be a movie star!"

The translator can also help the medical office understand a patient's culture. For example, a patient who stares at the floor during the entire conversation with the physician might give the physician the impression that she or he is depressed or disinterested, when actually the person is showing respect. Some cultures don't believe in germ-based illnesses; they believe that evil spirits cause illness, so an immunization shot that may cause a healthy child to become sick for a day doesn't make sense to them. Patience and understanding are the best tools to work with at times like this. No one said it would be easy meshing American-style medicine with various cultures, but it is interesting and rewarding.

Many agencies are available to help the office communicate with deaf patients also, who are legally entitled to a certified interpreter through the Americans with Disabilities Act of 1990. Schools for the deaf and agencies for the deaf can be of assistance in this situation.

PURCHASING POWER: BUYING EQUIPMENT, FURNITURE, AND OFFICE SUPPLIES

Control of Costs

"You do not need an MBA from Harvard to figure out how to lose money." —ROBERT LITTLE, CHAIRMAN, TEXTRON CORPORATION

Medical office managers should realize that a very important function should be to control costs. Some practices are charged for the amounts of electricity and water they use in their particular office space. Even if the office does not pay separately for these utilities, unwise use can increase these bills for the owner of the building, which will eventually be passed on to the office in the form of an increase in rent. Regardless of how the bills are divided, the office should be frugal about utilities.

Everyone should cut costs, because "costs" cost money! The office manager can cut costs by not spending a large amount on office decor and on equipment containing "bells and whistles" that might not be necessary. The medical office manager should make employees aware of the costs associated with the running of a medical practice and ask for their help in being as cost conscious as possible. The office manager can institute a few policies that will immediately save on office expenses:

- Purchase less expensive supplies by either buying off-brands or shopping around for a better price.
- Purchase stock when it is on sale. For instance, if computer paper is on sale this week at a very good price, purchase a few boxes and store for future consumption.
- Assess the staff to evaluate the need for the number of employees working there. Perhaps two tasks could be combined into one, which would reduce the payroll by one employee. However, *never* stress the employees to the point of breakdown in order to save money on payroll.
- Turn off utilities when not in use. When you are not using an examination room, keep the lights and equipment in there off and close the door to that room.
- Check expiration dates on vaccines and injectables. Many companies will give you credit on return and reorder.
- Maintain proper maintenance and cleaning of equipment—it will last longer.
- Cross-train employees so that you have flexibility when needed.
- Monitor inventory to prevent the need to pay for rushed delivery, shipments sent through Federal Express, or supplies that can be purchased quickly through local suppliers but at higher costs.
- Consider installing a computer as an alternative to increasing staff.
- Use part-time employees whenever possible to decrease payroll taxes and the costs of employee benefits. Job sharing works well.
- Know the cost of seeing a patient in the office and then do not participate in managed care programs that pay less than your costs.
- Look into employee benefits that are tax-free, perhaps in the form of a cafeteria plan for insurance.
- Terminate mediocre employees—the cost of nonproductive employees outweighs the cost of hiring and training a new employee.
- Decrease state unemployment taxes by reducing employee turnover.
- Pay income tax estimates on time.
- Avoid paying penalties for errors by knowing the Occupational Safety and Health Administration (OSHA) regulations, the *Current Procedural Terminology* and *International Classification of Diseases, Ninth Revision* codes, and the requirements of the Clinical Laboratory Improvements Amendments of 1988.
- Evaluate the necessity of having service contracts on equipment.
- Evaluate leasing versus purchasing equipment.
- Minimize the need for a collection agency by planning and implementing a collection system at the time of service.
- If the help of a collection agency is needed, shop around for one whose rates are acceptable.
- Submit insurance claims electronically to eliminate the cost of postage and employee time spent on billing.
- Computerize patient appointment scheduling to save staff's and the physician's time.
- Hire a competent accountant to help with budgeting, forecasting, and tax planning strategies.
- Choose a bank with competitive rates and good business packages.
- Ask the practice attorney to read over all contracts and agreements.

Bargain Shopping

Medical offices spend an average of 8% of their gross income on medical and office supplies. Depending on the type of specialty, it could be higher. The office manager should be bargain shopping whenever possible for best prices and discounts. There is much competition now, and many companies will negotiate prices with medical offices in order to be promised the account. Even desks and filing cabinets can be purchased inexpensively if they have a small dent or scratch. It is possible to negotiate deals in which the office can get as much as 50% off by buying equipment that is slightly dented or scratched.

You can also check with local medical suppliers to see if they have any used equipment for sale. If the practice is new, you and the physician might want to consider purchasing used equipment until the practice becomes profitable. The used equipment can then slowly be replaced with new equipment. Many young, new physicians today want to open an office with all new equipment. Try to dissuade them of this, explaining that it would be easier to start out with used equipment and replace it as the practice becomes more secure. Most new physicians are paying off multiple student loans and will appreciate the advice of a competent, seasoned office manager.

When you are looking for used equipment, it might be advantageous to check the county medical journals or local medical papers. Check journals for classified ads placed by physicians who are retiring or redecorating their offices and wish to sell their office furniture. In the yellow pages in the telephone book, under Business Furniture, Used, you might be able to find office equipment that you need. Avoid purchasing used furniture for the waiting room, however; this gives patients one of their earliest impressions of the medical office, and it should be clean, neat, and pleasant looking.

Leasing versus Buying

Most businesses today have the choice of either leasing or purchasing equipment. Each option has distinct advantages and disadvantages. Leasing helps keep expenses down and can also be used as a tax benefit. Leasing is popular with oncologists, ophthalmologists, and radiologists, because their technology changes so rapidly and is so expensive. The photocopier is always a popular item for leasing, because it gets so much use that the office will want to replace it every few years, rather than have costly repair bills and downtime.

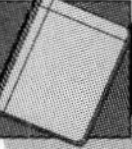

FROM THE EXPERT'S NOTEBOOK

If you plan on using a piece of equipment until it falls apart, buy it. Buying is cheaper than leasing because you may be able to deduct the depreciation.

If the office is preparing to purchase rather than lease, keep in mind the tax consequences of paying cash for the item. Leasing conserves office cash, and the interest paid on the lease offsets the taxable earnings. Medical equipment purchases are 100% depreciable over 5 years; office furniture can be fully written off over 7 years. The office is unable to depreciate equipment that is leased.

Leasing can be the most convenient way to obtain equipment, but it is not the cheapest way. If the office is having cash flow problems, leasing may be the only choice for obtaining the equipment needed.

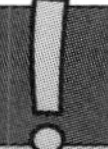

MANAGER'S ALERT

Watch out for leases that state you have the option to buy. The Internal Revenue Service (IRS) may take the position that you're buying the equipment, not leasing it.

It is always a good idea to have the practice lawyer read over all leases before signing them. Most physicians don't realize that personal liability is written into some leasing contracts. This is something that should be avoided if at all possible. The office manager must look for certain aspects of the lease to prevent problems with the Internal Revenue Service (IRS). There is a gray area between a lease and a purchase loan. To prevent any problems along this line, look for the following aspects:

- The leasing company must own at least 20% of the equity of the property during the term of the lease. If that is not the case, the IRS could consider the deal a purchase.
- The leasing company must show that it is making a profit, independent of its own tax benefits.
- At the end of the lease, the office cannot purchase the equipment at less than fair market value (bargain purchase option).
- It must be commercially feasible for someone else to use the equipment at the end of the lease.

Copiers

When you are shopping for a copier, you are shopping for more than just the copier itself. The service and actual downtime are very important factors to consider. For instance, if it is going to take the service technician 24 hours to get to the office to do a repair, you might want to consider a different brand of copier or a different dealership. An average acceptable time period for a technician to get to the office for a service call is 4 hours. Many dealers offer an even shorter time frame. The copier purchased should also have a generous warranty with it. Many companies are now offering generous warranties, enhanced service, and performance promises with every copier in order to obtain and keep their customer base.

The competition for these customers is fierce, so shop around and have an understanding of how the copier works before purchasing. Make a list of the features that your office will need. The following are some of the features available:

- Collator
- Sheet feeder
- Enlarge/reduce
- Automatic contrast
- Multiple paper trays
- Two-sided copying
- Sorter
- Zoom
- Shifting
- Dual-page copying
- Edge erase
- Single-color copying
- Booklet format
- Stapling

HOW TO GET THE MOST FROM YOUR COPIER

There are some basic rules to follow to ensure that you get the most from the copier you choose:

- Avoid placing the copier in direct sunlight or by a heating vent.
- Keep the copier out of drafts and make sure there is adequate circulation around it.
- Be careful when trying to save money by buying generic toners, copy cartridges, drum cartridges, and so on. These off-brands may damage the copier, and the repairs will cost more than you saved by buying an off-brand. As a side note, use of off-brands could also void your warranty. Check your manual before using these products.

- Use high-quality paper (at least 20-pound bond). When using transparencies, use only those specifically made for copiers.
- Make sure that paper remains dust free. Any paper dust can clog sensors and foul the mechanical parts.
- Keep the glass of the copier clean. This can be done easily with a glass cleaner or alcohol. This will help keep the quality of your copies high.
- Watch what you have near the copier; it doesn't digest foreign objects very well! Many is the time the technician has been called to the office for a "repair," only to extract a paperclip, a leaf from a plant, a staple, a pencil, a push pin, or a scrap of paper from inside the copier. *Never* leave a coffee cup or soda sitting on a copy machine. It can easily be knocked over; when liquid gets into the copier, it can cause major damage.
- Paper will curl in excessive heat. This can cause paper jams.
- Clear the exit tray regularly to avoid copy backups that will eventually cause a jam.
- When the paper is full of electricity and sticking together, spray the entire ream lightly with hairspray or static-removing spray.
- Schedule routine maintenance on a regular basis. It will extend the life of your copier.

The toner should be stored in a cool, dry place; otherwise, it will harden and form clumps. Gently shake the toner before installing it in the copier to remove clumping and clinging to the inside of the cartridge. Many toner companies now send mailing labels so that the empty toner cartridges can be returned for proper disposal or reuse.

COPY BANDITS

The need to control the use of the photocopier is essential in a medical office. It is the second most widely abused equipment in a medical office, the first, of course, being the telephone. It has been estimated that 20% of all copies made in an office are copies for personal use by the staff or physicians. Some of these copies are made just in case they are needed at a later date. This costs the medical practice in paper, toner, and wear and tear on the copy machine. Some companies sell copy "controllers" that monitor the number of copies produced, with the goal of controlling costs. The controllers are tied into a computer system that reads from them how many copies were made and by whom. Coin-operated copiers can also be purchased; however, these are the type seen in local libraries and post offices—and they are not very sophisticated. Some copiers contain a feature that only allows operation if you are assigned a specific code. These copiers are mainly found in large health systems and hospitals. One of the easiest ways to keep copy costs down is to make employees aware of the costs of the copier. If they are aware that management is monitoring the copies, they will tend to make fewer personal copies.

PAPER

The type of paper used in the copier can enhance the copies made. By buying quality paper, you will ensure that your copies come out clear and clean. In addition, keep all copy paper dry. This means do not store paper on a concrete floor in a basement. All paper should be stored on a shelf in a dry room.

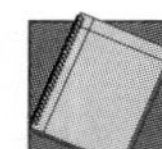

FROM THE EXPERT'S NOTEBOOK

Fan a ream of copy paper before inserting it into the copier tray. This will help eliminate jams and misfeeds.

Fax Machine

The fax machine has many uses in a medical office. If the practice has more than one location and does not have access to scanning and e-mailing, it can be extremely helpful to fax patients' records and test results between offices. Hospitals get into the act by faxing test results and information to the office when the office cannot wait for the regular mail and when the contents of the document are too complicated to explain over the telephone. Many practices today do not have e-mail, and therefore fax machines can make communication between the medical office and law offices and accountants' offices more convenient.

Some fax machines are more expensive than others because they offer features such as paper cutters, plain-paper usage, auto send/receive functions, programmable keys, and speed dialing. Some fax machines even offer additional memory to allow document storage and mailboxes for certain employees. Keep in mind that many of the uses for fax machines have been superseded by e-mail. An example of a basic fax cover sheet is shown in Figure 12-12.

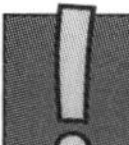

MANAGER'S ALERT

Be aware that if the practice uses a fax machine that has thermal paper, the paper will fade over time. It is best to use a plain paper fax.

Paper Shredder

The Environmental Protection Agency (EPA) has estimated that the typical employee throws away more than one-half pound of paper every day. Enter, the paper shredder. The paper shredder in a medical office cannot save the amount of paper waste, but for many office managers, it's a good

Facsimile Transmission Cover Sheet
Date:

To Name:
Location:
Phone number:
FAX number:

From Name:
Location:
Phone number:
FAX number:

Number of pages transmitted: ______________________ (including this cover sheet)

Special Instructions:

The information contained in this fax is intended only for the use of the individual or entity to which it is addressed and may contain information that is privileged, confidential, and exempt from disclosure under applicable law. If the reader of this message is not the intended recipient, or the employee or agent responsible for delivering the message to the intended recipient, you are hereby notified that any dissemination, distribution, or copying of this communication is strictly prohibited. If you have received this communication in error, please notify us immediately by telephone and return the original message to us at the above address via the U.S. Postal Service. Thank you.

FIGURE 12-12. Fax cover sheet.

place to start. Every business has records that shouldn't be seen by others, and a medical office is no different. Old payroll records, old telephone logs, old canceled checks, and old meeting minutes can be easily disposed of with a paper shredder. With the confidentiality issue so important, a paper shredder is a valuable asset to a medical office. Any paper with a patient name or identification number on it should be shredded when discarded. It is absolutely crucial to a medical practice to have a paper shredder.

Shredders come in a wide range of styles, prices, and capacities. There are personal-size shredders that sit on a trash can and large, centralized shredders. All can do the same job, but some fit the needs of the office more than others. One of the best shredders is a cross-cut shredder. It reduces the volume by five and absolutely destroys the document. It reduces the paper into a "confetti-like" size as opposed to regular shredders, which produce strips. When purchasing a paper shredder, be careful to check the warranty. Be sure that it includes the cutters and labor. Check to see what other parts are covered by the warranty.

Security System: A Must!

Every medical office needs a security system. It has been proven that burglars break into offices without alarms five times more often than they break into those with alarms.

Many factors must be considered when choosing a security system. One important thing to realize is that no security system is a substitute for a strong door with a deadbolt lock. When you are shopping for a burglar alarm, have a representative come to check over the office. Have the representative check the windows and doors for danger signs such as weak hinges, old wooden frames, poor outdoor lighting, and so on. Some police departments will do such an inspection at no cost to the office.

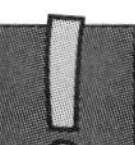

MANAGER'S ALERT

Remember, although alarm systems deter some burglars, no security company can give you a 100% guarantee that your office will be completely protected against a professional or determined burglar.

COMPONENTS OF THE SECURITY SYSTEM

There are three basic components of the security system: sensors and detectors, master controls, and alarm devices.

Sensors and Detectors

Perimeter protection is the first line of defense against a burglar. Perimeter sensors sense the intrusion on the property before the burglar is able to get inside. These can be found in the form of a door sensor, which sounds an alarm if the intruder attempts to open the door, or a window sensor, which sounds an alarm if the intruder attempts to break a window. Area protection is a scanner that scans a specific area, usually with a beam. When the beam is broken, an alarm sounds. This can sometimes be enough to scare away an intended burglar. It is best to install both perimeter and area protection alarms for complete coverage.

One of the most common types of perimeter sensors is a magnetic switch. This is the sensor that is placed on doors, windows, or any other moveable area. This type of sensor will not deter experienced intruders. They simply break the window and put a magnet next to the switch, which simulates that the area is closed. Also, an experienced intruder can cut the glass so as not to trip the switch and climb through the window without disturbing the magnetic switch. To prevent entry of the premises through broken glass, you can use a metal foil or audio sensor.

Area sensors are usually more sophisticated and more commonly chosen as the sensor of choice. Area sensors can be ultrasound, microwave, infrared, floor mat switches, or photoelectric beams. As you can see, protection systems can be elaborate or they can be kept simple, but effective.

Master Control

The master control is the part of the system that reads the information from the sensors and decides what action to take. This control is programmed by the owner and makes decisions according to what it has been told to do. The master control comes with a variety of features: lockup relay, set switches, automatic shutoff, and delay entry/exit circuits. The individual vendors of systems can explain in detail the features of each type of alarm system.

Security Devices

The last part of the security system is the actual alarm itself. There are sirens, bells, whistles, and flashing lights. Depending on the vicinity of the office, the physician might want to choose one type over another. The police will most probably suggest that a light be left outside of the office if the office is in a single-structure building. Alarm systems can also be connected to automatic telephone dialers that will call either a switchboard or the local police station. Self-installed alarm systems can be purchased and installed for between $150 and $2,000, depending on the type of system chosen. Professionally installed systems can cost between $500 and $3,000 for full office coverage, both outside and inside. If a system is chosen that involves a security company, be advised that the security company will charge you an additional $40 per month, on average, for its services. Alarm company decals are also a very popular item today. Many people purchase the decal for the window, without purchasing the actual alarm system. This does deter more inexperienced burglars, who will choose a location without a decal. However, professional burglars are likely to know what kind of system is in place by the name on the decal and are adept at bypassing the alarms. In this case, the decal would definitely be a disadvantage, rather than an advantage. Remember, burglary is a crime of opportunity, so don't make it easy for them!

BOX 12-7 How to Choose the Right Security System

1. Choose a company.
2. Ask your personal property insurance agent for a recommendation of qualified installers.
3. Contact the National Burglar and Fire Alarm Association in Bethesda, Maryland, for a list of its members in the area of your office.
4. Check with the Better Business Bureau for reputable companies.
5. Ask other physician offices about the companies they use.
6. Ask several security companies to survey the premises and submit a proposal.
7. Check Consumer Reports for their comments.

Once you have chosen a company, ask the following questions:

1. What types of alarms do you install?
2. Do you specialize in business or residential systems?
3. Are your employees bonded?
4. How long will it take to install the system?
5. What are the guarantees or warranties of the system?
6. How soon can the system be installed after the decision is made?
7. Does your company operate a monitoring station, or do you use a separate company?
8. What liability will you assume if the office is burglarized because of a system malfunction?
9. Does your system ever experience downtime?

When choosing the alarm system for the office, you need to consider various external factors (Box 12-7), such as the type of building that the office is located in—whether it is an office building or a single standing structure. If it is an office building, is it a high rise or a condominium style, with all offices on the ground floor? What type of neighborhood is it in? Is it on a busy highway with a lot of passer-by coverage? Is the neighborhood well lit, or is the office in a dark area of town? Is the office in a city or a small town? These factors are very important when assessing the needs of the office for a security system.

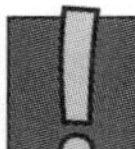

MANAGER'S ALERT

When buying an alarm system, don't forget to get a battery backup. If the burglars cut the electric line, the office will still be secure.

Desk Accessories

CONTAINERS

Most employees like to work at a desk that has color and personality. In the past, we have seen offices decorated in burgundy, mauve, navy, slate blue, forest green, and ecru.

Many brands of accessories come in these bold colors. Art deco, traditional wood, leather, and marble can still be found, but plastic comes in the widest range of colors. The look that seems to be in demand is plastic with rounded edges and bright colors, although wire has also found its way into the workplace in the form of coiled wire for wastebaskets, pencil holders, and so on. Some offices purchase employees' items of choice for them and allow free reign in selection of color and material. Other offices ask employees to purchase their own accessories for their desks and allow them the same openness. Regardless of who buys, allow some latitude in personal choices of accessories and the office environment will seem a more content one.

Stacking trays can be helpful on desks where limited space is available. Now, in our age of high technology, almost everyone has a computer on her or his desk. Couple that with an adding machine/calculator, stapler, tape dispenser, pen and pencil holder, desk calendar, and a Rolodex, and there is little room left for actual work. Desk drawer organizers can eliminate desk drawer clutter. They can hold a variety of items, such as paper clips, staplers, scissors, rulers, and other items. These trays come in letter size and legal size to accommodate all situations. The office should have staplers that provide stapling capabilities for various amounts of paper. At the very minimum, the office should have one regular stapler and one heavy-duty stapler. Office supply stores also have staplers for in-between amounts of paper. It is good to have a calculator with a tape or an adding machine for checking figures. These can be most helpful when completing the deposit slip or when manually totaling end-of-day sheets. There are several colors of highlighters that become problematic when copied or faxed. The highlighting shows up as a black mark, making it impossible to read what has been highlighted. Always use yellow highlighters because information highlighted with a yellow highlighter can be copied and faxed.

WRITING INSTRUMENTS

For more than 5,000 years, humans have been recording events by using some type of writing instrument. The Egyptians used hollow reeds, the Chinese used brushes, the Europeans used quills, and the Greeks used a metal stylus very similar to our metal-tipped pens of today. Even though we find ourselves in a high-tech world, we still have the need for a reliable pen and pencil. Each desk in the medical office should be equipped with the appropriate number of pens, pencils, and highlighters.

In 1884, Louis Waterman, from New York, patented the first fountain pen. This pen became very well known and is the pen of choice for most physicians today. The rest of the staff generally use ballpoint pens, which were introduced in 1945. However, there is still a place for the pencil. Pencil lead comes in a variety of colors, which the medical office can use to its advantage. Perhaps the office would like to record the physician's meetings in green pencil, the physician's lectures in red, the physician's personal appointments in blue, and so on. This can be very helpful in keeping schedules straight. In addition, pencils should always be used when scheduling patient appointments if the office is not using computerized scheduling. *Many* changes take place in the appointment book, so it is easier to use pencil only! Some hospital billers like to use mechanical pencils when doing their billing, because of the constant sharp point. Many bookkeepers also choose to use mechanical pencils. Check with your employees to find out their needs. If they have the equipment that they want, they will be happier and more productive.

Pharmaceutical representatives often offer pens and notepads in exchange for seeing the physician. Most office pens can be obtained through these reps, which helps to keep office supply costs down.

Supply Order Log

The inventory of supplies should be checked on a weekly basis. This task should be assigned to one person in the clinical area and one person in the clerical area. This person then assumes the responsibility of maintaining and ordering the supplies needed in each area.

Develop a log in which to track both medical and office supplies that have been ordered (see Figure 12-13 for a sample). This can be done very easily by using a three-ring binder or by computer database. Keep supply order forms in the front and a complete list of vendors' names, addresses, and telephone numbers. It might also be helpful to list the items that are ordered from each vendor, along with their prices. If ordering is done in this organized fashion, it can be done by staff members instead of you. Remember, it is important to delegate as many tasks as possible to give yourself time for more important duties. When items are delivered, it is important for the employee to check the supply order log and verify that the order is complete. Take special note of items that are backordered and check the office stock to ensure that the stock will not be depleted before the new stock arrives.

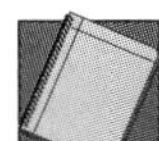

FROM THE EXPERT'S NOTEBOOK

Post a list in a convenient spot in the office where employees can list any supplies that they may need. It is easier than trying to "track down" the person who orders!

EMPLOYEE THEFT

Employee theft is a huge and growing problem. The goods and cash lost to theft are estimated to total $120 billion a year. Some workers plan to exploit their employer by some type of theft. Employee theft comes in a variety of

Date	Vendor	Item(s) Ordered	Date Items Received	Initials

FIGURE 12-13. Page from a supply log.

forms. It can be as simple as a pen, notepad, postage stamp, and tissues or as high level as petty cash and daily cash intakes.

The figures aren't good, and the office manager must take precautions to prevent as much theft as possible. By using personal interviews, credit checks, and reference checks, most office managers can ward off the "rough" employees. They can also make use of honesty tests. These tests cost approximately $10 to $20, which includes the scoring of the test. They can predict future behavior based on the test taker's attitudes and past conduct. Providers of these tests include the following companies:

- ReidLondon House
  www.reidlondonhouse.com
  1-800-221-8378
- Reid Psychological Systems
  www.reidsystems.com
  1-800-922-7343
- Association of Test Publishers
  www.testpublishers.org
  1-202-857-8444
- Pinkerton Services Group
  www.worklife.com/partners/pinkertn.htm
  1-800-528-5745

Although these tests were developed to show "core integrity," they can also forecast absenteeism, accidents, and other problems associated with employees. Use caution in choosing a company to supply such tests, because tests that do not meet the standards of reliability can leave the door open to lawsuits. A set of standards can be obtained from individual test publishers or from the Association of Test Publishers listed above.

One of the best ways to curtail employee theft is to promote positive feelings toward the office and the physician. Employees tend to steal more if they feel that the office has been unfair to them. Studies have shown that there are lower levels of employee theft in offices with low employee turnover and high performance on the job.

Setting up a formal chain of command in cash management can also discourage employee theft. This chain should be set up as follows:

- Employee 1 collects money from patients.
- Employee 2 processes these payments.
- Employee 3 deposits these payments.

If this system is established, it becomes difficult for one person to be able to steal. The report of payments posted for the day should match the daily deposit. Some offices deposit only on a weekly basis; this should be changed to daily if at all possible. If the office cannot change to daily depositing, the daily sheets should be totaled at the end of the week and should then match the weekly deposit.

Payments received through the mail should be tallied on a separate sheet, and a separate deposit should be made for these checks. On the deposit slip, write the word "mail" somewhere, so that the bookkeeper will know the source of these funds. The employee should also initial each daily sheet and mail sheet, so that it creates a paper trail in case of a problem.

A final way to decrease employee theft is to prosecute employees who steal. This has been proven to be one of the most effective deterrents. Although it costs money and takes time, the result is that the office gets restitution and doesn't suffer morale problems. Civil restitution is a popular way of recouping losses in a medical office. The physician and the employee work out an arrangement for the repayment of the theft. Many offices prefer to simply terminate the employee without any type of restitution or prosecution. This sets a bad example for the other employees who are still in the office. Any type of prosecution can send a strong message to others that the office will not tolerate that type of behavior. This can work to the advantage of the office, because any other employees who were stealing, or thinking about it, will soon stop.

One way to protect the office and the physician is to purchase dishonesty insurance. This insurance can be purchased as part of a package for office liability and personal property. It protects the office from any losses from employee theft. The office manager can also check into purchasing fidelity bonding on the employees who handle cash in the office. Fidelity bonding is a type of insurance that reimburses the practice in the event of employee theft. The employees who handle cash are asked by the insurance company to sign an application for bonding. The employees are then aware that they are being monitored, which tends to keep them honest.

WORKFORCE TESTING

The testing companies mentioned under the Employee Theft section perform a variety of tests involving employees. For example, ReidLondon House provides solutions for the following:

- Preemployment recruiting
- Leadership management development
- Aptitude tests
- Organizational surveys
- Human resource assessments
- Consulting services

Reid Psychological Systems has been an international human resources provider for the past 50 years. It provides such services as the following:

- Health care employee productivity report
- Health care risk avoidance profile
- Health care service relations profile
- Health care numeric skills profile
- Health care safety profile
- Caregiving attitudes profile
- Numeric skills profile
- Employee productivity report
- Management potential report

OTHER OFFICE INSURANCE

Everyone today focuses on malpractice insurance, giving little thought to other types of insurance needs. The office manager should shop around and compare insurance plans before choosing a policy for the office.

Injury Liability

Injuries from falls and bumps are always occurring in the medical office. All those in business are subject to liability every time an individual steps into their place of business. A medical office has an even greater risk, because many patients are ill and fragile.

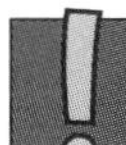

MANAGER'S ALERT

Patients can sue you successfully even when their injuries are partly their own fault!

The office manager should carefully walk through the office to evaluate any potential disasters that might cause a need for this additional insurance. The manager should also check to see exactly where the liability ends. If the office is located in a free-standing dwelling, liability extends to the edge of the property.

Personal Property Insurance

Evaluate and prepare a list of equipment for personal property insurance and make sure the coverage is ample for fire, theft, flood, or any other disaster that may hit the office. Planning for these types of events helps to make them less painful if they occur. Check into "continuing business coverage," so that in the event of disaster, the office can rent temporary accommodations and continue to see patients while repairs are being made. This coverage should also handle cleaning of the office. Some physicians ask colleagues about sharing space in their office in the event of an emergency situation. One of the most important things to remember is that if the office is computerized, copies of the daily, monthly, and yearly backup disks should be kept in a fireproof cabinet so that they are not lost. Finally, don't forget the patients! Someone should be designated to call the patients, explain the situation, and reschedule appointments at a designated time and place.

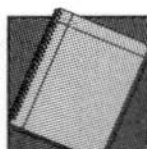

FROM THE EXPERT'S NOTEBOOK

One way to safeguard against loss of files in the computer in the event of disaster is to have the computer operator back up the files once a week and send them electronically to a server company. Some smaller offices back up the system and take a copy of the disk home at the end of the week. Some offices back up on a disk and deposit it in a safe-deposit box at the practice's bank for safekeeping.

Notify all vendors when disaster strikes. Postpone deliveries and possibly make payment arrangements for bills. As an extra note, have an engraved sign in the window or on the bottom of the door, stating "In case of an emergency, please notify..." That will ensure that someone from the office is notified immediately. You should have certain emergency telephone numbers at home and in your car. Having these numbers readily available will be of tremendous help when disaster strikes. The following is a list of people whose emergency telephone numbers you should have:

- Insurance agent
- Landlord
- Neighbors
- Emergency boarding-up service
- Staff at home
- Vendors, companies, and utilities
- Rental companies for furniture, equipment, and office space
- Public insurance adjusters

The physician pays top dollar to get excellent malpractice coverage, so don't skimp on this insurance; it is just as important!

THE FACILITY

Office Leases

Many private physicians lease office space, as opposed to buying. Ownership ties up capital and severely limits options regarding the future. There are real estate brokers who work solely with health care professionals. These brokers specialize in commercial and professional space.

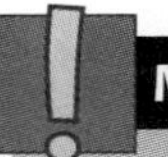

MANAGER'S ALERT

Never sign a lease without first having the attorney review it.

Leases for medical offices come with their own set of problems. Some brokers want signatures on leases that allow no sublet and assignment rights and provide no disability escape clause. Don't lease on impulse! Just because the office is in a pretty building doesn't mean it is the office for you. Evaluate the needs of the practice, the layout, and location you desire, and the price you can pay. Then have the broker meet and discuss these considerations. She or he will be able to find a space that fits your needs. Don't forget to inquire as to the stability of the owner of the building. The appropriate time frame for a relocation is about 1 year. In Chapter 8 there is a discussion on the ramifications of the Americans with American Disabilities Act for an office. A "workletter," which allows for construction or reconstruction of the office space to meet the tenant's needs, is a necessary part of any lease. Costs of modifying the office vary, depending on the location of the office. Because skilled labor is involved in the modification of a medical office, the cost will be high no matter where the office is located. Check with the landlord; often, she or he will give a cash contribution or discount on monthly rent to help with the changes.

A "triple net lease" is a lease whereby the tenant pays her or his share of the building's utilities, maintenance expenses, and real estate taxes. This lease comes with strings attached, in that "maintenance expenses" can include repair or replacement of heating or air conditioning. This is expensive, so beware!

Give the lease to the attorney for review before you sign it!

Planning Your Office Space

The office manager's main objective when a new facility is being planned is to design an office that "works." This means that each area of the office allows the practice to run efficiently, increasing productivity and profits, while allowing the delivery of quality care.

But, as office manager, you can be much more effective if you make use of the resources available to you when planning your office. Some furniture dealerships provide free design consultation and space planning as a part of their service, including both two-dimensional and three-dimensional computer-generated layouts of the space, giving you a good idea of what the office will look like before you order furniture. Make full use of the space planner, so that you can devote your valuable time to managing the day-to-day operations of the practice.

Before sitting down with the space planner, divide the office into sections, such as business, clinical, professional, and reception. Depending on the type of practice, there might be additional areas in the office, such as an anesthesia room. Once these areas have been identified, consult the employees of each area on what changes, if any, to the current design might help them perform their duties more effectively. Ask for ideas for how patient flow can be maintained and organization can be put into place. Make a list of everyone's ideas and then discuss each idea with the space planner and the physician. Remember, the new office design should not repeat mistakes made in the current office. Do not be afraid to make major changes in the layout.

Today, furniture has come a long way from the standard desk, file, and chair. The advent of computer use in every office has changed the way furniture looks. Furniture today is more ergonomic and modular in function. This will be useful for designing your space, because modular furniture is more adaptable to different sizes of offices. When selecting furniture for the office, keep the following things in mind:

- Get a desk that lets you look ahead. A modular desk is easy to set up initially and then reorganize or reconfigure later to adapt to future needs.
- Avoid tangles. Make sure your desk has at least one grommet hole to keep computer and telephone wires out of the way. A hutch should have a sweep that manages computer and telephone wires. Desks should have wire management troughs to allow smooth routing of cables with no aesthetic intrusion.
- Stacking file drawer systems will allow for future expansion. For example, most files, when filled, must be discarded if you need to put more file drawers in the same space. Some manufacturers offer stacking file cabinets, so a two-drawer cabinet can be converted to a three-drawer cabinet merely by ordering an additional drawer.
- Consider ergonomics. With OSHA standards in constant flux, and repetitive-stress injury claims by employees at an all-time high, a few dollars more spent on a chair or a keyboard tray with additional functions now could save thousands in potential claims and lost productivity down the road.
- Don't skimp on construction. There's a reason that one desk is $179 while another is $379, and going with the cheaper item may just mean that you will end up replacing it again in 3 years. Look for balanced construction: this means that the desk is completely sealed on all sides (top, underside, base, and edges) to prevent heat and moisture from destroying the core of the desk. Newer modular desk systems should feature a 3 mm ABS edge or a solid wood edge, both of which are practically indestructible. ABS is a resin composed of acrylonitrile, butadiene, and styrene that is used for toys, office furniture, cameras, etc. It is chosen because of its hardness, impact resistance, fatigue resistance, and gloss. Seating should use only commercial-grade fabrics and should be backed by a written warranty.
- Know your supplier. Lots of furniture and space-planning companies guarantee that they stand behind the product they sell. But a guarantee is only as good as the company who provides it. Ask questions. How long has the company been in business? What, exactly, does their "guarantee" cover? Are they willing to state their guarantee in writing?
- Plan ahead. Be sure to provide the furniture supplier with a date by which you need the furniture installed, and remember that the planning process could take some time. Allow time for revisions and selection of your office. Some furniture companies carry inventory that is available for quick shipment, but some items may need to be produced by manufacturers specifically for your office, which could take longer. Make sure your requirements are clearly articulated at the beginning of the process, not after you have selected chairs that will take 10 weeks when you have a grand opening a week from tomorrow!
- Get it in writing. Don't rely on verbal quotations from the furniture company. Make sure that the quotation includes shipping, delivery and setup (if needed), and all applicable taxes. Too often, when purchases are made on a "handshake agreement," the order can go very wrong. A written agreement protects both the practice and the furniture company. And, of course, unless you have the authority, never sign an agreement yourself. Lawyers will tell you, "If it's not written down it didn't happen."

Think Safety When Filing

Many workplace injuries are related to filing. It is important to position filing cabinets so that drawers do not open into aisles. One way to ensure safety is to purchase lateral files that do not allow you to open more than one drawer at a time. Close drawers when they are not in use, and when closing them, always use the handles to avoid catching fingers in the drawers! And what about heavy objects? Store all heavy objects in the bottom drawers and do not place heavy objects on the top of the filing cabinets. You may want to consider a stacking file system, which will conform to ADA standards, allowing locks to be accessed by a person in a wheelchair. *Never* move filing cabinets when they are loaded. If it is necessary to move them, always empty the drawers first. Cardboard filing boxes can be obtained from your office supplier, and each drawer can be kept intact by emptying a file drawer and placing it in a cardboard filing box with a label as to what drawer it is. This system will keep everything in an organized fashion.

Selecting the Right Workstation

When searching for the right workstation it is important to consider its purpose, which will be decided by the nature of your tasks. It is best to look for products that have been designed and engineered to help make your workspace more productive. This can be achieved in a variety of ways. As a guide, observe how your work flows through your office in a typical day. It is likely that you'll uncover a number of distinctive and repetitive task patterns. Once these patterns have been identified, organize them according to their intended use and the frequency of their use. Now you are ready to investigate the pertinent factors that will determine the workspace you eventually select. Some factors to keep in mind are the keyboard, monitor, monitor stand, and mouse:

- Keyboard
  - Has a palm rest, preferably gel-filled
  - Should have an attached mouse tray, which can be adjusted
  - Easily adjusts the angle of the keyboard
  - Easily adjusts the keyboard height
- Monitor
  - There should be a direct line from the center of the monitor to the "J" key on your keyboard, which should line up with your belt buckle
  - Position the monitor at arm's length
  - Make sure that the top of your monitor screen is slightly below eye level
  - A monitor stand may be used to achieve the height
- Monitor stand
  - Allows adjustment of the monitor to the level that is right for you
  - Results in less eye strain and less neck pain
- Mouse
  - Support your palm and your wrist in a neutral position
  - Avoid stretching; try to keep your arms close to your body
  - Use the whole arm movement; avoid quick wrist movements
  - Try to use hot keys and keystrokes instead of using the mouse
  - Try to place tasks that are performed regularly within arm's reach
  - Avoid unnecessary reaching and bending, which leads to fatigue and possible muscle strains and can reduce efficiency
  - Keep in mind other related tasks in your planning

How do I Select a Chair?

To ensure that you have chosen the correct chair for your needs, follow the eight simple rules of selecting a chair:

1. A **contoured backrest** will give your back the comfort and support it needs. Pick a chair shaped to match the natural contour of your spine.
2. **Backrests should be height adjustable,** providing your back with customized comfort and support.
3. **Don't go too soft.** For total comfort, seat and back foam must be dense enough to support your weight evenly and it should be sculpted to fit the human form.
4. **Look for "waterfall" seat cushions** that slope down at the front of the chair. This important ergonomic feature helps improve circulation to your lower legs.
5. **Rest your arms.** Armrests help keep your arms in a comfortable position, reducing shoulder, neck, and back strain. Height- and tilt-adjustable models are especially good.
6. The **pneumatic height adjustment** on a chair lets you alter your seating position throughout the day with a smooth, easy, one-touch action.
7. **Remain seated.** Make sure all adjustment controls can be reached from a seated position. Keep moving. Multitilt and operator mechanisms are important for data entry or computer work. They let you vary your position while maintaining maximum support.
8. **Good chairs have casters** for easy mobility. Be sure to get the right kind for your floor. Choose a chair with a choice of casters designed for carpets, hard surfaces, or a combination.

ERGONOMIC AND TASK CHAIRS

Task seating is an ideal choice for individuals spending large amounts of time seated at their workstations, dedicated to certain tasks. Task, or operator, chairs are "ergonomically" designed to work with you. Easily adjustable chair surfaces allow you to move around freely and help to maintain support for your back, legs, and arms as you change body positions. Task chairs can be the difference between absolute comfort and irritating distress.

MANAGEMENT CHAIRS

Management, or executive, office seating is designed to provide hours of comfort for the manager who is the sole user of her or his chair. Traditional managerial seating comes equipped with high, wide back, deep seat, and "ergonomic" features to facilitate the time spent at a desk, computer, or workstation. Modern work ethics require a comfortable chair, which will encourage the user to remain productive throughout the often long work week. Although management seating does not offer as many seating adjustment options as many other chairs, today's executives can take advantage of sophisticated knee-tilt and other tilter mechanisms. These will ensure that feet are kept flat on the floor for added comfort. For the executive, management seating is often covered in leather or upholstered in other quality fabrics.

CONFERENCE CHAIRS

Formal meetings, impromptu team gatherings, and presentations are typical business situations all requiring stylized, conference seating. The traditional boardroom setting is migrating toward conference meeting rooms flavored by the culture and traditions unique to the individual organization. These conference areas can be furnished with task, guest, or management seating—the choice is entirely yours!

GUEST CHAIRS

Guest seating or side chairs are generally offered with a sled base or as a four-legged chair without casters. Guest chairs often function as a comfortable seating solution for short periods of time, most commonly in a waiting area. Designed to complement executive and task seating, these chairs are usually available with or without arms. Most manufacturers commonly feature a side chair in each of their seating series to provide you with the best options possible for your needs.

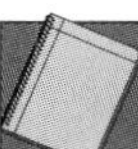

FROM THE EXPERT'S NOTEBOOK

The office should consider spraying new fabric chairs with a Scotchgard type of product to protect them and make them easier to clean.

Moving the Office

Everyone knows the hassles of moving. By using the concept of the moving team, your office can handle this project with ease. A staff member from each department is assigned the responsibility for her or his department and is a member of the team. The office manager keeps the employees advised at all times regarding changes in plans and their responsibilities. Each department representative plays a critical role in handling the issues that arise during this project.

- Management representative
  - Schedules meetings with members of the team, the office manager, and the architect.
  - Distributes memos to keep employees up to date regarding the move. This is crucial for morale in the office during this period of change.
  - Asks employees for suggestions regarding the move and allows them to voice any concerns.
- Accounting/bookkeeping representative
  - Prepares budget for moving expense and new equipment purchases.
- Computer systems representative
  - Obtains lockable space from contractor for new equipment that is being delivered.
  - Arranges for computer vendor to move computer to new space and install it there.
- Facilities representative
  - Holds regular on-site meetings with the office manager, physician, and architect.
  - On the first day in the new place, posts lists for employees to write suggestions and problems.
- Administration representative
  - Leases laptop computer for easier note taking and documentation during the move.

Building a New Facility

Growth and expansion are a way of life for a medical office. Practices grow, more physicians are hired, more office hours are needed, and so on.

PITFALLS TO AVOID

Even the most effective plan for building a new facility is likely to have some pitfalls. These pitfalls generally include the following:

- Poor location
- Inadequate time to properly plan, design, and construct a building
- Lack of attention to future expansion
- Misunderstandings about costs

Location

One of the most difficult and frustrating issues is location. Land is expensive, growth is unpredictable, and zoning is sometimes difficult. Perception is a major problem when talking about sites of offices. Sizes of lots can be deceiving, and land may appear adequate when it is actually too small to allow growth. Parking is a main consideration when constructing a new office; each municipality has zoning regulations regarding parking. Some townships require a designated number of parking spaces per square foot of office space. A multistory building requires two stairwells and an elevator shaft, which eliminates much-needed medical space. An elevator is also an extra added expense. Other site pitfalls include storm water runoff from the property, easements, height restrictions, and landscape requirements.

Time Allowance

Normally, no matter how much time is allotted for the building project, it will take longer. Planning and design can take as much time as the actual construction, if not more. Other time-consuming factors include the following:

- Searching for and actually purchasing the land
- Rezoning the land
- Obtaining approval from regulatory offices
- Allowing staff to review architectural drawings and cost estimates

Long-Term Perspective

Long-term needs are major considerations when building a new facility. Practice growth, additional services, an increase in physicians, expansion of surrounding areas, increased staffing, and space requirements need to be considered. When making these plans, it is best to project 5 to 10 years into the future.

Building Costs

Costs are always higher than expected. Inflation is almost never taken into consideration, and physicians tend to compare the costs of the new office to the costs of their homes. On a per-square-foot basis, the cost of a medical office is always more than that of any other building type. Costs are never clear-cut; it is always a guess as to what is included and what is excluded. The total project cost includes the following:

- Site work, such as excavation, paving, sidewalks, fencing, lighting, and curbing
- Fixtures, wall covering, and window treatments
- Architectural, engineering, and interior design fees
- Furniture and equipment

A design firm should be brought in to help the physician and the office manager with these decisions. Evaluate the firm's experience, references, reputation, and range of services before deciding to enlist its efforts. Make the firm aware of the office's budget so that planning takes it into consideration. A building design done quickly and with little thought will result in unnecessary costs, as well as inefficiencies. If the project is planned correctly and patiently, the medical office will probably be a more successful and productive office.

OFFICE BLUEPRINT

The office manager's main objective when a new facility is being planned is to design an office that "works." This means that each area of the office allows the practice to run efficiently, increasing productivity and profits, while allowing the delivery of quality care.

Decide what present equipment will be kept and what will be purchased new. By using an office furniture template (Figure 12-14), you can draw the furniture in various ways to check on availability of space. Try not to waste space; if there seems to be dead space somewhere, use it as a closet or for some type of storage. An office can never have too much storage! There are also commercial design kits that can be purchased for this project. Remember to allow enough space for everyone to move around easily. The following are questions you might ask yourself at this time:

- Do I want panel systems or individual desks in the business office?
- Would I be better off with computer stations than with individual desks?
- What type of filing requirements do I have in the business office?
- What arrangements do I need to make for patient files? Do I want a record room?
- Where will the employees eat?
- What types of appliances will I need electrical outlets for in the kitchen/lounge area?
- How many "dedicated" outlets will I need, if any?
- Where will I put the copier? Will it be too noisy in certain areas?
- Where will I put the computer? Will it be easily accessible to others? Will the printer be noisy?
- How should the examination tables be placed? Is it easy for the physician to access the patient that way?
- What is the best way to direct the flow of patient traffic?
- Is the waiting room friendly?
- Is there easy access to the receptionist's window?
- Is the billing manager situated in a private area, so that patients can discuss financial matters?
- Do we have enough storage areas for both clerical and clinical supplies?
- Does the transcriptionist have an area free of background noise?

All of these questions and more come up when designing a new office. A good office manager addresses these questions before finishing the plans and moving in! Once the office is situated, it becomes much more difficult and costly to make changes. There are price wars going on all the time in the office furniture business. Don't hesitate to try to negotiate with office furniture salespeople. Make sure everything is written down and both the supplier and the office have a copy. Don't rely on someone with a kind face saying, "Don't worry about that, I'll take care of it!" Many a nice relationship has soured over verbal deals such as these. Office furniture such as desks, chairs, computer stations, filing cabinets, bookcases, and credenzas can be found in catalogs at discounted prices. Check on shipping costs and the availability of the items before deciding to take this route.

Don't Move...Spruce It Up!

When the office size and location are suitable for the practice's needs, a coat of paint and some new furniture can change a rather dull office into a "showplace." Redecorating not only is less expensive than moving, but it has been proven to increase employee morale and therefore productivity.

The first thing to focus on when redecorating an office is the reception area. This is where the patients get their first impression of the practice. Soft wall colors, subdued wallpaper, tasteful pictures, healthy plants, and a quiet sound system with soothing music can do a world of good for a medical office. If the carpeting is poor, replace it. There are great new commercial carpets available that give that "warm and fuzzy" feeling to patients as they arrive at the office. Never buy couches. People generally do not like to sit next to others. They will always pick single chairs when choosing where to sit in the reception room. The best chairs are ones with arms that are approximately 18 inches deep and no deeper, because deep chairs are difficult for patients to get out of. Magazine racks are better than magazines arranged on a table. Magazines on a table always look messy, no matter how hard the staff try to keep them neat. Televisions are always a good idea in a reception area. Patients can watch the news or other shows, and will forget about the time passing. Remember to

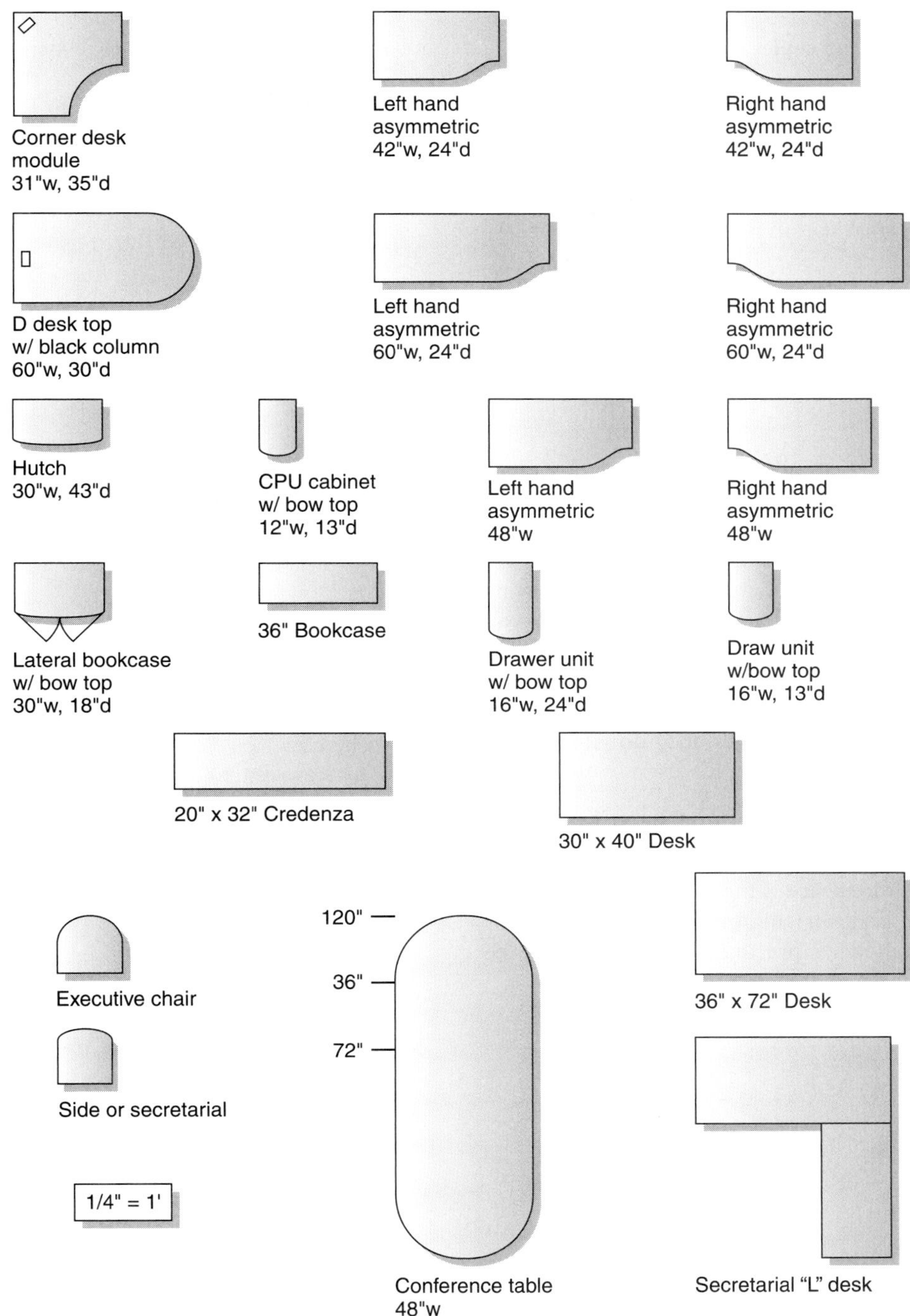

FIGURE 12-14. Template for arranging office furniture. (Courtesy of Lizell Office Furniture, 800-501-3375.)

keep the volume low so as not to disturb other patients. Studies have found that placing a television in a reception room decreases the number of complaints from patients in the reception room. The number of seats in the waiting room should be for three times the average number of patients seen in an hour. This will accommodate the drivers, family, and friends of patients, along with patients who have chosen to arrive an hour early for their scheduled appointment.

Many patients find the best recipes while sitting in the waiting room. Unfortunately, the magazine becomes tattered by patients tearing out those wonderful-sounding recipes. Place an index card on a table so that patients can copy the recipe without tearing it out of the magazine or bothering the receptionist for the copier or pen and paper.

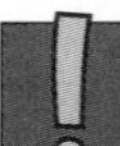

MANAGER'S ALERT

Make certain that all furniture ordered is delivered into the appropriate area within the office. Make sure that this is stated clearly at the time of purchase. Some companies state that they deliver only to the door. Delivery into the room will cost extra. Also make sure that assembly, if necessary, is included.

REVAMPING OF PRESENT SPACE

Limited remodeling and expansion can be done with a minimal amount of mess and can make employees and physicians happier. With just the smallest changes, patient flow and office efficiency can increase. By simply moving walls and decreasing space where it is not needed, you can open up additional rooms. For instance, by shaving off square footage on three examination rooms, a clinical room can be created for patients undergoing electrocardiograms and other special procedures that do not require much room. By creating this space, the examination room becomes free for the next patient. Revamping does not have to mean the moving of walls; it can be done simply by remodeling existing space and reorganizing. Getting the most from the office space is the most important issue. By using a space designer and/or an architect, major changes that will enhance practice productivity can be accomplished (Figure 12-15).

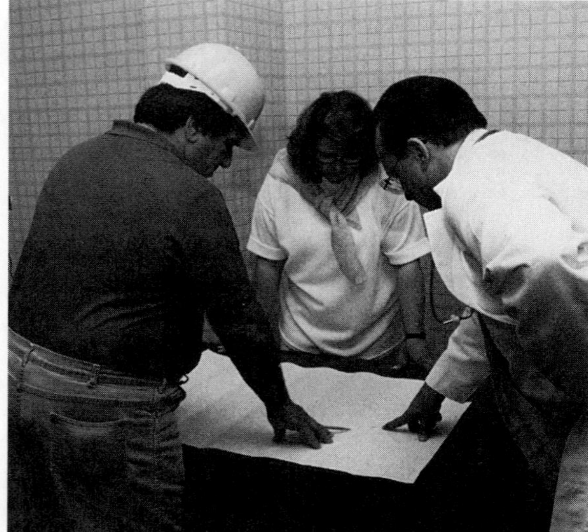

FIGURE 12-15. The architect, office manager, and physician should meet to establish the best design for the office.

Restrooms should be large enough so that patients do not hit their chin on their knees when they sit down!

As required by ADA regulations, there must be a restroom in the facility that will accommodate a wheelchair.

EXERCISES

MULTIPLE CHOICE

Choose the best *answer for each of the following questions.*

1. Which of the following is a characteristic of a creative manager?
   a. Caring for employees' psychologic health
   b. Seeing the big picture
   c. Dealing with employees' inflexibility
   d. All of the above
2. Directing strives to accomplish which of the following?
   a. Set plans for action
   b. Team up employees for set goals
   c. Encourage two-way communication
   d. None of the above
3. Examples of misconduct would be
   a. Physicians inappropriately touching patients
   b. Unusual breast examinations
   c. Hugging or kissing patients as part of therapy
   d. All of the above
4. Which of the following should not be continually evaluated during an operational review?
   a. Staffing ratios
   b. Physician's mileage
   c. Currently used forms
   d. Job descriptions
5. The National Practitioner Data Bank collects such information as
   a. Civil judgments
   b. Health care–related criminal convictions
   c. Number of patients in a practice
   d. Certification actions
6. Which of the following is a disadvantage to a practice merger?
   a. Group purchase discounts
   b. Centralized billing
   c. Inflexibility of personnel
   d. Overhead economies of scale
7. What are the characteristics of a good keyboard?
   a. Palm rest
   b. Good color
   c. Height and angle are easily adjusted
   d. Adjustable mouse tray
8. What style of seat cushion should you look for in a chair?
   a. Waterfall
   b. Dam
   c. Stream
   d. Pond

9. When building a new office, time-consuming factors can be
   a. Rezoning
   b. Obtaining approval from regulatory offices
   c. Searching for land
   d. All of the above
10. When selecting office furniture, which of the following things should be considered?
   a. Ergonomics
   b. Seating friends by friends
   c. Know your supplier
   d. Avoid tangles
11. Which of the following is not a true statement?
   a. Keep copy paper dry.
   b. Remove static from paper by using a small spray of Windex.
   c. Buy quality paper.
   d. Don't store paper on a concrete basement floor.
12. Which of the following is *not* a way to save on office expenses?
   a. Buy the best
   b. Maintain office equipment
   c. Evaluate leasing versus purchasing
   d. Use part-time employees whenever possible
13. Which is *not* a pitfall of building a new office?
   a. Poor location
   b. Lack of planning
   c. Employees don't like new building
   d. Misunderstanding about costs
14. The management principle that subscribes to "Where you stand depends on where you sit" is what principle?
   a. The Law of Effect
   b. Miles' Law
   c. Parkinson's Law
   d. None of the above
15. Which of the following is an important component of leadership?
   a. Skills
   b. Knowledge
   c. Talents
   d. All of the above
16. Skills that are essential to perform certain functions are
   a. Competencies
   b. Talents
   c. Knowledge
   d. None of the above
17. According to O'Malley, what percentage of employees are committed during their first year of employment?
   a. 15%
   b. 100%
   c. 43%
   d. 61%
18. Which of the following is *not* a characteristic of a committed employee?
   a. Pleasant
   b. Takes advantage of time off
   c. Hard working
   d. Productive
19. Behavior that is rewarded is likely to be repeated. What theory is this?
   a. Two-factor theory
   b. Learned need theory
   c. Reinforcement theory
   d. Expectancy theory
20. Which of Maslow's needs involves breathing, food, water, and sleep?
   a. Esteem
   b. Physiologic
   c. Psychologic
   d. Self-actualization

MATCHING

Match the following manager types.

1. ______ Problem manager	A. Does few things at office, then leaves.
2. ______ Novice manager	B. Corrects employees in front of others.
3. ______ Task master	C. Cannot deal with conflict.
4. ______ Phantom	D. Does not have necessary skills.
5. ______ Intimidator	E. More hours worked, or work done.

TRUE OR FALSE

1. ______ Hairspray is used to remove static from paper.
2. ______ The Family and Medical Leave Act is an employment law.
3. ______ The best paper shredder is the "cross-cut" shredder.
4. ______ Reid Psychiatric House is an employee testing company.
5. ______ The MGMA is an association for hospital administrators.
6. ______ For staff meetings, topics should be broad.
7. ______ Nail polish remover is used to clean copiers.
8. ______ Medical practices typically spend 20% of their gross income on medical and office supplies
9. ______ The leasing company must own at least 20% of the equity of the property during the term of the lease.
10. ______ Cell phones have replaced pagers in many instances.
11. ______ Credentialing physicians can be done rather quickly.
12. ______ Employee benefits should be included in a policy and procedure manual.
13. ______ Administering is a management style.
14. ______ Many bookkeepers use mechanical pencils.
15. ______ When using a mouse, avoid quick wrist movements.
16. ______ Leasing equipment keeps up-front expenses down.
17. ______ Copiers should be located in direct sunlight.
18. ______ Use 24-pound paper in the copier.
19. ______ When selecting a chair, make sure it is really soft.
20. ______ Safety is one of the needs in Maslow's theory.

THINKERS

1. List five major frustrations of the physician-administrator relationship.
2. Describe the four goals of an office manager.
3. Explain what an office manager should look for when purchasing a new chair.

REFERENCES

Associated Regional Accounting Firms. *First, Stop the Bleeding.* Norcross, GA: Author, 1993.

Astrachan, A. "Spruce up the Office—and Boost Your Earnings?" *Medical Economics,* January 1987, pp. 177-188.

Bernstein, A., & Rozen, S. *Dinosaur Brains.* New York: Ballantine Books, 1989.

Bliss, E. *Getting Things Done*: The ABC's of *Time Management.* New York: McGraw Hill, 1983.

Brown, S., Nelson, A., Bronkesh, S., & Wood, S. *Patient Satisfaction Pays.* Gaithersburg, MD: Aspen Publications, 1993.

Buss, D. "Ways To Curtail Employee Theft". *Nation's Business,* April 1993, pp. 36-38.

Calano, J., & Salzman, J. "The Careful Manager's Guide to Snap Decisions". *The Office,* May 1988, pp. 86-87.

Calero, L. "An Office Relocation Needs a Project Team". *The Office,* April 1992, pp. 52-53.

Demos, M.P. "What Every Physician Should Know about the National Practitioner Data Bank". *Archives of Internal Medicine,* September 1991, pp. 1708-1711.

Dolan, M. "Building New Facilities—What Planners Need to Know". *Group Practice Journal,* March/April 1993, pp. 40-42.

Dupree, M. *Leadership as an Art.* New York: Bantam Doubleday Dell, 1990.

Farber, L. *Encyclopedia of Practice and Financial Management.* Oradell, NJ: Medical Economics Company, 1988.

Green, W. "How to Run a Really Good Meeting". *US News & World Report,* October 12, 1987, pp. 80-82.

Grothe, M., Wylie, P. Problem *Bosses: Who They Are and How to Deal with Them.* New York: Fawcett Books, 1988.

Heller, W. "How Safe Is Your Bank?" *Physician's Management,* February 1992, pp. 149-170.

Jamison, K. *The Nibble Theory.* New York: Paulist Press, 1984.

Kahaner, L. "Security Systems: How to Pick the Best for Your Home and Office". *Physician's Management,* March 1992, pp. 175-188.

Ketchum, S. "Overcoming the Four Toughest Management Challenges". *Clinical Laboratory Management Association,* August 1991, pp. 246-263.

Krill, M. *Successful Partnerships for the Future.* Englewood, CO: Medical Group Management Association, 1995.

Lankford, N. "Copier Trends". *The Office,* January 1993, p. 60.

Lopez, J.A. "The Boss from Hell". *Working Woman,* December 1991, pp. 69-71.

LeBoeuf, W. "Writing a CV That Brings Interviews". *Medical Economics,* May 1992, pp. 127-130.

Le Gallee, J. "Copier Control Systems Do More Than Curb Waste". *The Office,* March 1992, pp. 61-88.

Lucash, P. *Medical Practice Change Management.* Burr Ridge, IL: Irwin Publishing, 1997.

Mackenzie, A. *The Time Trap.* New York: American Management Association.

Murray, D. "Coping with Tougher Times, Save Big on Equipment and Supplies". *Medical Economics,* September 1993, pp. 55-66.

O'Malley, M. *Creating Commitment: How to Attract and Retain Talented Employees by Building Relationships That Last.* New York: John Wiley & Sons, 2000.

Page, L. "Lost in the Translation". *American Medical News,* February 1993, pp. 31-32.

Peoples, D.A. *Presentation Plus.* New York: John Wiley & Sons, 1992.

Pepper, J. "Coping with Copiers". *Working Woman,* April 1990, p. 54.

Relman, A. "The Health Care Industry: Where Is It Taking Us?" *New England Journal of Medicine,* September 1991, pp. 20-21.

Simendinger, E.A. & Moore, T.F. "The Physician Administrator Relationship." *Hospital Forum Magazine,* Chicago: American Hospital Association, 1999.

Slomski, A. "Making Sure Your Care Doesn't Get Lost in Translation". *Medical Economics,* May 1993, pp. 122-139.

Smith, P. *Taking Charge: Making the Right Choices.* Wayne, NJ: Avery, 1988.

Spero, K. "Ten Ways to Evaluate an Accountant". *Physician's Management,* August 1991, pp. 138-150.

Tinsley, R. "Plan Ahead before Merging Medical Practices". *Group Practice Journal,* December 1993, pp. 28-32.

Tomasko, R. *Rethinking the Corporation.* New York: American Management Association, 1993.

Yerkes, L. "Making the Most of a Management Consultant". *Physician's Management,* July 1992, pp. 97-106.

13

OUTPATIENT SERVICES, AMBULATORY SURGERY CENTERS, AND HOSPITALS

CHAPTER OUTLINE

CHAPTER OBJECTIVES

After completing this chapter, you will be able to do the following:

- Cite examples of outpatient services
- Recognize the benefits of a physician office laboratory
- Define "Certificate of Waiver" and know what it is for
- Describe the concept of ambulatory care
- Purchase laboratory equipment
- Differentiate the types of hospitals, their structure, and their departments

OUTPATIENT SERVICES

Many forms of outpatient care are provided to patients: x-ray examinations, electrocardiograms (ECGs), ultrasonography, computed tomography (CT) scans, laboratory services, physical therapy, and home care (Figure 13-1). The health care system today is undergoing massive "cosmetic surgery," shifting from hospital care to outpatient care and ambulatory services. This shift is creating an environment in which physician offices can thrive by offering a variety of services to patients. Office managers must be aware of the many services physicians can provide patients, so that their staff can be trained to better assist the physician and patient during medical treatment (Figure 13-2).

Americans are hungry for medical testing as they strive to understand medicines, their own bodies, and wellness. People flock to health fairs, shopping centers, and drug stores in an effort to obtain free testing for various disorders. In fact, health fairs test approximately 20 million people every year for blood pressure, cholesterol, diabetes, or other tests. This type of patient, the "informed consumer," has created a demand for outpatient testing. These consumers are going to facilities where they get the best deal for their money. Since they have become more "in tune" with their bodies and how they function, they do not always rely on the first opinion they hear. They expect choices and will "doctor shop" until they find the right combination of caring, availability, and price.

Hospitals are promoting wellness by holding wellness clinics that provide preventive care. They offer senior citizens free blood pressure checks, low-cost eye examinations, and free cholesterol checks. More sophisticated programs offer chest x-rays, mammograms, ECGs, and Papanicolaou (Pap) smears. The cost of having these more sophisticated tests done at a wellness clinic is minimal compared with what they would cost if a private physician ordered them. Most physicians do not see this as an economic threat and recommend low-cost wellness clinics to their patients. Results of these tests can be sent to the family physician at the patient's request. Some hospital services are provided by hospital satellite facilities that offer a full range of primary care services for patients. Clinics are opening across the country in deprived urban areas. Physicians who do feel threatened by these clinics and satellites should offer more services to offset this "competition." This can be done by adding an x-ray unit, an office laboratory, physical therapy staff, or by just being more available. Physicians must remember that availability is one of the most important factors for patients when they are choosing a physician. Simply by extending weekday office hours or by adding Saturday hours, patients can be better accommodated and more content with the office.

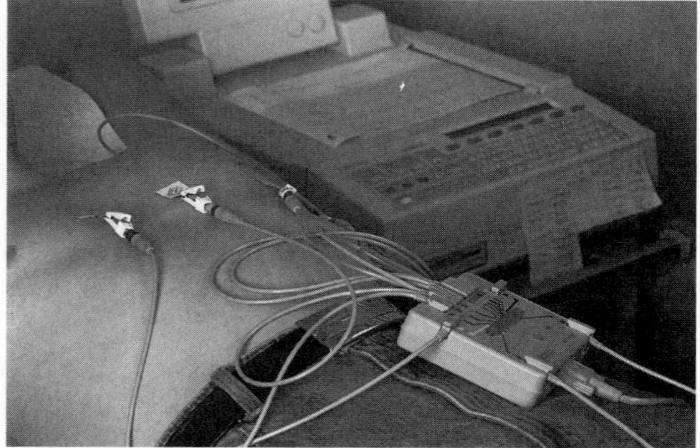

FIGURE 13-1. A patient with chest pain is able to have an electrocardiogram in the physician's office.

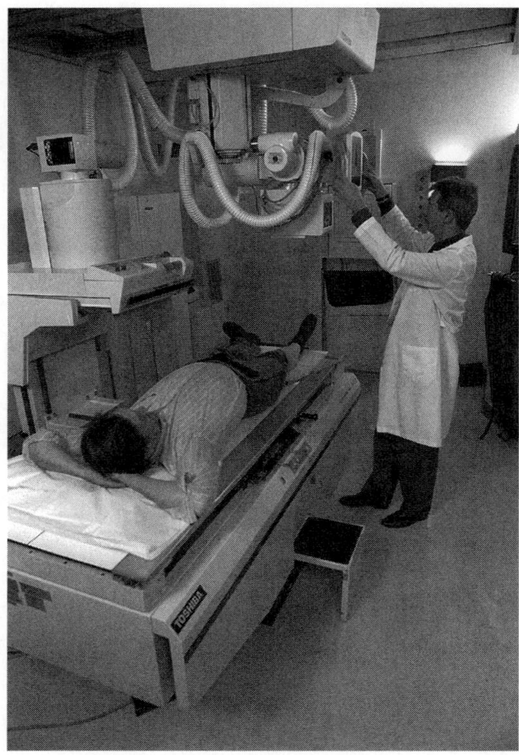

FIGURE 13-2. A patient receives an x-ray of his knee in his orthopedic surgeon's office.

Defensive medicine is another reason for an increase in outpatient testing. Because of the medical-legal environment, patients with simple cold symptoms will likely find themselves subjected to a battery of laboratory tests. The most common reason for extensive medical testing is not to diagnose disease, but to protect the physician from charges of negligence.

PHYSICIAN OFFICE LABORATORIES

As a result of the government's plan for "Medicare prospective payment," many physicians are setting up physician office laboratories (POLs) to cut the cost of preadmission

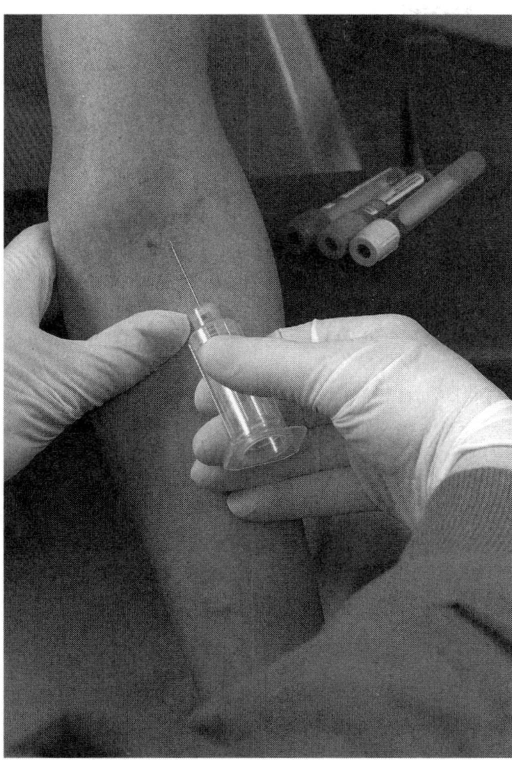

FIGURE 13-3. Patients can conveniently have laboratory tests done in their physician's office when there is an in-office laboratory.

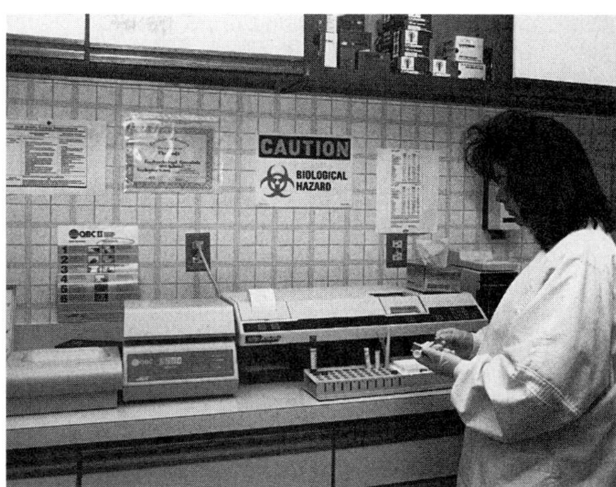

FIGURE 13-4. Physicians can obtain faster laboratory results for their patients when they have a laboratory in their office.

testing. The convenience to patients and the increased revenues that POLs generate create a win-win situation for everyone involved (Figure 13-3). As of June 2007, there were 106,982 registered POLs in the United States. Most physicians consider their testing equipment to be so user friendly and accurate that it can provide test results faster than traditional hospital laboratories (Figure 13-4), thus facilitating better patient care, which is a physician's main concern. In addition, POLs perform less costly tests than those performed by most independent or hospital laboratories. However, many physician's offices experience difficulty using their POL under the many different managed care plans. The American Academy of Family Physicians is attempting to help physicians with their POLs, and has endorsed a paper developed by the American Society of Internal Medicine titled "Assuring Appropriate Access to Laboratory Testing for Patients in Managed Health Care Plans." This paper can help physicians negotiate with health plans; it also contains recommendations for patient access to laboratory services.

Clinical Laboratory Improvement Act

Every facility that tests for the diagnosis and treatment of diseases must meet certain federal requirements. The practice is not only responsible for performing the tests, but also for maintaining records. Under the Clinical Laboratory Improvement Act (CLIA) regulations, POLs with a Certificate of Waiver (COW) may perform only those tests that have been classified as waived. POLs with a provider-performed microscopy (PPM) certificate may perform tests, using a microscope, during the course of a patient visit on specimens that cannot be transported easily. Laboratories that perform waived tests are required by CLIA to enroll in the program and follow the testing instructions by the manufacturer. Laboratories that perform PPM tests are required to enroll in the program and address certain quality and administrative requirements.

Clinical Laboratory Improvement Act Amendments of 1988

Amendments to the CLIA effective October 1, 1997, required all providers of laboratory services to obtain a certificate of registration. CLIA provides certification for either waived tests or physician-performed microscopy. A physician-performed certificate allows the physician to perform any tests in a POL that are of moderate or high complexity. This regulation requires that all POLs include their CLIA registration number for all tests performed. This number should be entered in Box 23 on the HCFA-1500 form (or the appropriate field for electronic submissions).

Waived Laboratories

Problems encountered in waived laboratories include the following:

- 32% Failed to have current manufacturer's instructions
- 32% Did not perform quality control (QC) as required by the manufacturer or the Centers for Disease Control and Prevention (CDC)
- 23% Had certificate issues (change of name, director, and/or address)

20% Cut occult blood cards and urine dipsticks
19% Had personnel who were neither trained nor evaluated
16% Failed to follow current manufacturer's instructions
9% Did not follow manufacturer's storage and handling instructions
7% Did not perform calibration as required by the manufacturer
6% Were using expired reagents

Problems encountered with PPM laboratories include the following:

38% Had no prothrombin time (did not evaluate test accuracy twice a year)
36% Had no microscope/centrifuge maintenance
28% Had no director-approved procedure manual
25% Did not document personnel competency
23% Had certificate issues

The checklist for waived testing compliance is as follows:

1. Use the most recent package insert of manufacturer's instructions. They may change from lot to lot.
2. Perform QC and/or calibrate as specified by the kit manufacturer.
3. Use the reagents in the form in which they are received.
4. Store and handle all test kits according to the manufacturer's instructions.
5. Never use outdated reagents.
6. Document training of all testing personnel.
7. Inform the POL's surveying agency when there is a change.
8. Follow all Occupational Safety and Health Administration (OSHA) regulations that pertain to laboratory testing.

The checklist for PPM testing compliance includes the above eight items, plus the following:

1. Perform either proficiency testing or quality assurance at least two times per year for documentation of accuracy of the procedures.
2. Perform and document microscope and centrifuge maintenance.
3. Develop and maintain a current procedure manual for all microscopy tests.
4. Inform the POL's surveying agency of any change in status of the laboratory.
5. Follow all OSHA regulations as they pertain to laboratory testing.

Categorization of CLIA Criteria

Every test is graded for complexity for seven specific criteria. A score of 1 indicates the lowest level of complexity, and a score of 3 indicates the highest level. Once these scores are totaled, tests with 12 points or less are categorized as moderate complexity and those receiving scores above 12 points are considered to be of high complexity. Tests can also be categorized as waived.

CATEGORIES

1. Knowledge
   Score 1. (A) Minimal scientific and technical knowledge is required to perform the test. (B) Knowledge required to perform the test may be obtained through on-the-job training.
   Score 3. Specialized scientific and technical knowledge is essential to perform preanalytic, analytic, or postanalytic phases of the testing.
2. Training and experience
   Score 1. (A) Minimal training is required for preanalytic, analytic, and postanalytic phases of the testing process. (B) Limited experience is required to perform the test.
   Score 3. (A) Specialized training is essential to perform the preanalytic, analytic, or postanalytic testing process. (B) Substantial experience may be necessary for analytic test performance.
3. Reagents and materials preparation
   Score 1. (A) Reagents and materials are generally stable and reliable. (B) Reagents and materials are prepackaged or premeasured, or require no special handling, precautions, or storage conditions.
   Score 3. (A) Reagents and materials may be labile (unstable) and may require special handling to ensure reliability. (B) Reagents and materials preparation may include manual steps such as gravimetric or volumetric measurements.
4. Characteristics of operational steps
   Score 1. Operational steps are either automatically executed (e.g., pipetting) or are easily controlled.
   Score 3. Operational steps in the testing process require close monitoring or control, and may require special specimen preparation, precise temperature control or timing of procedural steps, accurate pipetting, or extensive calculations.
5. Calibration, quality control, and proficiency testing materials
   Score 1. (A) Calibration materials are stable and readily available. (B) Quality control materials are stable and readily available. (C) External proficiency testing materials, if available, may be labile.
   Score 3. (A) Calibration materials, if available, may be labile. (B) Quality control materials may be labile, or not available. (C) External proficiency testing materials, if available, may be labile.
6. Test system troubleshooting and equipment maintenance
   Score 1. (A) Test system troubleshooting is automatic or self-correcting, or clearly described or requires minimal judgment. (B) Equipment maintenance is provided by

the manufacturer, is seldom needed, or can easily be performed.

Score 3. (A) Troubleshooting is not automatic and requires decision making and direct intervention to resolve most problems. (B) Maintenance requires special knowledge, skills, and abilities.

7. Interpretation and judgment

Score 1. (A) Minimal interpretation and judgment are required to perform preanalytic, analytic, and postanalytic processes. (B) Resolution of problems requires limited independent interpretation and judgment.

Score 3. (A) Extensive independent interpretation and judgment are required to perform the preanalytic, analytic, or postanalytic processes. (B) Resolution of problems requires extensive interpretation and judgment.

Certificate of Waiver

On February 28, 1992, regulations defined *waived tests* as simple laboratory examinations and procedures that are cleared by the Food and Drug Administration (FDA) for home use; employ methodologies that are so simple and accurate as to render the likelihood of erroneous results negligible; or pose no reasonable risk of harm to the patient if the test is performed incorrectly. The Clinical Laboratory Improvement Amendments of 1988 law identified testing requirements to be based on complexity and provided the provision for the "waived" test concept. This regulation can be found in the *Federal Register* at 42 CFR 493.15 (b) and 493.15 (c). Tests that are listed as waived are as follows:

- Dipstick or tablet reagent urinalysis (nonautomated) for the following:
  - Bilirubin
  - Glucose
  - Hemoglobin
  - Ketone
  - Leukocytes
  - Nitrite
  - pH
  - Protein
  - Specific gravity
  - Urobilinogen
- Fecal occult blood
- Ovulation tests (visual color comparison tests for luteinizing hormone)
- Urine pregnancy tests (visual color comparison tests)
- Erythrocyte sedimentation rate (nonautomated)
- Hemoglobin—copper sulfate (nonautomated)
- Blood glucose by glucose monitoring devices cleared by the FDA specifically for home use
- Spun microhematocrit
- Hemoglobin by single-analyte instruments with self-contained or component features to perform specimen/reagent interaction, providing direct measurement and readout

A waiver may be granted to any test listed in the regulation (as above), any test system for which the manufacturer applies for a waiver, or any test that is cleared by the FDA for home use.

Some examples of physician-performed microscopy tests are as follows:

- Wet mounts
- KOH preparations
- Pinworm
- Urine sediment examination
- Semen analysis

MANAGER'S ALERT

Don't let the wording of the phrase "physician-performed microscopy" tests fool you! These tests can be performed by physician assistants, nurse practitioners, and nurse-midwives.

Types of Laboratory Tests Performed by POLs

Five types of laboratory tests are performed by POLs:

1. Screening tests
2. Confirmatory tests
3. Monitoring tests
4. Stat tests
5. Preadmission tests

A screening test is performed to identify a disease process. Screening tests are generally quick and less expensive than most other laboratory tests. An example of a screening test is a "strep" test, which produces results within 5 minutes (Figure 13-5).

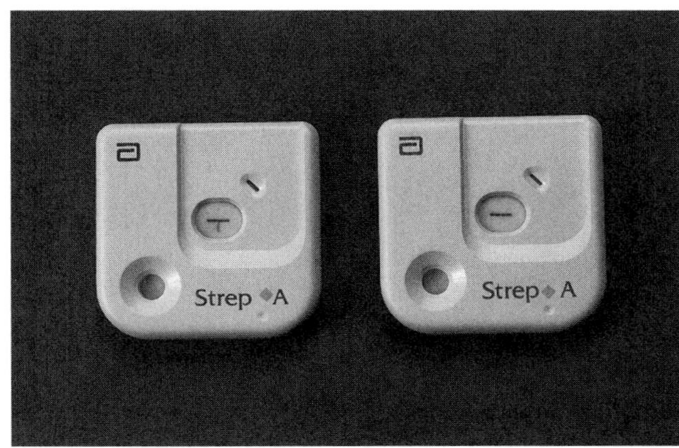

FIGURE 13-5. An example of a screening test for strep.

Positive screening tests are often followed by confirmatory testing to diagnose the patient accurately. Confirmatory tests are more expensive and require more time for processing. They provide more specific information and are more complex in nature. An example of a confirmatory test is a test for hepatitis.

Monitoring tests are continuous in nature and follow the patient through a course of treatment. They differ from other tests in that they are always performed on patients for whom a diagnosis has already been made. An example of a monitoring test is a complete blood count on a patient receiving chemotherapy drugs.

Stat tests are ordered on patients in emergency situations. They are most commonly used in the hospital setting. However, there are some instances in which stat tests are ordered in the physician's office. For example, when a patient arrives at the office with severe diabetic symptoms, the physician needs a glucose stat. It is important to identify whether the patient's glucose is too high or too low to treat the patient effectively.

Preadmission tests are usually nonurgent tests required for a patient to be admitted to the hospital, but they are also ordered for patients having outpatient surgery. These tests are screening tests designed to reveal any abnormalities that could affect the patient's hospitalization or procedure.

Billing

As for all medical services and procedures, the medical necessity of each laboratory test performed must be established. In addition to the tests processed for in-office patients, offices with POLs can also bill for laboratory tests run on samples drawn from patients in nursing facilities. The practice may also bill for travel to the nursing facility. Check with your carrier to obtain billing requirements, because some will reimburse a flat rate whereas others reimburse on a per mileage basis.

Equipment

The type of equipment purchased is of utmost importance to the success of a POL. Equipment must be easily maintained, have excellent service support, and be easy to use. When shopping for laboratory equipment, you should contact several vendors. Keep the following concerns in mind:

- Ease of use
- Technical support
- Downtime
- Interactive features
- Cost of equipment
- Cost of reagents/supplies
- Speed
- Maintenance costs

PREPARING FOR AN INSPECTION

The CLIA inspection regulations can be found in Subpart Q of the *Federal Register.* These regulations should be reviewed. To begin the preparation for a CLIA inspection, it is first necessary to gather all the required documents. These documents include the following:

- Personnel files
- Procedure manual
- Instrument maintenance logs
- Temperature logs
- Quality control logs
- Patient records
- Patient test management
- Calibration verification logs
- Quality assurance plan

The final preparations include all of the following:

- Make sure that everything that needs to be signed is signed.
- Make sure all the quality control records are up to date.
- Double check supplies for expiration dates.
- Make sure all supplies are stored properly.
- Make sure that all laboratory personnel are prepared to answer any questions the laboratory inspector may have.
- The day before the inspector comes, run through things once again; make sure the laboratory is spotless!
- Make sure that no one has stored any food in the laboratory.
- Do not argue with the inspector.
- Be pleasant, helpful, and polite.

The Inspection

Laboratories may be asked to do any of the following:

- Run test samples, perform procedures
- Permit interviews of all personnel
- Permit personnel to be observed while they are performing tests
- Permit Centers for Medicare and Medicaid Services (CMS) access to all areas covered by the certification, such as the specimen procurement and processing areas, storage facilities for specimen reagents, supplies, records, and testing and reporting areas
- Provide CMS with copies (exact duplicates) of all records and data it requires
- Have all data accessible and ready for review

There is an accreditation program that has helped countless POLs stay in compliance with CLIA. This organization is the Commission on Laboratory Accreditation (COLA). The Web site for this organization is as follows: www.cola.org/pol.

Opening a POL

So, you want to open a POL. Follow these steps and you will be on your way to POL testing. First, decide what level of complexity you want your laboratory to be. Do you want to perform waived tests only, do you want moderate or high complexity, or are you thinking about provider-performed microscopy procedures?

Once the complexity decision has been made, it is then necessary to obtain CMS Form 116, which is used to apply for CLIA certification. This form can be downloaded from the CMS Web site. Next complete the form based on the complexity of your proposed laboratory. Once the laboratory has been inspected, it will be billed by CMS for the certificate and inspection. Once the form has been completed, it must be submitted to the local state agency, along with any state-mandated paperwork that may be necessary. Certificate of Waiver laboratories will be charged a fee of $150, Certificate of Provider Performed Microscopy Procedures (PPMP) laboratories will be charged a fee of $200, and Certificate of Accreditation laboratories will be charged $100 for an interim certificate. The next step is to enroll in an approved proficiency testing program for all tests on your testing list. Set up the laboratory using the CLIA requirements. Schedule your inspection and correct any deficiencies that may have been pointed out. Maintain the CLIA certification and renew every 2 years.

Web sites that may be helpful with POLs include the following:

- List of waived tests—www.cms.hhs.gov/clia/downloads/cr5083.waivebl.pdf
- List of PPM procedures—www.cms.hhs.gov/clia/downloads/ppmp.list.pdf
- To determine the complexity of a test—www.accessdata.fda.gov/scripts/cdrh/cfdocs/cfCLIA/search.cfm
- CLIA requirements—www.phppo.cdc.gov/clia/regs/toc.aspx

AMBULATORY CARE

What Is Ambulatory Care?

The tremendous increase in ambulatory care facilities is a response to the ever-changing and expanding needs of the modern population. *Ambulatory care* is a broad term that refers to the delivery of outpatient services in a wide variety of settings. That may sound scary to some, and many would rather call these patients walking patients. However, ambulatory care fits right into the mold of the managed care model, providing medical services in an ambulatory setting with less cost.

Ambulatory care can be preventive, primary, or secondary. Preventive care focuses on the wellness of individuals and their efforts to avoid disease. Primary care focuses on the daily, routine, basic care that individuals require from health care professionals. Secondary care is the care provided to ambulatory patients who require more specialized diagnosis and treatment.

Although most ambulatory care is provided in physician offices, an increasing number of services are being provided in hospitals, ambulatory surgery centers (ASCs), and clinics. Hospitals, through increased use of short procedure units (SPUs), are continually increasing the number of procedures they provide on a "same-day surgery" basis. Chemotherapy, blood transfusions, kidney dialysis, and many other services have joined the ranks of ambulatory care. Most hospitals have responded to the need for ambulatory services and have redesigned their facilities to further expedite the treatment of individuals with ambulatory care needs. By promoting ambulatory care, hospitals have positioned themselves in managed care to negotiate for both inpatient and outpatient services, thus providing flexibility and opportunity for hospitals and managed care plans to effectively control costs.

Ambulatory Surgery Centers

Medicare defines an ASC as a center that is a distinct entity operating exclusively for the purpose of furnishing outpatient surgical services. It is a health care facility that specializes in providing surgery, pain management, and certain diagnostic services (e.g., colonoscopy, esophagogastroduodenoscopy [EGD], arthroscopy, etc.) in an outpatient setting. ASCs may be independent or may be owned and operated by a hospital. Some facilities are owned and operated solely by the physicians of a particular practice. Other centers have been opened by affiliations of several physician groups (usually from different specialties) that have pooled their resources in an effort to provide quality care at reduced costs. These joint ventures design and construct facilities to meet the needs of the ever-growing community. If an ASC is owned by a hospital, it has the option of either being covered by Medicare as an ASC or of continuing to be covered as a hospital-affiliated ASC. There are even hospitals involved in joint ventures with physicians to construct ASCs in an effort to maintain their standing in the health care marketplace.

The first ASC opened in Phoenix, Arizona. Its sole purpose was to provide "same-day" surgery care for patients who normally would be treated in hospitals. It was completely independent of a hospital and provided a wide range of services, including colonoscopies, gastroscopies, bronchoscopies, thallium stress testing, cataract surgeries, laparoscopies, vasectomies, oral surgeries, arthroscopies, cartilage repairs, and plastic surgeries. With society becoming more mobile and transient, ASCs provide a type of patient care that is vitally needed. Approximately 2,400 procedures have been approved by Medicare that can be performed in an ASC.

Medicare payment for services provided in an ASC are made by Part B. To receive payment for these services, the facility must be certified and meet the requirements for an ASC. There must be a written agreement between the facility and CMS stating that Medicare will pay for the procedures that it has identified as ASC facility services. This is known as the ASC list.

Factors contributing to the rise of ASCs are increased revenues by way of facility fee reimbursement, convenience to the physician and patient, efficient appointment scheduling, and a friendlier environment. Cost containment can also factor into the equation. Physicians are constantly looking for ways to maximize their efficiency. Developing an ASC can help them accomplish this while allowing them to continue to deliver quality care to patients. Quality assurance tends to be more thorough than in a hospital setting, and only patients whose health is generally good are scheduled for procedures in an ASC. Any patient considered at risk is scheduled to have his or her procedure performed in the usual hospital setting (Figure 13-6).

The effort to make surgical procedures more user friendly has resulted in an influx of some patient groups to ASCs. The success of this "mobile medical business" is based on factors such as the following:

- Increased demand for outpatient surgeries by cost-conscious patients

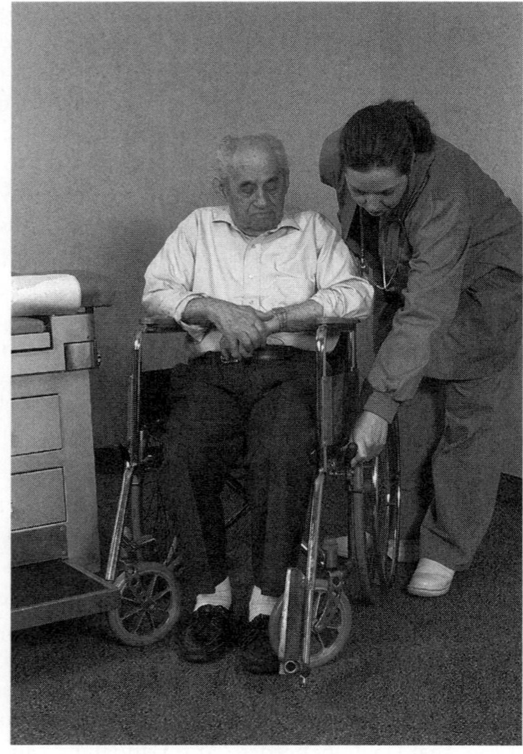

FIGURE 13-6. Care should be taken when discharging a patient after a procedure.

- Increased desire of third-party payers to purchase services while remaining cost conscious
- Increased incentives from third-party payers for same-day surgeries
- More flexible physician schedules, allowing for increased productivity, which ultimately increases revenue
- Incentives from Medicare for the development of ASCs
- Easing of previously strict regulations for the establishment of ASCs

More than 2 million surgical procedures are performed in ASCs every year, and the number keeps rising (Figure 13-7). Many ASCs in the United States provide surgical procedures that would cost 50% to 60% more if they were performed in a hospital operating room.

PAYMENT RATES

In 2003, Congress approved the Medicare Modernization Act of 2003 (MMA), which was to implement a new payment system for ASCs. In July 2007, CMS released the long overdue final rule for policy for the revised payment system for ASCs. The new payment system was effective on January 1, 2008. This new rule has encouraged quality and efficient care for patients in the ASC setting. It was also designed to align payment rates across all payers to eliminate any potential payment incentives that would favor one over another. Procedures performed in ASCs before January 2008 were classified into nine reimbursement categories. The new payment schedule was based on the outpatient prospective payment system (OPPS). CMS will use a significantly lower conversion factor multiplied by the ASC/OPPS relative weights to determine payment for an individual procedure. CMS estimates that under the new payment system, ASCs will be paid approximately 67% of what hospitals are paid for the same procedures in 2008.

Facility fees will cover the following:

- Nursing services
- Drugs, dressings, supplies
- Diagnostic items and services
- Blood and blood components
- Anesthesia supplies
- Intraocular lenses

A facility fee does not cover the following:

- Physician services
- Lease, sale, or rental of durable medical equipment
- Ambulance services
- Braces
- Laboratory services (independent)
- Artificial limbs and eyes

Transition Period

The ASC final rule provides for a 4-year transition period for implementation of the rates calculated using

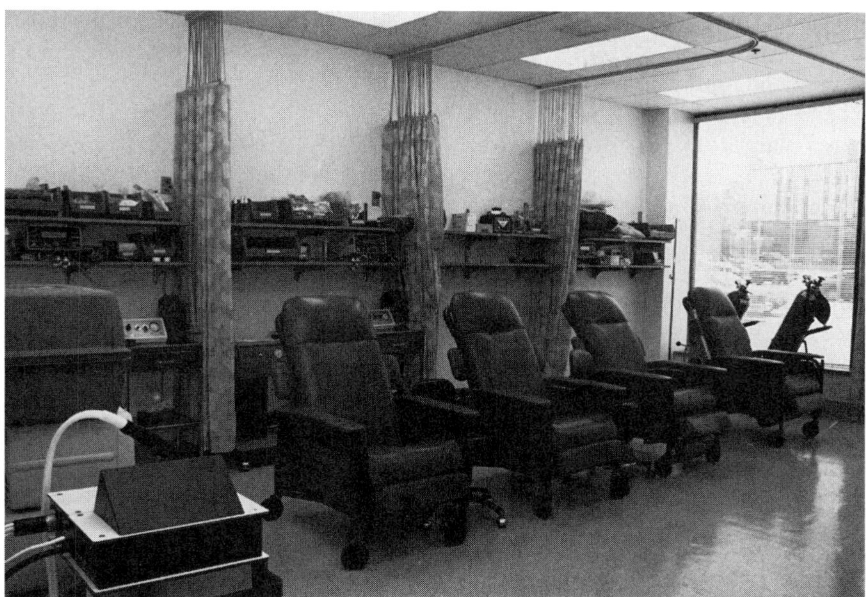

FIGURE 13-7. A recovery room in an ASC.

the methodology of the revised ASC payment system. It will implement the new ASC payment system on a blended percentage basis using both the new ASC payment rates and the current ASC rates.

ARE YOU READY FOR AN ASC?

Experience is usually the best teacher. Because many ASCs have been established throughout the country, it is best to learn from their experiences and try to avoid unnecessary aggravation. There are a few basic steps that your office must take before jumping into the ASC arena.

- Determine the purpose of the facility.
- Discuss organizational issues and produce a business plan.
- Develop a team.
- Determine the location.
- Address construction issues.
- Consider costs.

Purpose of Facility

The first step is to identify the purpose of developing the ASC. Is it being developed to increase physician revenues, or to provide physicians with greater flexibility? Greater flexibility would allow physicians to become more productive, which would allow them to see additional patients. Greater flexibility would also give physicians more leisure time. One of the most important and basic steps in this process is to identify physicians' needs. After physicians' needs have been established, you can begin assembling the building blocks necessary for this enormous undertaking.

Organizational Issues

Having a qualified and informed individual to schedule all procedures performed at the ASC is imperative. This person is key to the ASC's success. He or she should have clinical working knowledge of the procedures being performed; knowledge of physicians' preferences in sutures, equipment, anesthesia, and other supplies; and awareness of the length of time necessary to perform each procedure (including cleaning and preparation of the room and equipment). Having a highly competent person in this position should minimize turnaround time and maximize productivity.

A director can be appointed to oversee facility operations, or the office manager can do this. In either case, the ASC should be constantly monitored for patient satisfaction, referring physician satisfaction, and cost containment. The director or office manager should be concerned with streamlining any task that hasn't already been simplified and should use automation whenever possible. Computers and efficient use of forms can save time spent on documentation.

Development of a Team

Teamwork is of the utmost importance in developing an ASC. Job descriptions must be precise, cross-training must take place, and staff members must be aware of their roles. Staffing should be analyzed with regard to the ASC schedule to ensure efficient patient flow and quality care. Because supplies account for approximately 40% of ASC operating costs, one team member should be designated as the supplies controller. This person is responsible for the following:

- Monitoring and maintaining the medical supply inventory
- Standardizing equipment and supplies whenever possible
- Monitoring supply charges to be sure they are captured
- Negotiating price with supply vendors

Location

The ASC location depends heavily on whether it will be used solely by the medical office developing it or will be opened for use by other physician groups. If others are involved, the site should be close to all participants and the hospital. If the ASC is going to be used by only one physician group, choosing the location should not be a difficult task; it should be close to the office and hospital. Other considerations are parking, easy access, and traffic patterns.

Although some people believe that the ages of patients, where they live, and their genders have an effect on an ASC's success, patient demographics have little to no effect. Physician commitment is a far more important consideration.

Construction

Before construction takes place, it must be decided whether the facility will be applying for ASC certification. If certification is sought, there are extensive architectural regulations that must be followed. This, of course, increases construction costs; construction modifications to meet ASC requirements can go as high as $150,000 or more. It is best to use the expertise of a consultant to ensure that the proper steps are taken in complying with architectural regulations.

Costs

The two largest variable costs of running an ASC are personnel and medical supplies. Variable costs mean just that—they are variable and therefore can be negotiated. The two largest fixed costs in the operation of the ASC will be rent (or mortgage) and equipment. Fixed costs are set costs, and no amount of negotiating will change them.

"SIZING UP" THE PRACTICE

Before leaping into the world of ASCs, you must consider which of the following models the business will follow:

Model A:
- There are two to three physicians in the group.
- A minimum of 100 procedures are generated each month.
- The practice has a positive cash flow.
- There are 1,500 to 2,000 square feet available for a procedure room.

Model B:
- There are three to five physicians in the group.
- A minimum of 150 procedures are generated each month.
- The practice has a positive cash flow.
- The facility has two procedure rooms, each providing 2,000 square feet

Model C:
- There are at least five physicians in the group.
- A minimum of 200 procedures are generated each month.
- The practice has a positive cash flow.
- The facility has three procedure rooms, each providing 3,000 square feet.

The average cost of setting up an ASC, including development, construction, and operation, ranges between $250,000 and $500,000 per procedure room. In most states, a project will take 12 months from start to finish. In a few states with more stringent regulations, a project could take as long as 24 months. If the conditions in model A, model B, or model C cannot be met, it is not advisable to pursue the development of an ASC.

HIRE A CONSULTANT

It is a good idea to get help from professionals who have experience developing ASCs. The business plan can be completed before the consultant is hired; this is not difficult and will save the practice additional costs. However, if the practice feels incapable of developing a plan, it is always a good idea to seek the help of a consultant. Developing an ASC requires a high level of organizational and time management skills. Complying with licensing offices is just the tip of the iceberg. The following are other areas where consultants can help in this major undertaking:

- Design
- Evaluating equipment needed
- Obtaining a contractor
- Negotiating financial contracts
- Daily operations
- Negotiating contracts with third-party payers
- Recruiting professional personnel

Some consultants can help with all of these areas and can coordinate office personnel in daily, efficient operations once the project is completed. Some consultants provide ongoing facility management if needed. A consulting engagement that combines advice with a specific deliverable objective is referred to as *task orientation.* In other words, an architect might be consulted regarding the feasibility of an ASC's specific location. This same architect might be called on later to produce sketches and drawings of the proposed building. A broader consulting engagement, whereby the medical practice asks a consultant to address a variety of issues, is commonly referred to as a *comprehensive study.* The goals of this study are not always related; in fact, they usually are not. Most comprehensive studies are multi-issue studies.

For more information about ASCs, contact the American Association of Ambulatory Surgery Centers (AAASC).

This is the national association dedicated to advancing patient care through ASCs. Their Web site address is www.aaasc.org.

COST ANALYSIS OF ASC PROCEDURES

One of the most challenging projects an office manager will ever face is determining the cost of each procedure performed in the ASC. This analysis can be tedious, but its results are invaluable.

Start by making a list of all the items used for each procedure. Don't forget articles used for administering anesthetics (e.g., nasogastric tubes, syringes, and intravenous [IV] fluids). Now comes the "fun" part. Sit down and assign a cost to each item on the list. This is actually not a difficult task, because it can be accomplished simply by pulling invoices for medical supplies. For instance, if a bag of 10 nasal cannulas for oxygen costs $52.50, you know that the cost of each nasal cannula is $5.25. Do this with each item used in the procedure until a total item cost for the procedure is compiled.

Once you've tallied the total cost of supplies used in a procedure, it is time to figure out the cost of the personnel involved. This is an easy calculation. Take the monthly salary cost, including the cost of benefits, for all personnel and divide this figure by the number of procedures done that month. For instance, if the monthly total personnel costs were $12,466 and 74 procedures were performed that month, the personnel cost per procedure performed is $168.46. To find out if this cost is in line with personnel costs of other offices in the area, divide the monthly cost of the personnel net revenue for the month; for example, $12,466/$38,982 = 32%. Personnel costs generally run between 15% and 25% of each dollar made. Thus, in this example, personnel costs are running a little high.

Determine the total cost of supplies and personnel used for every procedure. By performing this calculation, you can assess the efficiency of the ASC and perhaps reevaluate what you're paying for supplies and personnel.

MANAGING THE ASC

For the successful operation of the ASC, you must wear the hats of the following managerial positions:

- Organizer
- Financial manager
- Facilities manager
- Human resources manager
- Director of patient services
- Director of operations

As the organizer, you must develop a system of organization that ensures quality patient care, productive use of the physicians' time, efficient use of personnel, and reduced costs. You must continually review daily operations for possible streamlining opportunities.

As the financial manager, you must be acutely aware of the financial operating systems of the facility. There must be a cash management policy; a system for collecting debt and managing accounts receivable; a continual audit of patient records to ensure accurate coding and billing; and, last but not least, a budget. This budget should provide the physician with such information as revenues and expenses, a cost analysis of services, and the projected costs of supplies and personnel. To perform your financial management duties effectively, you will need the following information:

- Income tax returns
- Information for income distribution
- Information for financial planning
- Information for decision making (e.g., staffing ratios, hours of operation)

This type of financial information is directly related to the control of the practice and is used for making practice growth decisions.

As the facilities manager, you are responsible for the physical operations of the facility. This is an essential role. Regular consideration must be given to expansion, redesign, and renovation of the current facility. Problems with parking, building access, and efficient patient flow require your attention. The need for replacement or additional equipment must also be assessed.

As the human resources manager, you must realize the importance of having highly trained and dedicated employees. Continuously evaluate the number of employees to ascertain whether the facility requires additional personnel or whether revision of job descriptions can eliminate unnecessary personnel. "Right-sizing" the staff will create more efficient use of the facility. Share your management philosophies with your staff and make sure the "vision" of the facility places employees in a positive environment. This role might also involve you in the procurement of physicians, nurse practitioners, physician assistants, and other skilled professionals. Physician recruitment can be aided by outside services that provide temporary or permanent physicians.

As the director of patient services, you are ultimately responsible for any function that involves patient care. The umbrella of patient services covers the following:

- Scheduling
- Patient referrals
- Ancillary services such as laboratory tests, x-ray examinations, ECGs, and physical therapy
- Patient education
- Medical records

Your role as director of operations involves you in the short- and long-term planning of the facility. You develop goals for the facility and make decisions regarding the facility in relationship to community needs. In the health care environment, preparing for the future is an important responsibility.

FACILITY DESIGN AND DEVELOPMENT

Designing and developing an ambulatory care facility requires much stamina and flexibility. You cannot appreciate the stress involved in such a project until you have been there. Before embarking on this project, find out your state's guidelines for the development of ASCs. Because health care regulations change so rapidly, it is imperative that you contact your state Department of Health for an up-to-date list of design requirements.

WHAT IS A CON?

Certificate of Need (CON) programs prevent rising health care costs and allow coordinated planning of new services and construction. Many states require a CON for Medicare certification of an ASC. The CON is a leftover from World War II when states imposed restrictions to minimize health care expenditures on facilities. In many states, these laws have not been updated and about 36 states retain some type of CON program. The basic belief of the CON is that facility overbuilding results in health care price inflation. When a facility has empty beds, the fixed costs must be met by charging more for the beds that are filled.

To be eligible to bill for a facility fee to Medicare, the ASC must be Medicare certified. This certification hinges on fulfilling the regulations of the following:

- The state
- Medicare
- The state fire marshal
- Federal life safety regulations

Even in states that do not require a CON, it is generally in the best interests of the practice to apply for a state license. States that do not require specific need criteria put the burden on the practice to show a need for an ASC. The following list contains states that have had the CON law repealed or there is not one in effect:

- Arizona
- California
- Colorado
- Idaho
- Indiana
- Kansas
- Minnesota
- New Mexico
- North Dakota
- Pennsylvania
- South Dakota
- Texas
- Utah
- Wyoming

For more information regarding CONs, the National Conference of State Legislature has a Web site that will provide valuable contact information: www.ncsl.org/public/leglinks.cfm

AMBULATORY CARE DOCUMENTATION AND FORMS

When developing an ASC, it is important to follow the documentation guidelines for each procedure performed. Generally, it is required that all medical records at an ASC contain the following forms:

- Consent for procedure
- History and physical form

Anesthesia records should contain the following:

- Consent for anesthesia
- Health history
- Anesthesia record
- Operative record
- Report of procedure
- Postprocedure instructions

These forms must be completely filled out, signed, and dated. Sample forms are provided in Figure 13-8.

URGENT CARE FACILITIES

Free-standing emergency centers have been popping up in every city to treat emergency ailments. These "Doc-in-a-Boxes" relieve hospitals of the burden of treating nonemergency patients who might otherwise go to the emergency department. They mainly provide primary care medicine with some additional emergency services, and are designed to handle the simple cuts, viral syndromes, and strains and sprains associated with daily community and family life. The increase in the number of urgent care facilities has taken some burden from hospital emergency departments, which provides shorter waiting periods and more treatment time for acutely ill or injured patients.

HOSPITALS

Physician practices and hospitals have shared resources for many years. From the information technology (IT) department to marketing, this bond is strong. Hospitals are well aware that physicians can send their patients to other hospitals and are therefore anxious to share their resources in an effort to maintain an ongoing relationship with each practice. If physicians provide quality care in a cost-effective way, many hospitals will seek them out. Physician practices in communities with more than one hospital find themselves in a very good position. The key to a good relationship with the hospital is for the physician and/or office manager to have a good relationship with the hospital leadership.

What Is a Hospital?

The oldest hospital in the United States, Pennsylvania Hospital, was founded in Philadelphia in 1756. A *hospital* is

1 I hereby authorize ______________________ and such assistants as may be selected by him or her to perform a special diagnostic procedure.

2 The procedure(s) necessary to treat/diagnose my condition (has, have) been explained to me by the physician and I understand it (them) to be:
Gastroscopy, Biopsy, or Heater Probe-passage of a flexible lighted instrument into the stomach, remove tissue/growth and cauterize blood vessels if needed.

3 It has been explained to me that during the course of the procedure, unforeseen conditions may be revealed that necessiate change or extension of the original procedure(s) or different procedure(s) than those already explained above. I therefore authorize and request that the above named physician and his or her assistants and designees perform such procedure(s) as are necessary and desirable in the exercise of his or her professional judgment. I understand that such conditions may cause a need for additonal surgery due to bleeding, perforation, or infection.

4 I have been made aware that there are risks and possible undesirable consequences associated with the treament and diagnosis of my illness, including (but not limied to) severe blood loss, bowel perforation, infection, heart complications, blood clots, or death, that are attendant to the performance of any surgical procedure and I understand these risks. I am aware that the practice of medicine and surgery is not an exact science, and I acknowledge that no quarantees have been made to me concerning the results of the operation, procedure, or treatment.

5 The items listed above have been explained to me by Dr. ______________________ , and I understand and consent to them.

____
(Witness)

______________________ ______________________
(Date) (Signature of patient/legal guardian)

FIGURE 13-8. **A,** Procedure Consent Form. (Courtesy of Gastrointestinal Specialists, Inc.)

defined as "an institution where the ill or injured may receive medical, surgical, or psychiatric treatment, nursing, food, and lodging during illness."

The American Hospital Association

The American Hospital Association (AHA) is the national organization that represents all types of hospitals, just as the American Medical Association (AMA) represents all specialties of physicians. There are approximately 5,000 hospitals and 37,000 individual members that are part of the AHA. This organization was founded in 1898 and provides educational programs and information on current issues and trends in health care. The Web site for this organization is www.aha.org. To search for a hospital in the United States, try "The Hospital Link" at www.hospitallink.com and "The American Hospital Directory" at www.ahd.com.

Hospital Classifications

Hospitals can be distinguished by a number of different attributes:

- Type of ownership (i.e., private or government)
- Type of problems they treat (e.g., tuberculosis, hypertension)
- Whether they play a role in physician education (i.e., teaching hospitals)
- Average length of stay (i.e., short term or long term)
- Type of medicine provided (i.e., medical or osteopathic)
- Size of the institution (i.e., number of beds)

HOSPITAL OWNERSHIP

There are three types of hospital ownership:

- Government or public
- Voluntary
- Proprietary

Government Ownership

Government ownership refers to hospitals owned by federal, state, or local governments. The following are examples of federally owned hospitals:

- Veterans Administration hospitals
- Military hospitals owned by the Department of Defense (e.g., Bethesda Naval Hospital in Bethesda, Maryland, and Walter Reed Army Hospital in Washington, D.C.)
- Federal prison hospitals, owned by the Department of Justice
- Hospitals owned by the Department of Health and Human Services (e.g., Gallup Indian Medical Center in Gallup, New Mexico, and St. Elizabeth's Hospital in Washington, D.C.)

The federal government operates military hospitals for the sole purpose of treating military personnel and their families. Some states operate a hospital system designed specifically to treat the mentally ill or mentally retarded. These hospitals are used by state residents who cannot afford care at another hospital. Some states also operate hospitals for the treatment of specific chronic illnesses,

Gastrointestinal Specialists, Inc,
History & Physical Form

Age: ________ Sex: ________ Race: ________ S.M.W.: ________

Allergies: ____

Purpose of procedure: ____

Chief complaint: ____

History of present illness: ____

Past medical history: ____

Review of symptoms: ____

Family & social history: ____

Date: ____________________________

Physical Examination:

TPR: ____________ BP: ____________ Weight: ____________

Diagnosis: ____

Signature: ____

FIGURE 13-8. **B,** History and Physical Form. (Courtesy of Gastrointestinal Specialists, Inc.)

such as tuberculosis. Other state-owned facilities are state university medical school hospitals and state prison hospitals.

Voluntary Ownership

Voluntary ownership refers to private, nonprofit ownership of a hospital. The following are examples of voluntary hospitals:

- Hospitals owned by churches (e.g., the Sisters of Mercy hospitals owned by the Roman Catholic Church)
- Shriner's hospitals
- Health maintenance organization (HMO) hospitals (e.g., Kaiser-Permanente Hospital)

Proprietary Ownership

Proprietary ownership refers to private, for-profit ownership of a hospital. Proprietary owners of hospitals range from corporations to individuals.

TYPES OF HOSPITALS

Teaching Hospitals

A teaching hospital has a physician residency training program. It has an agreement with a medical school to

R&P Anesthesia Associates
Important Information—Please Read

B. Paul Stewart, CRNA, B.A.
Ronald Burkitt, CRNA

For your comfort and safety, your surgeon has requested a Certified Registered Nurse Anesthetist to be with you during your surgery to administer the necessary medications and monitor your vital signs. The anesthetist will meet with you the morning of surgery, review your history, and ask you questions about your medical health in order to select the appropriate anesthetic for you and the procedure you are about to undergo. He or she will also answer any question you may have.

In the office operating suite there are generally two types of anesthesia which may be utilized. They are as follows:

1 Local anesthesia with IV sedation—This is the most common anesthesia in the office operating suite, and can be related to "twilight" sleep, wherein you are given a combination of medications that will make you very comfortable and will be generally unaware of what is happening. For example, patients are usually able to respond if spoken to, but will be asleep during the procecdure.
2 General anesthesia—In this instance, patients will be completely asleep. In some cases, when it is necessary to change the position of the patient, it will be necessary to place an endotracheal tube in the trachea (windpipe) to control the breathing.

In each case, the heart rate, blood pressure, electrocardiogram, arterial oxygen saturation, and respirations will be closely and continuously monitored by the anesthetist.

The anesthetist will remain with you throughout the procedure. After a suitable period of time, depending on the individual, you will be allowed to leave the facility in the company of a responsible adult. You will probably be sleepy and find that you will sleep for several hours after you return home. It is vitally important that you arrange to have someone with you for 24 hours after your surgery to help you to and from the bathroom, prepare liquids or soft foods for you to eat, assist with ice packs if ordered, and make sure you take your medications as they have been prescibed. You should not undertake any responsible activity, make any important decisions, or drive a car for a minimum of 24 hours after your surgery.

You may experience some mild nausea, sore throat, redness or bruising at the intravenous site, and a generalized feeling of being "washed out" for several days. Persistent or severe nause and vomiting, bleeding, or severe swelling should be reported to the doctor immediately.

You should understand there is always a slight risk when you undergo surgery and anesthesia, and results cannot be guaranteed. If you have any further questions before the anesthetist meets with you, please do not hesitate to call Paul Stewart or Ron Burkitt, at the above telephone numbers.

AUTHORIZATION FOR ANESTHESIA

I hereby authorize and request R&P ANESTHESIA ASSOCIATES to administer the necessary anesthetics to ____________________

(name) that in their opinion, may be deemed appropriate for the surgical procedure to be performed by Dr. ____________________

(physican's name) on (date) __________________

I certify that the nature of the anesthetic procedures, including risks and possible complications, have been explained to me and that I understand the purpose of this authorization form.

____

Date Signature

____

Date Witnesss

FIGURE 13-8. C, Anesthesia Consent Form. (Courtesy of R&P Anesthesia Assoc.)

provide student physicians the clinical experience needed to complete their degrees. Teaching hospitals also provide clinical experience for nurses and allied health personnel.

Community Hospitals

A community hospital has a very broad definition. A community hospital serves a particular locality and/or is open to anyone, as opposed to being open only to particular patient groups. Community hospitals are generally nonteaching hospitals. A community hospital may take the name of the town or locale in which it is located, such as Monroe County General Hospital, Doylestown Hospital, and Suburban General Hospital (Figure 13-9).

Osteopathic Hospitals

Osteopathic hospitals were started for the sole purpose of allowing osteopathic physicians to treat and hospitalize patients. Now osteopathic hospitals have a mixed staff (i.e., both medical and osteopathic physicians). An osteopathic physician is one who is trained in osteopathy, a

R&P Anesthesia Associates
HEALTH HISTORY

Name of patient: ________________________________

Date of birth: ______________________ Sex: M F Height: ____________________ Weight: _______________

1 Are you allergic to any medication? Yes No. If yes, please list.

2 Are you taking any medications? Yes No. If yes, please list, and include over-the-counter preparations such as aspirin or antihistamines.

3 Do you smoke? Yes No. If yes, how many packs per day?

4 Do you drink alcohol? Yes No. If yes, how much?

5 Do you or have you ever used recreational drugs? Yes No. If yes, when was the last time? Such as: marijuana, cocaine

6 Do you have a history of any of the following?

Asthma	Yes	No	Hiatal hernia	Yes	No
Bronchitis	Yes	No	Diabetes	Yes	No
High blood pressure	Yes	No	Seizures	Yes	No
Liver problems (hepatitis, mono)	Yes	No	Cancer	Yes	No
Kidney problems	Yes	No	Thyroid problems	Yes	No
Rheumatic fever	Yes	No	Arthritis	Yes	No
Bleeding problems	Yes	No	Anemia	Yes	No
Ulcers	Yes	No	Fainting spells	Yes	No
Heart problems or murmurs	Yes	No	Glaucoma	Yes	No

7 Have you ever had any surgery? If so, please explain.

____

____

8 Have you or any member of your immediate family had any problems with anesthesia? If so, please explain.

____

____

9 Is there a chance you might be pregnant?

10 Are you under the care of a physician? If so, please list name and address:

____

____

11 How would you describe your present health? Excellent Good Fair

12 Have you ever had a blood transfusion? Yes No

13 Do you have any dentures, partial plates, or capped teeth? Yes No

14 Are you bothered by motion sickness? Yes No

FIGURE 13-8. D, Anesthesia Health History Form. (Courtesy of R&P Anesthesia Assoc.)

Anesthesia Record Page

Operation ______________________________

____

Diagnosis ______________________________

Anesthestist ______________________________

Surgeon ______________________________

Date __________ Time X Started __________ Time X Finished __________ P.S. 1 2 3 4 5 E Allergies __________

Pre-anesthetic med. & time ____________________

or consent: ☐ Patient identified ☐ Premed. effect

Medications:

H/H 1

Weight:
Height:
Est. bld. vol.
Meal:
Monitor: B.P.
EEG Temp.

Preparation
I.V.
C.V.P.
Art.
L.P.
H.R. Resp. O_2
EKG

TIME														
O_2 L/min. (FIO_2)														
E.K.G.														
%SAO_2														
$ETCO_2$														

Maintenance:
Equipment ☐
Airway: Nat. O.P. N.P. Mask
Intub: OT N.T. Trach
Trauma:

Symbols
: BP
• HR
Respiration
○ Spont
Ø Assist
⊗ Control
◑ Mech
△ Temp
x Start anes
• Start surg
⊗ End surg
⊗ End anes
◐ To RR
VE
Position
Index

°C-220
38-200
36-180
34-160
32-140
120
100
80
60
40
20
00

FIGURE 13-8. E, Anesthesia Record. (Courtesy of R&P Anesthesia Assoc.)

Urine output	ml	Other fluids
Meas bld loss		
E.S.T. Bld loss	ml	Total blood loss
Replacement	ml	ml
	ml	Total blood repl
I.V. Fluids	ml	ml
	ml	**Total fluids**
	ml	

Agents	To R.R. ICU/PCU Room
Conc/dose	CNS: Awake, Sleepy, Respon, Unconsc; Airway: Nat, OP/NP, Intub, Trach; Resp: Spont, Assist, APNFIC
Tech/route	
	BP Pulse

FIGURE 13-8 (CONTINUED)

medical discipline founded by Andrew Taylor Still that is based on the theory that the body is capable of remedying itself when its structure is normal. Practitioners of this discipline use the same medicinal, physical, and surgical methods of diagnosis and treatment that medical physicians use, while maintaining the importance of normal body mechanics and manipulation. As seen in Figure 13-9, Suburban General Hospital is not only a community hospital, but an osteopathic hospital as well.

Specialty Hospitals

Specialty hospitals provide care only for patients with a particular type of disease (e.g., tuberculosis, orthopedic disease, or ophthalmologic disease). An example of a specialty hospital is the National Hospital for Orthopedics and Rehabilitation, located in Arlington, Virginia.

Medical Centers

Medical centers consist of either one or several hospitals that have come together as a complex in a geographic area. Medical centers are often associated with a medical school or university. They are generally known for their expertise in certain types of medical care, such as pediatric care or urgent care.

Tertiary Care Hospitals

Tertiary care hospitals are mainly university hospitals and work with the most complex patients. Many of their clientele are referred by other hospitals for special care. Examples of this type of hospital are the University of Pennsylvania and the University of Pittsburgh.

Private Hospitals

A private hospital is owned by an individual, a group of individuals, or a corporation. Examples of private hospitals are as follows:

- USA Medical Center (Alabama)
- Shriner's Hospital (Pennsylvania)
- Betty Ford Center (California)

Private hospitals are becoming increasingly popular as various HMOs and religious groups get involved in health care. Some private hospitals are owned by corporations for the care of their employees.

A private hospital may have for-profit or nonprofit ownership. A nonprofit, or voluntary, hospital is formed for the purpose of providing hospital care to members of a group or community. A for-profit hospital is owned by a physician, group of physicians, or corporation for the care of its patients.

General Hospitals

The general hospital is the most common type of hospital and accounts for the most admissions. A general hospital is run by a board of governors, which generally has 5 to 15 members. This board is divided into committees, such as the executive committee, the finance committee, and the fundraising committee. One of the functions of the executive committee is to approve physician appointments to the staff. The hospital administrator is appointed by the executive committee and is responsible for appointing

Patient identified: ______________________________

Diagnosis: ______________________________

Significant medical/surgical history: ______________________________

Allergies: ____________ Glaucoma: ____________ Pacemaker: ____________

Diabetes: ____________ Dentures: ____________ Heart disease: ____________

Current medications: ______________________________

Site of heplock or IV started: ______________________________

Procedure: ____________ Site of cautery return pad: ____________

Instrument used: ____________ Condition of return pad site: ____________

	Medication dosage, Route	To be given		Signature
		Date	Time	Title
Start procedure: ____________				
Finish procedure: ____________				
Time of discharge: ____________				
Accompanied by: ____________				
Mode of transportation: ____________				

Specimens: Pathology: ______________________________

Cytology: ____________ Microbiology: ____________

Time	Vital signs	Nurse's notes

Date: ______________________________

Signature: ______________________________

Nurse: ______________________________

FIGURE 13-8. **F,** Procedure form.

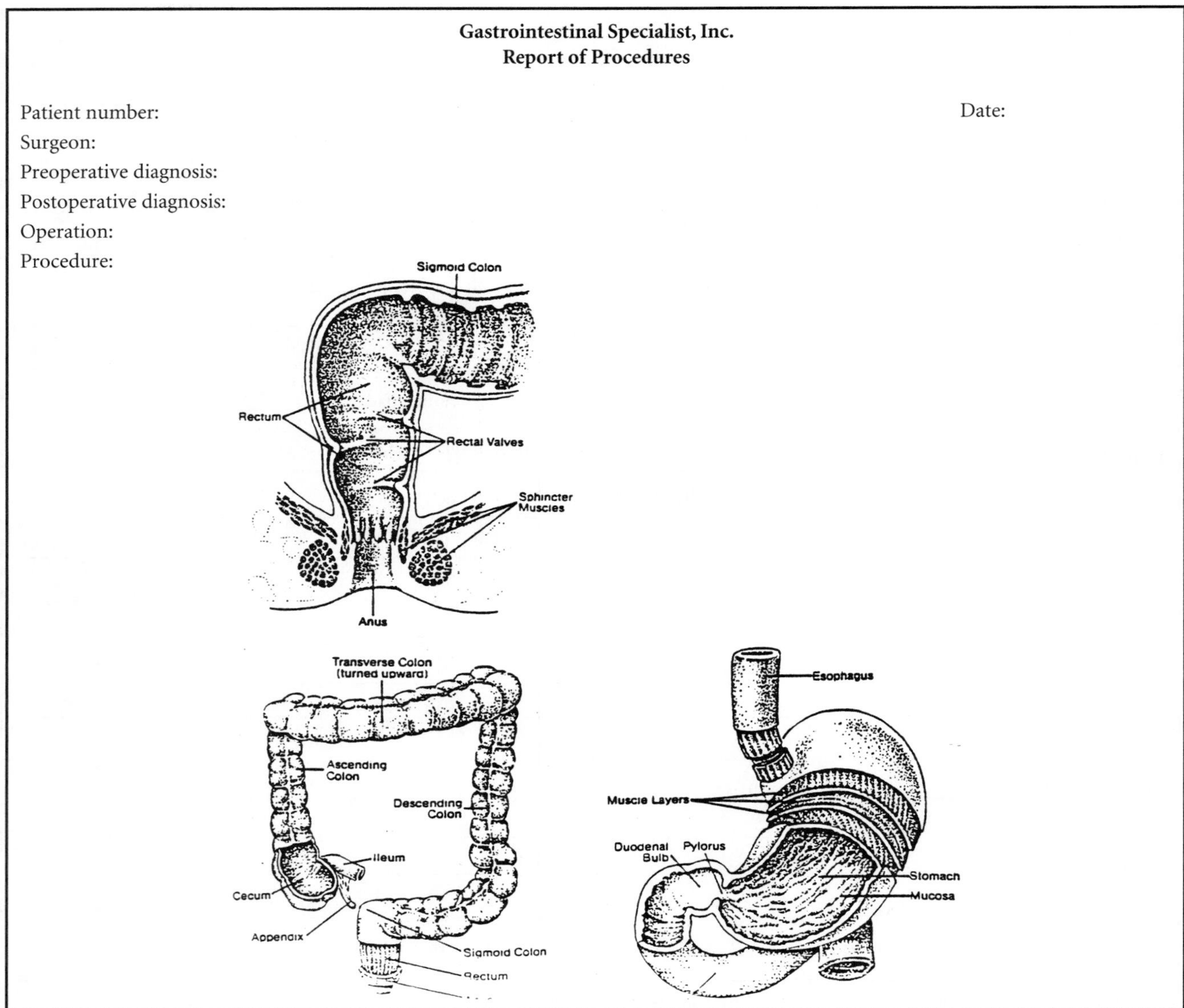

Gastrointestinal Specialist, Inc.
Report of Procedures

Patient number: Date:
Surgeon:
Preoperative diagnosis:
Postoperative diagnosis:
Operation:
Procedure:

FIGURE 13-8. **G,** Report of Procedure.

Postprocedure Instructions for Gastroscopy

1. You may not eat for 20 minutes after the procedure.
2. You may not drive for 6 hours after the procedure.
3. You may be drowsy. Do not operate any dangerous machinery or lift any heavy object.
4. If you have a sore throat, you may use a throat lozenge or cough drop.
5. Report to us if you develop a fever, chest or abdominal pain, or black or bloody stools.
6. If you have any questions or problems, do not hesitate to call our office at 555-9700.

FIGURE 13-8. **H,** Postprocedure Instructions. (Courtesy of Gastrointestinal Specialists, Inc.)

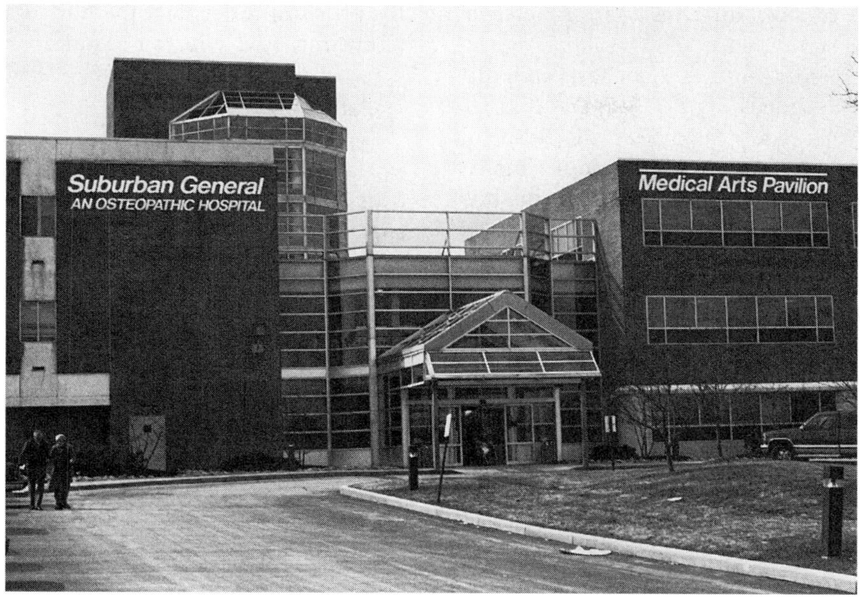

FIGURE 13-9. A community hospital in the suburbs of Philadelphia, Pennsylvania.

department heads. The components of a general hospital are as follows:

- Medical staff
- Nursing services
- Medical departments
- Support services
- Administrative services

Internal Structure of the Hospital

A hospital's governing body is the board of trustees, which is made up of approximately 20 members. They meet once a month, abide by their own bylaws, and elect their own officers. The board is divided into various committees, one of which is the executive committee. The executive committee is responsible for appointing the hospital administrator, physicians, and other health care professionals to the medical staff.

MEDICAL STAFF

The medical staff consists of physicians, dentists, podiatrists, psychologists, and physician extenders. A medical staff may be open or closed. When it is open, any physician can apply and, after approval, be admitted to the staff. When it is closed, the hospital is not allowing new physicians on staff at that time.

Several types of hospital staff membership are open to physicians. When you are recredentialing the physician, it is important to know in what capacity he or she wants to be on staff. The following categories are available:

- Active staff—regular membership
- Associate staff—physicians who are new on the staff or who do not want admitting privileges
- Consulting staff—physicians who are allowed to consult but cannot admit
- Courtesy staff—physicians who are allowed to use the hospital only on occasion
- Emeritus—physicians who are retired from the active staff
- House staff—residents
- Honorary staff—physicians of distinction who are not regularly involved in the hospital

Hospital bylaws govern each category. It is important to be aware of the rules and regulations associated with each type of staff membership so that the physician complies with them. Failure to comply can lead to termination of staff privileges.

The medical staff has an elected president, vice president, secretary, and treasurer. It is also represented by the following committees:

- Executive committee
- Utilization review committee
- Credentials committee
- Tissue committee
- Medical records committee
- Pharmacy committee
- Infection committee

The *executive committee,* which is made up of the various chiefs of service medicine (e.g., surgery, anesthesia), makes decisions regarding the medical staff and hospital.

The *utilization review committee* reviews all charts to establish the validity of hospital admissions.

The *credentials committee* consists of appointed staff physicians who review the applications of all current and new physicians for membership.

The *tissue committee* reviews surgeons' performance by checking specimens submitted.

The *medical records committee* ensures that charts are properly documented and signed.

The *pharmacy committee* regularly reviews the hospital's drug formulary. Changes are made at various times to update the types of pharmaceuticals carried in the hospital pharmacy.

The *infection committee* reviews all diagnoses of contagious diseases among patients and monitors the hospital's infection control procedures.

DEPARTMENT AND OFFICE INTERACTION

The hospital is organized into different departments that function together to provide the highest quality of care for patients. Typically, these departments are as follows:

- Nursing
- Medicine
- Surgery
- Pathology
- Radiology
- Physical therapy
- Anesthesiology
- Dietary
- Medical records
- Human resources
- Social services
- Central supply
- Housekeeping
- Physical plant operations
- Security
- Emergency medicine

Nursing Department

The nursing department is the largest department in the hospital. The medical office deals directly with floor nurses when the physician has patients in the hospital. Nurses can be found not only on the floors, or units, of the hospital, but also in operating room suites, recovery rooms, nurseries, delivery rooms, cardiac rehabilitation areas, and wellness units. The chain of command in the nursing department is as follows:

1. Director of nursing
2. Nursing supervisor
3. Head nurse/department head
4. Registered nurse
5. Licensed practical nurse
6. Nurse's aid
7. Unit clerk

The medical office will most likely have relationships with the registered nurses, licensed practical nurses, and unit clerks. If the office or physician has an unresolved problem with any of the nursing staff, it is appropriate for you or the physician to contact the nursing supervisor or director of nursing. Problems can be quickly resolved at this point.

Pathology Department

Another department important to the medical office is the pathology department. This is the department that performs tests on patients' blood, urine, and various tissues. This department is also responsible for performing autopsies (as discussed in Chapter 9). The pathology department is generally divided into subdepartments. The medical office commonly interacts with the following subdepartments:

- Chemistry
- Hematology
- Bacteriology/microbiology
- Cytology/histology
- Blood bank
- Immunology

The *chemistry department* analyzes blood for abnormalities involving the liver, pancreas, heart, kidney, thyroid, muscle, gallbladder, and so on. A chemistry analyzer performs all of these tests on one small sample of blood or serum.

The *hematology department* analyzes blood for abnormalities and anemias.

The *bacteriology/microbiology department* analyzes bacteria and their growth.

The *cytology/histology department* prepares tissue samples and bodily fluids for analysis of cell changes.

The *blood bank* maintains blood and blood products for patients who need transfusions.

The *immunology department* evaluates the function and structure of the immune system.

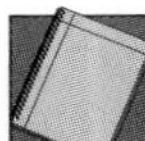

FROM THE EXPERT'S NOTEBOOK

Always have a professional contact in the laboratory and radiology departments. This contact may come in handy when you must schedule a patient for a test on a day on which there is no opening. It is easier to ask favors if you have already cultivated a relationship with someone in that department. It is nice to treat your contacts to lunch once in a while to show that you appreciate their help.

Radiology Department

The radiology department is another department that interacts closely with the medical office. This department performs x-ray studies of various parts of the human body. It reports such abnormalities as fractures, dislocations, masses, organ enlargements, ulcers, and any other abnormality seen on x-ray film.

Physical Therapy Department

The physical therapy department helps patients rehabilitate from both injury and illness. These very gifted people patiently help disabled patients relearn walking, talking, and other motor skills. Patients who have suffered a stroke or who have been in an automobile accident are referred to this department. Even patients with chronic back pain can benefit from services such as hot packs, cold packs, and massage.

Anesthesiology Department

The anesthesiology department maintains patients under anesthesia during minor and major operations. They may also be involved in pain relief management (e.g., nerve blocks) for patients who require treatment.

Personal Patient Services

A variety of personal services are available to patients in today's hospitals. Hospitals have become as service oriented as hotels! They understand that if they do not provide these services, patients will schedule their testing and hospitalizations at other facilities that do. Hospitals now commonly provide the following personal services:

- Pastoral care
- Communication services
- Hair care
- Automatic teller machines
- Gift shops
- Newspapers and book carts
- Televisions
- Notary public services
- Meals for visitors
- Valet parking
- Coffee and donuts in outpatient waiting areas
- Transportation
- Voice-to-voice communication system for patients living alone
- Pet therapy
- Community health education
- Sibling visitation

Hospital Accreditation

Every hospital must meet certain standards set forth by a professional association. The major accrediting body for hospitals is the Joint Commission on Accreditation of Healthcare Organizations (JCAHO). In 1917, the Third Clinical Congress of Surgeons of North America decided that a system of standardization of hospital equipment and wards was needed. However, it was not until 1951 that JCAHO was formed by the American College of Surgeons, American College of Physicians, American Hospital Association, American Medical Association, and Canadian Medical Association. The Canadians withdrew in 1959 and formed their own association.

JCAHO develops standards and provides advice to hospitals about meeting them. It also accredits long-term nursing care facilities, psychiatric facilities, and ambulatory care facilities. Many insurance plans will not provide reimbursement to facilities that are not JCAHO accredited. Educational grants and federal funding also hinge on this accreditation. Because of this agency, your office might occasionally receive panicky phone calls from a person in the hospital's medical records department asking that the physician finish his or her hospital charts because the hospital is being inspected the following day. This inspection is critical to the operations of the hospital.

Hospital Bills

Just as patients become confused with physician billing, patients are really confused when they receive page after page of hospital bill. Some of the entries on a hospital bill are self-explanatory, such as aspirin, "325 mg tablet." Other entries, such as "pathology—fungus smear" and "telemetry—semi," can be very confusing, leaving patients wondering if they really did receive all these things. According to The Patient's Advocate, a South Bend Indiana firm, 90% of all hospital bills have errors of some kind. Personnel at the medical practice may find themselves helping their patients who may not understand these bills. It may be necessary to look the bills over line-by-line to help the patients to understand. There is also a company called Medical Billing Advocates of America (www.billadvocates.com) that can help; however, there is a fee for this service.

Diagnosis-Related Groups

In 1980, a system of prospective reimbursement for hospital services based on diagnosis-related groups (DRGs) began to be used by the state of New Jersey. This system was used by all payers—Medicare, Medicaid, Blue Cross, and all other insurance plans. In 1983, this system was phased in nationwide under the Social Security Amendments of 1983. In this system, payment for care is fixed at a certain amount, regardless of whether the actual costs of care are over or below that amount. Each DRG is given a relative cost weight by which the dollar amount to be paid is determined, based on national cost averages. In other words, if Mrs. Smith is in the hospital for 5 days with pneumococcal pneumonia and Mr. Comer is confined for 7 days with the same ailment, both bills would be paid at the same rate, regardless of the number of days hospitalized. On April 12, 2006, CMS issued the hospital inpatient prospective system (IPPS) rule for fiscal year 2007, which proposed that a consolidated severity DRG system be adopted for fiscal year 2008.

Professional Standards Review Organizations

Hospital Professional Standards Review Organizations (PSROs) were mandated by the Social Security Amendments of 1972. The PSRO was to be an association of physicians who reviewed professional and institutional services covered by Medicare and Medicaid programs. It was intended to monitor both the cost and quality of care. Hospitals delegated their PSRO review functions to their utilization review committees. Because their effectiveness was not clear, PSROs were replaced in 1982 by Peer Review Organizations (PROs).

Peer Review Organizations

The Tax Equity and Fiscal Responsibility Act of 1982 led to the creation of PROs to regularly review the cost and quality of Medicare services. There were 54 PRO regions designated: one for each state, the District of Columbia, Puerto Rico, the Virgin Islands, and the Pacific territories. The major differences between PSROs and PROs are that PROs are statewide and their activities are carried out under performance-based contracts with the U.S. Department of Health and Human Services.

Physician-Hospital Relationship

The practice of medicine has changed a great deal in the last two decades. A climate of curtailed inpatient admissions and reimbursements is driving individual physician practices into extinction, and making it imperative for group medical practices and hospitals to rely on each other if they wish to thrive. Managed care policies are forcing the formation of key alliances between hospitals and clinics, between group medical practices and ambulatory surgical centers, and between HMOs and clinics. The rise of managed care has made patient satisfaction the shared goal of hospitals and medical practices. Both are striving to deliver quality care to each patient, increase patient safety and comfort, and improve the accuracy of diagnosis and treatment.

Hospitals and physicians are forming groups to negotiate better contracts with managed care companies. Hospitals are involving their medical staff in strategic decision making and are finding ways to accommodate the practical needs of physicians, including providing support for outpatient facilities.

Physicians who admit a higher number of patients wield more power than do physicians with minimal hospital admissions. They are better known by the hospital staff and their business is valuable enough to protect.

Most hospitals have a speaker's bureau that is used to market the hospital. Physicians can benefit from this goodwill by expressing intent to speak. The exposure for the physician practice can be great, and there may also be a mailing list of participants that the practice may obtain for its marketing efforts. The practice will receive "back-door" marketing through the hospital's promotion of these speeches.

EXERCISES

MULTIPLE CHOICE

Choose the best *answer for each of the following questions.*

1. Which of the following is *not* a type of hospital?
   a. Community
   b. Executive
   c. Tertiary
   d. Osteopathic
2. The accrediting body for a hospital is
   a. AHA
   b. JCAHO
   c. AMA
   d. VHA
3. ASC stands for
   a. Ambulatory surgery clinic
   b. Association of Surgery Centers
   c. Ambulatory surgery center
   d. Associated Surgery Clinics
4. The medical office does *not* interact with which hospital department?
   a. Central supply
   b. Laboratory
   c. Radiology
   d. Surgery
5. The regulations that must be followed for a CON are
   a. The state
   b. Medicare
   c. Fire marshal
   d. All of the above
6. The hospital's governing body is the
   a. Governing board
   b. Medical staff
   c. Administrative board
   d. Board of trustees
7. In an ASC, the facility fee covers
   a. Physician services
   b. Anesthesia supplies
   c. Ambulance service
   d. Braces
8. The ASC final rule allows for a transition period of
   a. 5 years
   b. 7 years
   c. 4 years
   d. 10 years
9. A strep test is what type of test?
   a. Preadmission
   b. Monitoring
   c. Screening
   d. Confirmatory

10. Which is *not* a POL certification?
    a. Minimal
    b. Moderate
    c. High
    d. Waived

TRUE OR FALSE

1. _____ The "CON" requirement is different from state to state.
2. _____ "POL" stands for "physician outpatient laboratory."
3. _____ Defensive medicine is the main reason for an increase in outpatient studies.
4. _____ A test containing the wording "physician-performed microscopy" means that only the physician can perform that test.
5. _____ Stat testing means that the test must be run when the patient is fasting.
6. _____ Consultants are often used in the development of an ASC.
7. _____ The executive committee of a hospital comprises leaders in the community.
8. _____ "Physical plant operations" is a department in the hospital.
9. _____ "DRGs" are used to reimburse the hospital for services rendered.
10. _____ A proprietary hospital is a private, for-profit hospital.

THINKERS

1. What are the steps that should be taken before committing to an ASC?
2. Describe the function of the executive committee.
3. What are the different attributes of hospitals?

REFERENCES

American Institute of Architects: *Guidelines for Design and Construction of Hospital and Health Care Facilities.* Washington, DC: AIA, 2001.

American Society of Internal Medicine. *Assuring Appropriate Access to Laboratory Testing for Patients in Managed Health Care Plans.* Philadelphia: ASIM, 2000.

Federal Register, CFR 42, 493.15(b), (c).

Federal Register, CFR 42, Volume Three, Parts 430.

Federal Register, CFR 42, 493.19.

Kobus, R.L., et al. *Building Type Basics for Healthcare Facilities.* New York: John Wiley & Sons, 2000.

MaGuire, N. *Part B Answer Book.* Rockville, MD: Part B News Group, 2002.

Malkin, J. *Medical and Dental Space Planning: A Comprehensive Guide to Design, Equipment, and Clinical Procedures,* 3rd edition. New York: John Wiley & Sons, 2002.

Miller, R., & Swensson, E. *Hospital and Healthcare Facility Design,* 2nd edition. New York: W.W. Norton, 2002.

Pozgar, G. *Legal Aspects of Health Care Administration,* 8th edition. Rockville, MD: Aspen, 2001.

Ross, A., Williams, S., & Schafer, E. *Ambulatory Care Management,* 3rd edition. Albany, NY: Delmar Publishers, 1998.

Speirs, L., Hicks, A., & Heppes, R. *Complete Guide to Part B Billing and Compliance.* Reston, VA: Ingenix, St. Anthony Publishing, 2002.

14

THE FINANCIAL SIDE

CHAPTER OUTLINE

CHAPTER OBJECTIVES

After completing this chapter, you will be able to do the following:

- Understand accounting basics
- Comprehend why financial statements are necessary and know how to read them
- Draw conclusions from financial ratios
- Discuss the purpose of cost analysis
- Know what to look for in choosing an accountant
- Understand banking practices
- Differentiate the types of bank accounts
- Identify the component parts of a check
- Understand how checks and endorsements are used
- Know how to prepare a deposit slip
- Understand the purpose of petty cash

INTRODUCTION TO ACCOUNTING

Fra Luca Pacioli, a scholar, mathematician, and Franciscan monk who lived in the fifteenth century, is known as the "Father of Accounting." He is credited as being the first to use the double-entry bookkeeping method (which had already been in use among Italian merchants for two centuries). The double-entry model has become the standard for accounting in the Western world.

Simply put, accounting is the art of interpreting, measuring, and describing economic activity. It is the system used to monitor the finances of a business. It is called the "language of business." We live in a time of accountability; a time of multinational corporations, banks, buyouts, and the growing realization that health care is a business. The purpose of accounting is to provide reliable financial information about an economic entity, such as a medical office.

An accounting system must be developed and implemented to communicate financial information. An accounting system consists of methods, procedures, and devices a business uses to keep track of its financial activities and to summarize them in an effort to make decisions. Three basic steps must be included in any accounting system: recording, classifying, and summarizing. Recording the daily office activities in terms of money is the first step. Any transactions that can be expressed in monetary terms must be entered into the accounting record. Classifying data into related groups or categories of transactions should be the second step. Summarizing the data in these categories is the third step in the process.

Cost accounting determines what it costs the medical office to perform a particular service. For example, the office manager should know what it costs the office to perform an x-ray examination. Cost accounting is valuable for understanding procedure costs, as well as patient office visit costs and hospital visit costs. It is often used to evaluate whether to participate in insurance plans. Knowing the cost of seeing a patient allows you to determine whether an insurance plan's reimbursement justifies your participation.

EARNED INCOME REPORTING SYSTEMS

Two systems are used for reporting earned income in a practice:

- Accrual basis
- Cash basis

The most common reporting system used in medical practices is cash basis. This method recognizes the cash when it is collected, as opposed to the accrual basis, where cash is realized at the time the charge takes place. Accrual basis accounting recognizes revenues when both conditions are met:

1. Revenue is earned
2. Revenue is realized

Revenue is earned when products are delivered or services are provided. Realized means cash is received. Cash basis accounting recognizes revenue when it is received.

FINANCIAL STATEMENTS

Two Major Financial Statements: The Balance Sheet and Income/Expense Statement

The financial statements of the practice should identify the amount of revenue of the practice, the amount of money that is owed to the practice, and the expenses that were incurred by the practice. The two financial statements most commonly used in a medical practice are the balance sheet and the income/expense statement.

BALANCE SHEET

A balance sheet is a financial statement showing the assets, liabilities, and owner's equity (also called capital) of the medical practice on a particular day. This information changes each time a transaction takes place. Assets are the economic resources owned by the practice, liabilities are the debts or financial obligations, and owner's equity is the owner's residual interest in the practice.

A ledger account is a device for recording increases or decreases in one financial statement item, such as a particular asset, a liability, or owner's equity. A ledger is an accounting record that includes ledger accounts for all items included in the practice's financial statements. A sample balance sheet is illustrated in Figure 14-1.

It is important to understand the differences between debits and credits:

- Increases in assets are recorded as debits.
- Decreases in assets are credits.
- Decreases in liabilities and owner's equity are recorded as debits.
- Increases in liabilities and owner's equity are recorded as credits.

Debit and credit rules are related to an account's location in the balance sheet. If the account appears on the left side of the balance sheet (assets), increases in the account balance are recorded by left-side entries (debits). If the account appears on the right side of the balance sheet (liabilities and owner's equity), increases are recorded by right-side entries. Every transaction is recorded by two sets of entries, hence the system is called the *double-entry system of accounting.* Debit and credit entries to one or more accounts make up this system. In recording any transaction,

NEALON MEDICAL PRACTICE, INC. Balance Sheet: December 31, 2008	
ASSETS	
Current Assets:	
Cash	$ 10,000
Other current assets	5,000
Total current assets	15,000
Equipment (net of accumulated depreciation of $5,000):	75,000
Total:	$ 90,000
LIABILITIES AND OWNER'S EQUITY	
Current Liabilities:	
Line of credit payable	$ 11,000
Current maturities of long-term debt	17,000
Retirement plan contributions payable	3,000
Total current liabilities	31,000
Long-Term Debt:	58,000
Total liabilities	89,000
Owner's Equity:	
Retained earnings	1,000
Total:	$ 90,000

FIGURE 14-1. Sample balance sheet. (Courtesy of Parente Randolph, LLC.)

NEALON MEDICAL PRACTICE, INC. Statement of Income and Expenses and Retained Earnings For the Year Ended December 31, 2008	
Revenues:	
Patient fees collected, net of refunds	$ 329,000
Other income	800
Interest income	200
Total revenues	330,000
Overhead Expenses:	157,000
Profit before Physicians' Expenses:	173,000
Physicians' Expenses:	
Salaries	125,000
Retirement plan contributions	22,500
Auto	8,000
Payroll taxes	7,000
Medical insurance	6,000
Travel	2,000
Meals and entertainment	1,500
Total physicians' expenses	172,000
Cumulative Profit This Year:	1,000
Retained Earnings, Beginning:	
Retained Earnings, Ending	$ 1,000

FIGURE 14-2. Sample statement of income and expenses. (Courtesy of Parente Randolph, LLC.)

the total dollar amount of debit entries must equal the total dollar amount of credit entries.

Journal entries must be made to record common business transactions. Each journal entry should include the following information:

1. Date of the transaction
2. Names of the ledger accounts affected
3. Dollar amounts of the changes in these accounts
4. Brief explanation of the transaction

INCOME/EXPENSE STATEMENT

The income/expense statement typically shows collected patient fees, paid overhead expenses, and year-end cumulative profit. It also provides total expenses paid for benefits. A sample statement can be seen in Figure 14-2; Figure 14-3 shows itemized overhead expenses.

By using this format, the office can track expenditures and easily spot trends. Other overhead expenditures that might be added to this statement are as follows:

- Equipment and improvements
- Employee benefits
- Employee retirement contributions
- Equipment lease payments
- Equipment repairs
- Office cleaning

The income/expense statement provides the following summary data:

- Total revenues
- Total overhead expenses
- Total physicians' expenses
- Cumulative profit

How to Read a Statement of Retained Earnings

If the income/expense statement reveals the office's cash inflows and outflows during a period, and the balance sheet shows a picture of the office's assets and liabilities on the ending date of that period, shouldn't this information reflect the financial health of the practice? It does. Net income for the period is added to an equity account called *retained earnings* to show that profits are reinvested into the company. Any profits paid to physician owners as dividends reduce retained earnings. Although this account reflects reinvested earnings, it does not represent cash. It is possible for an office with a growing clientele to experience financial problems. This is one reason why the office manager should have an understanding of cash flow mechanics. A *cash flow statement,* also called a *statement of income and expenses and retained earnings,* is commonly shown as a continuation of the income/expense statement. A sample cash flow statement can be seen in Figure 14-4.

NEALON MEDICAL PRACTICE, INC. Schedule of Overhead Expenses For the Year Ended December 31, 2008	
Personnel:	
Salaries and wages	$ 50,000
Retirement plan contributions	9,000
Employee benefits	8,000
Payroll taxes	5,000
Total personnel expenses	72,000
Other Overhead Expenses:	
Collection Fees	13,000
Medical Supplies	12,700
Rent	12,000
Malpractice insurance	10,000
Office supplies	7,000
Depreciation	5,000
Telephone, pagers, and answering service	5,000
Interest	3,500
Accounting and legal	3,000
Equipment lease	3,000
Cleaning	2,000
Utilities	1,600
Licenses and taxes	1,300
Insurance	1,200
Professional education	1,200
Advertising	1,000
Maintenance	800
Travel	600
Dues and subscriptions	500
Meals and entertainment	300
Equipment repairs	200
Miscellaneous expenses	100
Total Overhead Expenses:	$ 157,000

FIGURE 14-3. Sample schedule of overhead expenses. (Courtesy of Parente Randolph, LLC.)

NEALON MEDICAL PRACTICE, INC. Statement of Cash Flows For the Year Ended December 31, 2008	
Cash Flows from Operating Activities:	
Cumulative profit	$ 1,000
Adjustments to reconcile profit to net cash from operating activities:	
Depreciation	5,000
Changes in assets and liabilities:	
Other current assets	(5,000)
Retirement plan contribution payable	3,000
Total adjustments	3,000
Net cash from operating activities	4,000
Cash Flows Used in Investing Activities:	
Equipment acquisitions	(80,000)
Cash Flows from Financing Activities:	
Borrowings on line of credit	11,000
Proceeds from long-term debt	80,000
Principal repayment of long-term debt	(5,000)
Net provided by financing activities	86,000
Net Increase in Cash:	10,000
Cash, Beginning:	
Cash, Ending:	10,000

FIGURE 14-4. Sample cash flow statement. (Courtesy of Parente Randolph, LLC.)

Cash Flow Statements

Cash flow statements reveal not only the increase or decrease in collected cash for a given period, but the accounts, by category, that caused such changes. To read and understand a cash flow statement, you must start at the bottom of the statement where the increase or decrease in cash and the beginning and ending balances are revealed. It is important to understand the office's cash balance and how it changed during the periods that are being reviewed. Next, look at the total change in cash caused by the three major activities presented on this statement: operating, investing, and financing. To understand the medical office's daily cash flow fully, you need to analyze the increases and decreases in cash caused by changes in the working capital accounts and the revenue and expense accounts. Cash flows from operating activities can be presented using either the direct method or the indirect method. In the direct method, cash inflows and outflows are summarized for major categories, including the following:

- Cash received from customers
- Cash paid to employees
- Cash paid to suppliers
- Cash paid for interest
- Cash paid for taxes

Although the direct method is a more intuitive approach to understanding cash flows from operating activities, the indirect method is used in most annual reports.

The indirect method lists net income followed by a series of adjustments to remove the effects of accrual accounting. Accrual accounting is when revenue and expenses are recognized in the period in which they are earned and deducted. Most businesses use the accrual method of accounting; however, professions such as medicine and law tend to use the cash basis of accounting.

The first adjustment is to add back depreciation expense, because it is a noncash expense that was subtracted when determining net income. This subtotal is then added to or subtracted from the cash that was created or consumed by working capital accounts. The resulting cash flow from operating activities is one of the most important indicators of a company's performance. To review the statement of cash flows, you should have a general sense of the following:

- Amount of cash created or consumed by daily operations, including the cash effect from changes in working capital accounts
- Amount of cash invested in fixed or other assets
- Proceeds from the sale of stock or payments for dividends
- Increase or decrease in cash for the period

Because each financial statement presents a different focus on a practice's financial health—financial position versus operating performance versus cash flow—you must review them all to get a comprehensive picture.

FINANCIAL RATIOS TELL THE STORY

Financial ratios provide statistics and information that allow you to evaluate how well the medical practice is doing, and compare it with other practices in the same specialty or geographic area. You can also tell how well individual physicians are doing. Computing financial ratios entails converting raw numbers from the current year's and prior years' financial statements into ratios that highlight different financial characteristics, such as profitability and liquidity. However, before you rely completely on specific ratios, remember this advice: avoid drawing a strong conclusion from any one ratio, and always refer back to the specific accounts involved in the statements to see if the numbers confirm what the ratios suggest.

Accounts Receivable Distribution

Accounts receivable distribution (also called past due A/R) is a way of measuring how fast outstanding accounts are being paid. This analysis provides useful pictures of the status of collections and probable losses. The longer past due an account receivable becomes, the greater the likelihood that it will not be collected in full. Accounts receivable distribution is one of the most important "thermometers" of the practice's health. It is commonly referred to as an accounts receivable aging report. A practice that has good billing and insurance habits will have an accounts receivable aging report that looks like that found in Table 14-1. These figures are percentages of the total balance, and they will vary depending on the practice type and payer mix. You can use the accounts receivable aging in office meetings to show either the inefficiency or efficiency of the billing department.

TABLE 14-1 Sample Accounts Receivable Aging Report

CURRENT	31-60 DAYS	61-90 DAYS	91-120 DAYS	OVER 120 DAYS
75%	10%-12%	6%-7%	4%-5%	5%

Collection Ratio

A *collection ratio* calculates the percentage of outstanding debt collected. This is a good tool for instructing and motivating the collection department. This ratio is computed as follows:

$$\frac{\textbf{Total receipts}}{\textbf{Total charges}} = \textbf{Collection ratio (unadjusted)}$$

For example, if total receipts are $30,000 and total charges are $40,000, the unadjusted collection ratio is computed as follows:

$$\frac{\$30,000 \times 100}{\$40,000} = 75\% \textbf{ collection ratio (unadjusted)}$$

The *adjusted collection* ratio takes the following adjustments into consideration:

- Medicare
- Medicaid
- Workers' compensation
- Managed care
- Other adjustments

The adjusted collection ratio for the preceding example is computed as follows:

Total receipts = $30,000	
Add:	
Medicare adjusted	$2,000
Managed care adjusted	$3,000
Medicaid adjusted	$1,000
	$6,000 + $30,000 = $36,000

$$\frac{\$36,000 \times 100}{\$40,000} = 90\% \textbf{ collection ratio (adjusted)}$$

Billing Rate

The *billing rate* is an indicator of the average billing per patient. This is calculated by dividing the total billing per month by the total number of patients per month.

$$\frac{\textbf{Total billing}}{\textbf{Number of patients}} = \textbf{Average billing per patient}$$

For example, if the total billing for a month is $318,000 and the total number of patients is 3,700, the ratio is computed as follows:

$$\frac{\$318,000}{3,700 \textbf{ patients}} = \$85.94 \textbf{ average billing per patient}$$

Salary Rate

The *salary rate* is an indicator of the average amount of money a physician makes on a patient.

$$\frac{\textbf{Total salary}}{\textbf{Total patients}} = \textbf{Salary rate per patient}$$

For example, if Dr. Smith earns $40,000 in one month for seeing 525 patients, the salary rate for Dr. Smith is computed as follows:

$$\frac{\$40,000}{525\ \text{patients}} = \$76.19\ \text{per patient}$$

Overhead Ratio

The *overhead ratio* shows the cost of office overhead. It is calculated by taking total expenses, subtracting physician expenses, and then dividing by adjusted receipts. It is very important to monitor this figure monthly *and* year-to-year. This makes it easier to see trends in the cost of overhead. If the income/expense format detailed in this book is followed, the statement will be set up to provide the necessary information to calculate this ratio.

$$\frac{\text{Total expenses} - \text{Physician expenses}}{\text{Adjusted receipts}} = \text{Overhead expense}$$

Physician expenses consist of the following:

- Medical insurance
- Auto expenses
- Meals and entertainment
- Salary expenses and corresponding payroll taxes
- Travel
- Retirement plan contributions

For instance, a sample overhead ratio is computed as follows:

Physician expenses:	
Medical insurance	$500
Auto expenses	$500
Meals and entertainment	$250
Salary expenses	$8,750
Travel and lodging	$0
Total	$10,000

So, if there is $45,500 in total expenses, the overhead expense would be 88.7%:

$$\frac{\$45,500 - \$10,000 \times 100}{\$40,000(\text{Adjusted receipts})} = 88.7\%\ \text{cost of overhead expense}$$

Cost Ratio

To calculate the cost of performing a procedure or service in the office, divide the total expenses for 1 month by the number of procedures performed that month. The ratio is as follows:

$$\frac{\text{Total expenses}}{\text{Total no. of procedures}} = \text{Cost per procedure}$$

For example, if total expenses are $4,800 for 1 month and the total number of procedures is 24, the ratio is computed as follows:

$$\frac{\$4,800}{24} = \$200\ \text{cost per procedure}$$

Revenue Ratio

To calculate the *revenue ratio,* divide total revenue by the number of procedures performed in any given period. The ratio is as follows:

$$\frac{\text{Total revenue}}{\text{Total no. of procedures}} = \text{Revenue per procedure}$$

For example, if total revenue is $7,200 and the total number of procedures is 24, the ratio is computed as follows:

$$\frac{\$7,200}{24} = \$300\ \text{revenue per procedure}$$

Profit Ratio

The *profit ratio* is the amount of profit per procedure after total overhead and expenses are met. The ratio is as follows:

$$\text{Total revenue per procedure} - \text{Total costs per procedure} = \text{Profit}$$

$$\$300 - \$200 = \$100\ \text{profit on each procedure/service}$$

COST ANALYSIS

Cost, revenue, and profit ratios are used in many medical offices to evaluate the financial profitability of providing certain services in the office. For instance, an ophthalmologist might want to perform cataract surgery. After arriving at the total revenues from providing this service in the office and subtracting the total costs of providing this service, the ophthalmologist can determine whether the margin is enough to make it profitable. Some offices use cost, revenue, and profit ratios to determine whether simple laboratory studies or x-ray examinations should be done in their offices. By using these three ratios, the office is performing what is called a *cost analysis.*

Cost analysis is a very important aspect of practice accounting. It involves research and tedious amounts of work to determine exactly how much it costs the practice to provide a service. This same analysis is used by companies to set prices for their products. Two cost factors are involved in cost analysis: fixed costs and variable costs. *Fixed costs* are costs that do not change during a short period of time. Examples of fixed costs are mortgage payments, equipment lease payments, rent, depreciation of equipment, and insurance payments. *Variable costs* are costs that change regularly. Examples of variable costs are medical supplies, office supplies, electricity bills, billing services, and laboratory and x-ray services (Box 14-1).

The cost of treating each patient begins to add up when the patient enters the office. There are administrative costs associated with maintaining patient records and sending

BOX 14-1 Fixed and Variable Costs

Fixed Costs
- Mortgage payments
- Equipment lease payments
- Rent
- Insurance payments
- Depreciation of equipment

Variable Costs
- Medical supplies
- Office supplies
- Electric bills
- Billing service
- Laboratory and x-ray services

bills to patients. There are support personnel costs that arise from the care that the clinical staff provides to patients. There is the cost of capital equipment—supplies such as laboratory machines, gauze dressings, and alcohol pads—used on patients. Let's not forget the cost of the physician. The physician cost comprises the costs of malpractice insurance, interpreting tests, diagnosing a condition, and implementing treatment. Many office managers—and physicians for that matter—do not completely understand how much it costs a physician to see a patient in the office. By calculating and reviewing cost analyses, the office obtains information necessary to set fees and to market its services. Cost analyses help determine profit and monitor the practice's performance.

General practitioners and family practice physicians typically spend more on overhead than do such specialists as anesthesiologists and radiologists. It can cost the office many dollars if you wait until the end of the year to check on practice trends. A practical and easy way to control the office's finances is to estimate expenses and income for the next year. This can be done annually, quarterly, or even monthly.

FLASH REPORTS

A *flash report* is a series of calculations that can aid you and the physician in the financial management of the practice. This report should be distributed monthly to all physicians and should be discussed at monthly meetings. It essentially takes the pulse of the practice, showing trends in practice growth, expenses, and revenues. A sample flash report is shown in Figure 14-5.

COST CENTERS

Some larger practices set up cost centers within their practice, such as a laboratory, x-ray department, or satellite office, to identify expenses and revenues. To be an effective cost manager, the office manager must identify the relationship between the service or procedure and the costs that are incurred. A cost center does not serve patients directly; therefore only costs can be traced. A cost center measures the time spent and the quantity of resources consumed.

STEPS IN AN ACCOUNTING SYSTEM

The steps in an accounting system include the following:

1. Record transactions in a cash journal
2. Post information into ledger accounts
3. Prepare a trial balance
4. Prepare financial statements

Flash Report for ____________ (month)	____________
Total number of patients	____________
Total number of new patients	____________
Total charges	____________
Billing rate	____________
Collection rate (unadjusted)	____________
Collection rate (adjusted)	____________
Salary rate	____________
Accounts receivable ratio	____________
Overhead ratio	____________

FIGURE 14-5. Sample flash report.

In most computerized medical offices, steps 2 through 4 are done automatically by the computer.

Profits are the "bottom line" for every business. Not every physician is interested in all aspects of the financial reporting system, but every physician does want to know the bottom line—are we earning profits? If the practice's income is greater than its expenses, the answer to that question is yes. Profits are also called *net income.*

TYPES OF MEDICAL ACCOUNTING SYSTEMS

Different types of accounting systems exist, so it is important for you to identify your needs and evaluate how they may be met by the use of different systems. The two most common systems are

1. Computerized accounting systems
2. Pegboard systems

Not all medical offices have the same needs, and even though these two systems are based on the same principles, they differ somewhat in application.

Computerized Systems

Computerized accounting systems such as Quick Books, Quicken, and Peachtree are found in most offices today. By automating such functions as check writing, bank transfers, and account reconciliation, the office manager will have more time for other, more pressing issues. To use this system correctly, personnel must be trained in simple accounting and bookkeeping procedures. This system is based on the accounting principle that assets equal liabilities and capital. Each and every time a transaction is entered, it must be entered on both sides of the equation, and all transactions must remain in balance at all times. More can be found on computerized systems in Chapter 10.

Pegboard Systems

The pegboard system is a manual system that is easy to operate and makes the possibility of employee dishonesty less likely. It provides control over collections, payments, and charges. It provides a "running balance" on patient accounts and is easily used by office personnel. The initial cost of using this system might be higher than the initial cost of using other systems, but the ease of use and the control that it provides speak for themselves. To use this system, a pegboard and specially printed forms must be purchased. This pegboard is generally made of metal or plastic and contains a series of pegs down its left side for holding the forms in place. This system is a "one-write" system; by placing the forms in the correct manner on the board, the user simultaneously writes an entry on the daily sheet, the patient ledger card, and the patient's "walk-out" statement (Figure 14-6). The amount paid and the amount outstanding will be entered on each form. This system also eliminates errors that result from the need to make repetitive entries.

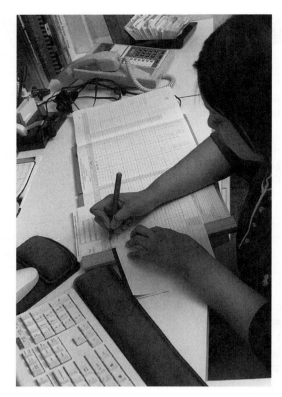

FIGURE 14-6. Preparing a walk-out statement or an encounter form for a patient using a pegboard system.

HOW TO CHOOSE AN ACCOUNTANT

Whom to hire as an accountant is one of the most crucial decisions the medical office manager makes. Thoroughly evaluate the office's needs and all candidates before deciding on an office accountant. It was once thought to be beneath a physician to consider his or her practice a business, and physicians perceived the business aspect of medicine as a hindrance. Few still think so today. However, perhaps as a carryover from the old days, many physicians view accountants simply as "number crunchers" and do not use their talents to the fullest. You can open the physician's eyes, if necessary, and help him or her choose an accountant who will strive for the best return on all the hard work the physician, you, and the staff do. Never just hire a friend, neighbor, or former classmate of the physician—or a friend of anyone's for that matter. An accountant is nothing less than a business investment. Choose the best!

Before beginning the search for an accountant, you need to determine the goals of the practice. Does the physician anticipate growth? Look to retire? Simply wish to skate by for the coming years? The physician who is looking for practice growth requires an accountant with expertise in business development and marketing. The physician who is facing retirement requires less financial planning (because most of this should already be done) and needs fewer accounting services. Discuss in detail with the physician his or her priorities and goals for the practice to help in evaluating an accountant.

Qualities of a Good Accountant

A good accountant is well versed in basic accounting knowledge. He or she is able to answer such simple questions as "Should we lease or purchase a photocopy machine?" "Should we incorporate?" and "What is the best method for obtaining financing?" It is good to know in advance the range of advice the accountant will be able to provide the office.

A good accountant interviews you as you are interviewing him or her. That is, the accountant wants to know and understand how your office works. A good accountant wants a list of the office's priorities so that it is easier to focus on relevant issues. An accountant who is really on the ball wants to know the source of office referrals. It is important to position the office so that it generates business in the manner the physician wants. Is the patient base referred by other doctors or the result of high visibility in the community?

A good accountant also wants to know the physician's future plans on a personal level. Does the physician plan to run for political office in the future? Is the physician's main goal in life to be an old-time "horse and buggy" type of doctor? Some physicians want to broaden their careers by devoting time to lecturing, networking, and serving on various boards, both professional and community based.

A good accountant has expertise in the intricacies of the medical profession. Check candidates' references to see if they have other clients in the health care profession. Ask candidates whether they are familiar with the problems associated with medical billing. Do they have an understanding of third-party billing? Do they understand coding and how it affects reimbursement?

A good accountant not only prepares monthly statements, but also sits and explains these statements to you and the physician in language you can understand. These reports become a valuable tool in troubleshooting. An easy way to understand accounting procedures is to think of a balance sheet as a snapshot of the practice's financial condition on a particular day. A balance sheet is a financial statement that indicates what assets the business owns and how those assets are financed in the form of liabilities or ownership interest. An income statement can be considered a video of the practice's financial condition over a particular time period. An income statement is a financial statement that measures the profitability of the business over a period of time. All expenses are subtracted from services to arrive at a net income. There are a variety of reports—an aged trial balance and an income statement analysis, for example—that should be run monthly. A good accountant explains what the various reports tell you about the practice (Figure 14-7). This accountant wants to see a financial statement so that he or she can analyze the whole picture, not just its parts.

A good accountant is knowledgeable about salaries, hiring and firing issues, health insurance plans, workers' compensation, and disability. You should be able to look to the accountant for advice when you are shopping around for health insurance for the employees. The accountant is not expected to know everything there is to know about each subject; however, he or she should know the basics and know where to go to get help if needed in these areas.

A good accountant can be consulted every time you buy new equipment. By way of a cost-benefit analysis, the accountant will tell you whether the ultimate benefit of the purchase will justify the cost. A good accountant is well versed in retirement plans. The physician will want a feasibility study done, with plans to install and carry out the necessary steps for retirement. If the accountant does not have expertise in financial planning, he or she should be able to recommend someone who does. Information regarding profit sharing and pension plans is highly important to most medical offices. The accountant should recommend the appropriate plan for an office of your size, number of employees, and cash flow.

A good accountant is aware of how new tax laws affect the medical office, and evaluates the office's tax situation, offering recommendations in a proactive way. Tax laws

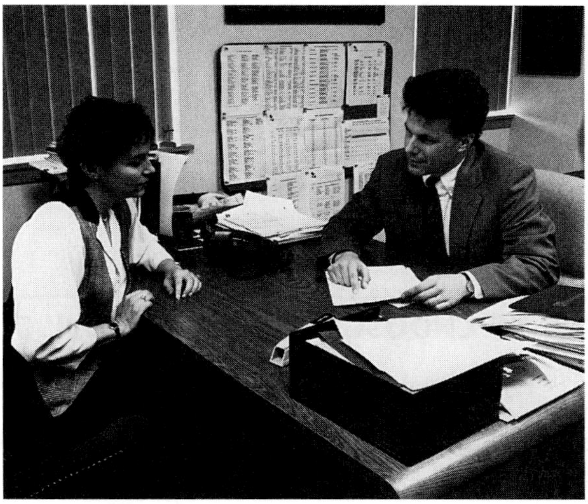

FIGURE 14-7. Meeting regularly with the accountant is important for the financial well-being of the practice.

are too complex for a black-and-white answer to exist for every question. They are subject to the interpretations of business owners and the Internal Revenue Service (IRS). The physician and the accountant should have similar philosophies regarding the interpretation of tax laws. Conservative or aggressive, the accountant should be in tune with the physician's general philosophy about taxes and understand how much "creativity" the physician wants him or her to use. As an example, whereas the uncreative accountant sees the physician's family members as dependency exemptions, the creative accountant sees them as avenues for income splitting to reduce taxes. It's not good to be too conservative. Ask candidates how many of their clients have been audited by the IRS. If the answer is none or very few, the candidate may be too conservative. In addition, be wary of any accountant who seems intimidated by the IRS. There is a difference between a conservative accountant and an accountant who is afraid to have his or her work examined.

There are three ways to handle a tax situation, and two of them are the wrong ways! The first is to lower your taxes and improve your cash flow. The second way is to overpay your taxes. The third way is to be challenged by the IRS and lose. The second and third ways should not even be considered! Meetings with the accountant should take place not only at tax time, but also throughout the year. You and the physician should be continually informed of financial, business, and tax strategies. Monthly financial statements should show a clear picture of the practice and serve as a springboard for ideas on how to improve the practice's bottom line, such as by lowering your taxes.

Accountants' Fees

The more contact the office has with the accountant, the higher the bills will be. When the bills reflect the quality of work done, the physician should be willing to authorize payment of these services. In general, an accounting firm will bill for services on an hourly rate commensurate with the level of the professional who performed the work. Fees can range from $65.00 to $250.00 an hour, depending on the complexity of the work done and the status of the accountant within the firm. A senior partner will come with a higher price tag than a new associate.

HOW TO CHOOSE A FINANCIAL ADVISOR

It is never an easy task to decide who to trust with profits. Financial advisors come in various shapes and sizes; however, there are a few questions that should help you select a good advisor:

- Tell me about your firm. How long have you been in business?
- What is your professional background?
- What qualifies you to advise me on these subjects?
- Describe your typical client.
- What is your investment philosophy? Is it conservative or aggressive?
- Do your clients rely solely on you for advice?
- Do your clients do a lot of their own homework?
- How often do you speak with your clients?
- How do you interact with your clients' other professional advisors?
- What sets you apart from others in your field?
- Why do you want to do business with me?

A financial advisor should want to understand the needs of the practice and meet them. He or she should always be there to guide the office in decision making and answer all questions that are raised. The most important concern is that the financial advisor should have the same philosophy as the office.

BANKING ON THE RIGHT BANK

The office manager should evaluate several banks before choosing one for the practice. To protect the office from losses that may be incurred if you choose an unstable bank, you can now call VERIBANC at 1-800-442-2657 to receive a report on the financial stability of each bank you are considering. VERIBANC (www.veribanc.com) is a bank rating and analysis firm in Massachusetts that reports any adverse financial conditions that might be found in a banking institution.

A bank that is insolvent is one whose liabilities are greater than the reasonable market value of its assets. With cost-containment measures being imposed on the health care profession today, the last thing the medical office wants to deal with is a troubled bank. You can also find out about problems with banks simply by reading articles in local newspapers regarding poor financial performance, management shake-ups, and regulatory examinations, or by checking with your accountant.

Choosing the Correct Bank Account

Banks offer a variety of services that can be used by the medical office (Figure 14-8). They offer four basic types of accounts: checking accounts, savings accounts, money market accounts, and certificates of deposit (CDs). Although most banks offer the same types of accounts, be certain to read the fine print when choosing an account. To open the office account, the physician should take the following items to the bank branch: money to deposit into the account, personal identification, a business license (some banks also ask to see a medical license), and his or her Social Security number or tax ID number.

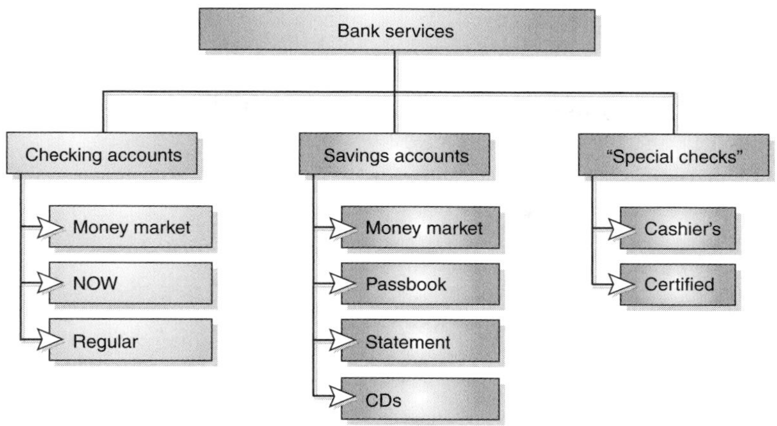

FIGURE 14-8. Services offered by most banks.

CHECKING ACCOUNTS

Checking accounts are the backbone of the banking system. Most people use checks to pay their bills. In fact, an average family writes approximately 20 checks in a month. When a staff member deposits a check into the office account, it is sent to the bank of the patient who wrote the check. The bank then takes money out of the patient's account and transfers it to the office account. How soon the office account will be credited depends on where the patient's or insurance company's bank is located. To be safe, always allow 2 to 5 days for the amount deposited to become available. Figure 14-9 shows the path of a check once it is issued to the physician's office. As discussed in Chapter 6, bank cards or debit cards are now linked to checking accounts. When these cards are used in place of writing a check, funds are immediately debited from the patient's checking account and credited to the office account.

If a staff member writes a check in error and the office wishes to stop payment on it, the bank will issue a "stop payment order" on the check for a fee. Most banks will ask that the office manager or another authorized employee sign the appropriate form in person. Some banks will allow individuals to arrange a stop payment order over the telephone. (Having a good working relationship with personnel at the bank comes in handy at times like this. Make sure that you become well known in the bank in which the office does its business.) The stop payment order is good for 6 months in most banks and is generally costly. This option should be used only when absolutely necessary.

If there is not enough cash in the office account to cover a check that the employer wrote, the bank can refuse to pay it. The office will be charged a fee for checks returned, and the individual to whom the check was issued will also be charged a fee.

The best way to avoid overdrafts on office checks is to apply for overdraft protection. This will prevent embarrassing situations with vendors and others if your bookkeeper should happen to make a mistake. The bank will

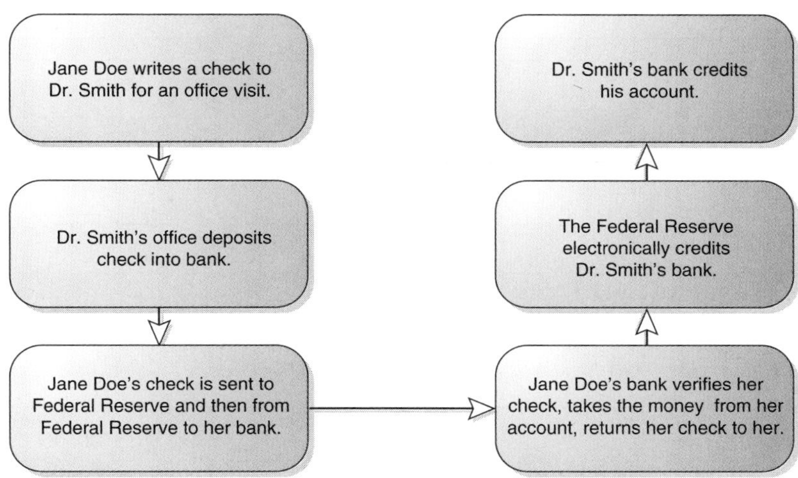

FIGURE 14-9. The life cycle of a check.

automatically transfer the necessary funds to cover the check. Overdraft protection saves the office money, embarrassment, and aggravation. Keep in mind that chronic bouncing of checks can affect the office's credit rating.

If a patient issues the office a bad check, the same fees apply. Some banks will not charge the practice's account if a patient's check is returned to him or her for nonsufficient funds.

Types of Checking Accounts

The three most common types of checking accounts are as follows:

1. Regular checking accounts
2. Interest-bearing checking accounts
3. Money market accounts

Regular checking accounts allow the office to write as many checks as necessary. The bank charges a fee for each check written on the account and a monthly service fee. There is no interest paid on the account. Interest-bearing checking accounts also allow the office to write as many checks as necessary. These accounts pay a small interest on the balance. These accounts generally come with added incentives, such as free traveler's checks, no annual fees for credit cards, and sometimes discounts on loans. These accounts generally require that a certain minimum balance be kept in the account at all times.

Money market accounts provide the office with an interest rate that changes on the basis of market conditions. A large minimum balance is required, and the fees for going below this balance can be severe. Some money market accounts limit the number of checks that may be written and limit the number of transfers per month.

The minimum balance is the smallest amount that can be kept in an account to qualify it for certain benefits, such as reduced fees or free checking. Some banks define the minimum as the combined amount in all of your accounts. If the office can take advantage of minimum balance options, it will save money. Ask your local bank what its requirements are.

Anatomy of a Check

Checks are an everyday part of any business, including the medical office. More than 90% of payments received in the medical office are checks. Most medical assistant training programs cover how to write a check and discuss a check's components. Others involved in health care have no formal training on this subject. Three different kinds of information are found on the front of a check. Some information is preprinted on the check, some is handwritten, and some is printed during processing at the bank. The following list describes a check's parts as numbered in Figure 14-10:

1. Name and address of the owner of the check
2. Date the check is written
3. Check number
4. Bank ID number
5. Name of the person or company to whom the check is written
6. Amount the check is written for
7. Name of the bank on which the check is drawn
8. Memo area where the reason for the check can be noted
9. Signature that authorizes the transaction (it must correspond to the bank signature card)
10. Check routing number (identifies the bank and the Federal Reserve in the area)
11. Check number, printed again when the check is processed
12. Amount of the transaction is printed at time of processing, so computers can scan it for accuracy

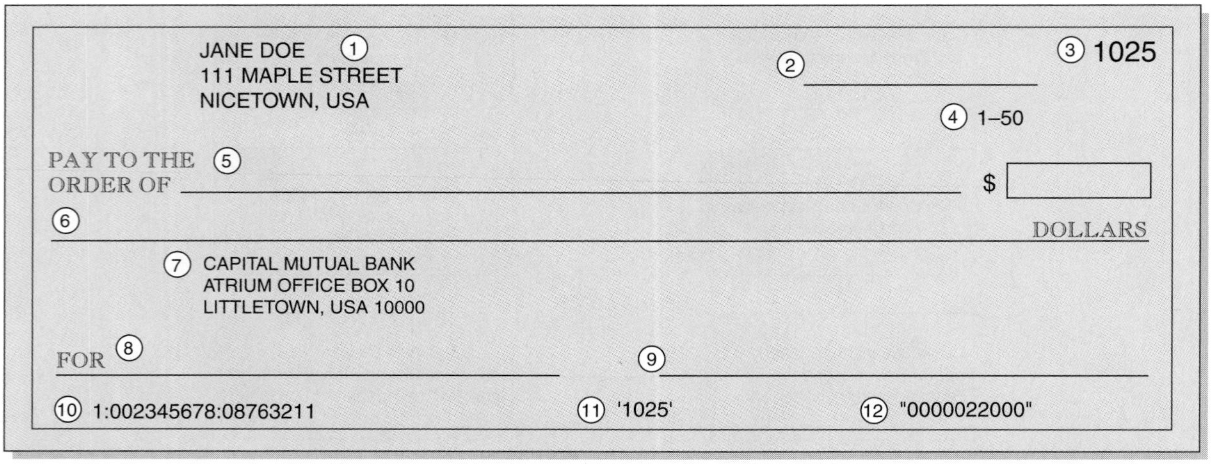

FIGURE 14-10. The parts of a check (see text for explanation of the numbered items).

Staff should be trained to make sure that a check is filled out completely by the patient before they accept it. Always make sure the patient has signed the check; there are times when patients are so distracted that they forget to sign. Some patients will even write out the check, sign it, and then close their checkbook and leave the office with the check in their checkbook. It is important to treat the financial part of the visit as carefully as the clinical part.

Check Endorsement

The endorsement of a check is an important step when accepting a check from a patient. The purpose of an endorsement is to transfer the rights in a check to another individual. The first step employees should take when accepting a check from a patient is to stamp the back of the check with a "For Deposit Only" stamp that includes the checking account number.

Patients may present the office with a check from a third-party payer that they would like to sign over to the office. This can be done, but certain steps must be followed for proper endorsement of this type of check. The patient, or guarantor, first signs the back of the check in ink. Then, under his or her signature, the patient writes "Pay to the order of" and the physician's name. The check may then be accepted by the office.

MANAGER'S ALERT

Never accept a postdated check from a patient. If a patient doesn't have sufficient funds in his or her account, have the patient date the check with the date of the visit, place the check in an envelope on which is written the date the check can be deposited, and place the envelope in a locked drawer until the date on the envelope.

Check Helpful Hints

Following are some points to keep in mind regarding checks:

- Do not accept checks with corrections on them. Ask patients to issue another check if they made an error when writing the first one.
- Do not accept a check marked "Payment in Full" if the check does not pay the account in full. Legally, you will not be able to collect the remaining balance.
- Accept checks only for the exact amount owed for the services rendered.
- Do not cash a check for a patient.
- Do not accept an out-of-town check unless it is from a family member of one of your patients.
- Do not accept third-party checks unless they are from an insurance carrier.

Bad Checks

Some checks that are issued to a physician's office do not clear the bank for one reason or another—a mix-up in bookkeeping on the patient's part, information missing from the check, or a stop payment order. In such situations, the office does not receive payment for that service. Banks will hold a check for 3 to 5 days before clearing it for deposit into the account. If you should call the bank to inquire about the account balance, the bank will generally offer two amounts: the balance and the currently available balance. The balance includes all deposits made by the office. The currently available balance, however, includes only deposited checks that have actually cleared. The difference between these two figures is the amount of the checks that have not yet cleared the bank, making the funds unavailable until they clear.

FROM THE EXPERT'S NOTEBOOK

When a patient issues a bad check, it is always a good idea to note that event either in the financial section of the patient's chart or in the computer. Some offices use a "colored dot" coding system that is placed on the patient chart to denote a financial problem.

How long it takes a check to clear the bank depends on where the check is drawn. If the check is drawn on the same bank that the office uses, the check amount will become available immediately. If the check is drawn on a different bank in town, the funds should be available no more than 2 days from the date of deposit. If the check is drawn on an out-of-town bank, it is usually cleared within 3 days. If the check is drawn on a bank in a different state, it is generally cleared within 5 days. Legislation in 1987 reduced the amount of time that a bank can hold a check to a maximum of 7 days from the date of deposit, but most banks clear a check within 5 days.

Special Checks

There are times when a business or personal check is not enough, and a certified check or cashier's check must be used. If an insurance company pays a patient instead of the office and the amount that the patient has to turn over to the office is large, the office may request to be paid with a certified check. A cashier's check is also called a bank check. A cashier's check is guaranteed because it is drawn against a bank's own account. It includes a carbon copy for the office to keep with its records. The charge for a cashier's check is less than the charge for a certified check.

A certified check is also a guaranteed check. It is a business check that the bank certifies as good. After the check is written, the bank freezes the account for the amount of the check and stamps the face of the check with the word "certified." There is a fee associated with purchasing a certified check.

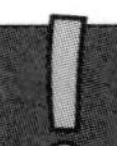

MANAGER'S ALERT

Once a cashier's check or certified check reaches its destination, you cannot put a stop payment order on it.

Traveler's checks and money orders also fall into the category of special checks. The office does not have any reason to purchase these checks; however, many patients use traveler's checks or money orders to pay for services in the office. Provide the front-desk staff with information about these checks so they know how to handle them.

Individuals who are traveling often use traveler's checks. They are issued by auto clubs, banks, and credit card companies, and come in various denominations. The purchaser must sign each check at the time of purchase and then again in front of the person to whom the purchaser is giving it.

Some patients pay their bills at the office with money orders. These are generally patients who do not have checking accounts. Money orders are to be accepted as cash. There is no risk involved in accepting money orders, and they should be included on the deposit slip as cash.

There are three types of savings accounts:

- Statement accounts
- Passbook accounts
- Money market accounts

Statement accounts are the type of savings account a person makes deposits on, withdraws from, and earns interest on. All the transactions for a month are reported on a statement (some banks issue quarterly statements instead of monthly statements). If the person also has a checking account with that bank, the statement savings account will show on the monthly checking account statement.

Passbook accounts are the old tried-and-true savings account. They are not very common today, most having been replaced with statement savings accounts; in fact, many banks no longer offer them. People with this type of account have a passbook that they take to the bank each time they conduct a transaction involving the account. When a transaction takes place, be it a deposit or withdrawal, it is recorded in the passbook. The frequency with which interest is added to the account depends on the number of transactions conducted.

Money market accounts are savings accounts with checking privileges. There is a limit on the number of checks that can be written each month. Money market accounts pay the most interest as long as a certain minimum balance is maintained. Many savings accounts can be tied into checking accounts to provide overdraft protection. Savings accounts do not pay as much interest as CDs or money market funds, but the money is more "liquid;" in other words, it is easier to retrieve if needed on short notice.

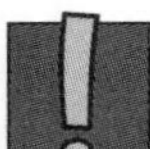

MANAGER'S ALERT

Be sure to check with the bank to see when it pays interest. Some accounts are credited quarterly, and if you withdraw before the quarter ends, you lose all the interest for that period.

Electronic Banking

The innovative banking methods available today allow the medical office to do its banking with the ease of a phone call. With electronic banking, the office can have its loan payments, mortgage or lease payments, insurance payments, and payments of utility and vendor bills automatically deducted from its checking account. When a bill arrives at the office, the bookkeeper simply calls the bank to authorize payment of the bill directly from the office's checking account. This method of electronic payments can also be prearranged, so that amounts are withdrawn automatically each month. Large offices find this especially helpful. You must sign a consent form to authorize the automatic payment of these bills. Banking can be done online by a simple click of computer keys—no more writing out checks and mailing them.

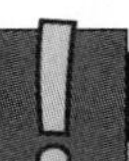

MANAGER'S ALERT

There are two ways in which bills are paid with electronic banking. Some banks pay bills through an electronic transfer of funds. Other banks send a paper check. The advantage of the electronic transfer of funds is that the bill is paid immediately. When the bank pays bills with a paper check, there is a 3- to 5-day waiting period before the payee receives the check.

End-of-Day Procedures

Whether you are computerized or using a manual system, it is important to run end-of-day reports. Offices that are computerized simply run a report at the end of the day that provides the following information:

- The number and type of transactions for the day
- The month-to-date and perhaps the year-to-date totals

Once the report is run or the end-of-day report is completed, all math in the totals column should balance. The report must total before the individual responsible leaves the office for the day. If the amount is able to be divided by nine, there is a good chance that the error is a result of transposed numbers. If the amount is able to be divided by two, there is a good chance that the error is a result of an incorrectly posted amount. Check each amount in each column to find the error. If there is still a problem, a co-worker or the office manager should check the numbers. Sometimes "fresh eyes" can find errors that have been looked at time and time again by the same person.

Deposits

DIRECT DEPOSITS

The office might want to consider direct deposit for its employees. Direct deposit can be used for payroll, pensions, and Social Security payments. Amounts are automatically deposited into the appropriate accounts on the designated day. The bank will do the rest. Most employees want the ease of direct deposits of their paychecks.

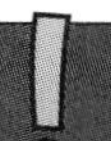

MANAGER'S ALERT

If employees make deposits in the night depository, be sure that it is well lit and that the bank branch is in a safe neighborhood. Safety is a must!

NIGHT DEPOSITORY

To maximize the office's cash flow, you should make sure that bank deposits are made daily. You can do this by using the night depository or going to the bank every day. Most medical offices use a night depository. To make night deposits, a night deposit bag must be purchased from the bank. The charge is nominal and provides you with a reusable bag, a key to lock the bag, and a key to open the night depository at the bank. Some banks now offer only disposable bags, which are more expensive, for night deposits. Try to avoid a bank with this type of system, because it can be costly for the practice.

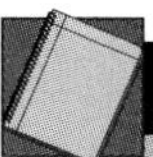

FROM THE EXPERT'S NOTEBOOK

Many banks are open on Saturdays and Sundays to be more available to their customers. Some are even open later in the evening, allowing practices with evening hours to make deposits without using a night depository bag.

PREPARING THE DEPOSIT SLIP

The bank will appreciate clients that know the proper way to prepare deposit slips. First, the cash should be counted and double-checked. The amount is then written on the deposit slip under "cash." Next, checks should be listed by inserting the bank number on the deposit slip in the block preceding the area where the amount of the check is written. Then the check amount is filled into the next block. An example of a deposit slip is shown in Figure 14-11.

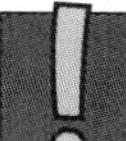

MANAGER'S ALERT

Do not get into the bad habit of making bank deposits only once a week. Remember that those checks will not earn interest if they are sitting in the office. The chance of lost checks or theft is also much higher when your receipts sit in a desk drawer. It is best to make deposits daily!

DATE ________

	DOLLARS	CENTS
CURRENCY		
COIN		
CHECKS		
1		
2		
3		
4		
5		
6		
7		
8		
9		
10		
11		
12		
13		
14		
15		
16		
17		
18		
19		
20		
21		
22		
23		
24		
25		
26		
PLEASE ENTER TOTAL		

TOTAL ITEMS

3-1
310

FIGURE 14-11. Sample deposit slip.

Reviewing the Bank Statement

Most practices have bookkeepers or accountants who handle the bank reconciliation each month. There are, however, some practices where this job falls on the office manager.

Each month, the bank sends a statement listing the deposits and checks written against the office account. It is important to reconcile this account monthly to ensure that the balance shown in the check register agrees with the bank's balance. Either the practice or the bank may make an error, and any error must be corrected. The following steps can be used to reconcile an office bank statement (Figure 14-12):

Step 1. Compare the account register to the account statement for unrecorded transactions. These transactions may be the use of an ATM card, interest earned, unrecorded deposits, or checks that haven't cleared. The new account register total should match the adjusted balance in line 6 (see Figure 14-12).

Step 2. Write in all deposits and interest, if applicable, that were made since the date of the statement.

Step 3. Add together the amounts listed in lines 2 and 3 in Figure 14-12.

Step 4. List and total all checks and withdrawals that were made and are not reflected on the account statement. This list will include any checks written after the date of the account statement, and may include checks written before that date that haven't yet found their way to your bank.

Step 5. Subtract the amount in line 5 (see Figure 14-12) from the amount in line 4. This is the adjusted balance and should match the balance in the account register.

DO YOU KNOW WHERE YOUR PETTY CASH IS?

Petty cash can be a problem in many offices. Money is kept in a petty cash box, and no one is accountable for it. The size of an office's petty cash fund is determined by several factors: the size of the office, the types of purchases made, and the frequency with which it is replenished.

The secret to a successful petty cash system is to appoint one staff member accountable for all transactions. This person can be the office manager or one of the other staff members. A voucher system should be used for all transactions. First, determine how much cash to keep in the box. Generally, if large purchases are not made with petty cash, a balance of $100 is more than adequate. When a staff member finds it necessary to make a purchase from petty cash, he or she must present a slip for the amount spent. This slip should specify the date and the item purchased. If it does not, the petty cash attendant must write this information on it. At the end of the month, the slips are totaled and presented to the bookkeeper or physician, who in turn writes a check to petty cash to replace the amount spent. An example is as follows:

Total starting amount	$100.00
Purchases:	
Coffee, cream, sugar	$10.61
Extension cord	$2.79
Light bulbs	$11.34
Total purchases	$24.74

When slips totaling $24.74 are presented to the bookkeeper, the bookkeeper writes a check for $24.74 to petty cash, the check is cashed, and the money is placed in the petty cash fund.

Bank Reconciliation

1. Compare balance in account register with balance on bank statement.
2. List closing balance on front of account statement. 3,125.60
3. List deposits made since this statement date.

Deposit:	830.00	Deposit:	5,324.00			
Deposit:	1,980.00	Deposit:	990.00			
Deposit:	476.00	Deposit:	3,170.00			
				TOTAL:	**12,770.00**	**12,770.00**

4. Add together lines 2 and 3. **15,895.60**
5. List all checks written since this statement date.

Check #	Amount	Check #	Amount			
555	538.20	558	430.00			
556	718.00	559	175.00			
557	2,018.00	600	950.00			
				TOTAL:	**4,829.20**	**4,829.20**

6. Subtract the amount in line 5 from the amount in line 4. **11,066.40**

The amount listed in line 6 represents the adjusted balance on the account statement. This should match the balance in the register. If it matches, the account has been reconciled. If it doesn't, there is a math error somewhere.

FIGURE 14-12. Sample bank reconciliation.

Some offices use petty cash to purchase stamps. This is not a good idea because it causes too much activity in the petty cash fund. Stamps should be purchased with a separate check. This creates a paper trail and makes tracking easier. There are occasions where there is postage due and petty cash can be used for that purpose.

CREDIT CARDS

Since more and more credit cards are being used today, it is good for office personnel to know how to process them. Medical practices mainly use banks to connect the credit card companies to the practice and permit the processing of credit card payments. This type of account is called a *merchant account.* This very convenient manner in which patients can pay for services does not come without a cost. Pricing for credit card transactions is based on a percentage of the transaction and a flat rate. When the card is swiped, the cost for the service is generally 1% to 3% of the transaction. The percentage can go up 1% on transactions that are keyed in via phone, mail, or Internet. In addition to the discount rate, there is a flat rate cost per transaction of approximately 10 cents. This translates to about 70 cents on a $20 co-pay. If the practice has a high total volume, it may be possible to obtain a lower rate.

Pricing for debit cards is a bit different. If the office processes a debit card payment by having the patient enter a personal identification number (PIN), you are charged only a flat rate. If the debit card is run through the machine like a credit card, the above payment scenario will exist. The practice must also purchase the terminal, which in most cases can be purchased from the bank that is going to service your merchant account. Equipment can cost from $100 to $400 depending on which equipment is chosen. If the practice is a busy one, there should be a terminal at each checkout clerk so that there is no delay in processing the patients.

The most expense credit cards for the office to handle are Discover and American Express. VISA and MasterCard tend to be more reasonable in fees. Merchant account providers can charge you extra charges, so shop around to be sure that you have the least expensive arrangement possible. Consider deals offered through the American Medical Association (AMA) and Medical Group Management Association (MGMA) before signing on the dotted line. As the future unfolds and various forms of credit and debit cards abound, payment cards will play an important role in how a medical office does business.

BUDGETS FOR MEDICAL PRACTICES

Budgets are an integral part of the decision-making process for a medical practice. “Can we afford a new computer system?” “Can we hire another staff member?” “Can we buy new carpeting this year?” Budgets help answer these questions. They help to set priorities, allocate resources, and monitor and control costs. Medical practices generally have limited cost management needs when compared with hospital systems; therefore their budget needs are generally simple.

Advantages to Budgets

There are several advantages to budgets, and the following list is just a few:

1. Budgets require management personnel to be organized.
2. Budgets help you coordinate long- and short-term planning.
3. Budgets help establish benchmarks for the group.

As an office manager, keep in mind that the success of your budget depends on the support of all physicians and managers within the group. This support transforms a simple report into a valuable management tool. The practice accountant can be a useful resource for preparing a budget.

EXERCISES

MULTIPLE CHOICE

Choose the best *answer for each of the following questions.*

1. Which of the following is a type of check that a medical office might see on occasion?
   a. Cashier's
   b. Traveler's
   c. Bank
   d. Certified
2. Which of the following should *not* be paid for using petty cash?
   a. Light bulbs
   b. Postage due
   c. Rent
   d. Coffee
3. The following information *cannot* be found on a patient's personal check:
   a. Check number
   b. Account balance
   c. Name of bank
   d. Bank identification number
4. The following is considered the routing number of a check:
   a. Identification number of bank
   b. Check number
   c. Number that identifies the bank and federal reserve area
   d. The amount of the transaction
5. Which of the following ratios illustrates the amount of money a physician makes per patient?
   a. Cost ratio
   b. Income ratio
   c. Salary rate
   d. Collection ratio

6. Profit and loss expenses for the month are found where?
   a. The balance sheet
   b. Cash flow statement
   c. Income/expense statement
   d. Cost/expense statement
7. Which of the following is *not* an example of a fixed cost?
   a. Rent
   b. Insurance payments
   c. Utility payments
   d. Equipment leases
8. A pegboard system is also known as a
   a. Double-entry system
   b. "One-write" system
   c. Duplicate system
   d. Copy system
9. If there is a possibility that a number has been transposed, the number in error should be divided by
   a. 5
   b. 10
   c. 9
   d. 3
10. The bank number on a check can be found
    a. In the bottom right
    b. In the top right
    c. In the bottom left
    d. None of the above
11. Which of the following is a reporting system?
    a. Accrual
    b. Dividend
    c. Check
    d. All of the above
12. To calculate the cost of performing a service or procedure, use which of the following?
    a. Revenue ratio
    b. Overhead ratio
    c. Collection ratio
    d. None of the above
13. To calculate the average billing per patient, one should use the
    a. Collection ration
    b. A/R ratio
    c. Salary rate
    d. Billing rate
14. Which of the following would *not* be paid for using petty cash?
    a. Stamps
    b. Electric bill
    c. Coffee, creamer, and sugar
    d. All of the above
15. Most of the payments made in the office are made by
    a. Credit card
    b. Cash
    c. Check
    d. None of the above
16. The following is *not* part of a check:
    a. Social Security number
    b. Check number
    c. Bank ID number
    d. Name of the bank
17. Checks used by individuals who are traveling are called
    a. Certified checks
    b. Traveler's checks
    c. Suitcase checks
    d. Mobile checks
18. To understand the office's daily cash flow fully, which of the following should be analyzed?
    a. Expense accounts
    b. Revenue accounts
    c. Capital accounts
    d. All of the above
19. An income/expense statement provides which of the following summary data?
    a. Total revenues
    b. Total overhead expenses
    c. Total physicians' expenses
    d. All of the above
20. Which of the following statements is *not* true?
    a. Increases in liabilities equal decreases in owner's equity.
    b. Increases in assets are recorded as debits.
    c. Decreases in assets are credits.
    d. Decreases in liabilities and owner's equity are recorded as debits.

TRUE OR FALSE

1. _____ Money market accounts do not pay interest to businesses.
2. _____ The routing number of a check is the person's bank account number.
3. _____ Medical offices always keep at least $500 in petty cash.
4. _____ A "cost center" is where the hospital keeps financial records of your practice.
5. _____ Budgets help to establish benchmarks for the practice.
6. _____ The accounts receivable ratio measures the average billing per patient.
7. _____ Increases in assets are recorded as credits.
8. _____ Increases in owner's equity are recorded as credits.
9. _____ A night depository can be used to make withdrawals for the practice.
10. _____ The profit ratio is the amount of profit before overhead.
11. _____ Cash basis reporting is most commonly used in medical offices.
12. _____ A/R stands for Aged Reporting.
13. _____ An example of a fixed cost would be a lease payment for medical equipment.
14. _____ Do not accept a check that is marked "payment in full" if the amount does not pay the account in full.
15. _____ A money market account is a type of checking account.

16. _____ Once a cashier's check reaches its destination, you cannot put a stop payment order on it.
17. _____ The passbook is a type of savings account.
18. _____ An end-of-day report contains the names of the patients.
19. _____ The bank bag used to make deposits after hours is called a night deposit bag.
20. _____ It is customary for money to sit in a desk drawer overnight.

THINKERS

1. Using a medical practice scenario provided by the instructor, construct an example of what the income/expense sheet may look like for your practice.
2. A new patient seeks care from your practice. On completion of the visit, the patient states that he is from out of town and is low on cash. He wants to write a check to pay for his visit. What would you say to him? Explain your decision.
3. You have a meeting scheduled with the physician to discuss the financial condition of the practice. Explain how you would prepare for this meeting and describe the reasons behind your preparations.
4. The physician feels that the office accountant is not providing the services that are needed. He does not have many health care clients and therefore does not always understand the needs of a medical practice. How would you interview for a new accountant? Explain what you feel is important for the practice in selecting a new accountant.

REFERENCES

Gapenski, L.C. *Cases in Healthcare Finance.* Chicago: Health Administration Press, 1999.

Gapenski, L.C. *Healthcare Finance: An Introduction to Accounting and Financial Management.* Chicago: Health Administration Press, 2001.

Gapenski, L.C. *Understanding Healthcare Financial Management,* 3rd edition. Chicago: Health Administration Press, 2001.

Lee, R.H. *Economics for Healthcare Managers.* Chicago: Health Administration Press, 2000.

Nowicki, M. *Financial Management of Hospitals and Healthcare Organizations,* 2nd edition. Chicago: Health Administration Press, 2001.

Zelman, W., et al. *Financial Management of Health Care Organizations: An Introduction to Fundamental Tools, Concepts, and Applications,* 2nd edition. London: Blackwell, 2002.

15

MEDICAL MARKETING

CHAPTER OUTLINE

CHAPTER OBJECTIVES

After completing this chapter, you will be able to do the following:

- Discuss the methods of marketing a medical practice
- Differentiate between advertising and marketing
- Define *quality service*
- Understand the importance of patient satisfaction
- Comprehend how patient perception and expectation affect a medical practice
- Draw conclusions from referring physician surveys
- Know how to access and present patient educational subjects
- Develop ways to market a new physician
- Comprehend the effect of managed care on marketing

MARKETING—IT'S EVERYWHERE

Marketing is found everywhere in our economy and it affects everyone. Marketing is more than just a business activity; it is something that everyone participates in, whether they be a marketer or customer. *Marketing* can be defined as the process of developing and selling ideas, goods, and services that satisfy customers using the principles of pricing, promotion, and distribution. *Service marketing* falls into the category of marketing of intangible products that offer financial, legal, medical, recreational, or any other benefits to the consumer. Throughout this chapter you will often see the words *patient satisfaction* and *consumers.* The concept that patients are consumers who must be satisfied is the core concept of marketing in the health care field.

SELLING THE PRACTICE'S SERVICES

"Be it furniture, clothes or health care, many industries today are marketing nothing more than commodities—no more, no less. What will make the difference in the long run is the care and feeding of the customers."

—MICHAEL AND TIMOTHY MESCON, HOW TO WIN CUSTOMERS AND KEEP THEM FOR LIFE

The first step in selling a practice is marketing its services via advertising, newsletters, seminars, direct mail, and mall and health fairs. Some practices go so far as to have a marketing and promotions company make up key chains and refrigerator magnets. One primary care practice made telephone labels for emergency numbers, which also contained the name and phone number of the physician and practice. The idea was that each time a member of the household picked up that phone, they would see the doctor's name.

As a medical office manager, you need to sell the practice's services just as a salesperson sells cars. Know your product! This is what they teach in sales school, and the same goes for a medical practice. You should have enough knowledge to be able to discuss in detail everything about the practice, and sell it.

The practice should be marketed to the following:

- Insurance companies
- Local companies
- Churches
- The community

Companies are looking to cut insurance costs and provide wellness care to their employees. This is an area where a physician's office can market itself easily and effectively. Make appointments with benefits managers at local companies to promote the practice's wellness and social programs such as drug and alcohol awareness. This is a great practice booster. You may want to suggest the following programs:

- Stress management
- Nutrition and diet
- Weight reduction
- Alcohol awareness
- Drug awareness
- Women's health issues
- Smoking cessation
- Acquired immunodeficiency syndrome (AIDS) awareness
- Cardiopulmonary resuscitation (CPR)
- Fitness and exercise
- Wellness (e.g., blood pressure monitoring, cholesterol monitoring, rheumatoid arthritis)

This benefits the practice and the company, because employee morale rises when a company institutes programs for their general well-being. The company can institute such programs at a low cost but with a high yield in employee satisfaction.

Most hospitals also provide wellness lectures for the community. A simple title for a lecture series may be "Come Meet the Doctor." Physicians of different specialties can speak each month. Some malls and department stores offer community health fairs and ask local physicians to speak on various topics.

BUILDING CUSTOMER SERVICE

We have established that patients are consumers, or customers, who want quality service. Customer service will help attract new patients and retain the current ones. Better customer service should be a priority, from the physician to the employees. It should be in the front of everyone's thoughts as they care for patients within the practice. Information and documentation are critical components of building customer service. The practice should continually generate reports that will provide them with tracking information that can be used to identify the changing needs of the practice. The practice should use the most up-to-date information because this will provide a format for quality care. To build customer service among your patients, it is important to not only recognize these factors, but to put them into play.

PLAN OF THREES

All businesses, and health care is no exception, must follow the plan of threes in order to be successful. The plan of threes consists of the following:

1. Business plan
2. Strategic plan
3. Marketing plan

It is an important basic foundation for a medical practice to have a business plan. This plan will outline the direction of the practice and will follow a mission statement that is prepared by the practice. It will provide a roadmap of the direction the practice plans to take in the future and may even provide the financial picture for future projects.

The strategic plan takes this information and uses it to take a look at the goals and objectives. It will point out strengths, weaknesses, and opportunities for the practice. It consists of a detailed plan that outlines expected results. The marketing plan consists of an outline of how the practice will market itself. It discusses in detail the various methods that will be used, the image that you want to project, and the expected results for success. These plans should contain marketing objectives the practice may have. These objectives may be such goals as to increase patient awareness and satisfaction, increase revenues and profitability for the practice, and increase the number of referring physicians, to name a few. It should contain a listing of possible target markets such as workers' compensation panels, referring physicians, community organizations, nursing homes, and so on. A marketing plan should consist of the following six parts:

Part One: Executive Summary. This part is generally completed last. It contains answers to who, what, where, when, and how with respect to marketing objectives and strategies.

Part Two: Industry Analysis. This part consists of the industry insights into competitors, regulatory environment, patients, and the place the practice holds within the industry (based on specialty, size, location, etc). The following two companies provide industry analyses: SWOT and Porter's. A *SWOT* analysis details the *strengths, weaknesses, opportunities,* and *threats* in health care. To complete a SWOT analysis, go to the following Web site: www.websitemarketingplan.com/marketing_managment/SWOT. *Porter's 5 Forces Analysis* analyzes the dynamics between and activities of current and future competitors; the practice; substitutes for the services the practice provides; the industry suppliers; and patients. To find out more about this company, go to the following Web site: www.websitemarketingplan.com/marketing_management/marketing_strategy.

Part Three: Products/Services and Corresponding Target Markets. Use this section to describe the products and services along with the target audiences for each. For each product or service, include the following information:
- Target market demographics such as income levels, age ranges, geographic locations, and so on
- Industry or societal trends that affect the practice
- The practice's target audience's needs and wants and corresponding benefits received from each

Part Four: Marketing Strategy. Consists of overall marketing objectives and the mission statement of the practice. Address each of the following:
- The product/service positioning relative to the competition
- The general strategies that will be used to reach the objectives
- The product's/service's marketing mix (address the "four P's" of marketing)

Part Five: Measurements. This part consists of building success metrics into each marketing program, including intermediate measures and how they will be used to monitor the progress of the marketing plan.

Part Six: Forecasts and Financial Analyses. This part consists of an explanation of the size of your target markets, market shares, and growth projections by month. It also includes financial analyses such as the following:
- Profit-and-loss statements
- Breakeven analysis

The Short List for Successful Marketing of Medical Practices

1. Identify the target audience.
2. Identify competition.
3. Implement a patient satisfaction survey.
4. Develop/revise a business plan, a strategic plan, and a marketing plan.
5. Practices with limited resources should start with only one marketing project at a time.
6. Whatever marketing project you use, track the progress of the plan to be sure the practice goals are being met.
7. Recognize the importance of internal marketing (i.e., patient satisfaction, pleasant surroundings, friendly staff, etc.).
8. As discussed in Chapter 3, greet all patients by their name within 20 seconds of them entering the office.
9. Develop a patient handbook that will answer most questions about the practice.
10. Develop a newsletter to include such articles as "Don't Forget Your Flu Shot," as well as informative articles about Crohn's disease, diabetes mellitus, and other health-related information.
11. Consider a bulletin board in the waiting room that could contain interesting articles such as a new specialist in town or the expansion of the local community hospital.
12. Thank patients for other patient referrals; thank new patients for choosing your office for care. It provides a great personal touch.
13. Regular reassessment of your availability and your office hours will ensure that you are meeting the needs of your patient population.

14. Always take calls from other physicians in the community.
15. Always return calls to patients. Place the policy on return phone calls in the patient handbook.
16. Consider involvement in research projects to better care for your patients.
17. Renew staff enthusiasm on a regular basis.
18. Emphasize the importance of teamwork.
19. Get out into the community; join community-minded groups such as the Lions, Rotary, Kiwanis, Elks, Moose, Soroptimists, Shriner's, and so on.
20. Sponsor children's sport's teams such as soccer, baseball, and midget football and perhaps even help coach as a great practice builder.
21. Volunteer as the school doctor for the local schools.
22. Provide comments on health issues for the local newspaper, radio, or television.
23. Develop a practice Web site.

Perform a Marketing Assessment

Some offices perform an internal marketing assessment to gain insight into the practice. Each employee and each physician should complete this assessment. Once completed, the office manager should compile the information by placing it into a spreadsheet. A marketing meeting should then be held to discuss the results.

A marketing assessment should include some of the following questions:

- What do you see as the strengths of the practice?
- What do you see as the weaknesses of the practice?
- What ideas do you have for possible opportunities for the practice?
- Do you know of any roadblocks for your practice?
- What is the most common service provided by the practice?
- Are there opportunities for new services to be offered?
- Based on patient volumes, do you know who your number one referring doctor is?
- Do you have any ideas for additional referrals into the practice?
- Do you see a need for change in physician availability or office hours?
- Do you know what the patient mix of your practice is? By gender? By age? By payer?
- Do you see the patient mix changing within the next 2 years? If so, why?
- Can you think of any patients who have left the practice within the past 2 years?
- Do you know why they left?
- Do you currently contribute to the marketing of the practice? If so, how?
- Do you know of any way in which you could help to market the practice?
- Do you see a need for a change from hospital-based procedures to ambulatory surgery centers (ASCs) or outpatient procedures?
- Are there any ASCs in the community?
- Do you have interest in an association with this ASC?
- What procedures would they be?
- If you are a specialty office, do you educate physicians within the community on the services you provide?
- Do you know the demographics of the community in which you practice?
- Do you know how to get them?
- Do you know the value of this information?
- Do you, as an individual, belong to any community organizations?
- Can this association help to market the practice?
- Do you have a need for additional physicians within your practice?
- Do you have a need for physician extenders within the practice?
- Would it be prudent to join the staff of another hospital?
- What do you currently do that enhances patient satisfaction?
- What do you think you should do to better serve the patient?
- What marketing have you done in the past?
- Do you think it was successful?
- Are you active within your individual professional group?
- Is teamwork important?
- Do you think your practice employees have a "teamwork" mentality?
- Does your practice have access to the Internet? How is it currently used?
- If not, do you think it could benefit from this access?
- How would it be used?
- Do you think the practice is successful?
- Do you think it can be even more successful?
- What do you think the practice needs to do to achieve this success?
- What can you do to help the practice to be successful?

ADVERTISING VERSUS MARKETING

Remember that advertising and marketing are two different things. Many types of advertising are discussed later in this chapter. Marketing involves analyzing the practice and its potential market. Only after this analysis is completed is an advertising campaign started. Physician offices that go straight into advertising before performing market analyses are wasting money and not being effective.

There are two types of marketing: external and internal. External marketing is the type that we see outside the office (e.g., an advertisement for Dr. Jones's Chiropractic Clinic). Even more important than external marketing is internal marketing—what the office does as an integral part of daily operations to promote itself.

INTERNAL MARKETING

Internal marketing includes the following activities:

- Ensuring patient satisfaction
- Conducting patient satisfaction surveys
- Conducting referring physician surveys
- Providing patient education programs and materials
- Distributing patient information handbooks

It is crucial to understand what can be done from inside the medical practice to make it grow. Internal marketing is the most important marketing that can be done for a medical office.

Perception Is Reality

Perception is reality for some patients. Ninety-five percent of unhappy patients will not tell a physician that they are unhappy. Up to 80% of patients who leave a practice do so because of the people who work there, not because of their displeasure with the physician. Understanding the importance of patient/customer perception is an important factor in all lines of business. Companies such as Disney, Wal-Mart, Federal Express, and Marriott have built successful businesses by understanding this concept. Now health care organizations realize the importance of patient perception and focus on measuring quality; managed care companies poll their members with "physician report cards," a practice that upsets some physicians.

Efforts to evaluate patients' satisfaction focus on their perceptions of their treatment and outcome. Most patients are not passive; they are knowledgeable consumers—educated, demanding, and involved in their own care. The role of the patient has changed.

A simple exercise will increase employees' awareness of the various things that can go wrong for patients during an office visit. Have the staff call out the steps a patient takes when he or she arrives at the office door, and have a staff member write each step down on a Post-It note. For instance:

Patient enters the office
Patient registers with the receptionist
Patient sits in waiting room (and so on)

Line the Post-It notes across the office wall. Then have the staff talk about what could go wrong at each step along the way. Write each possibility on a Post-It note and place everyone's suggestions directly under each step. You may end up with many Post-It notes. Remind employees that the purpose of this exercise is not to poke fun at the practice, but to point out what incidents may turn a patient away from the office. Be aware that some staff members may take offense, thinking co-workers are talking about them. Figure 15-1 shows an example of how to set up this exercise. Figure 15-2 takes the exercise to the next level, listing some of the things that can go wrong at various stages in the office visit, thus creating a dissatisfied patient.

To bring about patient satisfaction, physicians and staff must be willing to change their attitudes toward health care. It is important that you understand the value of improving practice processes and interaction with patients. Some office managers recognize that efficient and consistent service creates patient satisfaction and therefore practice success. Other office managers are more businesslike and view good service as simply a business principle. Change is part of life—both professional and personal life. Today, people have choices in many areas of their lives, including their health care. Patients and insurance companies make choices every day that will affect the future of health care. The successful office accepts change, putting patients and their needs first and constantly striving for patient satisfaction.

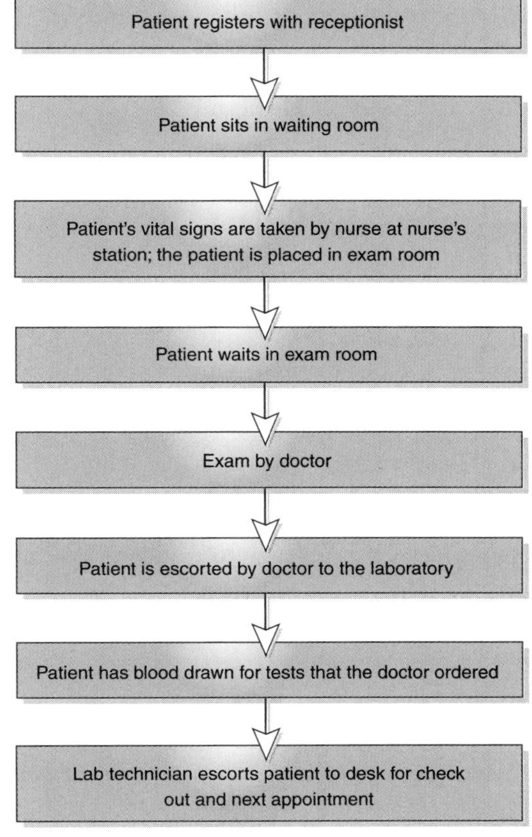

FIGURE 15-1. Patient flow chart for the medical office.

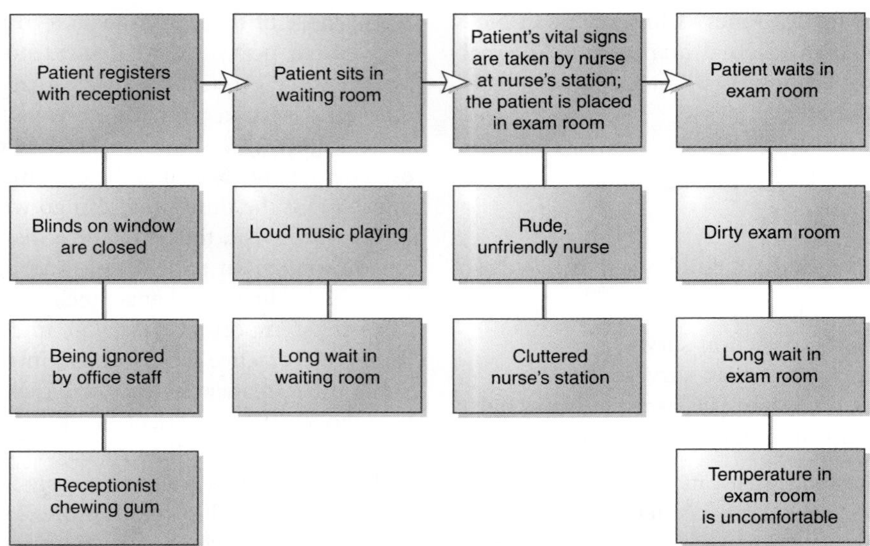

FIGURE 15-2. Things that should not occur during patient flow.

QUALITY SERVICE

Creating rapport with patients is easily done once they reach the office, but what about the following external factors that can influence patients before they reach the office?

- Word-of-mouth reports from other patients
- Newspaper, radio, or TV ads
- Word-of-mouth reports from co-workers
- Comments by other physicians

A medical office must deal with three important concepts:

1. Patient expectation
2. Patient experience
3. Patient perception

Patient expectation refers to patients' expectations regarding what will take place during an office visit. *Patient experience* is the circle of events that actually take place during an office visit. *Patient perception* is how a patient rates an office visit. Remember that the staff's perception of how a patient's office visit went can be very different from the patient's. A personal touch for every patient is very important in the outcome of an office visit. Patients must feel that they are cared for.

Expectation + Experience = Perception

Elements of Quality Service

Quality means a degree of excellence. An office's main goal should be to ensure that each patient feels that he or she has received high-quality service. There are four key elements to the delivery of quality service:

1. *The customer:* Without the customer (patient), there is no need to strive for quality service. There is also no need for the staff to come to work!
2. *Staff commitment:* Without the commitment of the office manager, physician, and staff, quality service will fall by the wayside.
3. *Patient expectations:* If the office does not attempt to fulfill patient expectations, it stands no chance of satisfying patients.
4. *Continuity of service:* Quality service requires consistency.

The coming together of these four elements results in patient satisfaction, staff motivation, professional fulfillment, and the practice's success.

Obstacles to Quality Service

The office as a whole must believe in quality service not just as a fashionable topic of discussion but as an attitude infusing every activity. An office's commitment to quality will be the driving force that makes it work; without it, quality service will not be delivered (Box 15-1). Deep commitment to quality service is a sure route to a successful practice!

BOX 15-1 Roadblocks to the Delivery of Quality Service

Lack of commitment
Doing too much too fast
Misplaced priorities
Disorganization

BOX 15-2 The Patient Creed

The patient is our reason for being here.
It takes months to find a patient, seconds to lose one.
Always be courteous and polite during each patient contact.
Always do more than is expected when you handle a patient's problem.
Never promise more than you can deliver.
Continually look to improve quality care and service to your patients.

Continuity of Service

Continuity means persistence without essential change. By instituting a continuity system, you ensure that quality service is given continuous, consistent attention. With continuity, service gets better day after day. Continuity doesn't mean that no change can take place. It requires flexibility and continuous vigilance. Continuity of service means continuing to do the very best that can be done for patients, while constantly looking for ways to improve. You cannot institute this system of continuity alone; it requires the commitment of physicians and staff to succeed! The patient creed in Box 15-2 sums up this idea.

Consumers

It is not so much what we do for our patients, but how we do it that matters!
—UNKNOWN

It has always been difficult for medical practices to perceive patients as consumers. The reality is that patients are indeed consumers—consumers who are shopping for a service—and they must be thought of in that respect. Everyone who works in a medical office knows that some patients are demanding, annoying, and loud; others are understanding, pleasant, and easygoing; still others are timid, soft-spoken, and unassertive. Too many offices perceive and talk about patients as if they were diseases (e.g., "The peptic ulcer in Room 4 needs lab work"). This type of office chatter demonstrates a lack of respect for a patient; the patient has been pigeon-holed as a disease category. That "peptic ulcer" in Room 4 has a name.

Rule #1: If we don't take care of the patient, someone else will!

Commitment

STAFF

Commitment to quality service must start at the top. Physicians must make a commitment to patients before staff can do so. A commitment is a pledge to provide a certain course of action. It carries with it a certain depth and sincerity. This commitment must be total; in other words, everyone on staff must be 100% committed to providing quality service to their patients. As the office manager, you are considered the physician's surrogate when it comes to management issues, and this principle must be conveyed to and understood by all employees.

The Credit Belongs

The credit belongs to those who
are actually in the arena who strive
valiantly; who know the great
enthusiasms, the great devotions,
and spend themselves in a worthy cause;
who at the best, know the triumph
of high achievement; and who,
at the worst, if they fail, fail
while daring greatly, so that their
place shall never be with those cold
and timid souls who know neither
victory nor defeat.

Theodore Roosevelt

OFFICE MANAGER

There are several fundamental practices that should be followed closely to facilitate commitment to quality service, including the following:

- Have a solid vision or reachable goal
- Have conviction in what the office is doing
- Be visible and available
- Learn and grow every day
- Reward staff for a job well done
- Review the office's progress at least once a year

A COMMITMENT EXERCISE

You may want to do the following commitment exercise at one of your regularly scheduled staff meetings. Hand a legal pad to each employee and ask him or her to respond to the following questions:

- What business are we in?
- Why are we in this business?
- Who are our patients?
- What type of patients do we want?
- What are our patients' expectations?
- How can we meet the expectations of our patients?
- What type of image do we want to portray?

Remind employees that there may be more than one answer to each question. They should feel free to write down all possible answers, and the questions should be answered honestly. This exercise can be done confidentially if staff members choose. You may wish to ask the physician to also answer these questions and then compare answers. The results can be interesting and eye-opening!

This exercise can also be done with a flip chart or blackboard. It can be a brainstorming session in which employees call out answers to each question, and all answers are written down to be discussed at the end of the session. Brainstorming is a method of encouraging free thinking and creative ideas within a group. During brainstorming sessions, make sure all employees are given time to think about each issue or question. Remind them that no idea is stupid! There can be no criticism and ideas should focus on processes, not people. Ideas should be spontaneous, and shy or quiet employees should be encouraged to participate. Once this information has been collected, use it to improve how the practice feels about itself and its patients.

Patient Satisfaction

It is a well-known fact that patients are the foundation of a medical practice. They are the base that health care professionals build on. What is this buzzword *patient satisfaction*? How is it defined? There are a variety of books and articles on the subject, and each defines it differently. Patients themselves define it differently, because each person's needs are different. No generic statement can be made about patient satisfaction; patients must be satisfied individually.

Patient satisfaction is made up of quality medical care and quality service:

Quality medical care + Quality service = Patient satisfaction

All physicians know that they are providing their patients with the best possible medical care; however, are they providing top-notch service?

Patient satisfaction rewards the practice with the following:

- Increased productivity
- Higher profitability
- More patient referrals
- Improved employee morale
- Increased collection rate
- Decreased employee turnover
- Lower risk of malpractice suits

Patient dissatisfaction results in losses for a practice. Leonard Abramson, past president of Aetna U.S. Healthcare (a large managed care company), once said, "Dissatisfied patients have feet—they'll walk away!" Statistics have shown that revenues lost through the loss of one patient are $238,000 over the life of a practice. From 27% to 52% of patients fail to keep appointments, often as a result of dissatisfaction. Missed appointments, of course, directly affect practice revenues. Not only is a patient lost, but also any referrals that the patient might have made in the future are gone. It is good practice to send patients thank-you notes when they refer new patients to the office. A note such as the one shown in Figure 15-3 can be used.

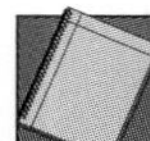

FROM THE EXPERT'S NOTEBOOK

It has been said that if you lose 1 patient, you actually lose 11, because 1 patient will influence 10 more!

The need to provide good service is not news to businesses that have long recognized the importance of service. Companies such as Federal Express, the Ritz-Carlton, Wal-Mart, and Disney have prided themselves on providing excellent customer service in a very competitive society. Health care facilities are now realizing that they, too, are

Dear ________________________:

Today, I was pleased to provide care to someone you referred to our office. I know how important it is for the friends and family members of our patients to get encouragement to come to us for their health care needs. When someone is looking for a doctor, that person wants to know that the doctor and staff are competent and that he or she will receive personalized attention. Thank you for trusting that my staff and I will meet the expectations of your friends and relatives.

If you have any health questions or concerns, please feel free to call our office. Also, if there is anything we need to know to improve our ability to serve you, I hope you will be direct in providing me with any suggestions that you might have. I value your perspective and know that there may be others you will send for diagnosis and treatment.

Thank you again for recommending my office. I value your participation in our practice.

Wishing you the best of health,

Alexander Babinetz, M.D.

FIGURE 15-3. Referral thank-you letter to a nonphysician.

businesses. Many health care institutions, such as Prudential, U.S. Healthcare, Cleveland Clinic, and Hospital Corporation of America, have begun to recognize the importance of the "customer satisfaction" credo and are now establishing patient satisfaction programs. Some insurance companies are now rating physicians who participate in their plans. Members are sent patient satisfaction forms and asked to complete them fully. Statistics are compiled from these forms, and "report cards" on physicians are sent to members. On these report cards, physicians are graded on appropriateness, cost, outcomes of care, and, of course, patient satisfaction. Today's patients are more educated and quality oriented than patients of the past. They want good service and quality care for their dollar. Sometimes a patient's primary concern is not money, but how he or she was treated!

Attitude is everything!

There are several areas in which a patient can become dissatisfied with a medical office:

- The office's automated telephone system is difficult to use
- The patient is unable to get an appointment when she or he wants one
- An injection is forgotten and the patient must return to the office
- The patient is waiting too long
- The office is too cold
- There is no parking
- Too many tests are ordered
- Staff are more interested in payment than in the patient
- Too many medications are prescribed
- Staff are unfriendly
- The physician is too hurried and appears disinterested
- And the list goes on and on!

PATIENT SATISFACTION FORM

A smart office manager obtains feedback from patients to make sure the office is doing a good job. A patient satisfaction form can be designed and distributed to patients to complete. This form can be distributed in various ways:

- The form can be handed to patients on a clipboard in the waiting room.
- Patients can be asked to complete the form while they are in the waiting room and place it in a box there.
- Have the form printed on a postcard with a flap so it can be taken home by patients and easily be mailed back with privacy maintained.

A sample patient satisfaction form is shown in Figure 15-4. It can be copied and used as is, or changed to better meet the needs of your practice. Once this information is collected from patients, schedule a meeting with staff to discuss the results and how the practice can better address patient needs.

WORD OF MOUTH

Every patient who knows you also knows 300 or 400 other people! Most physicians believe in word-of-mouth marketing. Each of your patients probably knows three or four dozen people well enough to speak with them often, and each of these other people regularly talks with three or four dozen other people. Making use of this communication network is called *market leverage.* It is easy to tap into the grapevine and use it to your marketing advantage. About 90% of all new patients (not referred by physicians) are nonetheless referred by someone. About 70% of all those people use information from friends, family, co-workers, and neighbors to select a physician. Another 15% to 20% come to a practice as a result of information obtained from a health care professional.

Two issues are involved in word-of-mouth marketing:

1. Stop negative word of mouth (as much as possible)
2. Promote positive word of mouth (always)

If your practice is providing merely adequate experiences, patients will not say anything, negative or positive. If you exceed their expectations, they will be pleasantly surprised and discuss how great you are at the next senior citizen's meeting or at the country club pool. If you don't meet their expectations, watch out! Dissatisfied people talk. They will complain to everyone they meet within the next 2 weeks!

As an office manager, it is important to observe and understand two facets of the practice: your office systems and the people skills of your personnel. These are the most likely problem areas. Review the office systems you have in place to identify any problems. Listen to your employees as they interact with patients. Listen for any interactions that may cause frustration, anxiety, disappointment, or irritation among patients.

Word-of-mouth marketing is usually a face-to-face interaction, which is the most powerful form of communication. Word-of-mouth marketers are generally well received and persuasive, because they are perceived as having nothing to gain from their communication. And finally, word-of-mouth marketing is never finished. It is not a process you complete once and walk away from; it is a constant, unceasing opportunity to build a practice.

PATIENTS SPEAK OUT

Patients want a physician who demonstrates the following characteristics:

- Is knowledgeable
- Is interested in patients
- Explains things clearly, in easy-to-understand terms
- Asks appropriate questions
- Offers practical solutions for problems
- Spends the necessary time with patients

Please rate our office by using the following grading system. Circle the appropriate number.

1 very dissatisfied   2 dissatisfied   3 satisfied   4 very satisfied

Were we able to give you an appointment in a timely manner?

1   2   3   4

Comments:

Once in our office, were you seen in a timely manner?

1   2   3   4

Comments:

Was our staff pleasant and eager to help you?

1   2   3   4

Comments:

Did you have any problems with our billing department?

1   2   3   4

Comments:

Were you satisfied with your total experience in our office?

1   2   3   4

Comments:

Did you have trouble finding our office?

1   2   3   4

Comments:

Would you recommend this office to others?

1   2   3   4

Comments:

FIGURE 15-4. Sample patient satisfaction form.

Patients want a medical office that provides the following:

- Patients want to be able to reach the office when they need to.
- They want a courteous office staff; they want the phone answered by a person with a friendly voice who understands.
- They want to know how long it will take for someone to return a phone call.
- They want on-time appointment schedules and appointments when needed.
- They want responsiveness to problems.
- They want informed information about their insurance, services and procedures, and coverage.

It is important to listen to what people are saying about you. Take this information and let it guide the office in how to do things better.

THAT WARM AND FUZZY FEELING

Make patients feel comfortable and special. Use their name several times when talking with them. A smile is great, but not enough. Be enthusiastic when greeting them. For new patients, take the time to provide them with a summary of how the office works. Ask how they heard about the practice. Give new patients a tour of the office, pointing out the restroom should they need it. When patients leave the office, thank them for choosing your office for their care. Send new patients a letter thanking them for selecting your office as their health care provider. A sample letter can be found in Figure 15-5.

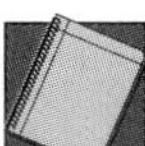

FROM THE EXPERT'S NOTEBOOK

Remember: You can be the best physician, and you can have equally good colleagues, but if you're not paying attention to service issues and concerns, you have a chance of losing patients.

Patient Satisfaction Checklist

Successful physician practices ask themselves the following questions about their reception area:

- Is the reception room pleasant and clean?
- Is coffee or juice available for the patients?
- Are the magazines up to date (no more than 90 days old) and is there a wide selection of topics?
- Is there information about the practice and/or the physician in the reception room?
- Are patient educational materials available?
- Are tissues available?
- Is there a suggestion box where patients can provide feedback?
- Are there toys and books appropriate for pediatric patients?
- Is the waiting period less than 15 minutes?

Use this list as a basis for preparing your own checklist for the patient.

PATIENT EXPECTATIONS

It is important that communication among physicians, staff, and patients be clear. After all, if staff are unaware of what a patient wants and needs, it is impossible for them to provide satisfaction. The examples listed in Box 15-3 illustrate common complaints of patients. Many employees know their patients well because they have been patients for many years. Some patients feel that the doctor's staff is like "family." In cases where a close relationship exists between office staff and patients, the staff is more aware of their needs and expectations. Employees who are not in tune with patients must try harder to understand their needs and make an effort to satisfy them. These expectations must be determined and immediately addressed.

Expectations differ from patient to patient. Various factors affect what a patient expects of an office visit, including the patient's age, sex, mood, life problems, the time of day, and the day of the week. In other words, there is no standard for patient expectations. You can, however, get to know patients to have a better idea of what their needs

Dear Mr. McNamara:

Thank you for coming to our office today. We are pleased to have had the opportunity to serve your health care needs. Our goal is to provide you with the kind of competent and personalized attention you need to enhance good health. If you have any questions about the office or about your visit, please do not hesitate to call me personally.

Many of our patients are recommended to us by their friends or families. We sincerely hope you received the type of care you would recommend to a friend. Please let me know if there is anything we can do to improve our office policies and procedures.

Wishing you good health,

Alexander Babinetz, M.D.

FIGURE 15-5. Sample thank-you letter.

BOX 15-3 Common Complaints of Dissatisfied Patients

- "I had to wait 2 hours before I was seen."
- "I had to put on that paper gown and sit in a cold exam room for 25 minutes, waiting for the doctor to come in."
- "The doctor kept getting interrupted by the telephone."
- "The doctor ordered all these tests and never told me what was wrong."
- "The doctor wasn't listening to me! He acted like he didn't care about what I was saying."
- "All that office was worried about was the money."
- "The doctor never returned my telephone calls."
- "The nurse was talking to another nurse about her date last night, instead of concentrating on giving me my shot."

may be. Understand their needs, be flexible, and gently manage unrealistic expectations through patient education. In Figure 15-6, a member of the physician's staff is taking the time to distract a child by entertaining him with a puppet.

PATIENT EDUCATION PROGRAMS

Patients love to read about illnesses! Whether it is their own or someone else's, they are often intrigued by various disorders. Patient education is an important part of patient satisfaction and is also monitored by insurance companies. They want their patients to be well informed and find that patients are more at ease when procedures and illnesses are explained thoroughly. Brochures and pamphlets can be purchased through a variety of vendors, but you might want to develop educational materials relating specifically to your office. For instance, an orthopedist might offer a pamphlet entitled "Saving Your Back. . .How to Lift Properly." A pediatrician's office might offer a pamphlet entitled "How to Choose a Qualified Day Care." Patient education materials from a gastroenterology office are presented in Box 15-4 and Figure 15-7.

BOX 15-4 Patient Education Material about Colonoscopy

About a Colonoscopy Procedure:
You will be asked to lie on the examination table and turn on your left side. The doctor will examine your rectum with a gloved finger and then insert the flexible colonoscopy tube gently into your rectum. He will advance the tube slowly through your colon, examining the lining thoroughly. You may feel some abdominal cramping from the air that the doctor injects into your colon. You may also be asked to change position slightly to help the passage of the scope.

Biopsies (tiny bits of tissue) may be taken for microscopic examination, but these should not cause you any pain or discomfort.

The colonoscopic examination takes about 20 minutes to 1 hour. After the procedure, you will be moved to a quiet room to rest until the effect of any medication wears off. You may feel some bloating from the air that remains in the colon. You may be more comfortable if you expel this air, but it is not advisable to force this.

It is very important that you be escorted home after the examination and that you remain home resting until the next day.

Web-enabled networks are a popular way to meet patient education needs. Many Web sites contain information that is clear and easy to follow, offering outcomes of studies and medical news that patients can use in everyday life. Many consumers will print out information

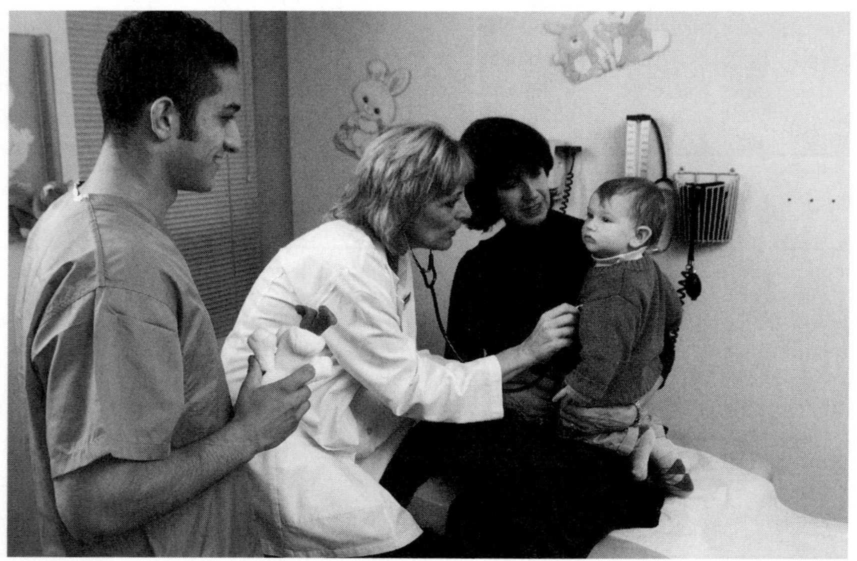

FIGURE 15-6. It is sometimes helpful to distract a child during an office visit.

- You are scheduled for a colonoscopy on: ________________
- Do not take any food or liquid by mouth after midnight the night before the procedure.
- You may take your medications with a sip of water the morning of the procedure.
- The day before the procedure, you should maintain a clear liquid diet. This can include Jell-O, tea, clear broths, or apple juice.
- On ______________________ start to take Golytely. This is one gallon of fluid. Drink one glass (8 oz) every 10 to 15 minutes until the entire contents have been consumed.
- Report to the office at Community General Hospital, Suite 20, on: ________________________ at ________________________

Because you will probably receive an anesthetic, it is important to bring someone with you to drive you home. If you have any questions, please call the office at (000) 111-1111.

Signed: ______________________________
Patient

Signed: ______________________________
Person Giving Instructions

Date: ______________________________

FIGURE 15-7. Patient instructions: preparing for a colonoscopy.

downloaded from the Web to take to their physicians for discussion. Even older Americans (those over 50 years of age) access the Internet an average of 14 days each month. The Internet provides unlimited possibilities for patients who crave information.

PATIENT INFORMATION HANDBOOK

A patient information handbook can be fun to design and a valuable tool when used correctly. A handbook can contain a wealth of information regarding the practice, such as its hours, how appointments are scheduled, and where its offices are located. Staff can hold regular meetings to develop this manual. Everyone's input is important!

Distributing the handbook to patients can eliminate many patient phone calls. Many misunderstandings can be eliminated if patients have their handbook to refer to regarding office policies and procedures. These handbooks can either be mailed to new patients before they arrive at the office or handed to them on their first visit. See Appendix E for an example of a simple patient information handbook.

REFERRING PHYSICIAN SURVEY

Referring physicians are an important factor for a practice. If you work for a specialty practice, referring physicians may be its lifeblood. One of the most important responsibilities of the medical office manager is to be aware of any problems that might occur between your office and the referring physician's office. A solid working relationship should be in place at all times. The referring practice's happiness (satisfaction) is a critical issue for the specialist practice. Some offices send surveys to their referring physicians to find out how they can better serve their needs. A more productive approach is for you to visit each referring physician's office, speak with the office manager to establish a common ground, and inquire about any problems that might be occurring between offices. This information can be extremely helpful for both practices. You can then take a minute (doctors are always busy and will appreciate your recognition of this fact) of the referring physician's time to introduce yourself and ask how your office can better accommodate his or her needs. A referring physician's satisfaction survey is shown in Figure 15-8 for copying or customizing.

Staff Satisfaction

A medical office staff has certain basic needs: good benefits, pleasant work environment, and competitive salaries. They also have another agenda of needs: recognition, appreciation, and participation. Staff satisfaction directly relates to patient satisfaction.

Happy staff = Happy office = Happy patients

Everyone wins in this situation. Every type of motivation works on someone at some time. It takes the proper mix of ingredients to provide staff satisfaction:

- Appreciation of their work
- Job security
- Good working conditions
- Loyalty from the management
- Competitive salaries
- An understanding office manager
- Participation in office decisions

Six factors influence job satisfaction:

1. Achievement
2. Recognition

Date: ______________________________

Name of Referring Physician: ______________________________

Name of Office Manager: ______________________________

Patient Comments:

Referring Physician Staff Comments:

Referring Physician Comments:

Did you receive an appointment for your patient in a timely manner? ______ Y ______ N

Did you receive a patient report in a timely manner? ______ Y ______ N

How can we improve our service to you?

FIGURE 15-8. Referring physician satisfaction survey.

3. The work itself
4. Responsibility
5. Advancement
6. Growth

The following extrinsic factors also affect job satisfaction:

1. Company policy
2. Supervision
3. Work conditions
4. Salary
5. Relationship with peers and subordinates
6. Status
7. Personal life
8. Security

Employees should find their positions meaningful and enriching. The best form of motivation is the kind that gets people involved with what they do, making them feel that their efforts result in worthwhile contributions to the organization. Encourage your employees to provide ideas on change that would benefit the office. When an employee offers a valuable suggestion or change, reward him or her. There are various ways to reward employees for achievement:

- An instant reward, such as a plant, flowers, or a gift certificate
- An incentive reward, such as immediate verbal recognition, a letter of thanks, or business cards for staff members
- Success celebrations, such as a half-day off with pay or a gift certificate for two at a local restaurant
- Team incentives, such as buying lunch for the office or having a casual-dress day once a week
- Financial rewards, such as salary increases, bonuses, better benefits, or a reduced workweek

Staff who feel appreciated are more productive, create a calm environment, and do the very best they can. People who show passion for and conviction in their work inspire others. People respond to enthusiasm and positive feedback. This type of atmosphere spills over onto patients, and the office becomes a warm, friendly, and caring place to be.

A Word about Competence

Unlike patients of the past, today's patients shop around for their doctors. They use stiff criteria, and their main concern is the skill and competence of both the physician and staff. All contact between patients and staff is critical, and courtesy is key. Many patients' unhappiness with a practice has its roots in dissatisfaction with the office staff. If patients feel neglected or become annoyed by office staff, they will not bother meeting the doctor.

Importance of a Mission Statement

What should be mentioned in a mission statement? Each practice has its own ideas about what should be addressed in its mission statement, including the following:

- Quality care
- Quality service
- Coordinated care
- Responsiveness to needs
- Enhanced quality of life for patients
- Recognition of patient, insurance company, hospital, staff member, and physician roles in care
- Need for a competent and trained staff
- Importance of wellness care

You should display your office's mission statement or vision, making it available for patients to read. Some offices have their mission statement professionally printed, framed, and hung in each examination room. Some offices hang it in the waiting room. Others have it printed on the back of their appointment cards. All offices should make their mission statement a part of their patient handbook. This is a great internal marketing tool and should be used whenever possible. This statement serves as the foundation for practice growth. It should demonstrate a solid commitment to patients, the practice, and community service. This statement says who you are, what you are, and what you intend to do. Box 15-5 presents a sample mission statement.

BOX 15-5 Sample Mission Statement

Quality patient care and patient satisfaction are the main goals of our practice. We believe the enthusiasm and efficiency of our staff are important aspects of achieving these goals. Because of our commitment to quality patient care, we hire staff that share in our commitment by exhibiting motivation, cooperation, productivity, and care. The physicians and staff at Central City Cardiology share in that commitment, which reflects the philosophy and direction of our practice.

Practice Newsletters

A practice newsletter can be either a gold mine or a ton of useless rock! A well-done practice newsletter generates income by attracting new patients and providing the proper amount of media exposure. With today's focus on patient satisfaction and education, a newsletter can be a handy means of providing professional information to patients in a friendly way. It can contain valuable information regarding the practice and its policies, which can save time for office staff. The downside is that depending on the demographics of the practice, some newsletters go unread.

PERSONALIZING THE NEWSLETTER

First you must decide on the newsletter's format and the type of information to include. It should look as though it is unique to the practice. It should convey the feeling that it was developed strictly for educating patients in your office. This will give a sense of personalization, which is very important these days. The following tips will help you keep your newsletter personal:

- Write the newsletter exclusively for your practice, not for a wide range of practices.
- The office manager should control the content.
- Write stories that reflect your physician's or office's personal philosophy.

You and your staff can easily put together a one-page newsletter on the computer. This entails simply inputting the copy and formatting it on the computer. You can then print it on either plain or colored paper. Fold the paper in thirds, staple it at the top, stamp it, and apply an address label. With today's computer resources, there is no need for costly printing, typesetting, and designing services. Even self-taught computer users can design and develop newsletters and brochures.

To make sure the newsletter looks professional, use a good desktop publishing program and a good printer (preferably laser). Make sure to pick a vibrant-colored paper to catch the reader's eye, or use a color printer if one is available to you. Look at magazines and newspapers for format and content ideas. If the newsletter cannot be produced in the office without looking shoddy, then by all means have it done professionally.

You also must commit to producing the newsletter regularly. Decide whether it should be released monthly, bimonthly, or quarterly, and set up a year's schedule of production dates based on that. If it cannot be produced at least quarterly, it should not be done. Don't be afraid to repeat certain important information—repetition pays off over time.

The following are some tips for producing a newsletter for your practice:

- Keep it dignified, professional, and honest.
- Stimulate inquiries by discussing symptoms of certain illnesses.
- Define the goals of the newsletter.
- Be sure to reflect the practice: let the newsletter mirror your perception of the practice.
- If you are unable to write engaging articles, seek professional writing help.
- Make the message subtle: give important facts about the practice along with health information.
- Have the physician give his or her thoughts on certain medicines and treatments.
- Be committed to the newsletter. Send it regularly and keep in mind that it isn't advertising—it's marketing!
- Mail the newsletter by first-class mail to distinguish it from junk mail. Be sure to put the return address on the top left corner.
- Consider mailing the newsletter to others besides your patients—for example, to pharmaceutical representatives, the media, hospital departments, and community organizations.
- Leave copies of the newsletter in the waiting room for new patients to pick up.
- Ask patients what they are interested in so you can easily pick popular topics for future discussion.

GETTING THE MARKETING EDGE

It may be a good idea to get involved with another office for the purpose of sharing the expense of a newsletter. This can be an opportunity to get greater exposure and can also be a practice builder. By splitting costs, each office gets more pages and more information for less. For instance, cooperation between an obstetrics/gynecology (OB/GYN) practice and an expectant-mothers group could be a perfect match. Even such specialists as cardiologists and ophthalmologists can create a newsletter that works for everyone. If you're working for a small, struggling practice, you might check with local newspapers to see if they are interested in running your newsletter as a community awareness article.

Most American companies today are concerned with the wellness and education of their employees. Such companies might be interested in helping finance your newsletter as a service to their employees. They may provide financial help if their employees receive copies of the newsletter when it is distributed. This can act as a growth tool, because some employees may wish to come see the physician who wrote that great article in last month's issue!

There are various ways to use the newsletter to benefit both the community and practice. Every community has bulletin boards. Mount copies of the newsletter on bulletin boards with staples or tacks so that individuals can easily take one. The newsletter can also be exhibited at health fairs and screenings in pharmacies, stores, and shopping malls. Place copies in adult day care centers, senior centers, and any other community buildings. Ask local nursing homes if you can place some of your newsletters in their waiting areas. Make copies available to schools, libraries, and medical supply stores. Offer copies to referring physicians for their waiting rooms and offer to place their newsletters in yours. This becomes a win-win situation for both offices.

MARKETING

No-Cost, Low-Cost Marketing Tools

Use the patient billing statement to your advantage! At the bottom of each statement, print a message that will bring in patients. For example, at the bottom of the July statement, print the message, "Don't forget about your children's back-to-school physicals!" This can be a standard message for a family practice or pediatrician's office. An August statement from an internist's office can read, "Flu season is approaching. Call for your flu shot today!" An ophthalmologist's billing statement for any month could read, "Glaucoma is a silent stealer of eyesight—have your eyes checked!" An internist's office could print the message, "Hypertension is the silent killer. When did you last have your blood pressure checked?" You can develop a set of "wellness" messages that can automatically be printed on each patient statement. This is a great way to show patients you care. It takes only a few minutes to implement this system, it doesn't cost any more in postage or stationery, and it can be very productive. If your office is like most offices today, you have a computer system—so why not use it?

You might want to suggest to the physician that he or she hold monthly lunches for referring physicians. This is a good way for the physician to develop rapport with referring physicians whom he or she doesn't see often. The lunch can be a simple buffet at a restaurant near the hospital. Monthly lunches with referring practices can be held for staff members, too. It never hurts to build good working relationships with your referring practices. These staff luncheons can be held in the office and can be either catered or potluck. Give the other office's staff members a tour of the facility, and perhaps point out any new equipment that was just purchased for special procedures. The staff will undoubtedly pass this information on to their physician when they return from lunch!

The diploma is a marketing tool in its own quiet way. One office covered a complete wall with its physician's diplomas. The massive "wall hanging" of diplomas and certificates looked very impressive. Other offices scatter the physician's diplomas and certificates around the examination rooms for patients to look at while they wait for the physician. Evaluate your office and decide which arrangement will work best. Whichever way you decide to do it, make sure that the physician's diplomas are in a highly visible place in the office.

Service Marketing

Service marketing differs from marketing in general because there is no product to market—rather, a service is made available to consumers. Service marketing has four unique characteristics:

1. *Intangibility:* The consumer cannot evaluate what is being marketed with sensory means such as sight, hearing, touch, or taste.
2. *Inseparability:* Performance of the service cannot be separated from consumption, which means that the consumer must be present at the time the service is performed.
3. *Perishability:* Services cannot be stored.
4. *Heterogeneity:* Performance of the service can vary.

There are five major classifications of services:

1. Profit: either nonprofit or for profit
2. Customer type: consumer or organization
3. Labor and equipment needs: labor based or equipment based
4. Customer contact: high or low degree
5. Provider skill level: professional or nonprofessional

Obviously, health care falls under the professional category of "provider skill level," which presents a couple of marketing challenges. First, services that are based on a high level of skill are hard to prove, even after the service is performed. This requires that consumer education be an integral part of the marketing scheme, because the benefits of some skilled services may be unclear to health care consumers. Second, services involving higher skill levels usually encounter more regulation from professional organizations. For example, health care professionals' services are regulated by the government and influenced by such groups as the American Medical Association.

Cooperative Marketing

The health care field is currently in the midst of incredible change: hospital mergers, declining reimbursement, hospital closings, medical practice mergers, layoffs, and hiring freezes. It is very difficult to compete as a single medical office. A first-class marketing and advertising campaign is needed. There is one problem with a first-class marketing and ad campaign, however: it costs a fortune! As a result, some practices are looking into the concept of "cooperative marketing." This concept can be an important tool for solo practitioners and group practices alike. It allows physicians to engage in marketing activities with other physicians and institutions while keeping their practices independent. Participating in community health fairs, forming joint ventures, and opening a free-standing ambulatory care center are just some of the activities that can be shared. The power that group marketing provides allows for the cost-effective delivery of quality care. Independent offices that join in cooperative marketing keep a strong presence and thrive with little or no sacrifice. By participating in cooperative marketing, the office can tap into a wider range of resources and can successfully compete with large offices and practices that have resulted from mergers.

An obstacle to cooperative marketing is that many physicians fear collaboration. This fear results from the tough competition for grades and facilities they experienced all through medical school. Ask the following important questions to determine whether cooperative marketing is right for your office:

1. Are the physician's services different from those of other physicians in the same type of practice?
2. Does your office do any special procedures that are not provided by other offices?
3. How do most of your new patients hear about the practice? Are they being referred? If so, by whom?
4. Do most of your patients come from a certain zip code?
5. Can your office afford to become involved in a marketing plan?
6. What new services can your office add that might benefit new patients?
7. How much time can your office give to a marketing plan?
8. What type of return are you looking for?
9. What services, if any, might your patients need in the future that your office can provide?

Cooperative marketing works best when accompanied by a long-range plan. The physician should be asked what long-range plans he or she has for the office. These plans and the physician's personal agenda can have a decisive influence on how aggressive a marketing plan should be. Call other office managers who work closely with your office to ask whether they have a marketing plan. It is crucial for you to be aware of what the competition is doing and to determine whether these efforts might be something that your office should be undertaking.

One way in which the office can use a cooperative marketing plan is to join in a cross-referral venture with other offices. This is a much more complex system than the ordinary referral programs. Physicians participating in a cross-referral system should clearly define duties and obligations and maintain an open and honest relationship with one another. All offices involved should train their staff to make them aware of specific referral procedures that must be followed.

An example of a joint marketing venture would be the mailing of brochures to current and prospective patients to describe any special services that the office might provide. Several physician offices may join together to create a community newsletter and share the cost of producing it. A family practice might contribute an article on ear infections and the upcoming swimming season; an OB/GYN practice might submit an article advising women on breast cancer and the importance of mammography; an allergist's practice might submit an article on the approaching allergy season; and an orthopedist's practice might contribute a piece on the many injuries being treated because of "in-line" skates. Other community-oriented issues are cataracts, glaucoma, colon cancer, and vasectomies. It is important that each cooperative marketing plan be designed to serve the specific community needs the offices want to target. Organizing and implementing such a program can be a big job for the office manager. Local hospitals, community organizations, and the Chamber of Commerce can be called on for guidance and human power. Don't hesitate to call them!

Sharing is a unique concept in a medical office and will probably bring the physician right to his or her feet when you start to discuss it. It actually is a very clever way to increase services at no extra cost to patients. All patients love the concept of one-stop shopping! They are happy to have an appointment and their laboratory work done in one office and then walk next door for an x-ray examination. Sharing special services and technologies between offices can be very beneficial. Billing services, legal services, and a variety of other services can be shared. By sharing technologies, offices can obtain state-of-the-art equipment and split the expense. Cooperative marketing is the only way some physicians can become involved in a highly professional, yet affordable, marketing plan. In today's competitive health care field, cooperative marketing can mean the difference between an office that is just treading water and an office that is swimming briskly upstream.

Marketing Your New Physician

Successful marketing of a new physician is a major impetus to the growth of a practice. Keep in mind the cost of marketing a new physician; don't spend more than the office can afford. Weigh the benefits of several marketing plans before choosing one. Marketing a new physician need not consist of big-ticket items such as a professionally designed and written announcement. The office must absorb some printing fees, but they can be kept at an acceptable level. The following paragraphs illustrate a few ways in which you can introduce your new physician.

To properly introduce a new associate, send out an announcement that you either designed on the computer or bought as a standard item through a catalog. Be sure to mention any special skills or education the physician might have. Send the announcement to physician members of the hospital staff, departments in the hospital, and some community members. Also send it to pharmacists, optometrists, opticians, dentists, psychologists, and solo physical therapists. It might also be beneficial to mail the announcement to any local community organizations and the Chamber of Commerce. It is a relatively inexpensive way to introduce a new physician and simultaneously advertise the practice.

Have a copy of the announcement printed in the local newspaper for about 2 weeks. Perhaps the newspaper would be willing to do a human-interest piece on this new addition to the practice. Maybe the physician has an interesting side to his or her personal life that can be mentioned, such as teaching blind persons how to ski or repairing old violins. This makes great reading and human-interest material.

A new physician should introduce himself or herself at local pharmacies. Building rapport with pharmacists is a good idea. They refer many customers to physicians—so why not your practice?

Some offices purchase local radio advertising to introduce their new associates. Television spots are unnecessary and expensive, and actually do not provide the kind of marketing that you need. Arrange for the new physician to meet social and community organizations. Advise the new physician that it would be prudent for him or her to join the local medical society and any other community group, such as the American Cancer Society, the American Red Cross, or the Diabetes Support Group. Have the new physician visit dentists in the area. You might want to enlist the expertise of a public relations firm to help you promote the new physician. The firm can provide you with tips on how to market the physician successfully, but it may be costly. Large practices usually use a public relations firm. Smaller practices usually cannot afford their rates. One practice formed the idea of throwing a "Welcome New Physician" party!

Geoecometric Marketing

If nothing else, the term *geoecometric* itself is impressive! Think of it as selective marketing. Just as patients today are shopping around for physicians, physicians should be selecting the best patient candidates. With geoecometric marketing, physicians can reach their ideal patients using whatever selection process they choose. This type of marketing, developed by Sansum Medical Clinic in Santa Barbara, California, is based on the concept that when ideal patients for a specific practice are targeted, good outcomes and patient satisfaction are a sure bet. Although it is expensive, this marketing style attracts patients who require more sophisticated diagnosis and treatment, and therefore leads to increased practice revenues.

It is no secret that there are more than 500,000 private physicians in the United States and that the reimbursement provided by insurance companies is shrinking. This is what is called pressure. The basis on which geoecometric marketing is founded is that certain characteristics identify the most desirable prospective patients. These characteristics encompass patient demographics such as age, sex, income, and education. In addition, there are certain motivational factors that cause people to do what they do. Those who are predisposed to take advantage of personalized service and can afford to do so are widely dispersed throughout the population. These patients can be found, however, by accessing a wide range of databases. It is imperative to analyze data concerning major disease categories within prescribed groups. Often, this research will identify a new service niche that the office can fill.

For example, one office purchased a mailing list from a magazine on fine dining and sent mailings regarding nutrition and diet and the services that the office provided along those lines. The goal of this office was to introduce itself to this targeted group of individuals. A mailing of 250,000 marketing pieces was done each quarter. The information in the marketing piece was designed to trigger responses. That is, an offer was made for interested individuals to be placed on a regular mailing list to receive the office's newsletter. This office received between 4% and 24% returns on their mailings; the average on normal mailings is 1%.

This marketing strategy has demonstrated that professional-services marketing can be cost-effective and can lead to an increase in revenues. The key to the success of this marketing is establishing positive, long-term relationships and maintaining the correct patient mix.

ADVERTISING

Gone are the days when a physician didn't dare advertise for fear of being thought unprofessional and unethical. Although there is still a slight stigma to medical advertising, most physicians now advertise. This doesn't mean that every medical practice must advertise, however. Depending on the type of practice, advertising can be a great help or a total waste of money. If the practice is a specialty practice such as cardiology or urology, most patients are referred by other physicians. However, if the practice is a family medicine, internal medicine, or plastic surgery practice, it is necessary to work a bit harder to attract patients. When patients look for a family or internal medicine practice, they usually seek recommendations from family, friends, and co-workers; look in the phone book, local newspaper, or on the Internet; ask a physician referral service; or jot down the name of a practice advertised on the radio. Physicians who use elaborate advertising techniques generally do not recover the costs of such advertising. The physicians who are most involved with advertising are those who want to promote special services or products. For example, a physician with expertise in sports medicine may do extensive advertising to gain public awareness.

Community Involvement

One of the best ways to advertise a practice is to get physicians involved in the community. If the physician joins any social or civic organization, he or she will become known. For example, one family practice physician agreed to become the physician for the school football team. It was not long before many players were coming to the office for non–football-related ailments and bringing their families with them. Have the physician volunteer at Little League games or join an adult softball team in the community. The physician might also want to organize a local chapter of a health organization in his or her specialty, such as the American Liver Foundation, the Diabetes Association, the American Cancer Society, the American Lung Association, or the Ileitis and Colitis Foundation. If the physician is interested in the arts, he or she might find that involvement in a local theater group or museum produces results for the practice. By volunteering to speak to local community groups such as the community garden club, the local nurses association, or the Moose or Elks club, or by providing a free lecture once a month at the local hospital on topics associated with his or her specialty, the physician will also benefit the practice.

A good office manager is constantly making time in the physician's schedule for promotional activities. Schedule Tuesday's appointments to end a little early so that the physician can visit local pharmacies. Making the physician aware of the importance of this type of marketing may be a challenge; however, it can be one of the most important aspects of your job as a medical office manager!

An Advertising Plan

An advertising plan should be developed and maintained. This plan should have specific objectives based on the physician's goals for the practice. What exactly does the physician want to accomplish with this campaign? There are many different reasons for advertising, including the following:

- An OB/GYN physician wants to discontinue the OB part of the practice.
- A physician who will be retiring soon wants to maintain a steady flow of patients without much growth.
- A young family practice physician wants to build his or her practice and is hoping to stimulate growth.

The Medium

After the objectives of advertising are clear, it is necessary to decide the medium in which to advertise. One deciding factor is cost. Many advertising options can be costly to medical practices. Consider the following advertising options:

- Internet/Web page
- Local newspaper
- City magazine
- Radio
- Direct mail
- Television
- Telephone book
- Newspapers and magazines
- Playbills from local school or community productions
- Programs for sporting events or community fairs

INTERNET/WEB PAGES

Many physicians have their own Web pages that give a personal history, provide an overview of the practice, and often provide information regarding specialty-specific topics. Finding the time and commitment to develop a marketing plan for the Internet can pose problems. The Web site marketing strategies should be a part of the overall business marketing plan. By aligning online marketing with offline efforts, the practice can better achieve its objectives. If the practice already has a site, you can use it to focus on marketing. If the practice does not have a site, the creation of this site should be part of the strategic plan. The online marketing plan includes such things as developing action plans that can help the practice to achieve its goals. As with any other marketing plan, it contains an objective, a marketing strategy, and a marketing tactic. These elements, however, are smaller in scope when addressing Web site marketing.

The *objective* answers the question of how to overcome any marketing challenges that may exist. If the practice's challenge is to figure out how to use the Web site to build the practice, the objective would be to enhance online client service and to build awareness for patients. The *marketing strategy* supports the objective. So, for the example given in the objective, the marketing strategy would be to improve online communication and interaction, information, and education. It should be to build awareness and interest in your physicians and practices and to communicate the Web site's existence and availability. The *marketing tactic* (action plan) is where the action actually takes place. It consists of a list of things that you will do to make this marketing strategy work for the practice. This can be done through an e-mail newsletter and perhaps even listing the site with search engines and directories. The explosion of information via the Web is beyond phenomenal!

RADIO

Radio advertising is a bit more costly and somewhat narrows the audience. An all-news station is the best bet for your money, because this type of station gets the most listeners. The office must decide when and how many times the advertisement should be aired. Should it be aired during the morning rush hour, when people are anxiously listening for traffic reports? Should it be aired in the evening, when people are home cooking dinner? These questions are best answered by the radio station. Ask for statistics regarding advertising and the targeting of certain individuals.

DIRECT MAIL

Direct mail allows the office to target a certain type of people or certain zip codes. This can be done inexpensively or expensively, depending on how direct mailings are targeted and the quality of the paper and printing used.

TELEVISION

Television is very expensive, doesn't target many people well, and is out of the financial reach of most medical offices. The total cost of air time, ad agencies, and preparation of material can be costly.

YELLOW PAGES

The yellow pages of the local phone book offer a variety of options to physicians' offices today. Studies have found that the public views the yellow pages as the most appropriate advertising medium for health care professionals, with the highest praise going to physicians who provide a lot of information in their listing. It has been found that 84% of people who refer to the yellow pages follow up their research with action. Few physicians today can afford not to have a prominent presence in the yellow pages directory.

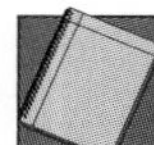

FROM THE EXPERT'S NOTEBOOK

Even in this high-tech world, the yellow pages are still the initial source when seeking services and are the most widely used form of advertising.

A listing in the yellow pages can be simple or elaborate, depending on the philosophy and needs of the practice. The following are a few possible types of yellow pages listings:

- The physician's name, address, telephone number, and specialty in the alphabetic listings
- The physician's name, address, telephone number, and specialty, with the physician's name and specialty in bold print, in the alphabetic listings
- The physician's name, address, telephone number, and specialty in the alphabetic listings, coupled with the same listing in a specialty section of the yellow pages
- An in-column ad of one eighth, one fourth, or one half of a page, with additional information such as hours and special procedures

- A display ad ranging from one column to a whole page (this is generally expensive)
- An in-column ad with two-color printing (this also can be expensive)

An in-column ad is a relatively modest way of providing information about the practice. It has the advantage of being relatively low cost while setting the practice apart from other listings in the section. This type of listing can be made distinctive through the use of a practice logo.

The display ad has become the norm for many large group practices in metropolitan areas of the country. This ad can be extremely helpful to potential clients, providing information such as what medical problems the practice specializes in and services it offers, what payment options are available, and whether the practice takes Medicare assignment or will file insurance. It can also explain the appointment policy along with the physician hours. A small map can even be included in the ad to aid patients in finding the office.

Ad Agencies

Ad agencies are another possibility for larger medical offices. If your office decides to use an agency, make sure that it has experience with health care advertising. Check fees carefully before hiring an agency, because there can be hidden costs, such as paying the person who writes the copy, the person who places the ads, and the person who sits and works with the printer. Find out from the agency just how the fee structure is set up, and make sure everything is written down in the contract.

MANAGED CARE FACTOR

We must plan for the future, because people who stay in the present will remain in the past. —ABRAHAM LINCOLN

Medicine is moving in the direction of managed care in many areas of the country. This is having an enormous effect on the medical office and the practice of medicine. Many offices where patients have been treated for years are now finding that employers' decisions to change insurance companies are snatching patients from the practice and placing them under the care of a participating physician of the employer's insurance plan. This is a traumatic situation not only for the patient, but also the office. Two issues have resulted from the continued growth of managed care:

1. The need for physicians to understand that patient satisfaction is critical to the success of the medical practice
2. The need for the physician and staff to understand the importance of a healthy relationship between the patient and the physician

To establish whether your office is ready for managed care, there are a few questions you and the physician must ask yourselves:

- Are you willing to accept capitation?
- Do you understand its cost structure?
- Are you willing to accept the outcomes of managed care?
- Do you measure your utilization rates?
- Is patient education a strong component of your practice?
- Are efforts to ensure patient satisfaction an integral part of your practice?
- Do you have quality management procedures in place?
- Do you have the capability to assess potential networks?
- Do you have a practice strategy in place?

Managed care covers most but not all parts of the country. If you answered "yes" to all of these questions, your office will be better prepared to face managed care should it come to your area.

EXERCISES

MULTIPLE CHOICE

Choose the best *answer for each of the following questions.*

1. Physician practices should be marketed to which of the following?
   a. The community
   b. Insurance companies
   c. Churches
   d. All of the above
2. Practices can boost their patient volumes by adding which of the following to their list of programs?
   a. Weight reduction programs
   b. Smoking cessation
   c. CPR
   d. Stress management
3. Which of the following is critical to building customer service?
   a. Information
   b. Color of the building
   c. Type of reception room chairs
   d. All of the above
4. Which of the following is *not* part of the plan of threes?
   a. Strategic plan
   b. Marketing plan
   c. Executive plan
   d. Business plan
5. Which of the following is *not* part of the marketing plan?
   a. Opportunities for the practice
   b. Various methods that will be used
   c. The image
   d. Expected results

6. Which of the following is part of the forecasts and financial analysis?
   a. Budget statement
   b. Profit-and-loss statement
   c. Cost ratio analysis
   d. Retained earnings statement
7. Which of the following is *not* part of a marketing assessment?
   a. Patient mix
   b. Number of employees
   c. Patient volumes
   d. Opportunities
8. Included in internal marketing is
   a. Patient satisfaction
   b. Referring physician surveys
   c. Patient education programs
   d. All of the above
9. There are two types of marketing. They are
   a. Intrinsic and extrinsic
   b. Administrative and clinical
   c. Internal and external
   d. None of the above
10. What percentage of patients leave a practice because of the staff, not the physician?
   a. 75%
   b. 25%
   c. 80%
   d. 50%
11. A medical office must deal with three important concepts. Which of the following is *not* one of these concepts?
   a. Patient expectation
   b. Patient experience
   c. Patient evaluation
   d. Patient perception
12. Which of the following is *not* an element of quality service?
   a. Hospital affiliation
   b. The customer
   c. Staff commitment
   d. Patient expectations
13. Some rewards of patient satisfaction are
   a. Increased productivity
   b. Higher profitability
   c. Lower risk of malpractice
   d. All of the above
14. Statistics show that the loss of one patient will cost the practice what amount in revenues over the life of the practice?
   a. $115,000
   b. $238,000
   c. $450,000
   d. $32,000
15. Which of the following is *not* an area of discontentment for patients?
   a. Telephone system
   b. Doctor's hairstyle
   c. Color of building
   d. All of the above
16. About what percentage of new patients are referred by other patients?
   a. 50%
   b. 30%
   c. 90%
   d. 63%
17. A patient information handbook should contain all of the following information *except*
   a. Office hours
   b. Information about the physicians
   c. Full names of the staff
   d. Office parking
18. Which of the following is a factor that influences job satisfaction?
   a. Recognition
   b. Growth
   c. Advancement
   d. All of the above
19. Which of the following should *not* be included in a mission statement?
   a. Responsiveness to patient needs
   b. Appointment scheduling
   c. Coordinated care
   d. Quality care
20. Which of the following is an advertising medium that can be used for physician practice marketing?
   a. Newspaper
   b. Radio
   c. Playbills from local school or community productions
   d. All of the above

TRUE OR FALSE

1. ______ Labor and equipment needs are one classification of service.
2. ______ The telephone is a major source of discontentment in a medical office.
3. ______ Patient dissatisfaction results in losses for the practice.
4. ______ Collaboration is an obstacle to cooperative marketing.
5. ______ A practice newsletter should contain only information about parking.
6. ______ An example of internal marketing is referring physician surveys.
7. ______ Public relations firms are not expensive to use.
8. ______ Community involvement is beneficial in marketing a physician.
9. ______ Practice newsletters must be professionally printed.
10. ______ Reminders in the form of messages on patient statements are not considered to be good marketing.
11. ______ Involving a physician in community activities is a great marketing strategy.
12. ______ Hanging a physician's diplomas on the wall is not considered marketing.
13. ______ Costs are generally not recovered on elaborate advertising schemes.
14. ______ A great place to market a practice is the video rental store.
15. ______ It is not important for a practice to focus on patient expectations.

16. ______ Teamwork is not important for marketing.
17. ______ Attitude is everything!
18. ______ Dissatisfied patients talk.
19. ______ Word-of-mouth marketing is usually a face-to-face interaction.
20. ______ Patient expectations are the same from patient to patient.

THINKERS

1. Your practice has hired a new physician. Describe and explain your ideas on how you would advertise and market this new physician.
2. A physician has decided to publish a practice newsletter. Develop an outline for articles and prepare a plan as to how this will be distributed.
3. Using a medical practice scenario provided by the instructor, describe what marketing tools you would use for your practice and why.

REFERENCES

Abbott, R.F. *A Manager's Guide to Newsletters: Communicating for Results.* Alberta, CA: World Engines Press, 2001.

Baird, K. *Customer Service in Health Care: A Grassroots Approach to Creating a Culture of Service Excellence.* New York: John Wiley & Sons, 2000.

Baker, S.K. *Managing Patient Expectation: The Art of Finding and Keeping Loyal Patients.* San Francisco: Jossey-Bass, 1998.

Baum, N., & Henkel, G. *Marketing your Clinical Practice: Ethically, Effectively, Economically,* 2nd edition. Rockville, MD: Aspen, 2000.

Brown, N., & Bronkesh, W. *Satisfaction Pays.* Rockville, MD: Aspen, 1993.

Colvin, G. "The Changing Art of Becoming Unbeatable." *Fortune,* November 24, 1997, pp. 299-300.

Gross, T.S. *Positively Outrageous Service.* New York: Matermedia Limited, 1991.

Herzlinger, R.E. *Market-Driven Healthcare: Who Wins, Who Loses in the Transformation of America's Largest Service Industry.* Cambridge, MA: Perseus Press, 1999.

Leebov, W., & Scott, G. *The Indispensable Health Care Manager: Success Strategies for a Changing Environment.* San Francisco: Jossey-Bass, 2002.

Leebov, W., et al. *Achieving Impressive Customer Service: 7 Strategies for the Health Care Manager.* San Francisco: Jossey-Bass, 2000.

MacStravic, R.S. *Creating Consumer Loyalty in Healthcare.* Chicago: Health Administration Press, 2002.

Marlowe, D. *Healthcare Marketing Plans that Work.* Chicago: Health Administration Press, 1999.

Nelson, A.M., et al. *Improving Patient Satisfaction Now: How to Earn Patient and Payer Loyalty.* Rockville, MD: Aspen, 1997.

O'Malley, J.F. *Healthcare Marketing Sales and Service: An Executive Companion.* Chicago: Health Administration Press, 2001.

Peters, T. *The Pursuit of WOW!* New York: Vintage Books, 1994.

Sherman, S.G. *Total Customer Satisfaction: A Comprehensive Approach for Health Care Providers.* San Francisco: Jossey-Bass, 1999.

Street, R., & Street, R. *Creative Newsletters and Annual Reports.* Gloucester, MA: Rockport Publishers, 2001.

Sturm, A. *The New Rules of Healthcare Marketing: 23 Strategies for Success.* Chicago: Health Administration Press, 1998.

APPENDIX A: SAMPLE EMPLOYEE PENSION PLAN BOOKLET

ARTICLE I: PARTICIPATION IN YOUR PLAN

Before you become a participant in the plan, there are certain eligibility and participation requirements that you must meet. These requirements are explained in this section.

Eligible Employees

All of your employer's employees are considered eligible employees and may participate in the plan once they meet the eligibility and participation requirements. This is with the exception of members of a collective bargaining unit and nonresident aliens.

Eligibility Requirements

You will be eligible to participate in the plan on the first entry date after you have attained age 20.5, completed 6 months of service, and been credited with 1,000 hours of service during the eligibility computation period.

The eligibility computation period is the 12-month period that begins with the date you were hired. If you don't meet the service requirements during the first year following your date of hire, the eligibility computation period becomes the plan year. You may then meet the requirements during any plan year.

Entry Dates

Participation in the plan can begin only on an entry date. Your first entry date will be the first day of the next plan year, January 1, after you meet the eligibility requirements.

Rehired Employees

If you satisfied the eligibility requirements before you terminated employment, you will become a participant immediately on the date you are rehired, if your rehire date is on or after your first entry date as defined above. Otherwise, you will be eligible to participate on the next entry date.

If you had not yet satisfied the eligibility requirements at the time you terminated employment, you must meet the eligibility requirements as if you were a new employee.

ARTICLE II: CONTRIBUTIONS

Employer Contribution

Each year, your employer will make a contribution to the plan on the behalf of the eligible plan participants. To receive the employer's contribution, you must have worked 1,000 hours during the plan year and be employed on the last day of the plan year. If you do not meet the hours requirement or are not employed on the last day of the plan year because you have become disabled or died, you or your estate will still receive a contribution.

The amount of the employer's contribution is 10% of your total compensation plus 5.7% of your compensation in excess of a fixed level amount. The fixed compensation level is defined as the Social Security wage base in effect on the first day of the plan year.

For example, you might receive 2% of your total pay plus another 2% of pay in excess of the fixed level. If your pay was \$20,000 and the level amount was \$10,000, your share would be:

$$\$20,000 \times .02 \text{ plus } (\$20,000 - \$10,000) \times .02 = \$600$$

If the level amount was \$10,000 and your compensation was \$9,000, your share would be:

$$\$9,000 \times .02 = \$180$$

Other Required Contributions

In certain situations, your employer may be required to change the amount of the contributions to the plan. If the plan is top-heavy (see Article IX), your employer may have to take corrective action. This action could result in either a reduction in the contributions for highly compensated participants or an additional employer contribution.

ARTICLE III: VESTING

The term *vesting* refers to the percentage of your employer contribution account that you are entitled to receive if your employment is terminated. If you terminate employment before you meet the requirements for retirement (see Article VII), the distribution from the employer account will be limited to the vested portion. Your vesting percentage grows with your years of service. Article VI explains how years of service are credited.

Vesting Schedule

Years of Service	*Percent Vested*
Less than 1	0
1 but less than 2	0
2 but less than 3	20
3 but less than 4	40
4 but less than 5	60
5 but less than 6	80
6 or more	100

You will also become 100% vested at normal retirement or if you become disabled or die. See Article VII for information on retirement, disability, and death.

ARTICLE IV: SERVICE RULES

Year of Service

You will earn a year of service for vesting if you are credited with 1,000 hours of service during a plan year or if you are credited with 1,000 hours during your first year of employment. However, you cannot earn more than 1 year of service credit during any plan year. Years of employment before age 18 will not be considered in determining your years of service.

If you terminate employment and are later rehired by the employer, your years of service after reemployment may be added to the years of service you had accumulated when you left. For the two periods of service to be added together, you must return to work within 5 years of your termination date.

Hours of Service

You will be credited with the actual number of hours you work for service and vesting purposes.

Break-in-Service Rules

For vesting, a break in service occurs whenever you fail to complete at least 501 hours during the plan year. Thus, in any year in which you work less than 501 hours (approximately 3 months), you will incur a break in service.

However, in certain circumstances your plan is required to credit you with 501 hours, even though you didn't actually work 501 hours. This credit is primarily used for employees who take time off to have, adopt, or care for a child for a period immediately following birth or adoption. You will receive this credit only for the purpose of determining whether you have incurred a break in service; it will not affect your vesting schedule or your eligibility for employer contributions.

ARTICLE V: COMPENSATION

Throughout this summary plan description, the words *compensation* and *pay* are used to define contribution amounts. *Pay* and *compensation* refer to the total wages paid to you by your employer for the plan year.

In no event shall compensation in excess of $200,000 (as adjusted for changes in the Consumer Price Index: $209,200 for 2002) be taken into account for any participant in this plan.

Your compensation for the first plan year in which you participate shall be your compensation from the employer from the time you became a participant through the end of the plan year.

ARTICLE VI: PARTICIPANTS' ACCOUNTS

Under the money purchase pension plan, your employer contributions are placed into investment accounts, which are credited with gains and losses at each valuation date. The valuation date for your pension plan occurs on the anniversary date.

Forfeitures

In addition to contributions, the employer contribution account is credited with forfeitures if they occur. Forfeitures are amounts that could not be paid to terminated participants because they were not 100% vested when they separated from service with the employer.

Rollover and Voluntary Accounts

Your plan may allow employees who had retirement accounts with a previous employer to transfer the previous account balance to their new plans. This is a segregated "rollover" account, and it is always 100% vested. In order to avoid taxes on your "rollover" money, you must transfer the money from your old plan to this plan within 60 days after receiving the money.

Also, your prior plan (if any) may have allowed you to make voluntary after-tax contributions to your plan. (You can no longer do so under this plan.) If you elected to make voluntary contributions under the prior plan, you also have a "voluntary" account.

Investments

All of the money deposited into the plan by your employer will be invested by the trustees.

The trustees are fiduciaries of the plan, which means that they have a responsibility to you to invest the plan assets prudently.

Crediting Your Accounts with Gain or Loss

Each investment account is credited with investment gain or loss as of each valuation date. Earnings or losses are allocated on the basis of the ratio your account balance bears to the total account balances of all participants in the same investment. You are then credited with that percentage of earnings or losses.

ARTICLE VII: BENEFITS UNDER YOUR PLAN

Normal Retirement Benefits

The normal retirement age for the plan is the later of age 65 or your age on the fifth anniversary of your participation in the plan. Your normal retirement date is the first day of the month coincident with or next following the date you reach normal retirement age. At your normal retirement date, you will be entitled to 100% of your account balance. Payment of your benefits will begin as soon as practicable after you've retired (see Article VIII).

Late Retirement Benefits

If you decide to work past your normal retirement date, you can defer payment of your benefits until your retirement date. Payment of your retirement benefits will commence as soon as practicable following your late retirement date.

Death Benefits

Should you die before retirement, your spouse or beneficiary will be entitled to 100% of your account balance.

If you are married at the time of your death, your spouse will be the beneficiary of your death benefits, unless you otherwise elect in writing on a form provided by the plan administrator. IF YOU WISH TO DESIGNATE A BENEFICIARY OTHER THAN YOUR SPOUSE AS YOUR BENEFICIARY, YOUR SPOUSE MUST CONSENT TO WAIVE HIS OR HER RIGHT TO RECEIVE DEATH BENEFITS UNDER THE PLAN. YOUR SPOUSE'S CONSENT MUST BE IN WRITING AND WITNESSED BY A NOTARY OR A PLAN REPRESENTATIVE.

If you are married and die before retiring, your spouse's benefits will usually be paid in the form of a "preretirement survivor annuity," a life annuity for your spouse. The amount of the annuity will depend on your account balance at the time of your death. Also, your spouse may be able to select another form of payment, depending on the options available at the time of your death.

If you want to designate someone other than your spouse as your beneficiary, you have the option of waiving the preretirement survivor annuity, with your spouse's consent. This waiver can be made at any time after the beginning of the plan year in which you reach age 35. The administrator will provide you with a detailed explanation of the preretirement survivor annuity before you reach age 35. This explanation will be given to you at some point during the 3-year period beginning on the first day of the plan year in which you reach age 32, or during your first 3 years of participation if you enter the plan after age 32. To receive this information in a timely manner, you should inform the plan administrator when you reach age 32.

If your spouse has consented to a valid waiver of any rights to the death benefit, or your spouse cannot be located, or you are single at the time of your death, then your death benefit will be paid to any beneficiary you may chose. The plan administrator will supply you with a beneficiary designation form.

Because your spouse has certain rights under your plan, you should immediately inform the plan administrator of any changes in your marital status.

Disability Benefits

Should you become permanently disabled while a participant under this plan, you will receive 100% of your account balance. Disability means a medically determinable physical or mental impairment that may be expected to result in death or to last at least a year and that renders you incapable of performing your duties with your employer. A determination of disability will be made by the plan administrator in a uniform, nondiscriminatory manner on the basis of medical evidence.

If it is determined that you are disabled, your payments will begin on or before the anniversary date following the date you were determined to be disabled.

Benefits on Termination

If your employment is terminated for any reason other than retirement or death, you will be entitled only to that portion of your employer accounts in which you are vested. (You are always entitled to 100% of the account balance of any voluntary contribution money you contributed to your plan.)

Vesting refers to the percentage of your account balance you are entitled to at any point in time. For each year you remain a participant in the plan, you become vested with a higher percentage of your employer account balance (see Article III).

If your benefit is over $3,500, you may, at your option and with your spouse's consent, request the plan administrator to distribute your benefit to you before your retirement date. However, you must incur a break in service before you can receive a distribution.

If your benefit is $3,500 or less, the plan administrator may distribute your benefit early. No spousal consent is needed for distributions of $3,500 or less.

Distributions Pursuant to a Domestic Relations Order

In general, contributions made by you or your employer for your retirement are not subject to alienation. This means they cannot be sold, used as collateral for a loan, given away, or otherwise transferred. They are not subject to the claims of your creditors. However, they may be subject to claims under a qualified domestic relations order (QDRO).

The administrator may be required by law to recognize obligations you incur as a result of court-ordered child support or alimony payments. The administrator must honor a QDRO, which is defined as a decree or order issued by a court that obligates you to pay child support or alimony or otherwise allocates a portion of your assets in the plan to your spouse, child, or other dependent. If a QDRO is received by the administrator, all or portions of your benefits may be used to satisfy the obligation. It is the plan administrator's responsibility to determine the validity of a QDRO.

Taxation of Distributions

The benefits you receive from the plan will be subject to ordinary income tax in the year in which you receive the payment, unless you defer taxation by a rollover of your distribution into another qualified plan or an IRA. Also, in certain circumstances your tax may be reduced by special tax treatment such as "5-year forward averaging."

In addition to ordinary income tax, you may be subject to a 10% tax penalty if you receive a "premature" distribution. If you receive a distribution on terminating employment before age 55 and you don't receive the payment as a life annuity, you will be subject to the 10% penalty unless you roll over your payment. There is no penalty for payments made because of your death or disability.

The rules concerning rollovers and the taxation of benefits are complex; please consult your tax advisor before making a withdrawal or requesting a distribution from the plan. The plan administrator will provide you with a brief explanation of the rules concerning rollovers if you request a distribution that is eligible for a rollover.

ARTICLE VIII: BENEFIT PAYMENT OPTIONS

Several different payment options are available under your plan. The method of payment you will receive depends on your marital status at the time you receive payment and the elections you and your spouse make. All payments under your plan are "equivalent." This means that, after making adjustments for longer or shorter periods, or for payments continuing to a beneficiary or spouse after your death, all payments are actuarially equal to one another.

If you have been married for at least 1 year at the time of your retirement, the normal payment option under your plan is 50% joint and survivor annuity. That means if you die before your spouse, your spouse will receive, after your death, 50% of the benefit you were receiving at the time of your death. You may elect another joint and survivor annuity or you may elect another form of payment, with your spouse's consent. However, electing another option will affect the payments made to you and your spouse. You should consult your tax advisor before making any election.

If you are unmarried or have been married for less than 1 year at the time of retirement, or if you and your spouse reject the joint and survivor annuity, you may choose to receive payment in the form of a lump-sum distribution of your total account balances, a life annuity, or any other form of payment that may be permitted under your plan, at the time of your distribution. Consult your plan administrator for other options of payment.

When you are near retirement, the plan administrator will furnish you with explanations of the joint and survivor and life annuities. You will be given the option of waiving the joint and survivor annuity during the 90-day period before the annuity payment is to begin. If you are married and decide to waive the joint and survivor annuity, your spouse must consent to the waiver. Your spouse's consent must be signed before a notary public or a plan representative. Any waiver you make can be revoked later. However, your spouse cannot revoke his or her consent to the waiver without your permission. The plan administrator will provide you with the necessary forms to waive the joint and survivor annuity.

The plan administrator may delay payment to you for a reasonable time for administrative convenience. However, unless you choose to defer receipt of your distribution, the plan must begin your payments within 60 days after the close of the plan year following the latest of the following:

- Date on which you reached your normal retirement age
- Tenth anniversary of the year in which you became a participant in the plan
- Date you terminated employment with the employer

In any event, the law requires that your distributions begin no later than April 1 of the year following the date you reach age 70.

ARTICLE IX: TOP-HEAVY RULES

A plan becomes top-heavy when the total of the key employees' account balances make up 60% or more of the total of all account balances in the plan. Key employees are certain highly compensated officers or owners/shareholders.

If your plan is top-heavy, plan participants who are not "key" must receive a minimum contribution. This minimum contribution is the smaller of the percentage of pay contributed by the employer to key employees, or 3% of the non–key employee's compensation. If the employer contribution allocated to your account for the top-heavy year is equal to or more than this minimum contribution, no additional employer contribution would be needed to meet the top-heavy rules.

ARTICLE X: MISCELLANEOUS

Protection of Benefits

Your plan benefits are not subject to claims, indebtedness, execution, garnishment, or other similar legal or equitable process. Also, you cannot voluntarily (or involuntarily) assign your benefits under this plan.

Loans

Loans are not permitted under this plan.

Amendment and Termination

The employer has reserved the right to amend or terminate your plan. However, no amendment can take away any benefits you have already earned. If your plan is terminated, you will be entitled to the full amount in your account as of the date of termination, regardless of the percent you are vested at the time of termination.

Pension Benefit Guaranty Corporation

The Pension Benefit Guaranty Corporation (PBGC) provides plan termination insurance for defined benefit pension plans. In your money purchase pension plan (a defined contribution plan), all of the contributions and investment earnings are allocated to participants' accounts. PBGC insurance is not needed and does not apply.

Claims

When you request a distribution of all or any part of your account, you will contact the plan administrator, who will provide you with the proper forms to make your claim for benefits.

Your claim for benefits will be given a full and fair review. However, if your claim is denied, in whole or in part, the plan administrator will notify you of the denial within 90 days of the date your claim for benefits was received, unless special circumstances delay the notification. If a delay occurs, you will be given a written notice of the reason for the delay and a date by which a final decision will be given (not more than 180 days after the receipt of your claim.)

Notification of a denial of claims will include the specific reasons for the denial; references to the plan provisions on which the denial is based; a description of any additional material necessary to correct your claim and an explanation of why the material is necessary; and an explanation of the steps to follow to appeal the denial, including notification that you (or your beneficiary) must file your appeal within 60 days of the date you receive the denial notice.

If you or your beneficiary do not file an appeal within the 60-day period, the denial will stand. If you do file an appeal within the 60 days, your employer will review the facts and hold hearings, if necessary, to reach a final decision. Your employer's decision will be made within 60 days of receipt of the notice of your appeal, unless an extension is needed due to special circumstances. In any event, your employer will make a decision within 120 days of the receipt of your appeal.

APPENDIX B: MEDICARE CARRIERS

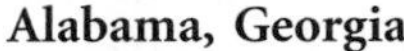

Alabama, Georgia
BC/BS of Alabama
PO Box 830170
Birmingham, AL 35283
Phone: 866-539-5598

Alaska, Arizona, Colorado, Hawaii, Iowa, American Samoa, Guam
Noridian Mutual Insurance Co.
430513 th Avenue, SW
Fargo, ND 58103
Phone: 701-282-1439

Arkansas
Arkansas BC/BS
601 Gaines Street
Little Rock, AR 72201
Phone: 501-378-2585

California (Northern)
National Heritage Insurance Co.
PO Box 602
Maryville, CA 95901
Phone: 877-591-1587

California (Southern)
National Heritage Insurance Co.
PO Box 60560
Los Angeles, CA 90060
Phone: 866-502-9054

Connecticut
First Coast Service Options, Inc.
321 Research Parkway
Meridian, CT 06450
Phone: 866-419-9455

Delaware
Trailblazer Health Enterprises, LLC
8330 LBJ Freeway
Dallas, TX 75243
Phone: 972-766-6900

Florida
BC/BS of Florida, Inc.
PO Box 44021
Jacksonville, FL 32231
Phone: 877-847-4992

Georgia
Cahaba GBA
PO Box 3018
Savannah, GA 31402
Phone: 866-582-3246

Idaho
Connecticut General Life Insurance Co.
2 Vantage Way
Nashville, TN 37228
Phone: 615-782-4511

Illinois, Michigan
Wisconsin Physicians Service Insurance
1601 Engel Street
Madison, WI 53713
Phone: 608-221-4711

Indiana
AdminaStar Federal, Inc.
8115 Knue Road
Indianapolis, IN 46250
Phone: 317-841-4633

Kansas
BC/BS of Kansas, Inc.
1133 Topeka Avenue
PO Box 239
Topeka, KS 66601
Phone: 785-291-4126

Kentucky
Administar Federal
9901 Linn Station Road, Suite 200
Louisville, KY 40223
Phone: 502-329-8604

Louisiana
Arkansas BC/BS
PO Box 83860
Baton Rouge, LA 70884
Phone: 800-462-9666

Maine
National Heritage Insurance NE
75 William Terry Drive
Hingham, MA 02043
Phone: 877-567-3129

Maryland; Washington, DC; Northern Virginia (counties of Arlington, Fairfax, and City of Alexandria)
TrailBlazer Health Enterprises, LLC
PO Box 5858
Timonium, MD 21094
Phone: 410-229-5454

Massachusetts
National Heritage Insurance NE
75 William Terry Drive
Hingham, MA 02043
Phone: 866-539-5595

Minnesota
Wisconsin Physicians Service
8120 Penn Avenue, South
Bloomington, MI 55430
Phone: 866-564-0315

Mississippi
Cahaba GBA
PO Box 22545
Jackson, MS 39225
Phone: 601-977-5764

Missouri
Arkansas BC/BS
601 Gaines Street
Little Rock, AK 72201
Phone: 501-378-2242

Missouri, Nebraska
BC/BS of Kansas, Inc.
1133 Topeka Avenue
Topeka, KS 66629
Phone: 785-291-7000

Montana
BC/BS of Montana, Inc.
PO Box 4310
340 North Last Chance Gulch
Helena, MT 59604
Phone: 877-567-7203

Nevada, Northern Mariana Islands, North Dakota, Oregon, South Dakota, Washington, Wyoming
Noridian Government Services
4305 13th Avenue South
Fargo, ND 58103
Phone: 877-908-8431

New Hampshire
National Heritage Insurance NE
75 William Terry Drive
Hingham, MA 02043
Phone: 877-567-3130

New Jersey
Empire Medicare Services—NJ
300 East Park Drive
Harrisburg, PA 17111
Phone: 877-567-9235

New Mexico
Arkansas BC/BS
701 NW 63rd Street, Suite 300
Oklahoma City, OK 73116
Phone: 405-841-6723

New York
Empire Medicare Services—NY
PO Box 1200
Crompond, NY 10517
Phone: 877-869-6504
Healthnow New York, Inc.
Upstate Medicare Division Operations
33 Lewis Road, PO Box 80
Binghampton, NY 13905
Phone: 607-766-6000
Group Health, Inc.
PO Box 1569
New York, NY 10023
Phone: 646-458-6618

County of Queens
Group Health, Inc.
25 Broadway
New York, NY 10004
Phone: 888-632-5572

North Carolina
CGLIC
PO Box 25226
Nashville, TN 37202
Phone: 615-782-4509

Ohio, West Virginia
Nationwide Insurance Co.
3400 Southpark Place, Suite F
Grove City, OH 43123
Phone: 614-277-7171

Oklahoma
Arkansas BC/BS
701 NW 63rd Street, Suite 300
Oklahoma City, OK 73116
Phone: 866-539-5596

Pennsylvania
Highmark Medicare Services
PO Box 890157
Camp Hill, PA 17089
Phone: 866-488-0549

Puerto Rico, Virgin Island
Triple-S, Inc.
PO Box 71391
San Juan, PR 00936
Phone: 787-749-4232

Rhode Island
BC/BS of Rhode Island
444 Westminster Street
Providence, RI 02903
Phone: 401-459-1719

South Carolina
Palmetto GBA
PO Box 100190
Columbia, SC 29202
Phone: 866-238-9654

Tennessee
Cigna-Part B Medicare
2 Vantage Way
Nashville, TN 37228
Phone: 615-782-4509

Texas
TrailBlazer Health Enterprises
PO Box 833928
Richardson, TX 75083
Phone: 469-372-2609

Utah
Regence BS of Utah
PO Box 30270
Salt Lake City, UT 84130
Phone: 801-333-2440

Vermont
National Heritage Insurance Co.
75 William Terry Drive
Hingham, MA 02043
Phone: 781-741-3122

Virginia (excluding counties of Arlington, Fairfax, and City of Alexandria)
TrailBlazer Health Enterprises, LLC
PO Box 26463
Richmond, VA 23261
Phone: 804-327-2043

Wisconsin
PO Box 8248
Madison, WI 53708
Phone: 877-908-8476

APPENDIX C: INTERNET WEBSITES FOR HEALTH CARE PROFESSIONALS

ORGANIZATIONS, ASSOCIATIONS, AND SOCIETIES

American Medical Specialty Organization, Inc. (a managed care company)	www.amso.com
National Center for Health Statistics	www.cdc.gov/nchs/
National Institutes of Health	www.nih.gov
American College of Healthcare Executives	www.ache.org
American Health Information Management Association	www.ahima.org
American Medical Informatics Association	www.amia.org
Medical Group Management Association	www.mgma.com
Health Care Compliance Association	www.hcca-info.org
Healthcare Information and Management Systems Society	www.himss.org
World Health Organization	www.who.int
American Medical Association	www.amasolutions.com
Medical Association of Billers	www.physicianswebsites.com
American Academy of Professional Coders	www.aapcnatl.org
American Informatics Association (e-mail guidelines for patients)	www.amia.org
American Academy of Family Physicians	www.aafp.org
American College of Legal Medicine	www.aclm.org/
American Health Lawyers Association	www.healthlawyers.org
Joint Commission on Accreditation of Healthcare Organizations	www.jcaho.org
U.S. Department of Health and Human Services	www.os.dhhs.gov
National Committee for Quality Assurance	www.ncqa.org
American College of Physicians	www.acponline.org

BILLING AND CODING

The Coding Institute (breaking news on CMS changes, etc.)	www.codinginstitute.com
Centers for Medicare and Medicaid Services (CMS)	www.cms.gov
Medical Association of Billers	www.physicianswebsites.com
American Academy of Professional Coders	www.aapcnatl.org
ICD-9 information (National Center for Health Statistics)	www.cdc.gov/nchs/icd9.htm
Code of Federal Regulations (U.S. Government Printing Office)	www.gpo.gov/nara/cfr/index.html
Federal Register (U.S. Government Printing Office)	www.access.gpo.gov/su_docs/aces/aces140.html

LAW, REGULATIONS, COMPLIANCE, AND GOVERNMENT

Legal resources	www.findlaw.com
U.S. Department of Justice	www.usdoj.gov
Links to law pages	www.lawlinks.com
U.S. General Accounting Office	www.gao.gov
American College of Legal Medicine	www.aclm.org/
American Health Lawyers Association	www.healthlawyers.org
Code of Federal Regulations (U.S. Government Printing Office)	www.access.gpo.gov/nara/cfr
U.S. Government Printing Office	www.gpo.gov
Joint Commission on Accreditation of Healthcare Organizations	www.jcaho.org
U.S. Department of Health and Human Services	www.os.dhhs.gov
National Committee for Quality Assurance	www.ncqa.org
HCFA publications and forms	www.hcfa.gov/pubforms/default.htm
Office of the Inspector General	www.oig.hhs.gov
Agency for Healthcare Research and Quality	www.ahcpr.gov
Americans with Disabilities Act	www.usdoj.gov/disabilities.htm

PHYSICIANS

The Center for Professional Well-Being (promotes physician retention, health, etc.)	www.cpwb.org
American College of Physicians (ACP)	www.acponline.org/counseling/physcomp.htm
Physician reimbursement models and physician contracting with Medicare	www.acponline.org/hpp/pospaper/privcont.htm
Managed Care Management Services (data management and reporting solutions for managed care)	www.managedcare.com

COMMERCIAL MEDICAL SITES

Medscape (free physician reference, free physician home pages)	www.Medscape.com
WebMD (services helping physicians, providers, patients, and health plans; contains physician practice management software)	www.webmd.com

MISCELLANEOUS

Patient education	www.scrippshealth.org
Journal of Medical Internet Research (research using the Internet)	www.jmir.org/index.html
American Academy of Family Physicians (patient satisfaction, improve productivity)	www.aafp.org/fpm
The Conflict Resolution Information Source	www.crinfo.org
Mayo Clinic (consumer content and bookstore)	www.mayoclinic.com

APPENDIX D: ABBREVIATIONS AND SYMBOLS USED IN THE MEDICAL OFFICE

aa: of each
A&W: alive and well
abd: abdomen
ac: before meals
ad: right ear
ant: anterior
as: left ear
ASA: aspirin
au: both ears
b: brother
bid: twice a day
BP: blood pressure
BS: breath sounds
c̄: with
Ca: carcinoma
cap: capsule
cath: catheter
CBC: complete blood count
CCU: coronary care unit
Chemo: chemotherapy
cm: centimeter
c/o: complains of
CPR: cardiopulmonary resuscitation
CXR: chest x-ray
d: daughter, died, dorsal
dev: deviated
dexter: right
diff dx: differential diagnosis
dx: diagnosis
ECG, EKG: electrocardiogram
ENT: ears, nose, and throat
et: and
ext: extremities
f: father
FH: family history
FU: follow-up
FUO: fever of unknown origin
g, gm: gram
GI: gastrointestinal
gtt(s): drop(s)
h: hour
Hct: hematocrit
Hgb: hemoglobin
h/o: history of
HR: heart rate
h.s.: at bedtime
Ht: height
Hx: history
ICU: intensive care unit
IM: intramuscular
IV: intravenous
L&A: light and accommodation
Lat: lateral
LL: left lower
LLQ: left lower quadrant
LU: left upper
LUQ: left upper quadrant
m: mother
M: heart murmur
med: medial, medication
meds: medications
mEq: milliequivalents
mg: milligram
mm: millimeter
N&V: nausea and vomiting
neg: negative
neuro: neurologic
NR: no repeat, no refill
occ: occasional
OD: right eye
OS: left eye
OU: both eyes
P: pulse
p: palmar surface, palm
pc: after meals
PE: physical examination
PERRLA: pupils equal, round, reactive to light and accommodation
Pes: foot
po: by mouth
pos: positive
post: posterior
pp: postprandial
prn: as needed

pt: patient
PT: physical therapy
q6 h: every 6 hours (can be any number)
qd: every day
qid: four times a day
qod: every other day
qs: as much as necessary
ret: return
r/o: rule out
rt: right
RL: right lower
RLQ: right lower quadrant
RRR: regular, rate, rhythm
RU: right upper
RUQ: right upper quadrant
Rx: treatment, prescription
s̄: sister
s: without
sib: sibling
Sig: directions for a prescription
sm: small
SOB: shortness of breath
ss: one half
Stat: immediately
sub Q: subcutaneous
Sx: symptoms
T: temperature
tab: tablet
tid: three times a day
Tx: treatment
UA: urinalysis, uric acid
ut dict: as directed
VS: vital signs
Wt, W: weight
WNL: within normal limits
↓: low, decreased
↑: high, increased
1 °: primary
2 °: secondary
3 °: tertiary
II: two
I: one
l/d: once a day

APPENDIX E: PATIENT INFORMATION HANDBOOK FOR CENTRAL CITY GASTROENTEROLOGY ASSOCIATES

TO OUR PATIENTS

We appreciate you selecting this office to serve your health care needs. Our office will do everything possible to provide you with the very best care. We have prepared this patient information handbook to acquaint you with the office and its policies. We believe that the more you know about our policies and methods of practice, the more we can be of service to you, and thus annoyances and frustrations arising from misunderstandings can be avoided.

WELCOME TO OUR PRACTICE!

What Is a Gastroenterologist?

A gastroenterologist is a physician who specializes in the evaluation and treatment of problems of the digestive tract, including the stomach, intestine, colon, liver, and pancreas. Procedures sometimes performed by a gastroenterologist are sigmoidoscopy, colonoscopy, gastroscopy, and biopsy.

OUR VISION

Quality patient care and patient satisfaction are the two main goals of our practice. The enthusiasm and efficiency of our staff are key elements in obtaining these goals. Because of our commitment to quality patient care, our staff exhibits motivation, cooperation, productivity, and caring. The physicians and staff at Central City Gastroenterology Associates share in that total commitment, exemplifying the philosophy and direction of our practice.

ABOUT OUR PRACTICE

Our practice is an academic-based practice with three offices in the Allentown area. We are a group practice of five physicians who specialize in gastroenterology. The physicians in our group are:

- Olivia Gentilezza, M.D.
- James Kelly, M.D.
- Steven Mensch, D.O.
- John Nealon, M.D.
- Maureen Smith, D.O.

All of our physicians are board certified in both internal medicine and gastroenterology. They regularly attend medical conferences and workshops designed to provide them with the latest in current therapies, practices, and procedures. Our physicians participate in lectures and courses for other physicians and actively teach interns, residents, and staff physicians.

Our physicians are affiliated with the following hospitals:

- Suburban Hospital, Doylestown
- Community General Hospital, Portland, Maine
- Medical College of Boise, Idaho

Our offices are located at:

Plaza Office
Two Plaza Place
Suite One
Philadelphia, PA
555-111-1234
Office Hours:
Monday: 9:00 AM to 4:00 PM
Tuesday: 9:00 AM to 3:00 PM
Wednesday: 8:30 AM to 6:00 PM
Thursday: 12:00 PM to 4:00 PM

Hills Office
Woody Hills Complex
Suite 110
Scranton, PA
720-123-2222
Office Hours:
Monday: 12:00 PM to 5:00 PM
Thursday: 8:30 AM to 2:00 PM

ABOUT APPOINTMENTS

Our offices are open during the hours listed above. We are closed on the following holidays:

- New Year's Day
- Good Friday
- Memorial Day
- Fourth of July
- Labor Day
- Thanksgiving Day
- Day after Thanksgiving
- Christmas Day

Office visits at either of our offices are by appointment only. We urge you to call as far in advance as possible for your appointments. If you must cancel an appointment, please give us as much notice as possible so that we may offer your appointment time to another patient. We will be happy to reschedule your appointment. If you have a problem and do not have a scheduled appointment, we will attempt to see you as quickly as possible, with proper respect to other patients. We ask that our patients do their best to be on time for their appointments. Being late is unfair to other patients who are being seen that day. Occasionally, our physicians will have emergencies that will delay their arrival at the office. We ask your patience and understanding at times like this.

OFFICE TELEPHONES

Normally, our office telephone lines are open during our office hours. When you call any of our offices, kindly explain your problem to our receptionists. We have instructed them to handle all incoming calls and to refer your call to the appropriate person. If there is an emergency, they will contact a physician immediately. If the doctor cannot speak with you at the time of your call for routine questions, our staff will take your number and have the doctor call you at some point during office hours. Our trained staff will efficiently gather the information to expedite the return call. Please cooperate with our staff by providing them with all the information necessary.

When calling the office for a prescription renewal, kindly have the following information available:

- Name of medicine needed
- srength of medicine and dosage
- Your telephone number
- Your pharmacy's name and telephone number

This information will allow our office to process your request in a timely manner. If there is a holiday approaching, please check your medication in advance so any necessary renewal can be handled before that holiday.

YOUR FIRST VISIT TO THE OFFICE

When you arrive at our office for the first time, you will be asked to fill out a Patient Registration Form. We would appreciate it if you would complete both sides of this standard form as thoroughly as possible. This information will aid our staff in processing your bills and insurance forms efficiently. Please bring your insurance cards to the office, so that we can make copies of them. The information you provide on the Patient Registration Form will also help us contact you when necessary.

If you have recently had x-ray studies, laboratory work, or any other testing done, please obtain copies of these tests and bring them with you to our office. This will prevent the needless repetition of tests that have already been done.

YOU AND YOUR DOCTOR

During evenings, weekends, and holidays, one of our physicians is always on call and available to handle emergencies. The physician on call is the physician who will treat you if you call during off hours. If you need urgent care, arrangements will be made for you to see a physician. If your physician is away at a medical conference or unavailable for any reason, you will be notified either by phone or by mail that your appointment needs to be changed. There is always a physician in our group who is ready to take care of your medical needs. Our physicians always work closely with your referring physician.

RELEASE OF MEDICAL INFORMATION

Should you require the release of any of your medical records, it is our office policy that you submit, in writing with your signature, a request that your records be forwarded. If you are near any of our offices, we have a Records Release Form that you may come in and fill out. Either method is satisfactory in obtaining a release.

TEST RESULTS

When inquiring about recent test results, please help our staff by telling them the type of test that was done, the date it was done, and where it was done. Our staff will obtain the results and have your physician return your call. Some tests may take a few days for us to obtain the results, so please be patient. Unfortunately, this delay is out of our control.

Note: Please call the office at which you were seen to obtain your test results. Your results will be sent to that particular office when completed.

PAYMENT FOR SERVICES

At the end of your visit, your physician will fill out a fee slip that will contain your diagnosis and your charges for the visit. Give this slip to the receptionist at the front desk for processing. If you need to have laboratory tests done, our medical assistants will show you to our laboratory. After completion of laboratory work, you will be guided to our front desk. The receptionist will then schedule your next appointment.

Our policy is that payment for services be made at the time of an office visit. If you have Medicare or a managed care policy that covers office visits, we will submit the entire bill to that insurance company. Any testing or procedure done during the office visit will be automatically billed to your insurance company as a courtesy to you. We do ask that you pay the office visit portion of your bill at the time of the visit. You will be given a receipt that you can submit to any major medical plan to which you may belong. These plans generally reimburse patients a portion of the office visit fee. Our fee for the office visit varies, depending on the length of the visit and the complexity of the diagnosis and treatment procedures. These fees are established by the physicians and not by the staff.

If your account becomes past due, our billing manager will contact you regarding setting up a workable payment plan. If we do not hear from you, our policy dictates that legal collection proceedings will be initiated. It is important to speak with the billing manager if you are having a problem paying your account. This will prevent further action on our part and save you needless worry.

INSURANCE PAYMENTS

The insurance contract is ultimately between you and your insurance company. Our office participates in many insurance plans that allow us to complete the insurance form for you. We will complete insurance forms for any testing done in the office and for hospital care. The office visit is paid for at the time of service. It is important for you to provide our staff with correct and complete insurance information. After we submit your insurance form, the payment generally comes directly to the office. In the event that the insurance company sends the payment to you, please call our office for directions on how to handle this situation. Your insurance company will not always cover the entire fee for service, because of the nature of the plan or the deductible. Thus sometimes you are responsible for an unpaid balance. Our office will send a statement to you showing the amount due.

MANAGED CARE PATIENTS (HMOs/PPOs)

Managed care patients must obtain a referral from their primary physician before coming to our office. Your insurance company will not pay for services at our office without a referral. Your insurance company has instructed us to reschedule any patient who arrives without a referral, until a referral can be obtained. These regulations are specified by your insurance company and not by our office. Your insurance manual explains the importance of this referral. It is important for you to remember that if you carry this type of insurance, you cannot be seen anywhere without a referral.

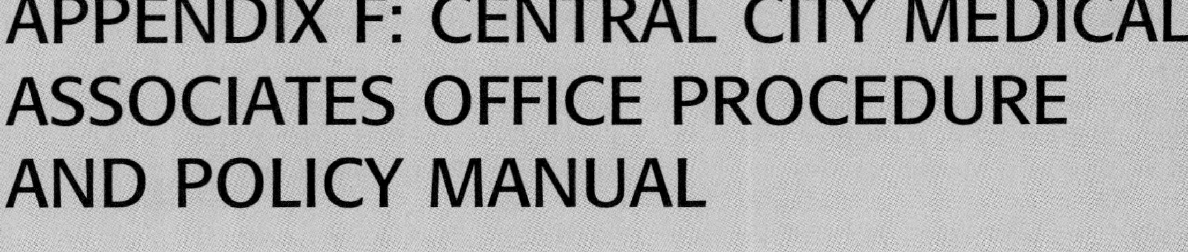

APPENDIX F: CENTRAL CITY MEDICAL ASSOCIATES OFFICE PROCEDURE AND POLICY MANUAL

MISSION STATEMENT

Quality patient care and patient satisfaction are the main goals of our practice. The enthusiasm and efficiency of our staff are key factors in achieving these goals. Because of our commitment to quality patient care, we hire staff who share in our commitment by exhibiting motivation, cooperation, productivity, and caring. This manual will help us all to understand that commitment and reflects the philosophy and direction of our practice.

ABOUT THE PRACTICE

Our practice is an academic-based practice with two offices in the Central City area. We have a group practice of four physicians who specialize in cardiology. Our doctors are affiliated with the following hospitals:

- Medical College of California
- Community General Hospital

Our offices are located at:

Suite One
100 Pine Street
Carson, CA 12345

and

111 Central Avenue
Central City, CA 24689

CONDUCT AND APPEARANCE

Our aim is to provide quality medical care to the patients we serve. What you say, what you do, and how you say and do it will either contribute substantially to the care of the patient or keep us from doing the best possible job. We strive for a continuously cooperative and friendly office environment, with the importance of personal growth recognized. Openness and support for co-workers are critical factors in our practice.

Many patients come to the office in less than a good mood. They are worried about their condition or depressed because their recovery might be slow. It is part of your job to be cheerful, tactful, and patient with our patients, even if their dispositions sometimes cause them to be impatient with you.

Your personal appearance is important, too. It can inspire confidence in both you and the entire practice. Neatness and cleanliness are, of course, particularly important in a doctor's office. We ask that our personnel wear clean, neat clothing with shoes that are clean and in good condition. Sandals and open-toed shoes are not permitted. T-shirts with advertising logos are not permitted. Employees should not wear sweat suits, low-cut tops, or skirts that are shorter than 2 inches above the knee. Because some of our patients have allergies and/or respiratory conditions, employees should refrain from wearing heavy colognes, perfumes, and/or aftershaves. Makeup should be in good taste.

Employees with facial hair, such as mustaches and beards, should keep it neatly trimmed and clean. Jewelry should be kept at a minimum and should be in good taste. Body piercings such as pierced tongues, eyebrows, and/or noses are not permitted on employees who have patient contact.

GOOD EMPLOYEE MANNERS

Patients form quick and lasting impressions of all of us as we conduct our daily business on the telephone, in writing, or in person. Always be courteous. When answering the telephone, always give your name, so the caller will know whom he or she is talking to. Remember that courtesy pays off.

CONFIDENTIALITY

As an employee of this office, you're bound by medical ethics. This means that you must keep confidential any information entrusted to you regarding patients, doctors, your fellow employees, or any office matter. You should never mention a patient's name outside the office. All of us are legally responsible for guarding privileged information and can be subject to legal action if we divulge it. We are all professionals.

DISCIPLINE

Discipline is important to ensure that we meet our goal of quality patient care. Time at the office is for office-related work. A nonsmoking office is what we prefer; if you find it necessary to smoke, we ask that you do it outside the office building. Some buildings have designated areas for smokers.

Personal calls should be kept to a minimum, and incoming calls should be discouraged.

EMPLOYEE WARNING NOTICE

Notice will be given to employees who have not acted within the guidelines of our practice. After the second warning, the employee will be placed on probation. After the third warning, the employee's employment with our practice will be terminated. A copy of the notice form can be found at the end of this manual.

GOSSIP

Gossip can be poisonous, and we sincerely hope that no employee will ever be guilty of repeating any gossip concerning a fellow employee, patient, physician, or any other person associated with our office. Any violation can be grounds for dismissal.

TRAINING PERIOD

Your first 3 months of employment are considered a learning period. Your response to training, ability to do the job assigned, general attitude, and ability to work with other people will be evaluated, and continued employment will be based on this evaluation.

If it is determined that your performance at any time during this 3-month period does not meet the established standards of the office, you may be dismissed. At the end of the learning period, if it is determined that your progress has been satisfactory, you will be considered for permanent employment.

JOB DESCRIPTION AND TEAMWORK

Each employee has been given a written job description for which he or she is responsible. Each position is given a job level that reflects the knowledge and responsibility required of the position. This in no way reflects the philosophy that teamwork is not important. We expect all employees to work together with initiative and cooperation. We ask that teamwork be recognized and practiced by all employees.

EMPLOYEE EVALUATIONS

Employee evaluations help the office manager determine periodic adjustments in each employee's salary. A copy of the employee evaluation form is presented at the end of this manual for your review. Employee evaluations take place annually before the end of the year. At this time, each employee meets with the practice manager to discuss the duties and responsibilities of each job and the results anticipated. The purpose of this evaluation is to help the employee meet the expectations of the practice, practice manager, and physicians. Each employee is rated on a set of factors that our medical practice believes to be critical to overall performance of the group.

BREAKS

All full-time employees are entitled to a 15-minute break in the morning, a half-hour lunch, and a 15-minute break in the afternoon. The lunch period is paid. Part-time employees are entitled to a half-hour break. This can be used as a lunch break or can be divided into two 15-minute breaks.

HOURS

All employees are expected to be in the office at their designated times. To ensure smooth flow of patients in the office, it is necessary for personnel to work on their designated days. Any changes must be approved by the practice manager. If a part-time employee needs a different day off, it is best to use vacation time so as not to interrupt the general flow of the office. Employee hours may sometimes be staggered to accommodate office needs. The office has the right to change an employee's work schedule and assignment when it is in the best interests of patient flow and quality care.

PART-TIME EMPLOYEES

A part-time employee is one who works fewer than 30 hours per week. Part-time employees are paid hourly. Part-time employees are eligible for sick leave in proportion to the hours that they work. A part-time employee who works 16 hours a week is therefore eligible for 16 hours of sick leave per year. After 1 full year of employment, part-time employees are eligible to take paid vacation time in proportion to the amount of hours they work. A part-time employee who works 16 hours per week is eligible, after 1 year's employment, to 4 days of paid vacation time per year. Because of the guidelines of the insurance company, part-time employees are not eligible for health insurance benefits if they work fewer than 30 hours per week. There will not be an increase in eligible vacation days for part-time employees.

PERSONAL TIME AND EMERGENCIES

Each full-time employee is given 2 personal days. Part-time employees are not given personal days. If a family emergency requires additional personal time, the matter will have to be discussed with the office manager. It is customary for employees to use vacation time for this.

TERMINATION

If it becomes necessary for a staff member's employment to be terminated, he or she will be given 2 weeks' notice. We expect that employees who end their employment with the office will provide the same courtesy, giving 2 weeks' notice in writing to the office manager.

SALARY/PAYROLL

Your salary is a confidential matter and should never be discussed with other employees. If you have a question regarding your salary, you should speak directly with the practice manager. Your salary will be reviewed when an employee evaluation takes place. At this time, adjustments will be granted or denied on the basis of the quality and quantity of work performed, progress, attitude, attendance, and the general state of the office economy. Payroll is biweekly and is distributed on Thursdays for your banking convenience.

SCHEDULING OF PATIENTS

Patients who call our office are often ill and generally need to be seen quickly. If there is a difficulty in giving them an appointment quickly, the doctor in the office should be asked when he or she feels the patient should be scheduled.

Of course, we should always schedule emergency patients immediately. With the medical-legal situation the way it is today, we cannot take the risk of making an emergency patient wait. Always advise the doctor of any conversation that you have with a patient who feels he or she is having an emergency. If there is no doctor in the office at the time of the call, tell the patient you need to review the schedule and will call him or her back in a few minutes. Immediately page the doctor nearest your vicinity to advise him or her of the situation so that he or she can decide when and where to see the patient. Always advise the physician when he or she gets behind in this office schedule. No one likes to wait an excessive amount of time, and the doctors certainly do not want to keep their patients waiting. This situation causes everyone—patient, doctor, and office staff—to become anxious. If the physicians are made aware of the situation, they will try their best to catch up.

TELEPHONE TIPS

If patients call for test results, always pull their chart to make sure the results are available, and tell them you will have the physician call them. If the results are not in the chart and you think that it has been a reasonable amount of time in which to receive a report, you should call the appropriate place and obtain the report for the physician.

Do not give results over the phone unless you have been instructed to do so by the physician.

DOCTOR'S PHONE CALLS

When physicians call the office to speak with one of our physicians, put them through immediately. If there is no physician in the office, ask the caller for his or her name and number and tell them you will gladly contact the doctor for them.

Regarding calls from patients, check with each doctor at the beginning of hours to see whether he or she wants to return some calls during hours or wishes to wait until the end of hours. Remember, doctors have their own style; we must respect that and be flexible.

BILLING

Refer all billing questions to the billing manager at the Central City office. Do not attempt to answer these questions yourself. There are many insurance carriers today, and each offers several plans. It is impossible for the front-desk staff to be knowledgeable about all the different plans. It is better to let the billing manager at the Central City office answer all billing questions.

RELEASE OF RECORDS

If patients call and request that their records be sent to another physician, you must pull their chart and give it to the physician in our office who treated them. The physician will instruct you on what to copy and send to the new physician. This, of course, requires the patient's signature on a Records Release Form. If we are sending records to a specialist to whom we referred the patient, we do not require the patient's signature; however, you must still pull the chart and ask what records the doctor would like to have sent.

HOLIDAYS

The following holidays are designated for employees each year:

- New Year's Day
- Good Friday
- Memorial Day
- Independence Day
- Labor Day
- Thanksgiving Day
- Christmas Day

SICK LEAVE

Sick leave with pay is granted to employees who have an illness that keeps them from doing their job. It is not to be considered something to which one is entitled for any other reason. The number of sick days allotted to a full-time employee is 5. Any day beyond this number will be considered a vacation day or will be deducted from that week's salary.

VACATION

Upon completion of 1 year of full-time continuous service, you will be eligible for 2 weeks of vacation with full pay. Persons with 5 consecutive years of full-time service will receive 3 weeks of vacation with full pay. Vacation will be arranged as nearly as possible to the employee's satisfaction, subject to the best interests of the office.

PENSION/PROFIT SHARING

At the present time, each employee is automatically enrolled in the pension/profit-sharing program after 1,100 hours of service. After the first year, the employee is 20% vested. After the second year, the employee is 40% vested, and so on. At the end of 5 years, the employee is 100% vested. Any other questions regarding these plans should be directed to the practice manager. Contributions to the plan are made each year by the physician officers of the practice and are in addition to the employee's salary. The plan is intended to reward devoted employees for their service.

MEDICAL CARE

One of the benefits of working in a medical office is that all employees receive free medical care from our staff of physicians. This benefit covers the immediate families of our employees also. It does not extend to hospital, drug expense, or medical equipment.

HEALTH INSURANCE

Health insurance through the practice is offered to all full-time employees after a 3-month waiting period, full-time being defined as 30 hours per week or more. This insurance benefit will be continued as long as it is financially feasible for the corporation to do so. Employees have arranged for additional coverage on their own for a prescription plan. The amount for this coverage may be deducted once a month from employees' checks, if they request it.

PREGNANCY

Maternity benefits will be handled on an individual basis. Length of service and potential for return to work will be considered. If complications dictate a longer leave, the situation will have to be discussed with the practice manager and perhaps family medical leave should be used.

COMPASSION LEAVE

Each full-time employee is entitled to 3 paid days of leave for the death of an immediate family member. Immediate family members are mother, father, sister, brother, child, and spouse. One day of leave is permitted for the death of a more distant relative. Employees become eligible for this leave after 1 year of employment.

GENERAL QUESTIONS

If you ever have any questions or problems, please feel free to contact the practice manager.

APPENDIX G: ANSWERS TO CHAPTER EXERCISES

CHAPTER ONE

Multiple Choice

1. b
2. c
3. c
4. b
5. b
6. a
7. c
8. d
9. b
10. a

Matching

PHYSICIAN SPECIALTIES

1. H
2. J
3. C
4. K
5. L
6. E
7. N
8. F
9. G
10. D
11. M
12. A
13. I
14. B

PROFESSIONS

1. C
2. D
3. F
4. B
5. A

True or False

1. F
2. F
3. F
4. T
5. F
6. T
7. F
8. T
9. T
10. T
11. F
12. F
13. T
14. T
15. F

Thinkers

1. List the five stages of a medical practice life cycle.
   a. Introduction
   b. Growth
   c. Maturity
   d. Decline
   e. Revitalization
2. List three disadvantages of a partnership.
   a. Interpersonal problems can arise.
   b. Management problems can occur.
   c. Life of the practice is limited.
3. List five traits of a professional.
   a. Highly skilled
   b. Competent
   c. Expert
   d. Specialist
   e. Experienced

CHAPTER TWO

Multiple Choice

1. d
2. d
3. d
4. c
5. c
6. d
7. d
8. d
9. b
10. a
11. b
12. d
13. a
14. b
15. a
16. c
17. d
18. b
19. d
20. a

Matching

1. A
2. C
3. C
4. A
5. A
6. B
7. C
8. C
9. A
10. C
11. C
12. B
13. C
14. B

True or False

1. T
2. T
3. F
4. F
5. T
6. F
7. T
8. F
9. F
10. F
11. F
12. T

13. F
14. F
15. F
16. F
17. F
18. F
19. T
20. F
21. F
22. T
23. F
24. F
25. F
26. T
27. T
28. T
29. F
30. T

Thinkers

1. Describe "Pragmatists" and how they work with other personality types.

   Pragmatists are task-oriented individuals who direct their action to an immediate goal. They are known for their belief in the trial-and-error method and take calculated risks when necessary. Pragmatists often act on principle and are excellent negotiators. They have a real need for achievement and are assertive and controlling. Their co-workers often perceive them as manipulative and exploitative. Pragmatists usually do not work well with others and may have difficulty with interpersonal relationships.
2. List three elements of an employment application and the reason for their importance.

   Any three of the following:

   - Education history
   - Employment history
   - Salary from last employment
   - Special qualifications
   - Reason for leaving previous position
   - Current salary requested
   - Long-range professional goals
   - Flexibility of applicant
   - Date of availability
3. Describe "Houdini."

   One concern of the office manager is the employee who is the "disappearing act." When employees leave their work area without mentioning to anyone where they are going, problems can occur. It should be a common practice in the office that employees inform each other, or the office manager, when they are leaving, where they are going, and when they expect to return. All employees should be held responsible for this, even if they are leaving their area for only a minute. One minute sometimes stretches to fifteen, and office flow should not be interrupted while someone frantically searches for the missing employee.
4. List four articles of clothing that would not be acceptable in a medical office.

   Any four of the following: T-shirts, shorts, jeans, hats, clothing with advertising logos such as sport's teams, beers, or a favorite race car driver, sweat suits, short skirts (shorter than 2 inches above the knee), low-cut tops, and any clothing that is acid-washed, faded, stained, ragged, dirty, or wrinkled does not belong in a medical practice.

CHAPTER THREE

Multiple Choice

1. a
2. a
3. b
4. c
5. c
6. b
7. c
8. d
9. a
10. c
11. d
12. d
13. c
14. c
15. d
16. d
17. d
18. d
19. a

True or False

1. T
2. T
3. T
4. T
5. F
6. F
7. T
8. T
9. F
10. T
11. F
12. F
13. T
14. F
15. F
16. F
17. F
18. T
19. T
20. T

Matching

1. I
2. G
3. H
4. J
5. F
6. C
7. E
8. D
9. B
10. K

Thinkers

1. Compare the difference between wave and modified wave appointment scheduling.

   The wave appointment scheduling approach is characterized by the scheduling of multiple patients in each hour. All patients are assigned the time of the top of the hour, that is, 10:00 AM, 11:00 AM, and so on. There may be four patients scheduled for 10:00 AM, another four patients may be scheduled with an appointment time of 11:00 AM, and so on. This type of scheduling creates a more even flow for the physician and staff. This scheduling approach is not as affected by no-shows as the standard or stream approach. If three of the four patients scheduled at 10:00 AM arrive at the same time, there are always patients to be prepped and seen. The fact that the fourth patient did not show for an appointment does not affect the staff or the physician. This approach is not always the best for the patient, however, because many patients have to wait longer for their appointment since it is on a first come, first served basis. The fourth patient to arrive for a 10:00 AM appointment will have to wait a significant period of time before he or she is seen. So by loading all the patients at the front end of the hour, the office schedule runs very efficiently.

The modified wave scheduling approach takes the wave scheduling approach and improves on it. It not only works well for the office, but is also more patient friendly. In a modified wave schedule, two patients are scheduled at the top of the hour, for example, two patients at 10:00 AM, two patients at 10:15 AM, one at 10:30 AM, and none at 10:45 AM as this is used as a catch-up slot. With this type of schedule, the physician can see more patients with only a small wait. Each office should identify the correct modified wave schedule for its practice. Since wave scheduling is so flexible, it can be used for portions of the day, hours in the day, or for all day every day. To determine the right scheduling for your practice, sit with the physician to identify how this will be set up. First, decide how many patient can be seen in an hour. Begin by scheduling half of the patients at the beginning of the hour and then the remaining patients through the second half of the hour.

2. List the six LISTEN techniques used to achieve telephone effectiveness.
   Let others speak
   Intend to hear what they are saying
   Speak when the caller has finished
   Talk with them, not at them
   Empathetically respond to patient's with a problem
   Never speak when the other person is talking
3. List ways to make a reception area "friendly."

   Noisy children playing should be asked to play quietly, loud patients should be asked to talk quietly, and patients should be reminded that there is no smoking, eating, or drinking in the office.

   This area should be a reflection on the practice and should not be cluttered or dirty. Although there are no tried and true cures for the reception room "blues," there are some things you can do to reduce anxiety as patients wait for their name to be called.

   Many offices have installed a television and some even use a VCR or DVD player to show movies throughout the day. Even though the physician is late in seeing the patient, the patient becomes engrossed in a television program or movie and does not realize the time. Other practices, such as some ophthalmology practices, use low lights and soft music. Whatever the preference of the physician, it should be a pleasant area.

   For patients who like to become better acquainted with their illnesses, or even read about what their friends have, it is a good idea to keep various educational brochures available in the reception room. For instance, a pamphlet on toilet training is of interest to a new mother and may be found in a family practice, obstetrics/gynecology, or pediatric reception room. A family practice or an internal medicine office may display brochures on hypertension, diabetes, arthritis, or high cholesterol. These brochures are sometimes provided by pharmaceutical companies, but if not, they can be purchased at a nominal price per copy. Some physicians like to personalize them by writing up their own pamphlets. Other practices develop 8 1/2 by 11 inch information sheets on various types of illnesses and/or injuries. They then print across the top, "WAITING ROOM COPY. DO NOT REMOVE." They print them on brightly colored paper and have them laminated. Patients can pick them up and read them while they wait. By having them laminated, it provides a more durable sheet. Keep in mind that some of these information sheets may "grow legs and walk away." It is a good idea to make a few sets of them.
4. Define the difference between a new patient and an established patient.

   A new patient is one who has not been seen in the office or hospital by the physician, or one of her or his colleagues of the same specialty, within the last 3 years. This distinction is not based on the diagnosis for the visit.

CHAPTER FOUR

Multiple Choice

1. c
2. c
3. d
4. d
5. a
6. d
7. c
8. b
9. d
10. b
11. b
12. a
13. d
14. b
15. a
16. b
17. c
18. d
19. a
20. a

True or False

1. F
2. F
3. T
4. T
5. F
6. T
7. F
8. T
9. T
10. T
11. T
12. T
13. F
14. T
15. F
16. F
17. T
18. F
19. T
20. T

Matching

1. D
2. E
3. I
4. H
5. B
6. J
7. C
8. A
9. G
10. F

Thinkers

1. The office has developed an office newsletter for its patients. The newsletter will be mailed to all of the practice's patients. What class of mail should be used and why?

   Standard mail consists of flyers, circulars, advertising, newsletters, bulletins, catalogs, and small parcels. All standard mail rates are bulk rates, and each mailing must meet a minimum quantity of 200 pieces or 50 pounds of mail to qualify. This is a great way to mail newsletters that the practice may want to send out to patients because it is the least costly mailing option.
2. Prepare an e-mail policy for the employee handbook.

   The practice e-mail policy should include the following:
   - Basic rules and regulations of the practice on how to compose an e-mail.
   - The amount of time that should be allowed to elapse before an e-mail should be answered. Some practices use 24 hours, others use 4 hours.
   - When e-mails should be sent with "high priority."
   - How to handle spam. There is software that can be purchased that will contain spam.
   - Cartoons, jokes, chain e-mails, and so on.
   - Personal use.
   - Newsletters and Listservs that are going to be permitted by the practice.
3. Describe the different types of postal mail.

   First class is the most common method of mailing and is used to mail most business envelopes, postcards, note cards, flats, parcels that meet the weight requirements, and business reply mail. The maximum weight of a first class mailing is 13 ounces. First class mail delivery includes forwarding and return services.

   Standard mail consists of flyers, circulars, advertising, newsletters, bulletins, catalogs, and small parcels. All standard mail rates are bulk rates, and each mailing must meet a minimum quantity of 200 pieces or 50 pounds of mail to qualify. This is a great way to mail newsletters that the practice may want to send out to patients because it is less costly than first class.

   Periodicals are a class of mail that consists of newspapers, magazines, and other publications. This is the mode of mail transportation that may deliver office and medical supply catalogs and books. The office manager should be aware that if the office needs to send books, they can be sent quite inexpensively with the fourth-class or book rate.

   Express mail is the fastest mail service offered by the U.S. Postal Service. It provides guaranteed expedited service that is offered 365 days a year, including Sundays and holidays. Express mail must be placed into an express mail container (envelope, box, or tube), which can be obtained at your local post office at no charge. The charge for this type of mail is based on the weight. A flat rate envelope is currently charged at $16.25.

   Priority mail consists of first-class mail that weighs over 13 ounces. If the practice wants the mail to get there fast, priority mail offers the best value. It includes forwarding and return services. Postage for priority mail weighing less than 1 pound is the same price, no matter where it is going. Mail over 1 pound is priced based on its destination (based on predetermined zones).

   Registered mail is first-class or priority mail. Any item of value that needs to be mailed should be sent via registered mail. This mail route is more expensive, but it is sometimes necessary. Each piece of registered mail is insured for up to $25,000 against loss or damage. With registered mail, the office manager can track the date and time of delivery online. This type of mail can also provide the sender with a receipt for an additional charge.

   Certified mail should be used when the office requires confirmation of a letter's or package's arrival at the specified address and acknowledgment of receipt at that address. This type of mail can also be tracked online. This is more expensive than regular mail, but it is commonly used in a medical office.
4. List the "six C's" of effective writing.
   a. Clear—Be clear about your objective for the communication.
   b. Coherent—Articulate consistent and accurate information.
   c. Concise—Make the point, short and snappy.
   d. Correct—Be accurate in statements.
   e. Courteous—Give consideration to the receiver.
   f. Confident—Be convinced and secure in what you are communicating.

CHAPTER FIVE

Multiple Choice

1. d
2. a
3. d
4. c
5. d
6. c
7. b
8. b
9. b
10. a
11. d
12. d
13. c
14. d
15. a
16. b
17. b
18. c
19. a
20. d

True or False

1. T
2. F
3. T
4. T
5. T
6. F
7. F
8. F
9. F
10. F
11. F
12. F
13. T
14. F
15. T
16. F
17. F
18. T
19. T
20. T

Thinkers

1. Define RFP and explain how it is used by the office manager.
   - Establish the needs of the practice.
   - Prepare a budget for the purchase.
   - Establish a time line for shopping, purchase, installation, and final implementation.
   - Prepare an RFP.
2. A clinical assistant has entered incorrect information into a patient's chart. She has used correction fluid, written "mistake" beside it, and initialed it. Is this the correct way to handle an error? If not, how should the correction be made?

   Draw a line through the error, write the word "error," date the entry, and place your initials.
3. Signature stamps can be very useful in a medical practice. They can also be a liability. Explain and offer examples.

   Signature stamps are helpful for the following:
   - Insurance forms
   - Membership applications to insurance companies
   - Notes for patients to return to work or school
   - Order forms for patient testing
   - Letters

   The downside of the signature stamp is the potential for abuse. The following suggestions will protect against misuse of signature stamps:
   - Assign the stamp to one employee who will be accountable for its use.
   - Have different stamps made and issue them to different employees. For example, the stamp "R. H. Hale, M.D." may be issued to one employee, the stamp "Robert H. Hale, M.D." assigned to another, and the stamp "Dr. Robert H. Hale" assigned to yet another. This way, you can track how each stamp is being used.
4. An office manager of a pediatric practice has purged medical records on patients who have "outgrown" a pediatrician. What should be done with the records and why?

   The length of time that a physician's office is legally required to keep a medical record varies from state to state. Each office manager should check with the practice's legal counsel or the local medical society to determine the statute of limitations for medical malpractice. This has a direct impact on the length of time the office must retain its patient records. From a strictly medical viewpoint, a medical office should retain medical records as long as the patient is active.

   Records should be retained indefinitely if the patient has undergone a procedure that could have an impact on him or her later in life.

   In most cases, medical records should be maintained for 7 to 15 years for patients who are no longer seeing the physician. For deceased patients, records should be maintained for 5 years from the date of their last service. Pediatric and family practices that treat children must maintain medical records for 7 to 10 years past majority (the age at which full civil rights are accorded). The age of majority differs from state to state; however, it is typically age 21. The office manager should check with state authorities or legal counsel to verify this age requirement. In other words, if you treat an infant and the infant's family moves out of town, the infant's medical record may be in your office for as long as 30 years! X-ray films of inactive patients should be maintained for 5 to 10 years after the patient is no longer active. Many consulting agencies will advise a medical office to condense the patient's chart if the patient has been inactive for 3 years. This means that not every piece of paper must be kept in the chart, but only pertinent information regarding medications, certain procedures, specific treatments and tests, and so on. If a copy of the patient's chart was sent to another physician, a copy of the record release authorization should also remain in the chart.

CHAPTER SIX

Multiple Choice

1. c
2. a
3. b
4. c
5. d
6. d
7. c
8. d
9. b
10. d
11. a
12. a
13. b
14. a
15. c
16. d
17. d
18. b
19. a
20. d

Matching

1. F
2. J
3. A
4. G
5. I
6. C
7. D
8. E
9. B
10. H

True or False

1. T
2. T
3. T
4. T
5. F
6. F
7. T
8. T
9. F
10. F
11. F
12. F
13. T
14. F
15. F
16. T
17. F
18. T
19. T
20. T

Thinkers

1. An overpayment has been made by Medicare for patient Josh Bok. Determine whether a refund should be made. If not, explain the reasoning behind your decision. If so, what steps should be taken to refund the overpayment?

   Yes, a refund should be made, otherwise you can be accused of fraud.

   Immediately notify the carrier as to how this overpayment occurred. Send notification by certified mail with a return receipt. If the check was only for that patient, write the word VOID across it, copy it for your records, and return that check. If the overpayment was made in part with other payments, cash the check and prepare a check from the practice in the amount of the overpayment. Make a copy of the check and then send it in to Medicare. Attach the EOB or the Remittance Advice to the letter. Include the patient's Social Security number; this identifies the patient and eliminates confusion and errors. Check the Medicare Web site because it may have an overpayment form that can be used.
2. Why is the reference remark important to a medical practice?

   The reference remark provides the practice with the reason that the claim was denied. Depending on the reason, the practice can then correct any error that may exist and resubmit the claim.
3. Develop a policy regarding ABNs and how they would be used in your medical practice.

   Be sure that the policy contains the necessary information from the chapter.
4. Design a patient encounter form for a medical practice (do not include ICD-9-CM or CPT codes).

   Be sure that the patient encounter form that is designed by each student contains the necessary information from the chapter.
5. A long-time patient of the practice has recently fallen on "hard times" and cannot pay the "patient balance due" after his surgery. How should the office manager handle this patient?

   The office manager should first speak with the doctor to get her or his comments. If the physician does not want to pursue collection of this balance, the policy in the manual should be followed. The patient should be asked to provide proof of income and should be required to complete the financial disclosure form. Once the practice has received these forms, the office manager should discuss them with the physician and a determination should be made. The patient should receive this determination by mail. The financial disclosure forms should be maintained in the office.

CHAPTER SEVEN

Multiple Choice

1. d
2. b
3. c
4. c
5. c
6. a
7. b
8. d
9. c
10. d
11. c
12. a
13. d
14. b
15. d

True or False

1. T
2. T
3. F
4. F
5. T
6. F
7. T
8. T
9. T
10. F

Thinkers

1. An office manager is new to a practice. She discovers that there are several credit balances on the books for a patient. Is it necessary for her to do anything about this discrepancy, or can she allow them to stay there until the patient returns to the office (to use up the credit)?

   All credit balances should be returned to the individual or carrier who paid for the service.
2. A good friend of the physician arrives for an office visit. The physician instructs the receptionist not to charge this individual. The receptionist comes to the office manager for guidance. How should the office manager handle this situation

   The office manager should approach the physician when he has finished with the patient and should explain why the office cannot provide these types of discounts and professional courtesies.?
3. Describe the self-disclosure program and how it may be used by a medical practice

   The self-disclosure program encourages anyone believing there are irregularities within their practice to disclose them using the self-disclosure protocol. Self-disclosure allows providers to reduce their costs, minimize the extent of the audit, negotiate settlements, and often avoid exclusion from governmental programs. There are times when the practice may be required to enter into an integrity agreement. A corporate integrity agreement is a corrective plan of action that is negotiated between carriers and medical practices. These contracts are used as part of a settlement to resolve violations of the civil False Claims Act and whistleblower suits. In this agreement, the physician practice does not accept liability or admit fault. Complete details of the self-disclosure protocol can be found on the OIG's Web site at www.hhs.gov/oig. Details can also be found in the *Federal Register,* Vol. 63, No. 210, page 58399.
4. Dr. Martin submits claims electronically for services that were not performed. What criminal statute(s) could this practice involve?

   False Statements Relating to Health Care Matters, Mail and Wire Fraud.

CHAPTER EIGHT

Multiple Choice

1. b
2. a
3. a
4. a
5. a
6. d
7. d
8. c
9. b
10. b
11. a
12. b
13. c
14. b
15. c
16. d
17. a
18. d
19. c
20. b

True or False

1. F
2. F
3. F
4. F
5. T
6. T
7. T
8. T
9. F
10. T
11. T
12. F
13. T
14. T
15. T
16. F
17. T
18. F
19. T
20. F

Thinkers

1. Compare and contrast the two documentation formats. Describe which format would be best for the medical practice scenario provided by your instructor.

   SOAP is a mnemonic used to recall a method of organized and comprehensive documentation. Documentation compiled under this method covers the following areas:
   - Subjective view of the case: Documentation includes patient complaints, history of injury or illness, answers to questions about organ systems, and past, family, and/or social history.
   - Objective data: Documentation includes findings on examination of the patient.
   - Assessment: Documentation includes prognosis and/or differential diagnosis of the patient and diagnostic studies.
   - Plan for treatment: Documentation includes patient instructions, prescriptions, testing to be performed, and next appointment.

   SNOCAMP is a mnemonic that is more closely related to the documentation guidelines.

- Subjective: Documentation includes patient complaints, history of injury or illness, answers to questions about organ systems, and past, family, and/or social history.
- Nature of presenting problem: A disease, illness, injury, symptom, or finding that relates to the chief complaint or reason for the visit.
- Objective: Documentation includes findings on examination of the patient.
- Counseling and/or coordination of care: Documentation includes patient encounters for which counseling and/or coordination of care constitute more than 50% of the visit.
- Assessment: Documentation includes prognosis and/or differential diagnosis of the patient and diagnostic studies.
- Medical decision making: Documentation includes complexity of the visit and the physician's thought process. This component is somewhat subjective and is based on the following three components:
  1. Number of diagnoses or management options
  2. Amount and/or complexity of data
  3. Risk of mortality/morbidity
- Plan: Documentation includes the treatment plan being considered for managing the patient's case. It should also include the rationale for ordering additional studies and/or procedures.

2. In the following scenario, determine whether the visit is a consultation or a new patient, and explain how you arrive at your decision.

   Kelly Mills was sent to Dr. Sara Class for evaluation of her abdominal pain. Her family physician, Dr. Babinetz, had seen Kelly in the office and needed the expert opinion of Dr. Class regarding her gastrointestinal (GI) complaints. Dr. Class reviewed the upper GI study that Kelly brought with her to his office. He did a thorough examination and ordered some additional studies. He believes that she has peptic ulcer disease. Dr. Class will see Kelly in follow-up in 3 weeks to discuss the results and her prognosis.

   This is an outpatient consultation 99241–99245. Diagnosis has not yet been made.
3. Describe what a medically unnecessary service is and provide an example of one.
   - It is a service that is not supported by the codes in the medical record.
   - Have student provide scenario.
4. List and define the two teaching physician modifiers.
   - -GC: This service is performed in part by a resident under the direction of a teaching physician. This modifier is to be used with all services provided by a teaching physician except where modifier -GE is appropriate. Use of this modifier acknowledges the presence of the teaching physician during the key portion of the service.
   - -GE: This service is performed by a resident without the presence of a teaching physician under the primary care exception. This modifier is used to indicate that the teaching physician was not present during the E&M service under the primary care exception being billed, but that the requirements for billing have been met.

CHAPTER NINE

Multiple Choice

1. a	**11.** a
2. a	**12.** d
3. c	**13.** b
4. b	**14.** c
5. d	**15.** a
6. d	**16.** b
7. d	**17.** c
8. c	**18.** d
9. b	**19.** a
10. b	**20.** d

Matching

1. B	**4.** A
2. E	**5.** D
3. C	

True or False

1. F	**11.** T
2. F	**12.** T
3. T	**13.** F
4. T	**14.** T
5. T	**15.** F
6. F	**16.** F
7. F	**17.** T
8. F	**18.** F
9. F	**19.** T
10. F	**20.** T

Thinkers

1. Mrs. Reynolds passed away during the night in the nursing home. What is the physician's responsibility, if any, at this point?

   Some physicians may go to the hospital when the nurse calls, but most will not. It is the physician's responsibility to complete a death certificate the next morning.

Most states will not allow the funeral director to pick up the body until there is a signed death certificate.

2. A patient has become noncompliant, failing to take prescribed medications and to go for requested testing. The physician feels that it is in the best interest of the patient to obtain a new physician to whom the patient will listen. How would the office manager handle this situation?

   The office manager would compose a letter of termination of the physician's service. The letter should state that the physician will provide emergency care for a set period of time while the patient obtains a new physician. This time period is generally 2 weeks to 1 month in length. The physician must sign the letter before it is sent. The letter should be sent via regular mail and also certified mail with a return receipt.

3. Someone from the sheriff's office has just served a subpoena duces tecum to the office. What is the office's responsibility at this point?

   A subpoena duces tecum is a written notification for records, documents, or other evidence described in a subpoena. Failure to bring the appropriate documents can also be considered contempt of court and carries with it a penalty of fines and/or imprisonment. If a subpoena is served to a physician or an employee of a practice, it is imperative to immediately contact the practice attorney. The attorney will provide guidance from there. Follow these guidelines:

   - IMMEDIATELY tell management (supervisor and/or physician) that you have received a subpoena. Don't ignore it; it is a legal document that can land you in jail or result in fines.
   - IMMEDIATELY, AT THE DIRECTION OF THE PHYSICIAN, CALL THE ATTORNEY FOR THE PRACTICE TO REPORT RECEIVING THE SUBPEONA.
   - DO NOT DESTROY any information, whether it be medical or financial in nature.
   - The receptionist who received the subpoena should note the date and time that it was served and how it was served.
   - The practice attorney will provide directions on how to handle this subpoena.

4. In a medical practice scenario provided by your instructor, list some ways in which you would use the practice attorney.

   This answer depends on the practice scenario that is provided by the instructor; however, it should cover the following areas:

   - Physician contracts
   - Retirement and profit-sharing plans
   - State and federal legislation
   - Health insurance plans
   - Partnership and corporation formation
   - Office and equipment leases
   - Managed care contracts
   - Representation of the physician in collection cases
   - Representation of the physician in hospital matters
   - Employment issues

5. Your office has interviewed an individual for a position at the front desk. This applicant is in a wheelchair. The assistant office manager tells you that you do not have to make special provisions for this applicant if you decide to hire him. What are your responsibilities to this applicant, if any? Explain your reasoning.

   Requirements set forth by the Americans with Disabilities Act provide guidance for the responsibilities of employers of disabled persons. This act can be found online at www.usdoj.gov/crt/ada/adahom1.htm.

CHAPTER TEN

Multiple Choice

1. c
2. d
3. a
4. c
5. a
6. b
7. c
8. d
9. a
10. d
11. b
12. d
13. b
14. d
15. c
16. c
17. a
18. a
19. a
20. b

True or False

1. T
2. F
3. F
4. T
5. F
6. F
7. F
8. F
9. T
10. F
11. T
12. T
13. F
14. F
15. F
16. T
17. T
18. T
19. F
20. T

Thinkers

1. Describe ways in which a physician or medical office can use the Internet.

   Many physicians and office managers use the Internet on a daily basis. Most professional or management journals can now be found online. Medical office personnel can simply print out the articles they want to read. But even with the Internet, it is time consuming to search for specific articles and information. The Internet provides not only research information, but information regarding new medications and techniques. Physicians and office managers can search for appropriate educational workshops that they may want to attend. They can print the conference information, such as hotels, agenda, dates and times, and so on. Once a decision has been made to attend, they can register online. They can then find a hotel and book a room, find a flight, if necessary, find a rental car, and find good restaurants, without leaving their chair.

2. Using the previously distributed medical practice scenarios, list the computer features that are important for your practice.

   This question involves the scenario distributed by the instructor and is based on each individual scenario. The computer features that are listed in the chapter should be followed, carefully choosing the ones appropriate for the student's scenario.

3. Using the previously distributed medical practice scenarios, design a patient encounter form for your practice.

   This question involves the scenario distributed by the instructor and is based on each individual scenario. The patient encounter form should be designed for each practice scenario using the information from the chapter that best suits the student's practice.

4. Explain the issues with e-discovery.

Attorneys are finding loopholes in electronic medical records (EMRs) that would not exist in a paper record. With the growth of EMRs, health care lawyers and health information technologists predict the number of e-discoveries to increase significantly in the next decade. E-discovery can reveal a lot about a record's reliability as evidence due to hidden time stamps that are embedded in the programming. E-discovery grants lawyers access deep into the malpractice case electronic records, which may provide information pertinent to a lawsuit. This data, referred to as digital Easter eggs, or metadata, is lying there waiting to be discovered. Metadata captures something that paper documents can't: the time that the entries themselves were made. Metadata can do more than capture the time entry; it can also show when a document was accessed, who looked at it, and if it was altered from its original format. It tells a lot about the integrity of the medical record and its reliability as evidence in the case. Because of this, e-discovery requests for metadata will increase as it becomes more widely known. The medical practice staff will need to familiarize themselves with this metadata and how to access it as the importance and availability of this type of data is discovered.

CHAPTER ELEVEN

Multiple Choice

1. b
2. b
3. c
4. d
5. d
6. a
7. b
8. d
9. a
10. b
11. d
12. b
13. d
14. c
15. d

True or False

1. F
2. T
3. F
4. T
5. F
6. F
7. F
8. F
9. T
10. F

Thinkers

1. List five policies that should be covered in the medical waste management plan.

   List five of these six:
   - Categories of waste
   - Disposal of sharps
   - In-service training
   - Medical waste containers
   - Preparation of medical waste for pickup
   - Weighing, storing, and tracking medical waste
2. There has been an explosion in a building on your block. The police have arrived at your office and state that the block must be evacuated. Identify the steps that you as the office manager should take after learning of this situation.
   - Identify potential risk
   - Store computer back-up tapes off-site
   - Store emergency supplies off-site
   - Develop an evacuation plan
   - Develop a plan for patient care off-site
   - Ensure that your insurance policy does not exclude certain disasters
   - Develop a plan for contacting patients, vendors, and employee's families
3. In preparation for an earthquake, what items should be in your disaster supply kit? Explain the reasons each item is necessary.
   - Insurance forms
   - Paper, pencils, pens
   - Petty cash

- Small kit of clinical equipment, including thermometer, blood-pressure cuff, stethoscope, Band-Aids, antibiotic creams, gauze and Ace bandages, tape, casting supplies (if you have them), *Physician's Desk Reference* (PDR), cell phone and charger, batteries of all sizes, patient list, flashlights, urine dip sticks, hurricane lamp with oil, hard candy, and samples of medications

4. An employee has accidentally stuck himself with a needle after drawing blood on a patient. The employee comes to you totally distraught. What does OSHA mandate that you do?

Exposure determination involves many components. Administration of HBV vaccine is one component of this category and is discussed in detail in Chapter 11. Should an exposure occur, a confidential medical examination and documentation are immediately required. The employee must identify the patient source, and that patient's blood must be tested as soon as possible after consent is obtained to determine HIV or HBV infectivity. Any information on the patient's HIV or HBV test must be provided to the evaluating physician. A copy of the OSHA guidelines must be on-site, readily available, and followed exactly.

CHAPTER TWELVE

Multiple Choice

1. d
2. a
3. d
4. b
5. c
6. c
7. b
8. a
9. d
10. b
11. b
12. a
13. c
14. b
15. d
16. a
17. c
18. b
19. c
20. b

Matching

1. C
2. D
3. E
4. A
5. B

True or False

1. T
2. T
3. T
4. T
5. F
6. F
7. F
8. F
9. T
10. T
11. F
12. T
13. F
14. T
15. T
16. T
17. F
18. F
19. F
20. T

Thinkers

1. List five major frustrations of the physician/administrator relationship.
- Problem solving and decision making at meetings
- Employees who do not follow office policy
- Interpersonal conflicts and communication problems
- The introduction of change
- Influencing decisions and policies
- Motivating the board

2. List four signs of a great office manager.
   a. Don't tolerate a slacker. Each employee has to hold her or his own and be accountable for her or his work.
   b. Refuse to pick favorites and ignore others. Employees should be rewarded based on a job well done, not because they are a friend of the office manager.
   c. Give and receive feed back on projects and ideas. Listen to how employees who are doing the job think it can be done better.
   d. Promote balance for each employee between work and home life. A good employee knows that the practice wants its employees to have a good balance.

3. Explain what an office manager should look for when purchasing a new chair.
   a. A contoured backrest will give your back the comfort and support it needs. Pick a chair shaped to match the natural contour of your spine.
   b. Backrests should be height adjustable, providing your back with customized comfort and support.
   c. Don't go too soft. For total comfort, seat and back foam must be dense enough to support your weight evenly and it should be sculpted to fit the human form.
   d. Look for "waterfall" seat cushions that slope down at the front of the chair. This important ergonomic feature helps improve circulation to your lower legs.
   e. Rest your arms. Armrests help keep your arms in a comfortable position, reducing shoulder, neck, and back strain. Height- and tilt-adjustable models are especially good.
   f. The pneumatic height adjustment on a chair lets you alter your seating position throughout the day with a smooth, easy, one-touch action.
   g. Remain seated. Make sure all adjustment controls can be reached from a seated position. Keep moving. Multitilt and operator mechanisms are important for data entry or computer work. They let you vary your position while maintaining maximum support.
   h. Good chairs have casters for easy mobility. Be sure to get the right kind for your floor. Choose a chair with a choice of casters designed for carpets, hard surfaces, or a combination.

CHAPTER THIRTEEN

Multiple Choice

1. b
2. b
3. c
4. a
5. d
6. d
7. b
8. c
9. c
10. a

True or False

1. T
2. F
3. T
4. F
5. F
6. T
7. F
8. T
9. T
10. T

Thinkers

1. What steps should be taken before committing to an ASC?

   Your office must take a few basic steps that before jumping into the ASC arena:
   - Determine the purpose of the facility
   - Discuss organizational issues and produce a business plan
   - Develop a team
   - Determine the location
   - Address construction issues
   - Consider costs
2. Describe the function of the executive committee.

   The executive committee, which is made up of the various chiefs of service medicine (e.g., surgery, anesthesia), makes decisions regarding the medical staff and hospital.
3. What are the different attributes of hospitals?
   - Type of ownership (i.e., private or government)
   - Type of problems they treat (e.g., tuberculosis, hypertension)
   - Whether they play a role in physician education (i.e., teaching hospitals)
   - Average length of stay (i.e., short term or long term)
   - Type of medicine provided (i.e., medical or osteopathic)
   - Size of the institution (i.e., number of beds)

CHAPTER FOURTEEN

Multiple Choice

1. b
2. c
3. b
4. c
5. b
6. c
7. c
8. b
9. c
10. b
11. a
12. d
13. d
14. b
15. c
16. a
17. b
18. d
19. d
20. a

True or False

1. F
2. F
3. F
4. F
5. F
6. F
7. F
8. T
9. F
10. F
11. T
12. F
13. T
14. T
15. T
16. T
17. T
18. T
19. T
20. F

Thinkers

1. Using a medical practice scenario provided by the instructor, construct an example of what the income/expense sheet may look like for your practice.

   This question involves the scenario distributed by the instructor and is based on each individual scenario. The income expense sheet may be different based on each practice scenario using the information from the chapter that best suits the student's practice. Students should be told to refer to this information in the chapter.
2. A new patient seeks care from your practice. On completion of the visit, the patient states that he is from out of town and is low on cash. He wants to write a check to pay for his visit. What would you say to him? Explain your decision.

   This answer should be based on information the student learned in this chapter and the student's own decision making.
3. You have a meeting scheduled with the physician to discuss the financial condition of the practice. Explain how you would prepare for this meeting and describe the reasons behind your preparations.

   Preparation for the meeting should be based on information such as the following:
   - The accounts receivable
   - Collection ratio
   - Billing rate
   - Overhead ratio
   - Salary rate
   - Cost analysis
   - Profit ratio
   - And so on

4. The physician feels that the office accountant is not providing the services that are needed. He does not have many health care clients and therefore does not always understand the needs of a medical practice. How would you interview for a new accountant? Explain what you feel is important for the practice in selecting a new accountant.

   Whom to hire as an accountant is one of the most crucial decisions the medical office manager makes. Thoroughly evaluate the office's needs and all candidates before deciding on an office accountant. It was once thought to be beneath a physician to consider his or her practice a business, and physicians perceived the business aspect of medicine as a hindrance. Few still think so today. However, perhaps as a carryover from the old days, many physicians view accountants simply as "number crunchers" and do not use their talents to the fullest. You can open the physician's eyes, if necessary, and help him or her choose an accountant who will strive for the best return on all the hard work the physician, you, and the staff do. Never just hire a friend, neighbor, or former classmate of the physician—or a friend of anyone's for that matter. An accountant is nothing less than a business investment. Choose the best!

   Before beginning the search for an accountant, you need to determine the goals of the practice. Does the physician anticipate growth? Look to retire? Simply wish to skate by for the coming years? The physician who is looking for practice growth requires an accountant with expertise in business development and marketing. The physician who is facing retirement requires less financial planning (because most of this should already be done) and needs fewer accounting services. Discuss in detail with the physician his or her priorities and goals for the practice to help in evaluating an accountant.

CHAPTER FIFTEEN

Multiple Choice

1. d	11. c
2. d	12. a
3. a	13. d
4. c	14. b
5. a	15. a
6. b	16. c
7. b	17. c
8. d	18. b
9. c	19. b
10. c	20. d

True or False

1. F	11. T
2. T	12. F
3. T	13. T
4. F	14. F
5. F	15. F
6. T	16. F
7. F	17. T
8. T	18. T
9. F	19. T
10. F	20. F

Thinkers

1. Your practice has hired a new physician. Describe and explain your ideas on how you would advertise and market this new physician.

   To properly introduce a new associate, send out an announcement that you either designed on the computer or bought as a standard item through a catalog. Be sure to mention any special skills or education the physician might have. Send the announcement to physician members of the hospital staff, departments in the hospital, and some community members. Also send it to pharmacists, optometrists, opticians, dentists, psychologists, and solo physical therapists. It might also be beneficial to mail the announcement to any local community organizations and the Chamber of Commerce. It is a relatively inexpensive way to introduce a new physician and simultaneously advertise the practice.

   Have a copy of the announcement printed in the local newspaper for about 2 weeks. Perhaps the newspaper would be willing to do a human-interest piece on this new addition to the practice. Maybe the physician has an interesting side to his or her personal life that can be mentioned, such as teaching blind persons how to ski or repairing old violins. This makes great reading and human-interest material.

   A new physician should introduce himself or herself at local pharmacies. Building rapport with pharmacists is a good idea. They refer many customers to physicians—so why not your practice?

   Some offices purchase local radio advertising to introduce their new associates. Television spots are unnecessary and expensive, and actually do not provide the kind of marketing that you need. Arrange for the new physician to meet social and community organizations. Advise the new physician that it would be prudent for him or her to join the local medical society and any other community groups, such as the American Cancer Society, the American Red Cross, or the Diabetes Support Group.

Have the new physician visit dentists in the area. You might want to enlist the expertise of a public relations firm to help you promote the new physician. The firm can provide you with tips on how to market the physician successfully, but it may be costly. Large practices usually use a public relations firm. Smaller practices usually cannot afford their rates. One practice formed the idea of throwing a "Welcome New Physician" party!

2. A physician has decided to publish a practice newsletter. Develop an outline for articles and prepare a plan as to how this will be distributed.

   Each student should follow the suggestions in this chapter and compose a newsletter for his or her practice. There is no right or wrong answer for this.

3. Using a medical practice scenario provided by the instructor, describe what marketing tools you would use for your practice and why.

   Using the practice scenario provided by the instructor, have each student prepare a marketing strategy for her or his practice. There is no right or wrong answer. Ask students to be creative, yet keeping in mind the costs involved.

APPENDIX H: SAMPLE ENCOUNTER FORM

SURGERY SPECIALISTS, INC.
111 Middle Street, Suite A1
Kinsley, KS

___ Patrick Henley, M.D. ___ William Scott, M.D. ___ Adam Crane, III, D.O. ___ Danelle Kelly, M. D.

DATE: ________ ACCT. NUMBER: ________ BIRTH DATE: ________

PATIENT: ________

ADDRESS: ________

HOME PHONE: ________ WORK PHONE: ________

(INSURANCE 1)
GRP # ______ ID # ______

(INSURANCE 2)
GRP # ______ ID # ______

OFFICE SERVICES

EVALUATION & MANAGEMENT SERVICES				
N/C OFFICE VISIT			99022	
POSTOP MAJOR N/C 90 MINOR 10			99024	
	OV NEW		**OV ESTAB**	
LEVEL 1	99201		99211	
2	99202		99212	
3	99203		99213	
4	99204		99214	
5	99205		99215	
CONSULTATIONS - OFFICE			**HOSPITAL**	
LEVEL 1	99241		99251	
2	99242		99252	
3	99243		99253	
4	99244		99254	
5	99245		99255	

OFFICE PROCEDURES		
Debridement Skin, Partial thickness	11040	
Debridement Skin, Full thickness	11041	
Unna Boot	29580	
I&D Simple	10060	
I&D Complicated	10061	
I&D Pilonidal Abscess, Simple	10080	
Incision & Removal Foreign Body, Simple	10120	
Incision & Removal Foreign Body, Complicated	10121	
I&D Hematoma	10140	
Incision Thrombosed Hemorrhoids	46083	
Rubber Band Ligation	46221	
Evacuation of Thrombosed Hemorrhoids	46320	
Sclerotherapy, One Vein	36470	
Scl. Multiple Veins - Same Leg	36471	
Scl. Multiple Veins - Both Legs	36471	
Aspiration of Breast Cyst	19000	
Each Additional Cyst	19001	

DIAGNOSIS: (print clearly or mark accordingly)

DIAGNOSIS CODES		
Cellulitis & Abscess	68_._	
(specify) ____		
Decubitus Ulcer	707.0	
Hidradenitis	705.83	
Ingrown Nail - Infected	703.0	
Lipoma	214._	
(specify) ____		
Sebaceous Cyst	706.2	
Goiter, Simple	240.0	
Hyperthyroidism	242.9 _	
(specify) ____		
Hyperparathyroidism	252.0	
Abnormal Mammogram	793.8	
Carcinoma, NEC Breast	174.8	
Cyst, Breast Benign	610.0	
Fat Necrosis of Breast	611.3	
Fibroadenoma, Adenosis Breast	610.2	
Fibrocystic Disease, Cystic Mastitis	610.1	
Mass Breast	611.72	
Mastodynia/Pain Breast	611.71	
Nipple Bleeding, Inversion, Discharge	611.79	
Gastroesophageal Reflux	530.81	
Abdominal Pain	789.0 _	
(specify) ____		
Fever	780.6	
Nausea Alone	787.02	
Nausea with Vomiting	787.01	
(specify) ____		
Cholelithiasis	574. _ _	
(specify) ____		
Pancreatitis, Acute	577.0	
Appendicitis	540.9	
Carcinoma, Colon	153. _	

Anal Rectal Stricture Stenosis	565.1	
Carcinoma, Rectum	154. _	
(specify) ____		
Hemorrhoids	455. _	
(specify) ____		
Pilonidal Cyst	685. _	
(specify) ____		
Hernia, Inguinal	550. _ _	
(specify) ____		
Hernia, Umbilical	55_._	
(specify) ____		
Hernia, Ventral	55_._ _	
(specify) ____		
Abdominal Aortic Aneurysm	441.4	
Aneurysm	442. _	
(specify) ____		
Aortoiliac Occlusive Disease	440.0	
Carotid Stenosis	443.1 _	
(specify) ____		
Chronic Renal Failure	585	
Occlusion Artery Lower Ext	444.22	
PVD	440.2 _	
(specify) ____		
Subclavian Steal Syndrome	435.2	
Varicose Veins	454. _	
(specify) ____		
CHF	428.0	
Other Comp Vascular Devices	996.74	
Other Comp Renal Dialysis Device	996.73	
Infection Amputation Stump	997.62	
Lymphadenopathy	785.6	
Lymphoma	202.8 _	
(specify) ____		

PATIENT BALANCE	INS. BALANCE	OTHER BALANCE	TOTAL BALANCE

APPENDIX I: AUDIT SUMMARY REPORT

MEDICAL RECORD DOCUMENTATION OFFICE
Audit No. 2
Completed 2/7/2008
Mason Green, M.D.

MEDICAL RECORD DOCUMENTATION AUDIT

Proper documentation is essential for quality patient care. The medical record is not only a tool used for quality patient care, but also a legal document and a vehicle by which health care services are reimbursed. Documentation in the medical record is transformed into a series of codes used for payment strategies by third-party payers. Solid and consistent documentation of the nature and extent of a patient encounter will result in accurate coding and reduce the possibility of audit liability.

Audit liability is measured by the content of documentation, or by what is missing in the documentation, in the medical record as it influences the possibility of a third-party audit. It is essential that physicians and health care facilities reduce their audit liability because doing so reduces the likelihood of any charge of fraud and abuse, fines, recoupment of previous payments, and deselection from third-party carriers.

This software has been designed to keep physician practices and health care facilities "out of the headlines" by alerting physicians and health care facilities of noncompliant areas within the medical record. The information provided in this report will not only identify areas of noncompliance, but can also be used as an educational tool for physicians and health care facilities.

DOWNCODING

Findings

Of the medical records reviewed, 14.29% were found to be downcoded.

Recommendations

We recommend that the physician and his support staff participate in educational training sessions to gain an understanding of the components necessary for choosing levels of evaluation and management services. All three components of history, examination, and medical decision making must be in the same level of evaluation and management service when choosing a new patient code. For an established patient, only two of the three components must be in the same level to choose the established patient code for that visit.

UPCODING

Findings

Of the medical records reviewed, 57.14% were found to be upcoded.

Recommendations

We recommend that the physician and his or her support staff participate in educational training sessions to gain an understanding of the components necessary for choosing the levels of evaluation and management services. All three key components of history, examination, and medical decision making must be in the same level of evaluation and management service when choosing a new patient code. For an established patient, only two of the three components must be in the same level to choose the established patient code for that visit. There must be documentation of each patient encounter to qualify as a billable service.

According to the Principles of Documentation released by the AMA and CMS in January of 1995, the chief complaint or reason for a patient visit is an integral part of documentation and must be present for each patient encounter. When documenting this element, avoid the use of nonspecific or vague language such as "checkup," "routine," or "follow-up." We recommend that the chief complaint or reason for the visit be documented to indicate the reason the patient sought care for that encounter. Documentation should be individualized for each patient and should "stand alone" so that other health care professionals will be able to continue patient care. If wording such as "follow-up" is used, support it by adding the reason a subsequent encounter is necessary. If these phrases must be used, it is important to support them with objective, precise documentation of the patient's condition; for example, "follow-up on left knee pain."

INCORRECT DIAGNOSIS CODE(S)

Findings

Of the medical records reviewed, 28.57% were found to be incorrect diagnosis code(s).

Recommendations

The diagnoses currently used must be reviewed, yearly at the very least, for accuracy. An ICD-9-CM code book should be purchased every year to ensure the use of the most valid diagnosis codes for billing. These codes should be changed not only in the diagnosis master file of the computer, but also on all billing forms.

USE OF RULE OUT, QUESTIONABLE, PROBABLE, AND SUSPECTED

Findings

Of the medical records reviewed, 14.29% were found to contain rule out, questionable, probable, and suspected.

Recommendations

Because rule out, questionable, probable, and suspected cannot be accurately coded, CMS advises using the codes in Chapter 16 of the ICD-9-CM code book for the coding of such conditions. The codes in Chapter 16 describe signs and symptoms that the patient presented during the patient encounter. These signs and symptoms codes should be reported when a definitive diagnosis is not available.

LACKING DOCUMENTATION OF MEDICAL DECISION MAKING

Findings

Of the medical records reviewed, 14.29% were found to be lacking documentation of medical decision making.

Recommendations

We recommend that the physician and support staff familiarize themselves with third-party documentation criteria governing coding for evaluation and management levels of medical decision making. If the medical decision-making portion of the patient encounter is not documented or is not legible, the service cannot be billed.

VAGUE DOCUMENTATION OF HISTORY OF PRESENT ILLNESS

Findings

Of the medical records reviewed, 14.29% were found to have vague documentation of history of present illness.

Recommendations

We recommend that a history of present illness be documented for each patient encounter. The documentation of history of present illness is required for every level of evaluation and management service. It should include such elements as the chronology of the illness, onset and duration, presenting symptoms, any complications, and character of the findings. Information such as changes in complaints, response to treatment, and any additional or new problem or complication can increase the accuracy of medical decision making and should be well documented.

DOCUMENTATION SUMMARY

The documentation found in the medical record is the only justification for payment of services. Documentation is the concrete evidence that illustrates and substantiates what services were performed.

Health care providers use specific language and codes on all claims billed to third-party carriers. These codes represent the procedures and services rendered and the applicable diagnoses. They represent a condensed version of your documentation in the medical record. Payment for these services rests on the assumption that all billed services are supported by the presence of equivalent, supporting written evidence in the medical record. For this reason, it is recommended that a medical record documentation audit be performed on a continual basis.

Proper reimbursement and medical record compliance often depends on proper documentation. The content of the medical record will become even more important in payment for services in the future. Managed care will continue to be a major component of health care delivery, and documentation will play a major role.

DOCUMENTATION SUGGESTIONS

Documentation that supports higher level of service:

Relevant Diagnoses, Symptoms and Conditions

When these affect medical decision making, document them! The guidelines relate to possible diagnoses (e.g., a patient with chest pain could have a number of possible diagnoses, such as myocardial infarction [MI], angina, pneumonia, rib fracture, etc.) It often helps to list some of the things you must eliminate, even if the final diagnosis is "indigestion."

Treatment Options

If a patient has shoulder pain, document the treatment that you considered (e.g., medications, hot packs, exercise, joint injections, etc.).

Test Results Reviewed (or To Be Reviewed)

Document all test results that you reviewed (e.g., laboratory tests, x-rays, ECGs, etc.). It is a good idea to initial each result after reviewing it. If you order additional studies based on results that you reviewed, write them down on the chart.

Consulting the *Physician's Desk Reference*

Document instances when you look up medications in the PDR or search a database for information.

If Another Physician Is Called

Document all calls to other physicians, including specialists such as radiologists, cardiologists, gastroenterologists, and so on.

Past Medical Records

Indicate if you reviewed past medical records from a hospital or another physician.

Communication with Family

Document any conversations with nursing homes, family members, other physicians, and so on regarding care and medical decision making for the patient.

Statements to Avoid

Avoid using phrases such as "patient feels fine," "patient has no complaints today," or "no change."

Medical Necessity

Medical necessity for all diagnostic tests should be clear. Indications include the following:

- Symptoms
- Monitoring of drug therapy
- Follow-up of abnormal test results
- Toxicity to certain medications

Family and Social History Documentation

Both family and social history must be included in notes to support certain levels of service.

Review of Systems

Document the review of systems thoroughly. Also document normal findings.

Risk Factors

Document any risk factors or multiple symptoms to justify a higher level of service.

From a professional liability standpoint, clear, concise, and accurate medical records will often prevent a potential plaintiff's attorney from filing a claim. Complications and unusual occurrences should normally be documented. Document any "issues" that might arise from patient's families. Document noncompliant patients, informed consent, telephone calls, and so on.

In this era of managed care, we will see an increasing emphasis on documentation and quality of care. Remember: If you don't document it, you didn't do it!

LOCUST STREET CLINIC: AUDIT RESULTS 2008 (MASON GREEN, M.D.)

PATIENT NAME	DATE OF SERVICE	LEVEL BILLED	LEVEL DERIVED	HISTORY COMPONENTS	EXAMINATION	MEDICAL DECISION MAKING	OTHER
Mollie Davis	1/31/07	99244	99243				3
Samuel Davis	2/2/07	99213	99213				
George Benson	2/4/07	99253	99221				4, 7
Florence Toth	2/5/07	99223	99221				3
Jason Hamilton	3/24/07	99274	99274				9
Gloria Frederick	5/8/07	99231	99232				2
William Cox	6/15/07	99202	99201				3, 8
Theresa Herst	7/3/07	99204	99202	5		6	3, 8

Legend:
1: Nonbillable service
2: Downcoded
3: Upcoded
4: Use of incorrect evaluation and management category
5: Vague documentation of history of present illness
6: Lacking documentation of medical decision making
7: Consultation-related issues
8: Incorrect diagnosis code(s)
9: Use of rule out, questionable, probable, and/or suspected

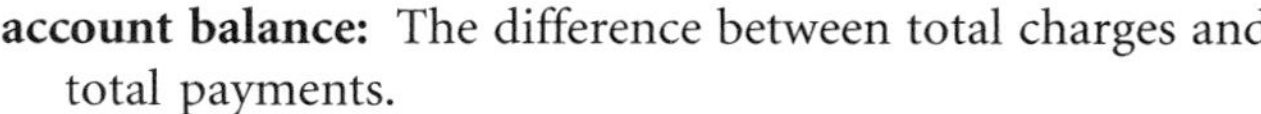

GLOSSARY

account balance: The difference between total charges and total payments.

accounts payable: Amount that has been charged but not yet paid.

accounts receivable ratio: Ratio that measures the amount of time it takes for accounts to be paid.

administrative: Dealing with managerial duties.

admissions: The number of patients accepted for hospital inpatient service during a set period of time.

advance directive: A statement in which a patient either expresses his or her choices about medical treatment or names the person who should make treatment choices if the patient becomes unable to do so.

against medical advice (AMA): When a patient in a hospital signs out against the advice of his or her physician.

AGPA: American Group Practice Association.

AHA: American Hospital Association.

allied health: Health-related personnel who perform functions necessary for assisting, facilitating, and complementing the work of physicians and other specialists.

alphanumeric: Consisting of both letters and numbers.

AMA: American Medical Association.

ambulatory care: Care given to patients at medical offices, outpatient departments, and freestanding health care centers.

analysis by aging: An analysis that classifies accounts by age.

ancillary: Supplementary; for example, x-ray technicians are considered ancillary staff.

AOA: American Osteopathic Association.

ART: Accredited record technician.

assignment of benefits: A signature that authorizes the insurance company to pay a fee directly to a patient's physician.

average length of stay (ALOS): The average stay, in days, of inpatients during a given time period.

BC: Blue Cross.

beneficiary: The person who receives benefits from an insurance policy.

BS: Blue Shield.

capital purchase: The purchase of a major piece of office equipment or furniture (for example, a photocopier).

capitation payment: A fixed monthly fee that an insurance company pays to a physician on behalf of its members, whether they received services or not.

CCU: Coronary care unit.

CDC: Centers for Disease Control.

census: The number of inpatients receiving care on an average day in a hospital.

CEO: Chief executive officer.

CHAMPVA: Civilian Health and Medical Program of the Veterans Administration.

chronological file: A filing system in which items are organized by date.

claim: A request by a physician or patient for services to be paid by an insurance company to either the physician or patient.

CMS: Centers for Medicare and Medicaid Services. The federal agency responsible for the administration of the Medicare and Medicaid programs.

co-insurance: A specific ratio of expenses due that are shared by the patient and insurance company for services rendered.

collection ratio: A ratio used to measure billing and collection activities.

CON: Certificate of Need.

contamination: The introduction of infectious or hazardous materials.

continuing education units (CEUs): Units applied to individuals attending approved educational seminars and workshops.

CPT: Current procedural terminology.

cross-reference: The specification in a file of another file in which the record may be found.

CT: Computed tomography.

DC: Doctor of chiropractic.

deductible: The amount an insurance company expects a patient to pay in a calendar year for medical services.

dictation: The process whereby patient records and letters are entered into a recording device (dictating unit).

direct filing system: A system based on itself, whereby an individual can locate information without having to check an alternate source.

disability: A condition resulting from illness or injury that prevents a person from working.

disbursement: Any type of money that is paid out.

DMD: Doctor of dental medicine.

DO: Doctor of osteopathy.

Drug Enforcement Agency (DEA): A federal agency under the Department of Justice that enforces laws regarding narcotics and other controlled substances.

dual pitch: The capability of a typewriter to switch from pica to elite type.

ED: Emergency department.

EEG: Electroencephalogram.

effective date: The date a patient's insurance becomes effective and can be used.

elective admission: A patient who can be admitted to the hospital on any day and whose delayed admission will not cause harm to the patient.

elite type: A type that generates 12 characters per inch.

emergency admission: A patient who must be admitted and treated immediately.

endorser: The person who signs over a check made out to him or her to another person.

ER: Emergency room.

EW: Emergency ward.

exclusion: A specification within a patient's insurance policy that exclude certain conditions not covered by the patient's plan.

expendable: Office supplies that are used on a daily basis (pencils, stamps, etc.).

extern: An individual allowed to gain experience in a medical office as part of an educational program.

FDA: Food and Drug Administration.

fee schedule: A list from an insurance company that states the specific amount it will pay for various types of medical procedures and visits to health care providers.

fee slip: A document, generally printed by a computer, that specifies the patient's demographics and lists codes and fees for medical services provided to the patient.

filing system: System for organizing records to ensure easy access at a later date.

FP: Family practice.

freestanding emergency center (FEC): A facility that is not a hospital but is equipped to handle medical emergencies.

ghost surgery: A situation in which a patient consents to surgery by one surgeon and later discovers that the surgery was performed by another surgeon.

GME: Graduate medical education.

GP: General practitioner.

group practice: A medical practice consisting of three or more physicians.

HCPCS: Healthcare Common Procedure Coding System.

Health Care Financing Administration (HCFA): Now known as the Centers for Medicare and Medicaid Services (CMS). The federal agency responsible for the administration of the Medicare and Medicaid programs.

health maintenance organization (HMO): A membership insurance company that provides payment for services at a fixed dollar amount.

ICD-9-CM: International Classification of Diseases, 9th revision, Clinical Modification.

ICU: Intensive care unit.

intermediate care facility (ICF): A facility that provides nursing care that must have a supervising registered nurse or licensed practical nurse on each day shift.

invasion of privacy: Unauthorized disclosure of information about a patient.

invoice: A statement received with delivered goods that describes the goods and specifies the amount due.

jargon: Vocabulary used by a specific group of people (for example, medical professionals).

JCAHO: Joint Commission on Accreditation of Healthcare Organizations.

liability: Financial or legal responsibility.

LOS: Length of stay.

LPN: Licensed practical nurse.

MD: Doctor of medicine.

Medicaid: A state and federally funded insurance carrier that provides health care for the medically indigent.

medically indigent: Unable to pay for basic medical care.

Medicare: A federally funded insurance carrier that provides coverage for a person receiving a Social Security check. Part A covers hospital services; Part B covers physician services.

member physician: A physician who has signed a contract with an insurance company to participate in that company's insurance plan and accept its reimbursements.

microfilming: A procedure by which records are reduced in size and stored on film.

MICU: Mobile intensive care unit.

MT: Medical technologist.

negligence: Failure to do what a reasonably prudent person would do under the same circumstances.

numeric filing: A filing system in which records are filed by number.

occupancy: The ratio of census beds to the number of beds in use in a medical facility.

Occupational Safety and Health Administration (OSHA): The federal agency under the Department of Labor that is responsible for industrial health and safety and the enforcement of related regulations.

OD: Doctor of optometry.

OR: Operating room.

orientation: A period of time in which a new employee is trained in the procedures of a specific medical office.

OTC: Over-the-counter.

PA: Physician's assistant.

packing slip: A slip enclosed in a supply carton listing the items it contains.

patient demographics: A patient's name, address, date of birth, Social Security number, telephone number, sex, employer, and so on.

patient statement: A document sent to patients requesting payment for services.

payable: Any amount that one individual owes to another.

payee: A person to whom a check is written.

payer: A person who writes a check.

PDR: *Physician's Desk Reference.*

pica type: A type that generates 10 characters per inch.

posting: Transferring information from one record to another.

power of attorney: A legal document authorizing an individual to act in the place of another individual.

PPC: Progressive patient care.

pre-existing condition: A condition that existed in a patient before he or she obtained a particular insurance policy.

preferred provider organization (PPO): An insurance company much like an HMO, with the exceptions that doctors are paid fees for service and patients may use non-network physicians.

PRO: Peer Review Organization.

professional courtesy: A reduction in fees-for-service that a physician may give to colleagues.

prognosis: A prediction of what course a patient's condition will take.

prudent: Demonstrating reasonable caution and judgment.

PT: Physical therapy.

purging: The process of removing inactive files from active records and placing them in a separate but accessible area.

reasonable prudence: The legal specification that a professional must exercise judgment in a manner similar to that exercised by his or her peers.

respondeat superior: "Let the master answer," a legal term meaning that employers are legally responsible for the consequences of their employees' actions when they are acting within the scope of their employment.

resume: A personal listing of education and work history that a person provides to a prospective employer.

RN: Registered nurse.

RPh: Registered pharmacist.

RVS: Relative Value Scale.

self-pay: Payment made by a patient directly, as opposed to payment through an insurance company.

seminar: A gathering of individuals for the purpose of education.

skilled nursing facility (SNF): A facility that provides 24-hour nursing care and has at least one registered nurse on each day shift.

SMA: Sequential multiple analyzer.

solo practitioner: A physician who maintains a medical practice alone.

SSA: Social Security Administration.

standard of care: A description of conduct that is expected of an individual in a given situation; a measure against which a defendant's conduct is compared.

stat: Immediately.

subscriber: A person who is named by an insurance company as the person holding the contract.

superbill: A document containing the information needed for payment of medical services.

third-party check: A check made out by one party to a second party, who offers it as payment to a third party.

third-party payer: A party other than the patient who is responsible for paying the patient's medical fees (for example, a lawyer or insurance company).

tickler file: A file in chronological order used for recalling patients at certain times of the year.

transcription: Translation of dictation into written form.

TRICARE: Health care plan formerly known as Champus, which covers the fees of civilian physicians to treat any illness or injury of military dependents.

UR: Utilization Review.

usual, customary, and reasonable: The system of price standards used for determining payment of insurance benefits.

VA: Veterans Administration.

VNA: Visiting Nurse Association.

INDEX

N

O

P

S